everyd

www.EverydayHealth.com

# MY **calorie** COUNTER

**Complete nutritional information on more than 8,000 popular brands, fast-food chains, and restaurant menus**

Jennifer Sucov and
Maureen Namkoong, MS, RD

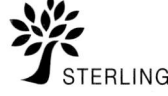

STERLING

New York / London
www.sterlingpublishing.com

Special thanks to Sheila Buff, the gang at Sterling Publishing and everyone else who contributed to this project: Lesley Alderman, Jennifer Bayliss, Irene Bayly, Tony Brancato, Shawn Crahan, Adrian Dunn, Richard Egan, Lori Flynn, Alexis Gentle, Sheri Iodice, Laura Klein, Kelly MacDonald, Deborah Meyer, Anne-Marie O'Neill, Steven Petrow, Jennifer Perciballi, Beth Piantoni, Darcie Sosa, Nancy Walker, and Karen Widrick

10  9  8  7  6  5  4  3  2  1

Published by Sterling Publishing Co., Inc.
387 Park Avenue South, New York, NY 10016
© 2011 by Everyday Health, Inc.

Nutritional data for Common Foods was obtained from the USDA Nutrient Data Laboratory

Distributed in Canada by Sterling Publishing
c/o Canadian Manda Group, 165 Dufferin Street
Toronto, Ontario, Canada M6K 3H6
Distributed in the United Kingdom by GMC Distribution Services
Castle Place, 166 High Street, Lewes, East Sussex, England BN7 1XU
Distributed in Australia by Capricorn Link (Australia) Pty. Ltd.
P.O. Box 704, Windsor, NSW 2756, Australia

Cover and interior design by Anna Christian

*Printed in the United States of America*
*All rights reserved*

Sterling ISBN 978-1-4027-8619-8

For information about custom editions, special sales, premium and corporate purchases, please contact Sterling Special Sales Department at 800-805-5489 or specialsales@sterlingpublishing.com.

# Contents

## The Secret to Losing Weight?

We all wish there was a magic formula for losing weight and keeping it off for good. But the "secret" to shedding unwanted pounds the healthy way isn't banishing carbs or eating gallons of cabbage soup. Doctors and nutritionists

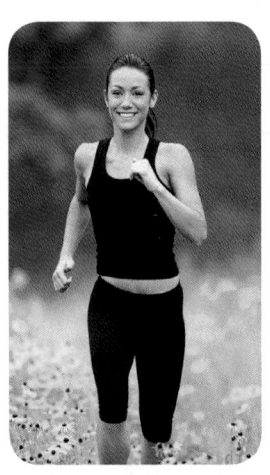

agree that sustained, healthy weight loss comes down to a pretty basic equation: fewer calories plus more exercise. By eating delicious, nutritious meals and snacks, and keeping track of how many calories you consume and burn every day, you can slim down, gain energy, and stave off a whole host of health problems.

Maintaining a healthy diet, however, isn't always easy. We're surrounded by super-size portions of tasty, high-calorie food that has little to no nutritional value—it's quick, it's cheap, and it tastes good. This is where *Everyday Health* can help. We provide the tools and the support you need to stick with your plan.

ONLINE ▶ Look for this icon to learn about weight-loss tools on EverydayHealth.com.

## HERE'S HOW IT ALL WORKS:

**Use this book** to look up the calories, portion sizes, and nutritional content (fat, sodium, carbohydrates, fiber, and protein) for thousands of foods and restaurant dishes.

It contains the most detailed, up-to-date information available, organized in three sections:

- Common Foods, such as vegetables, fruits, meats, grains, oils
- Store Brands, covering hundreds of common supermarket brands
- Restaurant and Fast Food menus, including appetizers, entrées, sides, drinks, and desserts

To get the most from *Everyday Health: My Calorie Counter*, start with this introductory section. You'll learn how to set realistic goals and find out why eating certain nutrients is key to successful weight loss.

**Keep a daily calorie journal** to stay on track. You can keep a notebook or log on to EverydayHealth.com and use the free *Food and Fitness Journal*. Enter a food you've eaten and the tool will tell you how many calories you consumed, as well as the number you have left for the day to stay within your target. It even factors in calories burned from exercise.

**Share your progress** (and pitfalls). Studies have shown that having a weight-loss buddy to encourage you when you falter, celebrate your weight-loss milestones, or just listen to a list of what you ate that day can help you stick to your goals. Log on to the groups on EverydayHealth.com to find a weight-loss buddy, get advice, or just vent.

 **ONLINE** Try the free *Food and Fitness Journal* and find support in the groups on EverydayHealth.com.

> ❝ *I knew I was going to need some help to lose weight—and I found all the help I could ever want at EverydayHealth.com. I've made friends and met people who understand the everyday struggle of losing weight, sticking to an eating plan, and finding time to work out with a busy schedule. I've lost 54 lbs, four sizes, and 30 inches.* ❞
>
> HEATHER F.

## Your Goal: A Healthy Weight

Don't be daunted by the number on the scale. Health professionals have found that if you're overweight, losing just five percent of your body weight can boost energy levels, relieve aching knees and hip joints, and improve serious health problems such as high blood pressure and Type 2 diabetes. Just as important is what losing weight can *prevent*, including:

- **Type 2 diabetes.** If you've been diagnosed with pre-diabetes, shedding pounds can keep you from developing the disease. And if you already have diabetes, you'll see improvements in blood sugar control and lower your risk of complications as you lose weight.

- **High blood pressure.** Losing weight can lower high blood pressure—the culprit behind many strokes and heart attacks—and you may undo some damage to your heart and blood vessels while you're at it.

- **Cancer.** That's right—slim down and your chance of getting many kinds of cancer drops. About half of all new cancer cases in women can be linked to being overweight or obese. For advanced breast cancer alone, overweight women are 10 percent more at risk than women who are a healthy weight; if you're obese that number jumps to 56 percent.

- **Osteoarthritis**. Overweight women are four times more likely to develop "wear and tear" arthritis than women in the healthy weight range. For men, the risk is five times greater. A recent study of overweight women showed that dropping just 11 pounds reduced their chances of developing knee arthritis by half.

If you're already at a healthy weight, calorie counting can help you stay there—for life. By tracking your calories using this book and the tools at EverydayHealth.com, you can immediately detect and avoid the empty calories that might creep into your daily diet, and continue to make healthy choices. When you're aware of calorie counts and portion sizes, it's much easier to keep your weight under control.

> **❝** *I started using the tools on the Everyday Health site three years ago at 580 lbs. Today I weigh 379 lbs. I have a ways to go, but it feels good to have reached that mark. It shows that anyone can do this and battle through the ups and downs.* **❞**
>
> BRIAN F.

## Getting Started

How do you know what a healthy weight is for you? It will only take a few minutes to assemble your stats. You'll need a measuring tape and a calculator. Or, use the calculators and tools on EverydayHealth.com.

### FIRST, FIGURE OUT YOUR BMI.

The body mass index (BMI) is a quick and easy way to see if your weight is within the normal range for your height—and, if it's not, to determine how many pounds you should lose to get it there.

Check the BMI chart opposite for your height and weight. Or, use this formula:

1. Multiply your weight by 703.
2. Divide that number by your height in inches.
3. Divide that number again by your height in inches.
   - If your BMI is between 18.5 and 24.9, you're normal weight.
   - If your BMI is between 25 and 29.9, you're overweight.
   - If your BMI is between 30 and 39.9, you're obese—very overweight.
   - If your BMI is 40 or over, you're dangerously obese (sometimes called morbidly obese).

| | | Height | | | | | | | | | | | | | |
|---|---|---|---|---|---|---|---|---|---|---|---|---|---|---|---|
| | | 5'0" | 5'1" | 5'2" | 5'3" | 5'4" | 5'5" | 5'6" | 5'7" | 5'8" | 5'9" | 5'10" | 5'11" | 6'0" | 6'2" |
| **Weight** | 100 | 20 | 19 | 18 | 18 | 17 | 17 | 16 | 16 | 15 | 15 | 14 | 14 | 14 | 13 |
| | 110 | 22 | 21 | 20 | 20 | 19 | 18 | 18 | 17 | 17 | 16 | 16 | 15 | 15 | 14 |
| | 120 | 23 | 23 | 22 | 21 | 21 | 20 | 19 | 19 | 18 | 18 | 17 | 17 | 16 | 15 |
| | 130 | 25 | 25 | 24 | 23 | 22 | 22 | 21 | 20 | 20 | 19 | 19 | 18 | 18 | 17 |
| | 140 | 27 | 27 | 26 | 25 | 24 | 23 | 23 | 22 | 21 | 21 | 20 | 20 | 19 | 18 |
| | 150 | 29 | 28 | 27 | 27 | 26 | 25 | 24 | 24 | 23 | 22 | 22 | 21 | 20 | 19 |
| | 160 | 31 | 30 | 29 | 28 | 28 | 27 | 26 | 25 | 24 | 24 | 23 | 22 | 22 | 21 |
| | 170 | 33 | 32 | 31 | 30 | 29 | 28 | 27 | 27 | 26 | 25 | 24 | 24 | 23 | 22 |
| | 180 | 35 | 34 | 33 | 32 | 31 | 30 | 29 | 28 | 27 | 27 | 26 | 25 | 24 | 23 |
| | 190 | 37 | 36 | 35 | 34 | 33 | 32 | 31 | 30 | 29 | 28 | 27 | 27 | 26 | 24 |
| | 200 | 39 | 38 | 37 | 36 | 34 | 33 | 32 | 31 | 30 | 30 | 29 | 28 | 27 | 26 |
| | 210 | 41 | 40 | 38 | 37 | 36 | 35 | 34 | 33 | 32 | 31 | 30 | 29 | 29 | 27 |
| | 220 | 43 | 42 | 40 | 39 | 38 | 37 | 36 | 35 | 34 | 33 | 32 | 31 | 30 | 28 |
| | 230 | 45 | 44 | 42 | 41 | 40 | 38 | 37 | 36 | 35 | 34 | 33 | 32 | 31 | 30 |

| Underweight | Healthy Weight | Overweight | Obese | Morbidly Obese |
|---|---|---|---|---|

To see how many pounds you need to lose to enter a healthy weight range:

Place a finger on the square that corresponds to your height and weight on the BMI chart. Now slide your finger up until you hit the first weight in the healthy range. Subtract that weight from your current weight.

Find your Body Mass Index using the BMI Calculator at EverydayHealth.com.

You may want to lose even more pounds to reach the middle or lower end of that healthy range, but this is a good starting point.

## NEXT, WORK OUT YOUR BODY FAT PERCENTAGE.

Your body needs a certain amount of fat to function well. Fat stores energy for times when you may not be able to eat (if you have had a bad stomach bug, for instance), it helps keep you warm, and it protects you from bruising and cushions your body's organs. But you can have too much of a good thing. This is why your body fat percentage is another indicator of whether you need to lose weight.

The calculation for figuring this one out is complex, so use the body fat calculator at EverydayHealth.com.

Enter your gender, height, and weight. Then, using your measuring tape, enter the circumference, in inches, of your neck (measure in the middle of your throat), waist (at its smallest, just above your bellybutton), and hips (at their widest, around the buttocks).

For optimal health, your body fat percentage should be in the range of 21 to 36 percent for a woman, 8 to 25 percent for a man.

## FINALLY, CONSIDER YOUR WAIST-TO-HIP RATIO.

Are you shaped like an apple or a pear? When it comes to health problems such as heart disease and Type 2 diabetes, where your body carries weight counts. If you're heavier around the abdomen—an apple—then you will need to be more vigilant about keeping your weight down. In general, women with a waist circumference of 35 inches or more are likely to develop weight-related health problems; for men, the number is 40 inches.

Pears aren't off the health-hook, of course. But their risk of developing heart disease is somewhat lower. Here's how to assess your WHR:

Step 1: Measure your hips at their widest, around your buttocks.

Step 2: Measure your waist at its smallest, just above your bellybutton.

Step 3: Divide your waist measurement by your hip measurement. Then use the chart on the next page to check your health risk level.

ONLINE To determine your Body Fat Percentage, use the Body Fat Calculator at EverydayHealth.com.

### Waist-to-Hip Ratio Health Risk

| Women | Men | Risk Based on WHR |
|---|---|---|
| 0.80 or below | 0.95 or below | low risk |
| 0.81 to 0.85 | 0.96 to 1.0 | moderate risk |
| 0.85 or higher | 1.0 or higher | high risk |

## How Many Calories Do You Need?

The answer depends on the body you're in and how active you are. About two-thirds of the calories you consume 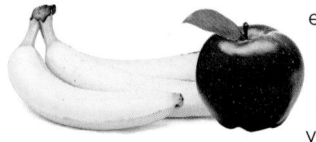 each day are used just to keep your systems functioning—your heart beating, your muscles moving, and so on. The rest of your calorie intake fuels your regular activities like walking around, exercising, typing an e-mail, doing a crossword. Anything left over is stored as fat. To work out how many calories you would need to maintain your current weight, let's do another quick calculation to find your base metabolic rate, or BMR.

Step 1: Women, multiply your weight by 10. Men, multiply by 11. This is your BMR.

Step 2: Now, add to that:

- 20 percent of your BMR if you have a sedentary lifestyle (you don't move around much).
- 30 percent if you are somewhat active.

- 40 percent if you are moderately active.
- 50 percent if you are very active.

**ONLINE** To figure out your Base Metabolic Rate, use the BMR Calculator at EverydayHealth.com.

So, let's say you're a somewhat active 145-pound woman. Your BMR is 1,450 calories a day, and your lifestyle quotient is 30 percent of that, or an additional 435 calories (1,450 x .30 = 435). Add them together, and you come up with a daily calorie total of 1,885 (1,450 + 435 = 1,885).

Now remember, this gives you the number of calories you need to consume each day to *stay at the weight you are now*. To lose weight, you'll need to cut calories, use some up by exercising, or both.

## Take It One Pound at a Time

Whatever your final goal, you should aim to lose about one pound each week. Most doctors caution against cutting your calories drastically. If you go below 1,200 calories a day for a woman or 1,500 calories a day for a man, it's difficult to get the nutrition you need, plus you'll feel hungry, tired, and grouchy. You'll also be at risk for some serious health problems, including gallstones and heart rhythm disruptions from the lack of minerals in your diet.

The good news: To lose one pound a week you only have to cut 500 calories from your diet each day. Why 500?

One pound of weight is the equivalent of approximately 3,500 calories that your body has stored but not used. If you cut 500 calories every day for seven days (500 x 7 = 3,500) your body will use up that pound.

The even *better* news: small changes make a big difference. Substitute diet drinks or water for regular sodas and you'll save about 150 calories per 12-ounce can. Swap your afternoon junk-food fix for a low-calorie snack, and you're well on your way to your goal—there are 250 calories in just two ounces of potato chips or one regular-size candy bar. Follow these tips for success:

## KEEP YOUR CALORIES IN CHECK.

- Start today. If you wait for a good time to begin, it may never come.
- Look up the number of calories for every food you eat and write it down. You could also use the *Food and Fitness Journal* on EverydayHealth.com or download the *My Calorie Counter* mobile app.
- Track your calories as soon after eating as you can. If you wait, you may forget a part of a meal or a snack.
- Be aware of portion size and track it accurately.
- Plan your meals using the calorie charts in this book and on EverydayHealth.com.
- Don't forget your exercise bonus! Add in half an hour of moderate walking each day and you can knock off about 100 calories from your daily total—as well as improve your blood sugar, blood pressure, and overall

## WHAT'S A CALORIE ANYWAY?

A calorie is simply a unit used to measure how much energy is contained in a particular food. The more calories a food has, the more energy it contains.

When you eat something, your body converts that food into energy to keep you alive and moving. If you consume more calories than you need to keep your body going, you'll gain weight. Why? Because the body stores all that excess energy as fat. If you take in fewer calories than you use, you'll lose weight as your body burns those fat stores to make up for the missing energy.

fitness. Did you move even more? The *Food and Fitness Journal* at EverydayHealth.com will calculate your calorie rebate based on the exercise type, speed, and time.

- Track your exercise soon after you do it. As with food, you may forget the details if you wait.
- Share your ups and downs. There's nothing like a diet buddy to give you an extra boost to keep going. Check in regularly with the groups on EverydayHealth.com.

> **66** *On the* Food and Fitness Journal *you can see whether you really did blow it on a particular day. Sometimes, when I thought I had eaten really badly, I was pleasantly surprised to see I hadn't consumed that much at all. I used to give up if I'd had one really bad day! I've now lost a total of 70 lbs.* **99**
>
> JULIE G.

# The Skinny on Carbs, Protein, Fat, and More...

To get the most out of calorie counting, it helps to have a basic understanding of what's in the food you eat. Once you know that, you can make good decisions about what types of calories to cut.

**Carbohydrates**

Carbs have gotten a bad rap lately. But they give you quick energy and they're an essential—and satisfying—part of any diet. The trick is to stick to the good ones—such

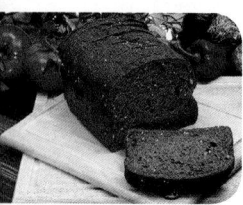 as whole grains, beans, vegetables, and fruit. These are what nutritionists call complex carbs: they take more time for the body to break down, so they keep you feeling full longer and give you a steady flow of energy. Refined carbs are the kind to avoid. They get absorbed quickly and give you a brief spike in energy, but that can be followed by an energy crash. You'll find the bad carbs in highly processed grains and sugars—which are the main ingredients in so many high-calorie, low-nutrition convenience foods and snacks—and in other white, starchy foods such as french fries.

One gram of any carbohydrate food contains 4 calories. That doesn't sound like much, but carb calories can add up fast. For instance, there are about 70 calories in a slice of bread and 285 calories in a large bagel. Cutting back on carbs, especially highly processed carbs that have little nutrition, can have a big impact on your daily calorie count. Aim to get about half your daily calorie intake from high-quality carbs.

## Protein

Protein comes from animal-based foods (meat, poultry, fish, eggs, and dairy products) and some plant-based foods (beans, soy, peas, nuts, and whole grains). Your body uses proteins to help build, maintain, and repair cells. Your body also uses proteins to help it produce hormones, enzymes, and many other chemical substances you need to function. With all the talk about high-protein diets, you may be surprised by how little you really need: the recommended daily intake for an adult woman is just 46 grams; for an adult man, 56 grams. To put that in perspective, two roasted chicken drumsticks contain about 25 grams of protein, a slice of American cheese about 5 grams, an egg around 6 grams.

## Fat

If you've ever been on any sort of diet, you've been told to cut back on fat. One gram of fat contains 9 calories, so eating less of it means consuming fewer calories. The problem: you're also cutting back on flavor and nutrition. Fat is what makes food taste good and satisfies your hunger. Cut back too much and you may end up consuming more calories than you save just to feel full. Plus, you could deplete your body's supplies of vitamin A, vitamin E, folic acid, calcium, iron, and zinc. So, how much do you need? Keep your fat intake to less than 30 percent of your daily calorie count. In a 2,000-calorie diet, that would mean roughly 600 fat calories or about 65 grams of fat a day. When choosing fats, go for the good ones: unsaturated or partially saturated fats that have no cholesterol. You'll find them in vegetable oils such as canola oil and olive oil, and in plant foods such as avocados and nuts. Another healthy food choice that is rich in healthy fats? Oily fish such as salmon and tuna. They are full of omega-3 fatty acids, which improve cardiovascular health.

Try to limit animal fats, such as butter, lard, and the fat found in meats, poultry, and dairy products. These are saturated fats that contain cholesterol, which can contribute to heart disease. The fat to avoid at all costs is trans fat, also known as partially hydrogenated vegetable oil. It's used in baked goods, in convenience and packaged foods, and as the oil for deep frying—and it has been linked to obesity, diabetes, and heart disease. Fortunately, many food manufacturers and restaurant chains have wised up to the health risks and stopped using trans fat, but check food labels to be sure.

### Fiber

Meet the calorie-counter's best friend. Dietary fiber is made up of all the parts of plant food that your body can't digest. Because it doesn't get broken down or absorbed, it passes right through your system—calorie-free. It gets even better: Fiber also makes you feel full. (Doctors agree, this does not involve magic.) Imagine eating six chocolate chip cookies in a row. All too easy, right? Now imagine eating six apples one after the other. Almost impossible, because just one or two apples would take a while to chew and would fill you up very quickly. Foods that are high in fiber tend to be low in calories—

there are 3 grams of fiber and only about 70 calories in a medium apple compared to 2 grams of fiber and 320 calories (162 of them from fat) in those six cookies. Because fiber sticks with you, eating a high-fiber snack in the late afternoon can keep you satisfied until supper. Similarly, starting your meal with a salad (use a low-calorie dressing) will help you avoid overeating later on.

Of course, fiber is also packed with healthy goodness. Apart from its famed ability to help prevent constipation and bowel problems such as hemorrhoids, fiber from foods like oatmeal, beans, peas, and bran can help lower your cholesterol and control your blood sugar.

You'd think we would all be gorging on this wonder food, yet most of us don't get the amount of dietary fiber that we need—studies show that only about 26 percent of all American adults eat 3 or more servings of vegetables each day. The Institute of Medicine suggests that women under age 50 should aim for 25 grams of daily fiber; for men the recommendation is 38 grams. Above age 50, women should aim for 21 grams daily, while men should aim for 30 grams.

### Sugar

You don't have to have a sweet tooth to overload on the stuff: it's in almost every packaged food, including salad dressing and savory sauces—even pizza.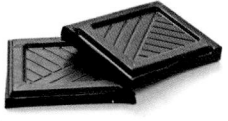
The USDA estimates that the average person consumes 31 teaspoons of sugar each day. There are 16 calories in one teaspoon, so that means you may be racking up 500 daily calories in sugar alone! According to the American Heart Association, women should be getting no more than

100 calories a day (about 6 teaspoons) from added sugar (as opposed to the natural sugar contained in whole foods like fruit); for men, it's 150 calories (about 9 teaspoons).

Clearly, there's plenty of opportunity to cut calories here. Simply skipping or eating smaller portions of sweet foods such as baked goods, fruit juice, and ice cream is a good start. Instead of adding sugar to your coffee or tea, try using a low-calorie sweetener. But beware of the sugar-free or reduced-sugar versions of sweet foods. Like low-fat alternatives, these may be just as high in calories as the regular version. The manufacturers simply bolster the flavor with other ingredients. Likewise, watch out for healthy-sounding sweeteners such as fruit juice concentrate; they have just as many calories as plain old sugar.

**Salt**

How can salt, which has no calories, be a big reason for excess weight? Because so many high-fat, high-calorie snack foods are salted. Take away the chips, pretzels, cheese curls, and other salty snacks, and you'll save a lot of calories. You'll also improve your health. Eating too much salt can raise your blood pressure, which in turn raises your risk of heart disease and stroke. The American Heart Association recommends taking in no more 1,500 milligrams of salt per day. That's just a bit more than half a teaspoon. The average American consumes about 3,500 milligrams a day, or close to 2 teaspoons.

Some of that comes from salt you add to food yourself, and about 12 percent comes from the salt that is naturally in food, but a whopping 77 percent of the salt in the

American diet comes from processed foods. That means salty snack foods and other products, such as tomato sauce, canned soups, and prepared mixes.

Because just about every doctor and health-related organization recommends limiting salt, many food manufacturers offer low- or reduced-salt options. It's the sodium in salt that raises your blood pressure, which is why the package labels often say sodium instead of salt. Read the label carefully. Some foods have less salt than the original version, but the total amount is still high.

**Vitamins and Minerals**
As long as you eat a wide variety of foods, you should get enough of all the essential nutrients your body needs. But on those days when you just can't manage to pull together a healthy or well-balanced meal, take a multivitamin with minerals.

As a calorie-counter, you should watch your calcium intake. Cutting back on full-fat dairy foods like cheese may keep you from getting the recommended 1000 milligrams a day of calcium. So be sure to swap those dairy calories for high-calcium, lower-calorie foods like low-fat dairy products, almonds, beans, spinach, and tofu. Check in with your doctor to see if you need a calcium supplement.

> 66 *I lost 21 lbs in 21 weeks. And I'll continue to keep to my diet, using* My Calorie Counter *at EverydayHealth.com, eating more fresh veggies and fruit, exercising, and drinking a lot of water. I wouldn't be able to do it without this website.* 99
> —Ashley H.

## THE NUTRITIONAL LABEL, DECODED

Knowing how to read all those tiny numbers and unpronounceable ingredients will help you make better choices and avoid overeating by accident.

**Serving Size:** The package might *look* like just one serving, but is it? It pays to check. Many 20-ounce drinks, for example, contain 2.5 8-ounce servings. The calories and other info on the nutritional label are for less than half the bottle, so you may be consuming more calories than you think.

**Nutrition Facts**

Serving Size 3 oz. (85g)

| Amount Per Serving | As Served |
|---|---|
| Calories 38 | Calories from Fat 0 |

| | % Daily Value |
|---|---|
| Total Fat 0g | 0% |
| Saturated Fat 0g | 0% |
| Cholesterol 0g | 0% |
| Sodium 0g | 2% |
| Total Carbohydrate 0g | 3% |
| Dietary Fiber 0g | 8% |
| Sugars 0g | |
| Protein 0g | |

| Vitamin A 270% | ¥ | Vitamin C 10% |
|---|---|---|
| Calcium 2% | ¥ | Iron 0% |

Percent Daily Values are based on a 2,000 calorie diet. Your daily values may be higher or lower depending on your calorie needs:

| | | Calories | 2,000 | 2,500 |
|---|---|---|---|---|
| Total Fat | Less than | | 65g | 80g |
| Sat Fat | Less than | | 20g | 80g |
| Cholesterol | Less than | | 300mg | 300mg |
| Sodium | Less than | | 2,400mg | 2,400mg |
| Total Carbohydrate | | | 300g | 375g |
| Dietary Fiber | | | 25g | 30g |

**Calories:** In general, less than 100 calories per serving is low, 100 to 400 calories per serving is moderate, and anything that's more than 400 calories per serving is high. Keep portions in mind—a couple servings of a low-calorie food still adds up.

**The Daily Value Column:** Use this as a rough guide. It's calculated for a 2,000-calorie diet. If your ideal calorie count is lower than that, adjust accordingly. In general, a DV of 5 percent or less is considered low for a particular ingredient. If the DV is 20 percent or more, it's considered high.

**Fat/Trans Fats/Sodium:** The lower the number and its DV the better. If a mid-morning snack promises to saddle you with 35 percent of your fat and sodium intake for the day, choose something else. Avoid trans fats altogether.

**Dietary Fiber:** The DV for fiber is 25 to 30 grams, though many experts feel this is on the low side and recommend more.

**Sugar:** Less is more—healthy, that is. (There is no DV for sugar.)

**Ingredients:** A good rule of thumb: the more ingredients a food has (especially unpronounceable ones), the more processed it is, and the more calories it contains. Ingredients are also listed by most to least, so make sure the first few are the healthiest.

## It's All in the Portions

In a world where Super-Size is the new Regular, it's easy to undercount your calories. Here are some tips to help you recognize standard serving sizes, and keep your portions under control.

Spend a half an hour in your kitchen with some measuring cups and a scale. Using uncooked rice or something similar, measure out a cup (the standard portion for milk, pasta, beans, and other foods) or three ounces (standard for meat, poultry, and fish). Pour it onto a dinner plate, a salad plate, into a soup bowl, and a drinking glass. You might be surprised by how little space a correct portion actually occupies.

- **Try not to eat right out of containers.** Measure out a small portion of a snack food and put it on a plate.

- **Ditch the desktop candy bowl.** Who on Earth can keep track of how many pieces they munch on during the day? (Your colleagues will also thank you.)

- **Spoil your appetite with a nutritious snack**—celery sticks with peanut butter, for example—an hour before mealtime. You'll eat less and feel more satisfied later. A recent study found that people who eat nuts throughout the day tend not to overeat at meals.

- **Use smaller plates and bowls.** A healthy portion looks lean and lonesome on an oversize plate but looks just right if you shrink its surroundings.

- **Divide your (smaller) plate.** Fill one half of the plate with vegetables and salad greens, one quarter with starchy foods—such as rice, beans, or potatoes—and one quarter with protein foods such as meat, poultry, or fish.

- **Think of a tennis ball.** That's about the size of 1 cup of food. Compare the correct portion of foods you eat regularly with something that's easy to remember.

> 66 *With the help of EverydayHealth.com, I set myself a daily calorie goal and began weighing and measuring portions. I have lost 50 lbs, and 9 inches off my hips alone.* 99

> KATHY S.

# THE USDA FOOD PYRAMID

The pyramid recommends the number of daily servings from each of six different nutrient-rich food groups suggested for good health. It's based on a diet of 2,000 calories a day and assumes you're basically healthy—use it as a guideline and modify it as needed if you have any dietary restrictions.

- Fruits: 4 daily servings, or 2 cups
- Vegetables: 5 daily servings, or 2.5 cups
- Grains: 6 daily servings, or 6 ounces. Aim to have half your servings be whole grains.
- Meat, poultry, fish, and beans: daily servings equal to 5.5 ounces
- Dairy: 3 cups or servings daily
- Fats and oils: Up to 6 teaspoons daily

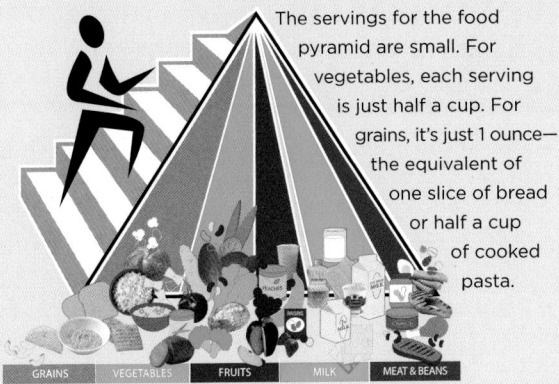

The servings for the food pyramid are small. For vegetables, each serving is just half a cup. For grains, it's just 1 ounce—the equivalent of one slice of bread or half a cup of cooked pasta.

| GRAINS | VEGETABLES | FRUITS | MILK | MEAT & BEANS |

You can learn more about using the food pyramid at www.mypyramid.gov.

# If at First You Don't Succeed...

When you first start counting calories, you'll probably lose weight steadily. After a few weeks, however, your weight loss is likely to slow as your body adjusts to eating less. Plateaus and stalls are nearly inevitable, as is the occasional binge or indulgence. Get back on track with these ideas:

- **Find a weight-loss buddy.** Counting calories with a friend provides mutual support, encouragement, and an incentive to stick with it.

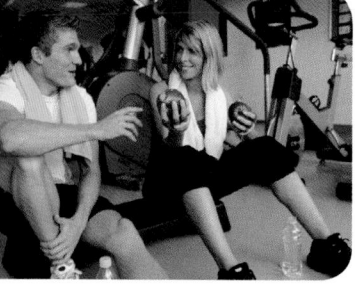

- **Eat more.** As in more low-calorie snacks between meals. It's hard to stay motivated when you're hungry. And healthy snacking helps you keep your mealtime choices and portions under control.

- **Plan ahead.** If you know you've got a busy week of deadlines coming up, stock up on healthy foods that are easy to prepare or can go in the microwave. You'll avoid the temptation to eat high-calorie fast food or take-out instead.

- **If you eat because you're bored,** find something else to do. Take up knitting, go for a walk, call a friend—anything that engages you and takes your mind off food.

- **If you're an emotional eater,** seek out other ways to cope with your feelings. Emotional eating is tough to overcome, but while you're working on it, surround yourself with low-calorie foods.

- **Enlist your family for support.** Explain that you want to lose weight to look and feel better and that you need their help. Ask them to understand your needs and not pressure you to eat more or eat foods you want to avoid.

- **Tap into a supportive weight-loss community.** As you learn to count calories and eat a healthier diet, you're bound to have lots of questions, moments to celebrate, and times when you need advice or some extra support. You can find all that and more on EverydayHealth.com.

## Now, You're Ready to Start Counting

You've set your goals, learned about calories, healthy nutrition, and portion control, and picked up some tips on how to stay motivated. So let's get counting!

Use the *Everyday Health: My Calorie Counter* to plan your grocery shopping trips and check out restaurant menus in advance. You can't always plan ahead, of course, which is why this book is portable. Keep it in your handbag: it's a handy, discreet way to find and track the calories in the foods you eat over the course of the day.

In the charts on the following pages, you'll find some 1,800 common food items, listed alphabetically by types (cheese, fruits, vegetables, etc.) and then names, like artichoke to zucchini.

There are also thousands of brand names listed alphabetically, so if you like to start your morning with Kellogg's Special K, just flip to Kellogg's to find the calorie count and nutritional content for your breakfast cereal.

Chances are you'll eat at least one meal away from home today—and that can be a real challenge when you're counting calories. So check out the Restaurant section that starts on page 175. Some 135 restaurants are listed alphabetically. Under each name, the menu items are then broken out alphabetically by category (salads, entrées, etc.) and then listed alphabetically by name.

For example:

**Burger King**
**BK SALAD COLLECTION**

| | | | | | | | | | |
|---|---|---|---|---|---|---|---|---|---|
| Garden Salad - No Chicken | 1 salad | 70 | 35 | 4 | 2.5 | 10 | 100 | 7 | 3 | 4 |
| Side Salad | 1 salad | 40 | 20 | 2 | 1 | 5 | 45 | 2 | 1 | 3 |
| Tendercrisp Chicken Salad | 1 salad | 410 | 200 | 23 | 6 | 65 | 1060 | 27 | 4 | 27 |
| Tendergrill Chicken Garden Salad | 1 salad | 230 | 70 | 8 | 3.5 | 85 | 930 | 9 | 3 | 34 |
| **BURGERS & SANDWICHES** | | | | | | | | | |
| Bacon Cheeseburger | 1 sandwich | 330 | 150 | 16 | 7 | 55 | 810 | 28 | 1 | 18 |
| BK Big Fish | 1 sandwich | 640 | 280 | 31 | 5 | 45 | 1560 | 67 | 3 | 23 |
| BK Double Stacker | 1 sandwich | 560 | 320 | 36 | 15 | 110 | 1040 | 29 | 1 | 30 |
| BK Quad Stacker | 1 sandwich | 920 | 570 | 63 | 28 | 220 | 1730 | 31 | 1 | 58 |

Remember all the info you just read about carbs, fat, protein, and salt? Along with calories, the charts in this book show how much of each of these nutrients is contained in every listed food. Armed with these details, and the great tools at EverydayHealth.com, you can make smarter choices every time you eat.

So turn the page, log on to EverydayHealth.com, and start your journey toward weight loss and better health.

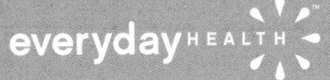

# common foods

# common foods

## Beverages
### ALCOHOLS

| | SERVING SIZE | CAL | CAL FAT | TOT FAT (G) | SAT FAT (G) | CHOL (MG) | SOD (MG) | CARB (G) | FIBER (G) | PROT (G) |
|---|---|---|---|---|---|---|---|---|---|---|
| *Beer* | | | | | | | | | | |
| Beer | 12 fl oz | 153 | 0 | 0 | 0 | 0 | 14 | 13 | 0 | 2 |
| Beer, Light | 12 fl oz | 103 | 0 | 0 | 0 | 0 | 14 | 6 | 0 | 1 |
| *Cocktails & Liqueurs* | | | | | | | | | | |
| Creme De Menthe, 72 Proof | 1 fl oz | 125 | 1 | 0 | 0 | 0 | 2 | 14 | 0 | 0 |
| Daiquiri, Canned | 7 fl oz | 259 | 0 | 0 | 0 | 0 | 83 | 32 | 0 | 0 |
| Daiquiri, Prepared from Recipe | 2 fl oz | 112 | 0 | 0 | 0 | 0 | 3 | 4 | 0 | 0 |
| Liqueur, Coffee with Cream, 34 Proof | 1 fl oz | 102 | 44 | 5 | 3 | 18 | 29 | 6 | 0 | 1 |
| Liqueur, Coffee, 53 Proof | 1 fl oz | 113 | 1 | 0 | 0 | 0 | 3 | 16 | 0 | 0 |
| Liqueur, Coffee, 63 Proof | 1 fl oz | 107 | 1 | 0 | 0 | 0 | 3 | 11 | 0 | 0 |
| Pina Colada, Canned | 7 fl oz | 526 | 152 | 17 | 15 | 0 | 158 | 61 | 0 | 1 |
| Pina Colada, Prepared from Recipe | 4-1/2 fl oz | 245 | 24 | 3 | 2 | 0 | 8 | 32 | 0 | 1 |
| Tequila Sunrise, Canned | 7 fl oz | 232 | 2 | 0 | 0 | 0 | 120 | 24 | 0 | 1 |
| Whiskey Sour, Canned | 7 fl oz | 249 | 0 | 0 | 0 | 0 | 92 | 28 | 0 | 0 |
| Whiskey Sour, Prep with Water, Whiskey, & Powder Mix | 1 packet | 169 | 0 | 0 | 0 | 0 | 48 | 16 | 0 | 0 |
| *Spirits* | | | | | | | | | | |
| Distilled, All (Gin, Rum, Vodka, Whiskey) 80 Proof | 1 fl oz | 64 | 0 | 0 | 0 | 0 | 0 | 0 | 0 | 0 |
| Distilled, All 86 Proof | 1 fl oz | 70 | 0 | 0 | 0 | 0 | 0 | 0 | 0 | 0 |
| Distilled, All 90 Proof | 1 fl oz | 73 | 0 | 0 | 0 | 0 | 0 | 0 | 0 | 0 |
| Distilled, All 94 Proof | 1 fl oz | 76 | 0 | 0 | 0 | 0 | 0 | 0 | 0 | 0 |
| Distilled, All 100 Proof | 1 fl oz | 82 | 0 | 0 | 0 | 0 | 0 | 0 | 0 | 0 |
| *Wine* | | | | | | | | | | |
| Cooking | 1 fl oz | 15 | 0 | 0 | 0 | 0 | 182 | 2 | 0 | 0 |
| Dessert, Dry | 3-1/2 fl oz | 157 | 0 | 0 | 0 | 0 | 9 | 12 | 0 | 0 |
| Dessert, Sweet | 3-1/2 fl oz | 165 | 0 | 0 | 0 | 0 | 9 | 14 | 0 | 0 |
| Red, Burgundy | 5 fl oz | 127 | 0 | 0 | 0 | 0 | 0 | 5 | 0 | 0 |
| Red, Cabernet Franc | 5 fl oz | 122 | 0 | 0 | 0 | 0 | 0 | 4 | 0 | 0 |
| Red, Cabernet Sauvignon | 5 fl oz | 122 | 0 | 0 | 0 | 0 | 0 | 4 | 0 | 0 |
| Red, Merlot | 5 fl oz | 122 | 0 | 0 | 0 | 0 | 6 | 4 | 0 | 0 |
| Red, Petite Sirah | 5 fl oz | 125 | 0 | 0 | 0 | 0 | 0 | 4 | 0 | 0 |
| Red, Pinot Noir | 5 fl oz | 121 | 0 | 0 | 0 | 0 | 0 | 3 | 0 | 0 |
| Red, Syrah | 5 fl oz | 122 | 0 | 0 | 0 | 0 | 0 | 4 | 0 | 0 |
| Red, Zinfandel | 5 fl oz | 129 | 0 | 0 | 0 | 0 | 0 | 4 | 0 | 0 |

| | SERVING SIZE | CAL | CAL FAT | TOT FAT (G) | SAT FAT (G) | CHOL (MG) | SOD (MG) | CARB (G) | FIBER (G) | PROT (G) |
|---|---|---|---|---|---|---|---|---|---|---|
| Sake | 1 fl oz | 39 | 0 | 0 | 0 | 0 | 1 | 1 | 0 | 0 |
| Table Wine, All | 5 fl oz | 123 | 0 | 0 | 0 | 0 | 7 | 4 | 0 | 0 |
| Wine, Table, Red | 5 fl oz | 125 | 0 | 0 | 0 | 0 | 6 | 4 | 0 | 0 |
| Wine, Table, White | 5 fl oz | 121 | 0 | 0 | 0 | 0 | 7 | 4 | 0 | 0 |
| White, Chenin Blanc | 5 fl oz | 118 | 0 | 0 | 0 | 0 | 0 | 5 | 0 | 0 |
| White, Fume Blanc | 5 fl oz | 120 | 0 | 0 | 0 | 0 | 0 | 3 | 0 | 0 |
| White, Gewurztraminer | 5 fl oz | 119 | 0 | 0 | 0 | 0 | 0 | 4 | 0 | 0 |
| White, Pinot Blanc | 5 fl oz | 119 | 0 | 0 | 0 | 0 | 0 | 3 | 0 | 0 |
| White, Pinot Gris (Grigio) | 5 fl oz | 122 | 0 | 0 | 0 | 0 | 0 | 3 | 0 | 0 |
| White, Riesling | 5 fl oz | 118 | 0 | 0 | 0 | 0 | 0 | 6 | 0 | 0 |
| White, Sauvignon Blanc | 5 fl oz | 119 | 0 | 0 | 0 | 0 | 0 | 3 | 0 | 0 |
| **CARBONATED BEVERAGES** | | | | | | | | | | |
| Club Soda | 16 fl oz | 0 | 0 | 0 | 0 | 0 | 100 | 0 | 0 | 0 |
| Cola, Contains Caffeine | 12 fl oz | 136 | 1 | 0 | 0 | 0 | 15 | 35 | 0 | 0 |
| Cola with Higher Caffeine | 12 fl oz | 151 | 0 | 0 | 0 | 0 | 15 | 39 | 0 | 0 |
| Cola without Caffeine | 12 fl oz | 151 | 0 | 0 | 0 | 0 | 15 | 39 | 0 | 0 |
| Ginger Ale | 16 fl oz | 166 | 0 | 0 | 0 | 0 | 34 | 43 | 0 | 0 |
| Soda, Chocolate-Flavored | 16 fl oz | 207 | 0 | 0 | 0 | 0 | 433 | 53 | 0 | 0 |
| Soda, Cream | 16 fl oz | 252 | 0 | 0 | 0 | 0 | 59 | 66 | 0 | 0 |
| Soda, Grape | 12 fl oz | 160 | 0 | 0 | 0 | 0 | 56 | 42 | 0 | 0 |
| Soda, Lemon-Lime, Contains Caffeine | 12 fl oz | 151 | 0 | 0 | 0 | 0 | 37 | 38 | 0 | 0 |
| Tonic Water | 11 fl oz | 114 | 0 | 0 | 0 | 0 | 40 | 30 | 0 | 0 |
| **COFFEES & TEAS** | | | | | | | | | | |
| Coffee, Brewed | 8 fl oz | 2 | 0 | 0 | 0 | 0 | 5 | 0 | 0 | 0 |
| Coffee, Brewed, Decaffeinated | 8 fl oz | 0 | 0 | 0 | 0 | 0 | 5 | 0 | 0 | 0 |
| Coffee, Brewed, Espresso | 1 fl oz | 1 | 0 | 0 | 0 | 0 | 4 | 0 | 0 | 0 |
| Coffee, Brewed, Espresso, Decaffeinated | 1 fl oz | 0 | 0 | 0 | 0 | 0 | 4 | 0 | 0 | 0 |
| Coffee, Instant | 1 tsp | 2 | 0 | 0 | 0 | 0 | 0 | 0 | 0 | 0 |
| Coffee, Instant, Decaffeinated | 6 fl oz | 4 | 0 | 0 | 0 | 0 | 7 | 1 | 0 | 0 |
| Coffee, Whitener, Reduced-Calorie | 1 tsp, dry | 9 | 5 | 0 | 0 | 0 | 14 | 1 | 0 | 0 |
| Tea, Brewed | 8 fl oz | 2 | 0 | 0 | 0 | 0 | 7 | 1 | 0 | 0 |
| Tea, Brewed, Decaffeinated | 6 fl oz | 2 | 0 | 0 | 0 | 0 | 5 | 1 | 0 | 0 |
| Tea, Herb, Brewed | 6 fl oz | 2 | 0 | 0 | 0 | 0 | 5 | 0 | 0 | 0 |
| **JUICES & NECTARS** | | | | | | | | | | |
| Fruit Punch Drink, Frozen Concentrate, Prepared with Water | 8 fl oz | 114 | 0 | 0 | 0 | 0 | 12 | 29 | 0 | 0 |
| Apple Juice, Unsweetened | 1 cup | 114 | 3 | 0 | 0 | 0 | 10 | 28 | 0 | 0 |

# common foods

| | SERVING SIZE | CAL | CAL FAT | TOT FAT (G) | SAT FAT (G) | CHOL (MG) | SOD (MG) | CARB (G) | FIBER (G) | PROT (G) |
|---|---|---|---|---|---|---|---|---|---|---|
| Blackberry Juice, Canned | 1 cup | 95 | 14 | 2 | 0 | 0 | 2 | 20 | 0 | 1 |
| Carrot Juice, Canned | 1 cup | 94 | 3 | 0 | 0 | 0 | 68 | 22 | 2 | 2 |
| Citrus Fruit Juice, Frozen Concentrate, Prepared with Water | 1 cup | 114 | 1 | 0 | 0 | 0 | 10 | 28 | 0 | 1 |
| Clam & Tomato Juice, Canned | 5-1/2 oz | 80 | 3 | 0 | 0 | 0 | 601 | 18 | 1 | 1 |
| Cranberry Juice Cocktail, Bottled | 1 cup | 137 | 2 | 0 | 0 | 0 | 5 | 34 | 0 | 0 |
| Cranberry Juice Cocktail, Bottled, Low Calorie | 1 cup | 45 | 0 | 0 | 0 | 0 | 7 | 11 | 0 | 0 |
| Cranberry Juice, Unsweetened | 1 cup | 116 | 3 | 0 | 0 | 0 | 5 | 31 | 0 | 1 |
| Cranberry-Apple Juice, Bottled | 1 cup | 154 | 2 | 0 | 0 | 0 | 5 | 39 | 0 | 0 |
| Cranberry-Apple Juice, Low Calorie | 1 cup | 46 | 0 | 0 | 0 | 0 | 12 | 11 | 0 | 0 |
| Grapefruit Juice, White, Canned, Sweetened | 1 cup | 115 | 2 | 0 | 0 | 0 | 5 | 28 | 0 | 1 |
| Grapefruit Juice, White/Pink, Raw | 1 cup | 96 | 2 | 0 | 0 | 0 | 2 | 23 | 0 | 1 |
| Guanabana Nectar, Canned | 1 cup | 148 | 4 | 0 | 0 | 0 | 20 | 37 | 0 | 0 |
| Guava Nectar, Canned | 1 cup | 143 | 1 | 0 | 0 | 0 | 18 | 37 | 3 | 0 |
| Lemonade, Frozen Concentrate, Pink, Prepared with Water | 1 cup | 106 | 3 | 0 | 0 | 0 | 10 | 27 | 0 | 0 |
| Lemonade, Frozen Concentrate, White, Prepared with Water | 1 cup | 99 | 1 | 0 | 0 | 0 | 10 | 26 | 0 | 0 |
| Mango Nectar, Canned | 1 cup | 128 | 1 | 0 | 0 | 0 | 13 | 33 | 1 | 0 |
| Orange Juice | 1 cup | 117 | 3 | 0 | 0 | 0 | 10 | 28 | 1 | 2 |
| Papaya Nectar, Canned | 1 cup | 143 | 3 | 0 | 0 | 0 | 13 | 36 | 2 | 0 |
| Peach Nectar, Canned | 1 cup | 142 | 0 | 0 | 0 | 0 | 17 | 35 | 2 | 1 |
| Pineapple Juice | 1 cup | 132 | 3 | 0 | 0 | 0 | 5 | 32 | 1 | 1 |
| Pomegranate Juice | 1 cup | 134 | 6 | 1 | 0 | 0 | 22 | 33 | 0 | 0 |
| Prune Juice | 1 cup | 182 | 1 | 0 | 0 | 0 | 10 | 45 | 3 | 2 |
| Tamarind Nectar, Canned | 1 cup | 143 | 3 | n/a | 0 | 0 | 18 | 37 | 1 | 0 |
| Vegetable & Fruit Blend Juice | 1 cup | 113 | 0 | 0 | 0 | 0 | 71 | 27 | 0 | 1 |
| **MALTED DRINK MIXES** | | | | | | | | | | |
| Chocolate, Powder | 3 tsp | 86 | 9 | 1 | 1 | 0 | 40 | 18 | 1 | 1 |
| Chocolate, Powder, Prepared with Whole Milk | 1 cup | 225 | 78 | 9 | 5 | 27 | 159 | 30 | 1 | 9 |
| **Bread & Bread Products** | | | | | | | | | | |
| **BAGELS** | | | | | | | | | | |
| Cinnamon-Raisin | 3" dia | 188 | 11 | 1 | 0 | 0 | 299 | 38 | 2 | 7 |
| Egg | 3" dia | 192 | 13 | 1 | 0 | 17 | 348 | 37 | 2 | 7 |
| Oat Bran | 3" dia | 176 | 7 | 1 | 0 | 0 | 407 | 37 | 2 | 7 |
| Plain, Onion, Poppy, Sesame | 3" dia | 177 | 10 | 1 | 0 | 0 | 357 | 35 | 2 | 7 |

| | SERVING SIZE | CAL | CAL FAT | TOT FAT (G) | SAT FAT (G) | CHOL (MG) | SOD (MG) | CARB (G) | FIBER (G) | PROT (G) |
|---|---|---|---|---|---|---|---|---|---|---|
| **BISCUITS** | | | | | | | | | | |
| Mixed Grain, Refrigerator Dough | 2-1/2" dia | 116 | 22 | 2 | 1 | 0 | 295 | 21 | 0 | 3 |
| Plain or Buttermilk, Commonly Baked | 1 biscuit | 128 | 52 | 6 | 1 | 0 | 276 | 17 | 0 | 2 |
| Plain or Buttermilk, Dry Mix | 1 cup | 548 | 177 | 20 | 5 | 3 | 1295 | 81 | 3 | 10 |
| Plain or Buttermilk, Dry Mix, Prepared | 1 oz | 95 | 31 | 3 | 1 | 1 | 271 | 14 | 1 | 2 |
| Plain or Buttermilk, Prepared from Recipe | 4" dia | 357 | 148 | 16 | 4 | 3 | 586 | 45 | 2 | 7 |
| Plain or Buttermilk, Refrigerator Dough, Higher Fat, Baked | 2-1/2" dia | 95 | 37 | 4 | 1 | 0 | 292 | 13 | 0 | 2 |
| Plain or Buttermilk, Refrigerator Dough, Lower Fat, Baked | 2-1/4" dia | 63 | 10 | 1 | 0 | 0 | 305 | 12 | 0 | 2 |
| **BREADS** | | | | | | | | | | |
| Banana Bread, Prepared from Recipe, Made w/Margarine | 1 oz | 92 | 27 | 3 | 1 | 12 | 86 | 15 | 0 | 1 |
| Boston Brown Bread, Canned | 1 slice | 88 | 6 | 1 | 0 | 0 | 284 | 19 | 2 | 2 |
| Bread Sticks, Plain | 4-1/4" long | 21 | 4 | 0 | 0 | 0 | 33 | 3 | 0 | 1 |
| Cornbread, Dry Mix | 8-1/2 oz | 1007 | 265 | 29 | 7 | 5 | 1969 | 167 | 16 | 17 |
| Cornbread, Dry Mix, Prepared | 1 piece | 188 | 54 | 6 | 1 | 37 | 467 | 29 | 1 | 4 |
| Cornbread, Prepared from Recipe, Made w/Reduced Fat (2%) Milk | 1 piece | 173 | 42 | 5 | 1 | 26 | 428 | 28 | 0 | 4 |
| Cracked-Wheat Bread | 1 oz | 74 | 10 | 1 | 0 | 0 | 153 | 14 | 2 | 2 |
| Egg Bread | 1 slice | 113 | 22 | 2 | 1 | 20 | 165 | 19 | 1 | 4 |
| French, Vienna, or Sourdough Bread | 1 slice | 185 | 11 | 1 | 0 | 0 | 328 | 36 | 2 | 8 |
| Irish Soda Bread, Prepared from Recipe | 1 oz | 82 | 13 | 1 | 0 | 5 | 113 | 16 | 1 | 2 |
| Italian Bread | 1 slice | 81 | 9 | 1 | 0 | 0 | 175 | 15 | 1 | 3 |
| Multi-Grain Bread (Includes Whole-Grain) | 1 slice | 69 | 10 | 1 | 0 | 0 | 111 | 11 | 3 | 4 |
| Oat Bran Bread | 1 slice | 71 | 12 | 1 | 0 | 0 | 122 | 12 | 1 | 3 |
| Oat Bran Bread, Reduced-Calorie | 1 slice | 46 | 7 | 1 | 0 | 0 | 132 | 9.5 | 3 | 2 |
| Oatmeal Bread | 1 slice | 73 | 11 | 1 | 0 | 0 | 127 | 13 | 1 | 2 |
| Oatmeal Bread, Reduced-Calorie | 1 slice | 48 | 7 | 1 | 0 | 0 | 89 | 10 | 0 | 2 |
| Pan Dulce, Sweet Yeast Bread | 1 slice | 231 | 66 | 7 | 1 | n/a | 144 | 36 | 1 | 6 |
| Pita, White | 6-1/2" dia | 165 | 6 | 1 | 0 | 0 | 322 | 33 | 1 | 5 |
| Pita, Whole-Wheat | 6-1/2" dia | 170 | 15 | 2 | 0 | 0 | 340 | 35 | 5 | 6 |
| Pumpernickel Bread | 1 slice | 65 | 7 | 1 | 0 | 0 | 174 | 12 | 2 | 2 |
| Raisin Bread | 1 slice | 88 | 13 | 1 | 0 | 0 | 125 | 17 | 1 | 3 |
| Rice Bran Bread | 1 slice | 66 | 11 | 1 | 0 | 0 | 119 | 82 | 1 | 2 |
| Rye Bread | 1 slice | 83 | 10 | 1 | 0 | 0 | 211 | 15 | 2 | 3 |
| Rye Bread, Reduced-Calorie | 1 slice | 47 | 6 | 1 | 0 | 0 | 118 | 9 | 3 | 2 |

| common foods | SERVING SIZE | CAL | CAL FAT | TOT FAT (G) | SAT FAT (G) | CHOL (MG) | SOD (MG) | CARB (G) | FIBER (G) | PROT (G) |
|---|---|---|---|---|---|---|---|---|---|---|
| Wheat Bread | 1 slice | 66 | 8 | 1 | 0 | 0 | 130 | 12 | 1 | 3 |
| Wheat Bread, Reduced Calorie | 1 slice | 46 | 5 | 1 | 0 | 0 | 118 | 10 | 3 | 2 |
| White Bread | 1 slice | 120 | 22 | 2 | 0 | 1 | 151 | 21 | 1 | 3 |
| White Bread, Reduced Calorie | 1 slice | 48 | 5 | 1 | 0 | 0 | 104 | 10 | 2 | 2 |
| Whole-Wheat Bread | 1 slice | 69 | 8 | 1 | 0 | 0 | 132 | 12 | 2 | 4 |
| **BREAD CRUMBS &** | | | | | | | | | | |
| **STUFFING** | | | | | | | | | | |
| Bread Crumbs, Dry, Plain | 1 cup | 427 | 52 | 6 | 1 | 0 | 791 | 78 | 5 | 14 |
| Bread Crumbs, Dry, Seasoned | 1 cup | 460 | 59 | 7 | 2 | 1 | 2111 | 82 | 6 | 17 |
| Bread Stuffing, Dry Mix | 6 oz | 656 | 52 | 6 | 1 | 2 | 2388 | 130 | 5 | 19 |
| Bread Stuffing, Dry Mix, Prepared | 1 oz | 50 | 22 | 2 | 0 | 0 | 149 | 6 | 1 | 1 |
| Cornbread Stuffing, Dry Mix | 6 oz | 661 | 64 | 7 | 2 | 0 | 2181 | 130 | 24 | 17 |
| Cornbread Stuffing, Dry Mix, Prepared | 1 oz | 51 | 22 | 2 | 0 | 0 | 129 | 6 | 1 | 1 |
| White Bread Crumbs, Prepared | 1 cup | 120 | 13 | 1 | 0 | 0 | 230 | 22 | 1 | 3 |
| **CRACKERS** | | | | | | | | | | |
| Cheese Crackers, Bite Size | 1 cup | 312 | 141 | 16 | 6 | 8 | 617 | 36 | 1 | 6 |
| Crispbread, Rye Crackers | 1 crispbread | 37 | 1 | 0 | 0 | 0 | 45 | 8 | 2 | 1 |
| Matzo, Egg | 1 matzo | 109 | 5 | 1 | 0 | 23 | 6 | 22 | 1 | 3 |
| Matzo, Egg & Onion | 1 matzo | 109 | 10 | 1 | 0 | 13 | 80 | 22 | 1 | 3 |
| Matzo, Plain | 1 matzo | 111 | 4 | 0 | 0 | 0 | 0 | 24 | 1 | 3 |
| Matzo, Whole-Wheat | 1 matzo | 98 | 4 | 0 | 0 | 0 | 1 | 22 | 3 | 4 |
| Melba Toast, Plain | 1 cup | 129 | 10 | 1 | 0 | 0 | 197 | 25 | 2 | 4 |
| Melba Toast, Rye or Pumpernickel | 1 toast | 19 | 2 | 0 | 0 | 0 | 45 | 4 | 0 | 1 |
| Melba Toast, Wheat | 1 toast | 19 | 1 | 0 | 0 | 0 | 42 | 4 | 0 | 1 |
| Milk Crackers | 1 cracker | 50 | 16 | 2 | 0 | 0 | 65 | 8 | 0 | 1 |
| Oyster/Soda/Soup Crackers | 5 crackers | 63 | 12 | 1 | 0 | 0 | 167 | 11 | 0 | 1 |
| Rusk Toast | 1 rusk | 41 | 6 | 1 | 0 | 8 | 25 | 7 | 0 | 1 |
| Rye Crackers, Sandwich-Type w/Cheese Filling | 1 sandwich | 34 | 14 | 2 | 0 | 1 | 73 | 4 | 0 | 1 |
| Rye Crackers, Wafers, Plain | 1 cracker | 37 | 1 | 0 | 0 | 0 | 61 | 9 | 3 | 1 |
| Rye Crackers, Wafers, Seasoned | 1 cracker | 84 | 18 | 2 | 0 | 0 | 195 | 16 | 5 | 2 |
| Sandwich-Type Crackers w/ Cheese Filling | 6 crackers | 191 | 86 | 10 | 0 | 2 | 342 | 23 | 1 | 3 |
| Sandwich-Type Crackers w/Peanut Butter Filling | 6 crackers | 193 | 88 | 10 | 2 | 0 | 356 | 22 | 1 | 5 |
| Snack-Type Crackers | 5 crackers | 81 | 37 | 4 | 1 | 0 | 138 | 10 | 0 | 1 |
| Whole-Wheat Crackers | 6 crackers | 120 | 36 | 4 | 1 | 0 | 169 | 19 | 3 | 3 |

| | SERVING SIZE | CAL | CAL FAT | TOT FAT (G) | SAT FAT (G) | CHOL (MG) | SOD (MG) | CARB (G) | FIBER (G) | PROT (G) |
|---|---|---|---|---|---|---|---|---|---|---|
| **ENGLISH MUFFINS** | | | | | | | | | | |
| Mixed-Grain or Granola | 1 muffin | 155 | 11 | 1 | 0 | 0 | 220 | 31 | 2 | 6 |
| Plain or Sourdough | 1 muffin | 134 | 9 | 1 | 0 | 0 | 264 | 26 | 2 | 4 |
| Raisin-Cinnamon or Apple-Cinnamon | 1 muffin | 137 | 9 | 1 | 0 | 0 | 158 | 27 | 1 | 5 |
| Wheat | 1 muffin | 127 | 10 | 1 | 0 | 0 | 218 | 26 | 3 | 5 |
| Whole Wheat | 1 muffin | 134 | 13 | 1 | 0 | 0 | 240 | 27 | 4 | 6 |
| **FRENCH TOAST** | | | | | | | | | | |
| French Toast, Frozen, Ready-to-Eat | 1 piece | 126 | 32 | 4 | 1 | 48 | 292 | 19 | 1 | 4 |
| French Toast, Prepared from Recipe, Made w/Reduced-Fat (2%) Milk | 1 slice | 149 | 63 | 7 | 2 | 75 | 311 | 16 | 0 | 5 |
| **MUFFINS** | | | | | | | | | | |
| Blueberry Muffin | 1 small | 259 | 114 | 13 | 2 | 26 | 230 | 33 | 1 | 3 |
| Blueberry Muffin, Dry Mix | 1 package | 1303 | 320 | 36 | 9 | 0 | 1951 | 225 | 0 | 17 |
| Blueberry Muffin, Low-Fat | 1 small | 181 | 27 | 3 | 1 | 20 | 293 | 36 | 3 | 3 |
| Corn Muffin | 1 small | 201 | 50 | 6 | 1 | 17 | 422 | 34 | 2 | 4 |
| Corn Muffin, Prepared from Recipe, Made w/Reduced-Fat (2%) Milk | 1 small | 180 | 63 | 7 | 1 | 24 | 333 | 25 | 0 | 4 |
| Oat Bran Muffin | 1 small | 178 | 44 | 5 | 1 | 0 | 259 | 32 | 3 | 5 |
| **OTHER BREAD PRODUCTS** | | | | | | | | | | |
| Phyllo Dough | 1 sheet | 57 | 10 | 1 | 0 | 0 | 92 | 10 | 0 | 1 |
| Popovers, Dry Mix | 6 oz | 631 | 66 | 7 | 2 | 0 | 1540 | 121 | 0 | 18 |
| **PANCAKES** | | | | | | | | | | |
| Blueberry Pancakes, Prepared from Recipe | 4" dia | 84 | 32 | 4 | 1 | 21 | 157 | 11 | 0 | 2 |
| Buttermilk Pancakes, Prepared from Recipe | 4" dia | 86 | 32 | 4 | 1 | 22 | 198 | 11 | 0 | 3 |
| Plain or Buttermilk Pancakes, Frozen, Ready-to-Heat | 6" dia | 164 | 34 | 4 | 1 | 13 | 369 | 29 | 2 | 4 |
| Plain Pancakes, Dry Mix, Prepared | 4" dia | 74 | 9 | 1 | 0 | 5 | 239 | 14 | 0 | 2 |
| Plain Pancakes, Prepared from Recipe | 4" dia | 86 | 33 | 4 | 1 | 22 | 167 | 11 | 0 | 2 |
| Whole-Wheat Pancakes, Dry Mix, Prepared | 4" dia | 92 | 26 | 3 | 1 | 27 | 252 | 13 | 1 | 4 |
| **ROLLS** | | | | | | | | | | |
| Dinner Roll, Egg | 1 roll | 107 | 20 | 2 | 1 | 18 | 161 | 18 | 1 | 3 |
| Dinner Roll, Oat Bran | 1 roll | 78 | 14 | 2 | 0 | 0 | 136 | 13 | 1 | 3 |
| Dinner Roll, Plain | 1 roll | 87 | 16 | 2 | 0 | 1 | 150 | 15 | 1 | 3 |
| Dinner Roll, Plain, Prepared from Recipe w/Reduced-Fat (2%) Milk, Medium | 1 roll | 136 | 28 | 3 | 1 | 15 | 178 | 23 | 1 | 4 |
| Dinner Roll, Rye, Medium | 1 roll | 103 | 11 | 1 | 0 | 0 | 234 | 19 | 2 | 4 |
| Dinner Roll, Wheat | 1 roll | 76 | 16 | 2 | 0 | 0 | 136 | 13 | 1 | 2 |

# common foods

| | SERVING SIZE | CAL | CAL FAT | TOT FAT (G) | SAT FAT (G) | CHOL (MG) | SOD (MG) | CARB (G) | FIBER (G) | PROT (G) |
|---|---|---|---|---|---|---|---|---|---|---|
| French Roll | 1 roll | 105 | 15 | 2 | 0 | 0 | 193 | 19 | 1 | 3 |
| Hamburger or Hot Dog Roll, Mixed-Grain | 1 roll | 113 | 23 | 3 | 1 | 0 | 197 | 19 | 2 | 4 |
| Hamburger or Hot Dog Roll, Plain | 1 roll | 120 | 17 | 2 | 0 | 0 | 206 | 21 | 1 | 4 |
| Hamburger or Hot Dog Roll, Reduced-Calorie | 1 roll | 84 | 8 | 1 | 0 | 0 | 190 | 18 | 3 | 4 |
| Hard/Kaiser Roll | 1 roll | 167 | 22 | 2 | 0 | 0 | 310 | 30 | 1 | 6 |
| Large Submarine/Hoagie Roll, Whole-Wheat | 1 roll | 359 | 57 | 6 | 1 | 0 | 645 | 69 | 10 | 4 |
| Pumpernickel Roll | 1 roll | 100 | 9 | 1 | 0 | 0 | 205 | 19 | 2 | 4 |
| **WAFFLES** | | | | | | | | | | |
| Buttermilk Waffle, Frozen, Ready-to-Heat | 1 waffle | 106 | 32 | 4 | 1 | 6 | 242 | 16 | 1 | 3 |
| Chocolate Chip Waffle, Frozen, Ready-to-Heat | 2 waffles | 195 | 63 | 7 | 2 | 15 | 380 | 29 | 1 | 4 |
| Plain Waffle, Frozen, Ready-to-Heat | 1 waffle | 100 | 31 | 3 | 1 | 5 | 223 | 15 | 1 | 2 |
| Plain Waffle, Prepared from Recipe | 1 waffle | 218 | 95 | 11 | 2 | 52 | 383 | 25 | n/a | 6 |

## Condiments & Sauces
### CONDIMENTS

| | SERVING SIZE | CAL | CAL FAT | TOT FAT (G) | SAT FAT (G) | CHOL (MG) | SOD (MG) | CARB (G) | FIBER (G) | PROT (G) |
|---|---|---|---|---|---|---|---|---|---|---|
| Catsup | 1 tbsp | 15 | 0 | 0 | 0 | 0 | 167 | 4 | 0 | 0 |
| Cranberry Sauce, Canned, Sweetened | 1 cup | 418 | 4 | 0 | 0 | 0 | 80 | 108 | 3 | 1 |
| Cranberry-Orange Relish, Canned | 1 cup | 490 | 2 | 0 | 0 | 0 | 88 | 127 | 0 | 1 |
| Croutons, Plain | 1 cup | 122 | 18 | 2 | 0 | 0 | 209 | 22 | 2 | 4 |
| Croutons, Seasoned | 1 cup | 186 | 66 | 7 | 2 | 3 | 436 | 25 | 2 | 4 |
| Fruit Butter, Apple | 1 tbsp | 29 | 0 | 0 | 0 | 0 | 3 | 7 | 0 | 0 |
| Guava Sauce, Cooked | 1 cup | 86 | 3 | 0 | 0 | 0 | 10 | 23 | 9 | 1 |
| Honey | 1 tbsp | 64 | 0 | 0 | 0 | 0 | 1 | 17 | 0 | 0 |
| Horseradish, Cooked with Salt | 1 cup, slices | 42 | 2 | 0 | 0 | 0 | 329 | 10 | 5 | 2 |
| Horseradish, Raw | 1 cup, slices | 37 | 2 | 0 | 0 | 0 | 42 | 9 | 3 | 2 |
| Jams & Preserves | 1 tbsp | 56 | 0 | 0 | 0 | 0 | 6 | 14 | 0 | 0 |
| Jams & Preserves, Apricot | 1 tbsp | 48 | 0 | 0 | 0 | 0 | 8 | 13 | 0 | 0 |
| Jams & Preserves, Diet, Any Flavor | 1 tbsp | 18 | 0 | 0 | 0 | 0 | 0 | 8 | 0 | 0 |
| Jellies | 1 tbsp | 56 | 0 | 0 | 0 | 0 | 6 | 15 | 0 | 0 |
| Jellies, Homemade | 1 tbsp | 34 | 0 | 0 | 0 | 0 | 0 | 9 | 0 | 0 |
| Lemon Juice, Canned or Bottled | 1 cup | 51 | 6 | 1 | 0 | 0 | 51 | 16 | 1 | 1 |
| Lemon Juice, Frozen, Unsweetened | 1 cup | 54 | 7 | 1 | 0 | 0 | 2 | 16 | 1 | 1 |
| Lemon Juice, Raw | 1 cup | 54 | 5 | 1 | 0 | 0 | 2 | 17 | 1 | 1 |
| Lemon Peel, Raw | 1 tbsp | 3 | 0 | 0 | 0 | 0 | 0 | 1 | 1 | 0 |
| Marmalade, Orange | 1 tbsp | 49 | 0 | 0 | 0 | 0 | 11 | 13 | 0 | 0 |
| Miso | 1 cup | 547 | 149 | 17 | 3 | 0 | 10252 | 73 | 15 | 32 |
| Molasses | 1 cup | 977 | 3 | 0 | 0 | 0 | 125 | 252 | 0 | 0 |

| | SERVING SIZE | CAL | CAL FAT | TOT FAT (G) | SAT FAT (G) | CHOL (MG) | SOD (MG) | CARB (G) | FIBER (G) | PROT (G) |
|---|---|---|---|---|---|---|---|---|---|---|
| Mustard, Prepared, Yellow | 1 tsp | 3 | 2 | 0 | 0 | 0 | 57 | 0 | 0 | 0 |
| Olives, Ripe, Canned, Jumbo | 1 olive | 7 | 5 | 1 | 0 | 0 | 61 | 0 | 0 | 0 |
| Olives, Ripe, Canned, Large | 1 olive | 5 | 4 | 0 | 0 | 0 | 32 | 0 | 0 | 0 |
| Orange Peel, Raw | 1 tbsp | 6 | 0 | 0 | 0 | 0 | 0 | 2 | 1 | 0 |
| Pickle Relish, Hamburger | 1 tbsp | 19 | 1 | 0 | 0 | 0 | 164 | 5 | 0 | 0 |
| Pickle Relish, Hot Dog | 1 tbsp | 14 | 1 | 0 | 0 | 0 | 164 | 4 | 0 | 0 |
| Pickle Relish, Sweet | 1 tbsp | 20 | 1 | 0 | 0 | 0 | 122 | 5 | 0 | 0 |
| Pimento, Canned | 1 tbsp | 3 | 0 | 0 | 0 | 0 | 2 | 1 | 0 | 0 |
| Prune Puree | 2 tbsp | 93 | 1 | 0 | 0 | 0 | 8 | 23 | 1 | 1 |
| Salsa | 1 cup | 70 | 4 | 0 | 0 | 0 | 1554 | 16 | 4 | 4 |
| Sauerkraut, Canned | 1 cup | 27 | 2 | 0 | 0 | 0 | 939 | 6 | 4 | 1 |
| Vanilla Extract | 1 tbsp | 37 | 0 | 0 | 0 | 0 | 1 | 2 | 0 | 0 |
| Vanilla Extract, Imitation, Alcohol | 1 tbsp | 31 | 0 | 0 | 0 | 0 | 1 | 0 | 0 | 0 |
| Vanilla Extract, Imitation, No Alcohol | 1 tbsp | 7 | 0 | 0 | 0 | 0 | 0 | 2 | 0 | 0 |
| Vinegar, Balsamic | 1 cup | 224 | 0 | 0 | 0 | 0 | 59 | 43 | 0 | 1 |
| Vinegar, Cider | 1 cup | 50 | 0 | 0 | 0 | 0 | 12 | 2 | 0 | 0 |
| Vinegar, Distilled | 1 cup | 43 | 0 | 0 | 0 | 0 | 5 | 0 | 0 | 0 |
| Vinegar, Red Wine | 1 cup | 45 | 0 | 0 | 0 | 0 | 19 | 1 | 0 | 0 |
| **GRAVIES** | | | | | | | | | | |
| Au Jus, Canned | 1 cup | 38 | 4 | 0 | 0 | 0 | 119 | 6 | 0 | 3 |
| Beef Gravy, Canned, Ready-to-Serve | 1 cup | 123 | 49 | 6 | 3 | 7 | 1305 | 11 | 1 | 9 |
| Chicken Gravy, Canned, Ready-to-Serve | 1 cup | 188 | 122 | 14 | 3 | 5 | 1009 | 13 | 1 | 5 |
| Mushroom Gravy, Canned | 1 cup | 119 | 58 | 6 | 1 | 0 | 1357 | 13 | 1 | 3 |
| Turkey Gravy, Canned, Ready-to-Serve | 1 cup | 122 | 45 | 5 | 1 | 5 | 1373 | 12 | 1 | 6 |
| **SAUCES** | | | | | | | | | | |
| Barbecue Sauce | 2 tbsp | 52 | 1 | 0 | 0 | 0 | 386 | 13 | 0 | 0 |
| Cheese Sauce | 1/4 cup | 110 | 75 | 8 | 4 | 18 | 522 | 4 | 0 | 4 |
| Chili, Peppers, Hot Sauce | 1 tbsp | 3 | 0 | 0 | 0 | 0 | 4 | 1 | 0 | 0 |
| Fish Sauce | 1 tbsp | 6 | 0 | 0 | 0 | 0 | 1413 | 1 | 0 | 1 |
| Hoisin Sauce | 1 tbsp | 35 | 5 | 1 | 0 | 0 | 258 | 7 | 0 | 1 |
| Mole Poblano Sauce, Dry Mix | 1 cup | 1513 | 991 | 110 | 0 | 0 | 3085 | 110 | 27 | 20 |
| Oyster Sauce | 1 tbsp | 9 | 0 | 0 | 0 | 0 | 492 | 2 | 0 | 0 |
| Pasta, Spaghetti/Marinara Sauce | 1/2 cup | 111 | 31 | 3 | 1 | 3 | 525 | 18 | 3 | 2 |
| Pepper or Hot Sauce | 1 tsp | 1 | 0 | 0 | 0 | 0 | 124 | 0 | 0 | 0 |
| Pizza Sauce | 1/4 cup | 34 | 7 | 1 | 0 | 2 | 117 | 5 | 1 | 1 |
| Plum Sauce | 1 cup | 561 | 29 | 3 | 0 | 0 | 1641 | 131 | 2 | 3 |
| Sofrito Sauce | 1/2 cup | 244 | 169 | 19 | 0 | 0 | 1179 | 6 | 2 | 13 |

# common foods

| | SERVING SIZE | CAL | CAL FAT | TOT FAT (G) | SAT FAT (G) | CHOL (MG) | SOD (MG) | CARB (G) | FIBER (G) | PROT (G) |
|---|---|---|---|---|---|---|---|---|---|---|
| Teriyaki Sauce | 1 cup | 256 | 1 | 0 | 0 | 0 | 11039 | 45 | 0 | 17 |
| Worcestershire Sauce | 1 cup | 214 | 0 | 0 | 0 | 0 | 2695 | 54 | 0 | 0 |

## Dairy
### CHEESES

| | SERVING SIZE | CAL | CAL FAT | TOT FAT (G) | SAT FAT (G) | CHOL (MG) | SOD (MG) | CARB (G) | FIBER (G) | PROT (G) |
|---|---|---|---|---|---|---|---|---|---|---|
| **American** | 1 oz | 94 | 62 | 7 | 4 | 18 | 274 | 2 | 0 | 6 |
| American or Cheddar, Fat-Free | 1 slice | 31 | 2 | 0 | 0 | 2 | 321 | 3 | 0 | 5 |
| American or Cheddar, Fat-Free | 1" cube | 24 | 1 | 0 | 0 | 2 | 244 | 2 | 0 | 4 |
| American, Low Fat, Diced | 1 cup | 252 | 89 | 10 | 6 | 49 | 2002 | 5 | 0 | 34 |
| American Spread | 1 oz | 82 | 54 | 6 | 4 | 16 | 381 | 2 | 0 | 5 |
| **Blue** | 1" cube | 60 | 45 | 5 | 3 | 13 | 237 | 0 | 0 | 4 |
| Blue | 1 oz | 100 | 73 | 8 | 5 | 21 | 395 | 1 | 0 | 6 |
| **Brick**, Diced | 1 cup | 490 | 353 | 39 | 25 | 124 | 739 | 4 | 0 | 31 |
| **Brie**, Sliced | 1 cup | 481 | 359 | 40 | 25 | 144 | 906 | 1 | 0 | 30 |
| **Camembert** | 1 oz | 85 | 62 | 7 | 4 | 20 | 239 | 0 | 0 | 6 |
| Camembert | 1 cup | 738 | 537 | 60 | 38 | 177 | 2071 | 1 | 0 | 49 |
| **Caraway** | 1 oz | 107 | 75 | 8 | 5 | 26 | 196 | 1 | 0 | 7 |
| **Cheddar**, Diced | 1 cup | 532 | 394 | 44 | 28 | 139 | 820 | 2 | 0 | 33 |
| Cheddar or Colby, Low Sodium, Diced | 1 cup | 525 | 388 | 43 | 27 | 132 | 28 | 3 | 0 | 32 |
| Cheddar or Colby, Low Fat, Diced | 1 cup | 228 | 83 | 9 | 6 | 28 | 808 | 3 | 0 | 32 |
| **Cheshire** | 1 oz | 110 | 78 | 9 | 6 | 29 | 198 | 1 | 0 | 7 |
| **Colby**, Diced | 1 cup | 520 | 381 | 42 | 27 | 125 | 797 | 3 | 0 | 31 |
| **Cottage**, with Fruit, (not packed) | 1 cup | 219 | 78 | 9 | 5 | 29 | 777 | 10 | 1 | 24 |
| Cottage, Low Fat, 1% Milk Fat, (not packed) | 1 cup | 163 | 21 | 2 | 1 | 9 | 918 | 6 | 0 | 28 |
| Cottage, Low Fat, 2% Milk Fat, (not packed) | 1 cup | 194 | 50 | 6 | 2 | 23 | 746 | 8 | 0 | 27 |
| Cottage, Nonfat, Uncreamed, Dry, Large or Small Curd, (not packed) | 1 cup | 104 | 4 | 0 | 0 | 10 | 478 | 10 | 0 | 15 |
| **Cream** | 1 tbsp | 50 | 45 | 5 | 3 | 16 | 47 | 1 | 0 | 1 |
| Cream | 1 cup | 793 | 715 | 79 | 45 | 255 | 745 | 9 | 0 | 14 |
| Cream, Low Fat | 1 tbsp | 30 | 21 | 2 | 1 | 8 | 70 | 1 | 0 | 1 |
| Cream, Low Fat | 1 cup | 482 | 330 | 37 | 22 | 130 | 1128 | 20 | 0 | 19 |
| **Edam** | 1 oz | 101 | 71 | 8 | 5 | 25 | 274 | 0 | 0 | 7 |
| **Feta** | 1 oz | 75 | 54 | 6 | 4 | 25 | 316 | 1 | 0 | 4 |
| Feta, Crumbled | 1 cup | 396 | 287 | 32 | 22 | 134 | 1674 | 6 | 0 | 21 |
| **Fondue** | 1/2 cup | 247 | 131 | 15 | 9 | 49 | 143 | 4 | 0 | 15 |
| **Fontina**, Diced | 1 cup | 513 | 370 | 41 | 25 | 153 | 1056 | 2 | 0 | 34 |
| **Gjetost** | 1 oz | 132 | 75 | 8 | 5 | 27 | 170 | 12 | 0 | 3 |
| **Goat**, Hard Type | 1 oz | 128 | 91 | 10 | 7 | 30 | 98 | 1 | 0 | 9 |

| | SERVING SIZE | CAL | CAL FAT | TOT FAT (G) | SAT FAT (G) | CHOL (MG) | SOD (MG) | CARB (G) | FIBER (G) | PROT (G) |
|---|---|---|---|---|---|---|---|---|---|---|
| Goat, Semisoft Type | 1 oz | 103 | 76 | 8 | 6 | 22 | 146 | 1 | 0 | 6 |
| Goat, Soft Type | 1 oz | 76 | 54 | 6 | 4 | 13 | 104 | 0 | 0 | 5 |
| **Gouda** | 1 oz | 101 | 70 | 8 | 5 | 32 | 232 | 1 | 0 | 7 |
| **Gruyere**, Diced | 1 cup | 545 | 384 | 43 | 25 | 145 | 444 | 0 | 0 | 39 |
| **Limburger** | 1 oz | 93 | 70 | 8 | 5 | 26 | 227 | 0 | 0 | 6 |
| Limburger, Crumbled | 1 cup | 438 | 329 | 37 | 22 | 121 | 1072 | 1 | 0 | 27 |
| **Monterey**, Diced | 1 cup | 492 | 360 | 40 | 25 | 117 | 708 | 1 | 0 | 32 |
| Monterey, Low Fat, Diced | 1 cup | 409 | 257 | 29 | 19 | 86 | 744 | 1 | 0 | 37 |
| **Mozzarella**, Nonfat, Shredded | 1 cup | 159 | 0 | 0 | 0 | 20 | 840 | 4 | 2 | 36 |
| Mozzarella, Part Skim Milk | 1 oz | 72 | 41 | 5 | 3 | 18 | 175 | 1 | 0 | 7 |
| Mozzarella, Part Skim Milk, Low Moisture, Diced | 1 cup | 399 | 238 | 26 | 14 | 71 | 861 | 5 | 0 | 34 |
| Mozzarella, Whole Milk | 1 oz | 85 | 57 | 6 | 4 | 22 | 178 | 1 | 0 | 6 |
| Mozzarella, Whole Milk, Shredded | 1 cup | 336 | 225 | 25 | 15 | 88 | 702 | 2 | 0 | 25 |
| Mozzarella, Whole Milk, Low Moisture | 1 oz | 90 | 63 | 7 | 4 | 25 | 118 | 1 | 0 | 6 |
| **Muenster**, Diced | 1 cup | 486 | 357 | 40 | 25 | 127 | 829 | 1 | 0 | 31 |
| Muenster, Low Fat | 1" cube | 49 | 28 | 3 | 2 | 11 | 108 | 1 | 0 | 4 |
| Muenster, Low Fat, Shredded | 1 cup | 306 | 179 | 20 | 12 | 71 | 678 | 4 | 0 | 28 |
| **Neufchatel** | 1 oz | 72 | 58 | 6 | 4 | 21 | 95 | 1 | 0 | 3 |
| **Parmesan**, Grated | 1 tbsp | 22 | 13 | 1 | 1 | 4 | 76 | 0 | 0 | 2 |
| Parmesan, Grated | 1 cup | 431 | 257 | 29 | 17 | 88 | 1529 | 4 | 0 | 38 |
| Parmesan, Hard | 1 oz | 111 | 66 | 7 | 5 | 19 | 454 | 1 | 0 | 10 |
| **Pimento**, Diced | 1 cup | 525 | 393 | 44 | 28 | 132 | 1999 | 2 | 0 | 31 |
| **Port De Salut**, Diced | 1 cup | 465 | 335 | 37 | 22 | 162 | 705 | 1 | 0 | 31 |
| **Provolone** | 1 oz | 100 | 68 | 8 | 5 | 20 | 248 | 1 | 0 | 7 |
| Provolone, Diced | 1 cup | 463 | 316 | 35 | 23 | 91 | 1156 | 3 | 0 | 34 |
| **Queso**, Anejo | 1 oz | 106 | 77 | 9 | 5 | 30 | 321 | 1 | 0 | 6 |
| Queso, Anejo, Crumbled | 1 cup | 492 | 356 | 40 | 25 | 139 | 1493 | 6 | 0 | 28 |
| **Ricotta**, Part Skim Milk | 1 oz | 39 | 20 | 2 | 1 | 9 | 35 | 1 | 0 | 3 |
| Ricotta, Part Skim Milk | 1 cup | 339 | 175 | 19 | 12 | 76 | 308 | 13 | 0 | 28 |
| Ricotta, Whole Milk | 1 cup | 428 | 287 | 32 | 20 | 125 | 207 | 7 | 0 | 28 |
| **Romano** | 1 oz | 110 | 69 | 8 | 5 | 29 | 340 | 1 | 0 | 9 |
| **Roquefort** | 1 oz | 105 | 78 | 9 | 5 | 26 | 513 | 1 | 0 | 6 |
| **Swiss** | 1 oz | 108 | 71 | 8 | 5 | 26 | 54 | 2 | 0 | 8 |
| Swiss, Diced | 1 cup | 502 | 330 | 37 | 23 | 121 | 253 | 7 | 0 | 36 |
| Swiss, Low Fat, Diced | 1 cup | 228 | 61 | 7 | 4 | 46 | 343 | 4 | 0 | 37 |
| **Tilsit** | 1 oz | 96 | 66 | 7 | 5 | 29 | 213 | 1 | 0 | 7 |

# common foods

| | SERVING SIZE | CAL | CAL FAT | TOT FAT (G) | SAT FAT (G) | CHOL (MG) | SOD (MG) | CARB (G) | FIBER (G) | PROT (G) |
|---|---|---|---|---|---|---|---|---|---|---|
| **FROZEN YOGURTS** | | | | | | | | | | |
| Chocolate, Soft-Serve | 1/2 cup | 115 | 39 | 4 | 3 | 4 | 71 | 18 | 2 | 3 |
| Vanilla, Soft-Serve | 1/2 cup | 114 | 36 | 4 | 2 | 1 | 63 | 17 | 0 | 3 |
| **ICE CREAMS** | | | | | | | | | | |
| Chocolate | 1/2 cup | 143 | 65 | 7 | 5 | 22 | 50 | 19 | 1 | 3 |
| Chocolate, Light | 1/2 cup | 127 | 44 | 5 | 3 | 19 | 48 | 18 | 0 | 3 |
| Chocolate, Light, No Sugar Added | 1/2 cup | 125 | 37 | 4 | 3 | 12 | 54 | 19 | 1 | 3 |
| Vanilla | 1/2 cup | 137 | 65 | 7 | 5 | 29 | 53 | 16 | 1 | 2 |
| Vanilla, French, Soft-Serve | 1/2 cup | 191 | 101 | 11 | 6 | 78 | 52 | 19 | 0 | 4 |
| Vanilla, Light | 1/2 cup | 137 | 33 | 4 | 2 | 21 | 56 | 22 | 0 | 4 |
| Vanilla, Light, No Sugar Added | 1/2 cup | 115 | 45 | 5 | 3 | 18 | 65 | 15 | 0 | 3 |
| Vanilla, Light, Soft-Serve | 1/2 cup | 111 | 21 | 2 | 1 | 11 | 62 | 19 | 0 | 4 |
| **MILKS** | | | | | | | | | | |
| Buttermilk, Low Fat | 1 cup | 98 | 19 | 2 | 1 | 10 | 257 | 12 | 0 | 8 |
| Condensed, Sweetened | 1 cup | 982 | 240 | 27 | 17 | 104 | 389 | 166 | 0 | 24 |
| Cream, Half & Half, Fat Free | 2 tbsp | 20 | 0 | 0 | 0 | 0 | 30 | 3 | 0 | <1 |
| Cream, Half & Half, Fat Free | 1 cup | 160 | 0 | 0 | 0 | 0 | 240 | 24 | 0 | 8 |
| Cream, Heavy Whipping, Fluid | 1 cup | 821 | 793 | 88 | 55 | 326 | 90 | 7 | 0 | 5 |
| Cream, Light (Coffee or Table Cream) | 1 tbsp | 29 | 26 | 3 | 2 | 10 | 6 | 1 | 0 | 0 |
| Cream, Light (Coffee or Table Cream) | 1 cup | 468 | 417 | 46 | 29 | 158 | 96 | 9 | 0 | 6 |
| Cream, Light Whipping, Fluid | 1 cup | 698 | 665 | 74 | 46 | 265 | 81 | 7 | 0 | 5 |
| Dry, Nonfat, Instant | 1 cup | 243 | 4 | 0 | 0 | 12 | 373 | 35 | 0 | 24 |
| Dry, Nonfat, Regular | 1 cup | 434 | 8 | 1 | 1 | 24 | 642 | 62 | 0 | 43 |
| Dry, Whole | 1 cup | 635 | 308 | 34 | 21 | 124 | 475 | 49 | 0 | 34 |
| Eggnog | 1 cup | 224 | 96 | 11 | 7 | 150 | 137 | 20 | 0 | 10 |
| Evaporated, Nonfat | 1 cup | 200 | 5 | 1 | 0 | 10 | 294 | 29 | 0 | 19 |
| Evaporated, Whole | 1 cup | 338 | 171 | 19 | 12 | 73 | 267 | 25 | 0 | 17 |
| Goat | 1 cup | 168 | 91 | 10 | 7 | 27 | 122 | 11 | 0 | 9 |
| Milk, Chocolate, Whole | 1 cup | 208 | 76 | 8 | 5 | 30 | 150 | 26 | 2 | 8 |
| Milk, Low Fat, 1% | 1 cup | 102 | 21 | 2 | 2 | 12 | 107 | 12 | 0 | 8 |
| Milk, Nonfat, (Fat Free/Skim) | 1 cup | 83 | 2 | 0 | 0 | 5 | 103 | 12 | 0 | 8 |
| Milk, Reduced Fat, 2% | 1 cup | 122 | 43 | 5 | 3 | 20 | 115 | 12 | 0 | 8 |
| Sheep | 1 cup | 265 | 154 | 17 | 11 | 66 | 108 | 13 | 0 | 15 |
| Whole | 1 cup | 149 | 71 | 8 | 5 | 24 | 105 | 12 | 0 | 8 |
| **MILK SHAKES** | | | | | | | | | | |
| Thick Chocolate | 10-1/2 oz | 357 | 73 | 8 | 5 | 33 | 333 | 63 | 1 | 9 |
| Thick Vanilla | 11 oz | 351 | 85 | 9 | 6 | 38 | 297 | 56 | 0 | 12 |

| | SERVING SIZE | CAL | CAL FAT | TOT FAT (G) | SAT FAT (G) | CHOL (MG) | SOD (MG) | CARB (G) | FIBER (G) | PROT (G) |
|---|---|---|---|---|---|---|---|---|---|---|
| **SOUR CREAMS** | | | | | | | | | | |
| Reduced Fat | 1 tbsp | 20 | 16 | 2 | 1 | 6 | 6 | 1 | 0 | 0 |
| Regular | 1 tbsp | 23 | 21 | 2 | 1 | 6 | 10 | 0 | 0 | 0 |
| **YOGURTS** | | | | | | | | | | |
| Fruit, Nonfat | 1 cup | 216 | 4 | 0 | 0 | 5 | 132 | 43 | 0 | 10 |
| Plain, Low Fat | 1 cup | 143 | 34 | 4 | 2 | 14 | 159 | 16 | 0 | 12 |
| Plain, Nonfat (Skim) | 1 cup | 127 | 4 | 0 | 0 | 5 | 175 | 17 | 0 | 13 |
| Plain, Whole | 1 cup | 149 | 66 | 8 | 5 | 32 | 113 | 11 | 0 | 9 |
| Vanilla, Low Fat | 1 cup | 193 | 26 | 3 | 2 | 11 | 150 | 31 | 0 | 11 |

## Dairy Alternatives

| | SERVING SIZE | CAL | CAL FAT | TOT FAT (G) | SAT FAT (G) | CHOL (MG) | SOD (MG) | CARB (G) | FIBER (G) | PROT (G) |
|---|---|---|---|---|---|---|---|---|---|---|
| **CHEESES** | | | | | | | | | | |
| Cheddar, Imitation | 1" cube | 42 | 22 | 2 | 2 | 6 | 235 | 2 | 0 | 3 |
| Cheddar, Imitation | 1 cup | 535 | 282 | 31 | 20 | 81 | 3013 | 26 | 0 | 37 |
| Mozzarella, Substitute | 1 oz | 70 | 31 | 3 | 1 | 0 | 194 | 7 | 0 | 3 |
| Mozzarella, Substitute, Shredded | 1 cup | 280 | 124 | 14 | 4 | 0 | 774 | 27 | 0 | 13 |
| **Imitation, Non-Soy Milks** | 1 cup | 112 | 44 | 5 | 1 | 0 | 134 | 13 | 0 | 4 |
| **SOYMILKS** | | | | | | | | | | |
| All Flavors | 1 cup | 109 | 44 | 5 | 1 | 0 | 122 | 8 | 1 | 7 |
| Fruit, Low Fat | 1 cup | 250 | 24 | 3 | 2 | 10 | 142 | 47 | 0 | 11 |
| Fruit, Low Fat, with Low-Calorie Sweetener | 1 cup | 257 | 31 | 3 | 2 | 15 | 142 | 46 | 0 | 12 |
| Fruit, Nonfat | 1 cup | 233 | 4 | 0 | 0 | 5 | 142 | 47 | 0 | 11 |
| Low Fat, All Flavors | 1 cup | 104 | 14 | 2 | 0 | 0 | 90 | 17 | 2 | 4 |
| Nonfat, All Flavors | 1 cup | 68 | 1 | 0 | 0 | 0 | 139 | 10 | 0 | 6 |
| Original/Vanilla, Light, Unsweetened | 1 cup | 83 | 19 | 2 | 0 | 0 | 153 | 9 | 1 | 6 |
| Plain, Nonfat | 1 cup | 137 | 4 | 0 | 0 | 5 | 189 | 19 | 0 | 14 |
| Plain, Whole Milk | 1 cup | 149 | 72 | 8 | 5 | 32 | 113 | 11 | 0 | 9 |
| Unsweetened, All Flavors | 1 cup | 80 | 35 | 4 | 1 | 0 | 90 | 4 | 1 | 7 |
| Vanilla, Low Fat | 1 cup | 208 | 28 | 3 | 2 | 12 | 162 | 34 | 0 | 12 |

## Desserts

| | SERVING SIZE | CAL | CAL FAT | TOT FAT (G) | SAT FAT (G) | CHOL (MG) | SOD (MG) | CARB (G) | FIBER (G) | PROT (G) |
|---|---|---|---|---|---|---|---|---|---|---|
| **Apple Crisp** | 1/2 cup | 227 | 44 | 5 | 1 | 0 | 495 | 43 | 2 | 2 |
| **Brownies** | 2-3/4" x 1" sq | 227 | 82 | 9 | 2 | 10 | 175 | 36 | 1 | 3 |
| **CAKES** | | | | | | | | | | |
| Angel Food | 1 piece | 73 | 2 | 0 | 0 | 0 | 212 | 16 | 0 | 2 |
| Boston Cream Pie | 1 piece | 232 | 70 | 8 | 2 | 34 | 234 | 39 | 1 | 2 |
| Cheesecake | 1 piece | 257 | 162 | 18 | 8 | 44 | 166 | 20 | 0 | 4 |
| Chocolate with Chocolate Frosting | 1 piece | 235 | 94 | 10 | 3 | 27 | 214 | 35 | 2 | 3 |
| Chocolate without Frosting | 1 piece | 352 | 129 | 14 | 5 | 55 | 299 | 51 | 2 | 5 |

# common foods

| | SERVING SIZE | CAL | CAL FAT | TOT FAT (G) | SAT FAT (G) | CHOL (MG) | SOD (MG) | CARB (G) | FIBER (G) | PROT (G) |
|---|---|---|---|---|---|---|---|---|---|---|
| Coffeecake, Cheese | 1 piece | 258 | 104 | 12 | 4 | 65 | 258 | 34 | 1 | 5 |
| Coffeecake, Cinnamon with Crumb Topping | 1 piece | 238 | 120 | 13 | 3 | 18 | 200 | 27 | 1 | 4 |
| Cupcakes, Chocolate with Frosting, Low Fat | 1 cupcake | 131 | 14 | 2 | 0 | 0 | 178 | 29 | 2 | 2 |
| Fruitcake | 1 piece | 139 | 35 | 4 | 0 | 2 | 116 | 26 | 2 | 1 |
| Gingerbread | 1 piece | 263 | 109 | 12 | 3 | 24 | 242 | 36 | 0 | 3 |
| Pineapple Upside-Down | 1 piece | 367 | 125 | 14 | 3 | 25 | 367 | 58 | 1 | 4 |
| Pound | 1 piece | 110 | 51 | 6 | 3 | 63 | 113 | 14 | 0 | 2 |
| Pound, Fat-Free | 1 cake | 962 | 37 | 4 | 1 | 0 | 1159 | 207 | 4 | 18 |
| Shortcake, Biscuit-Type | 1 oz | 98 | 36 | 4 | 1 | 1 | 143 | 14 | 0 | 2 |
| Sponge | 1 piece | 187 | 24 | 3 | 1 | 107 | 144 | 36 | 0 | 5 |
| White with Coconut Frosting | 1 piece | 399 | 104 | 12 | 4 | 1 | 318 | 71 | 1 | 5 |
| White without Frosting | 1 piece | 264 | 83 | 9 | 2 | 1 | 242 | 42 | 1 | 4 |
| Yellow with Chocolate or Vanilla Frosting | 1 piece | 243 | 100 | 11 | 3 | 35 | 216 | 35 | 1 | 2 |
| Yellow without Frosting | 1 piece | 245 | 89 | 10 | 3 | 37 | 233 | 36 | 0 | 4 |
| **COOKIES** | | | | | | | | | | |
| Butter | 1 cookie | 23 | 8 | 1 | 1 | 6 | 18 | 3 | 0 | 0 |
| Chocolate Chip | 1 cookie | 48 | 20 | 2 | 1 | 0 | 32 | 7 | 0 | 1 |
| Chocolate Wafers, Crumbs | 1 cup | 485 | 143 | 16 | 5 | 2 | 773 | 81 | 4 | 7 |
| Coconut Macaroons | 1 cookie | 97 | 27 | 3 | 3 | 0 | 59 | 17 | 0 | 1 |
| Fortune | 1 cookie | 30 | 2 | 0 | 0 | 0 | 22 | 7 | 0 | 0 |
| Gingersnaps | 1 cookie | 29 | 6 | 1 | 0 | 0 | 46 | 5 | 0 | 0 |
| Graham Crackers, Chocolate-Coated | 1 cracker | 68 | 29 | 3 | 2 | 0 | 41 | 9 | 0 | 1 |
| Graham Crackers, Plain/Honey/Cinnamon | 1 cup, crushed | 355 | 76 | 8 | 1 | 0 | 401 | 65 | 2 | 6 |
| Molasses | 1 cookie | 138 | 37 | 4 | 1 | 0 | 147 | 24 | 0 | 2 |
| Oatmeal with Raisins | 1 cookie | 65 | 22 | 2 | 0 | 5 | 81 | 10 | 0 | 1 |
| Oatmeal without Raisins | 1 cookie | 67 | 24 | 3 | 1 | 5 | 90 | 10 | 0 | 1 |
| Peanut Butter | 1 cookie | 72 | 32 | 4 | 1 | 0 | 62 | 9 | 0 | 1 |
| Shortbread, Plain | 1 cookie | 40 | 17 | 2 | 0 | 2 | 36 | 5 | 0 | 0 |
| Sugar Wafers with Crème Filling | 1 wafer | 46 | 20 | 2 | 0 | 0 | 13 | 6 | 0 | 0 |
| Vanilla Wafers | 1 wafer | 28 | 10 | 1 | 0 | 0 | 18 | 4 | 0 | 0 |
| **DOUGHNUTS** | | | | | | | | | | |
| Cake-Type, Chocolate | 1 doughnut | 250 | 107 | 12 | 3 | 34 | 204 | 34 | 1 | 3 |
| Cake-Type, Plain | 1 stick | 217 | 110 | 12 | 4 | 5 | 290 | 24 | 1 | 3 |
| Cake-Type, Plain, Chocolate Frosted | 1 doughnette | 82 | 41 | 5 | 2 | 3 | 75 | 9 | 0 | 1 |
| Crème Filled | 1 doughnut | 307 | 187 | 21 | 5 | 20 | 263 | 26 | 1 | 5 |
| French Crullers, Glazed | 1 cruller | 169 | 68 | 8 | 2 | 5 | 141 | 24 | 0 | 1 |

| | SERVING SIZE | CAL | CAL FAT | TOT FAT (G) | SAT FAT (G) | CHOL (MG) | SOD (MG) | CARB (G) | FIBER (G) | PROT (G) |
|---|---|---|---|---|---|---|---|---|---|---|
| Glazed | 1 hole | 52 | 22 | 2 | 1 | 4 | 50 | 7 | 0 | 1 |
| Jelly Filling | 1 doughnut | 289 | 143 | 16 | 4 | 22 | 249 | 33 | 1 | 5 |
| **FROZEN NOVELTIES** | | | | | | | | | | |
| Creamsicle Pops, No Sugar Added | 1 pop | 25 | 3 | 0 | 0 | 1 | 18 | 6 | 0 | 1 |
| Creamsicle Pops, Sugar Free | 2 pops | 39 | 17 | 2 | 2 | 0 | 5 | 10 | 6 | 1 |
| Fruit & Juice Bars | 2-1/2 fl oz | 67 | 1 | 0 | 0 | 0 | 3 | 16 | 1 | 1 |
| Fudgesicle Bars, Fat Free | 1 bar | 64 | 3 | 0 | 0 | 2 | 47 | 14 | 1 | 3 |
| Fudgesicle Pops, No Sugar Added | 1 pop | 88 | 7 | 1 | 0 | 2 | 86 | 19 | 1 | 3 |
| Ice Type, Fruit, No Sugar Added | 1 bar | 12 | 0 | 0 | 0 | 0 | 3 | 3 | 0 | 0 |
| Ice Cream Bar, Chocolate or Caramel Covered with Nuts | 1 bar | 171 | 98 | 11 | 7 | 1 | 50 | 17 | 0 | 2 |
| Popsicle, Sugar Free, Orange, Cherry, & Grape | 1-3/4 fl oz | 11 | 0 | 0 | 0 | 0 | 5 | 3 | 0 | 0 |
| **PASTRIES** | | | | | | | | | | |
| Cream Puffs with Custard Filling | 1 cream puff | 335 | 181 | 20 | 5 | 174 | 443 | 30 | 1 | 9 |
| Croissants, Apple | 1 medium | 145 | 45 | 5 | 3 | 18 | 156 | 21 | 1 | 4 |
| Croissants, Butter | 1 mini | 115 | 54 | 6 | 3 | 19 | 97 | 13 | 1 | 2 |
| Croissants, Cheese | 1 small | 174 | 79 | 9 | 4 | 24 | 152 | 20 | 1 | 4 |
| Danish, Cheese | 1 pastry | 266 | 140 | 16 | 5 | 16 | 229 | 26 | 1 | 6 |
| Danish, Fruit | 1 large | 527 | 236 | 26 | 7 | 162 | 503 | 68 | 3 | 8 |
| Éclairs, Custard-Filled with Chocolate Glaze | 1 éclair | 293 | 158 | 18 | 5 | 142 | 377 | 27 | 1 | 7 |
| Puff Pastry, Frozen, Rtb, Baked | 1 sheet | 1367 | 849 | 94 | 13 | 0 | 620 | 112 | 4 | 18 |
| **PIES, CRUSTS, & FILLINGS** | | | | | | | | | | |
| Crust, Cookie-Type, Chocolate, Ready Crust | 1 crust | 882 | 368 | 41 | 9 | 0 | 916 | 117 | 5 | 11 |
| Crust, Cookie-Type, Graham Cracker, Ready Crust | 1 crust | 915 | 408 | 45 | 9 | 0 | 604 | 117 | 3 | 9 |
| Crust, Standard-Type, Baked | 1 crust | 949 | 561 | 62 | 16 | 0 | 976 | 86 | 3 | 12 |
| Crust, Standard-Type, Frozen, Baked | 1 crust | 783 | 397 | 44 | 14 | 0 | 720 | 87 | 5 | 10 |
| Fillings, Apple, Canned | 21 oz | 595 | 5 | 1 | 0 | 0 | 280 | 155 | 6 | 1 |
| Fillings, Blueberry, Canned | 8 oz | 474 | 5 | 1 | 0 | 0 | 31 | 116 | 7 | 1 |
| Fillings, Cherry, Canned | 21 oz | 684 | 4 | 0 | 0 | 0 | 107 | 167 | 4 | 2 |
| Apple Pie | 1 piece | 411 | 174 | 19 | 5 | 0 | 327 | 58 | 0 | 4 |
| Blueberry Pie | 1 piece | 360 | 157 | 17 | 4 | 0 | 272 | 49 | 0 | 4 |
| Cherry Pie | 1 piece | 486 | 198 | 22 | 5 | 0 | 344 | 69 | 0 | 5 |
| Chocolate Crème Pie | 1 piece | 301 | 173 | 19 | 5 | 5 | 135 | 33 | 2 | 3 |
| Dutch Apple Pie | 1 piece | 398 | 142 | 16 | 3 | 0 | 274 | 61 | 2 | 3 |
| Egg Custard Pie | 1 piece | 221 | 110 | 12 | 2 | 35 | 158 | 22 | 2 | 6 |

# common foods

| | SERVING SIZE | CAL | CAL FAT | TOT FAT (G) | SAT FAT (G) | CHOL (MG) | SOD (MG) | CARB (G) | FIBER (G) | PROT (G) |
|---|---|---|---|---|---|---|---|---|---|---|
| Lemon Meringue Pie | 1 piece | 362 | 147 | 16 | 4 | 67 | 307 | 50 | 0 | 5 |
| Mince Pie | 1 piece | 477 | 160 | 18 | 4 | 0 | 419 | 79 | 4 | 4 |
| Peach Pie | 1 piece | 261 | 105 | 12 | 2 | 0 | 227 | 38 | 1 | 2 |
| Pecan Pie | 1 piece | 503 | 244 | 27 | 5 | 106 | 320 | 64 | 0 | 6 |
| Pumpkin Pie | 1 piece | 322 | 116 | 13 | 3 | 35 | 450 | 46 | 2 | 5 |
| **PUDDINGS & CUSTARDS** | | | | | | | | | | |
| Banana, Dry Mix, Instant | makes 1/2 cup | 92 | 1 | 0 | 0 | 0 | 375 | 23 | 0 | 0 |
| Chocolate, Dry Mix, Instant | makes 1/2 cup | 95 | 4 | 0 | 0 | 0 | 357 | 22 | 1 | 1 |
| Coconut Cream, Dry Mix, Instant | 1/2 cup | 97 | 5 | 1 | 1 | 0 | 260 | 23 | 1 | 0 |
| Flan, Caramel Custard | 1/2 cup | 222 | 55 | 6 | 3 | 138 | 81 | 35 | 0 | 7 |
| Lemon, Dry Mix, Instant, Prepared | makes 1/2 cup | 95 | 2 | 0 | 0 | 0 | 333 | 24 | 0 | 0 |
| Mousse, Chocolate | 1/2 cup | 455 | 291 | 32 | 18 | 283 | 77 | 32 | 1 | 8 |
| Rice Pudding | 4 oz | 134 | 27 | 3 | 2 | 20 | 139 | 22 | 1 | 4 |
| Tapioca, Dry Mix | makes 1/2 cup | 85 | 0 | 0 | 0 | 0 | 110 | 22 | 0 | 0 |
| Vanilla, Dry Mix, Instant | makes 1/2 cup | 94 | 1 | 0 | 0 | 0 | 360 | 23 | 0 | 0 |
| **TOPPINGS** | | | | | | | | | | |
| Butterscotch or Caramel | 2 tbsp | 103 | 0 | 0 | 0 | 0 | 143 | 27 | 0 | 1 |
| Dessert Topping, Pressurized | 1 tbsp | 11 | 8 | 1 | 1 | 0 | 2 | 1 | 0 | 0 |
| Dessert Topping, Semi Solid, Frozen | 1 tbsp | 13 | 9 | 1 | 1 | 0 | 1 | 1 | 0 | 0 |
| Frostings, Chocolate, Creamy, Ready-to-Eat | 2 tbsp | 164 | 65 | 7 | 2 | 0 | 75 | 26 | 0 | 0 |
| Frostings, Cream Cheese-Flavor, Ready-to-Eat | 2 tbsp | 135 | 51 | 6 | 1 | 0 | 62 | 22 | 0 | 0 |
| Nuts in Syrup | 2 tbsp | 184 | 81 | 9 | 1 | 0 | 17 | 24 | 1 | 2 |
| Pineapple | 2 tbsp | 106 | 0 | 0 | 0 | 0 | 18 | 28 | 0 | 0 |
| Strawberry | 2 tbsp | 107 | 0 | 0 | 0 | 0 | 9 | 28 | 0 | 0 |
| **Eggs** | | | | | | | | | | |
| Substitute, Liquid or Frozen, Fat Free | 1/4 cup | 29 | 0 | 0 | 0 | 0 | 119 | 1 | 0 | 6 |
| White, Dry Powder | 1 tbsp | 26 | 0 | 0 | 0 | 0 | 87 | 0 | 0 | 6 |
| White, Fresh | 1 large | 16 | 1 | 0 | 0 | 0 | 55 | 0 | 0 | 4 |
| Whole, Dried | 1 tbsp | 30 | 18 | 2 | 1 | 86 | 26 | 0 | 0 | 2 |
| Whole, Fresh | 1 ex large | 80 | 50 | 6 | 2 | 237 | 78 | 0 | 0 | 7 |
| Whole, Fried | 1 large | 90 | 63 | 7 | 2 | 210 | 94 | 0 | 0 | 6 |
| Whole, Hard-Boiled, Chopped | 1 cup | 211 | 130 | 14 | 4 | 577 | 169 | 2 | 0 | 17 |
| Whole, Poached | 1 large | 71 | 45 | 5 | 2 | 211 | 147 | 0 | 0 | 6 |
| Whole, Scrambled | 1 cup | 328 | 213 | 24 | 7 | 609 | 319 | 4 | 0 | 22 |
| Yolk, Dried | 1 tbsp | 27 | 20 | 2 | 1 | 93 | 5 | 0 | 0 | 1 |
| Yolk, Fresh | 1 large | 53 | 40 | 4 | 2 | 205 | 8 | 1 | 0 | 3 |

| | SERVING SIZE | CAL | CAL FAT | TOT FAT (G) | SAT FAT (G) | CHOL (MG) | SOD (MG) | CARB (G) | FIBER (G) | PROT (G) |
|---|---|---|---|---|---|---|---|---|---|---|
| **NON-CHICKEN EGGS** | | | | | | | | | | |
| Duck, Whole, Fresh | 1 egg | 130 | 87 | 10 | 3 | 619 | 102 | 1 | 0 | 9 |
| Goose, Whole, Fresh | 1 egg | 266 | 172 | 19 | 5 | 1227 | 199 | 2 | 0 | 20 |
| Quail, Whole, Fresh | 1 egg | 14 | 9 | 1 | 0 | 76 | 13 | 0 | 0 | 1 |
| Turkey, Whole, Fresh | 1 egg | 135 | 84 | 9 | 3 | 737 | 119 | 1 | 0 | 11 |
| **Fats, Oils, Spreads, & Dressings** | | | | | | | | | | |
| **BUTTER** | | | | | | | | | | |
| Butter | 1 tbsp | 102 | 104 | 12 | 7 | 31 | 2 | 0 | 0 | 0 |
| Butter, Whipped with Salt | 1 tbsp | 67 | 69 | 8 | 5 | 21 | 78 | 0 | 0 | 0 |
| Butter with Salt | 1 tbsp | 102 | 104 | 12 | 7 | 31 | 82 | 0 | 0 | 0 |
| **DRESSINGS** | | | | | | | | | | |
| Creamy, Made with Sour Cream &/or Buttermilk, Reduced Calorie | 1 tbsp | 24 | 19 | 2 | 0 | 0 | 153 | 1 | 0 | 0 |
| Creamy, Made with Sour Cream &/or Buttermilk, Reduced Calorie, Fat Free | 1 tbsp | 18 | 4 | 0 | 0 | 0 | 165 | 3 | 0 | 0 |
| Creamy, with Sour Cream &/or Buttermilk, Reduced Calorie, Cholesterol Free | 1 tbsp | 21 | 11 | 1 | 0 | 0 | 140 | 2 | 0 | 0 |
| 1000 Island Dressing | 1 tbsp | 58 | 49 | 5 | 1 | 4 | 135 | 2 | 0 | 0 |
| 1000 Island Dressing, Fat Free | 1 tbsp | 21 | 2 | 0 | 0 | 1 | 117 | 5 | 1 | 0 |
| 1000 Island Dressing, Reduced Fat | 1 tbsp | 30 | 16 | 2 | 0 | 2 | 127 | 4 | 0 | 0 |
| Bacon & Tomato Dressing | 1 tbsp | 49 | 47 | 5 | 1 | 1 | 163 | 0 | 0 | 0 |
| Blue or Roquefort Cheese Dressing | 1 tbsp | 73 | 70 | 8 | 1 | 5 | 142 | 1 | 0 | 0 |
| Blue or Roquefort Cheese Dressing, Fat Free | 1 tbsp | 19 | 2 | 0 | 0 | 0 | 135 | 4 | 0 | 0 |
| Blue or Roquefort Cheese Dressing, Low Calorie | 1 tbsp | 15 | 10 | 1 | 0 | 0 | 184 | 0 | 0 | 1 |
| Blue or Roquefort Cheese Dressing, Reduced Calorie | 1 tbsp | 13 | 4 | 0 | 0 | 2 | 150 | 2 | 0 | 0 |
| Buttermilk Dressing, Light | 1 tbsp | 30 | 17 | 2 | 0 | 2 | 136 | 3 | 0 | 0 |
| Caesar Dressing | 1 tbsp | 80 | 77 | 9 | 1 | 6 | 158 | 0 | 0 | 0 |
| Caesar Dressing, Low Calorie | 1 tbsp | 17 | 6 | 1 | 0 | 0 | 162 | 3 | 0 | 0 |
| Coleslaw | 1 tbsp | 61 | 47 | 5 | 1 | 4 | 111 | 4 | 0 | 0 |
| Coleslaw, Reduced Fat | 1 tbsp | 55 | 30 | 3 | 1 | 4 | 269 | 7 | 0 | 0 |
| French Dressing | 1 tbsp | 71 | 63 | 7 | 1 | 0 | 130 | 2 | 0 | 0 |
| French Dressing, Fat Free | 1 tbsp | 21 | 0 | 0 | 0 | 0 | 128 | 5 | 0 | 0 |
| French Dressing, Reduced Calorie | 1 tbsp | 32 | 19 | 2 | 0 | 0 | 162 | 4 | 0 | 0 |

# common foods

| | SERVING SIZE | CAL | CAL FAT | TOT FAT (G) | SAT FAT (G) | CHOL (MG) | SOD (MG) | CARB (G) | FIBER (G) | PROT (G) |
|---|---|---|---|---|---|---|---|---|---|---|
| French Dressing, Reduced Fat | 1 tbsp | 36 | 17 | 2 | 0 | 0 | 128 | 5 | 0 | 0 |
| Honey Mustard, Reduced Calorie | 2 tbsp | 62 | 27 | 3 | 0 | 0 | 270 | 9 | 0 | 0 |
| Italian Dressing | 1 tbsp | 43 | 38 | 4 | 1 | 0 | 150 | 2 | 0 | 0 |
| Italian Dressing, Fat Free | 1 tbsp | 7 | 1 | 0 | 0 | 0 | 158 | 1 | 0 | 0 |
| Italian Dressing, Reduced Calorie | 1 tbsp | 28 | 25 | 3 | 0 | 0 | 199 | 1 | 0 | 0 |
| Italian Dressing, Reduced Fat | 1 tbsp | 11 | 9 | 1 | 0 | 1 | 205 | 1 | 0 | 0 |
| Peppercorn Dressing | 1 tbsp | 76 | 74 | 8 | 1 | 7 | 143 | 0 | 0 | 0 |
| Ranch Dressing | 1 tbsp | 73 | 69 | 8 | 1 | 5 | 122 | 1 | 0 | 0 |
| Ranch Dressing, Fat Free | 1 tbsp | 17 | 2 | 0 | 0 | 1 | 106 | 4 | 0 | 0 |
| Ranch Dressing, Reduced Fat | 1 tbsp | 29 | 17 | 2 | 0 | 2 | 136 | 3 | 0 | 0 |
| Russian Dressing | 1 tbsp | 54 | 36 | 4 | 0 | 0 | 152 | 5 | 0 | 0 |
| Russian Dressing, Low Calorie | 1 tbsp | 23 | 6 | 1 | 0 | 1 | 141 | 4 | 0 | 0 |
| Sesame Dressing | 1 tbsp | 68 | 62 | 7 | 1 | 0 | 153 | 1 | 0 | 0 |
| Spray-Style Dressing, Assorted Flavors | 10 sprays | 13 | 8 | 1 | 0 | 0 | 88 | 1 | 0 | 0 |
| Sweet & Sour Dressing | 1 tbsp | 2 | 0 | 0 | 0 | 0 | 32 | 1 | 0 | 0 |
| **FATS** | | | | | | | | | | |
| Beef Tallow | 1 tbsp | 115 | 115 | 13 | 6 | 14 | 0 | 0 | 0 | 0 |
| Chicken Fat | 1 tbsp | 115 | 115 | 13 | 4 | 11 | 0 | 0 | 0 | 0 |
| Duck Fat | 1 tbsp | 113 | 115 | 13 | 4 | 13 | 0 | 0 | 0 | 0 |
| Goose Fat | 1 tbsp | 115 | 115 | 13 | 4 | 13 | 0 | 0 | 0 | 0 |
| Mutton Tallow | 1 tbsp | 115 | 115 | 13 | 6 | 13 | 0 | 0 | 0 | 0 |
| Turkey Fat | 1 tbsp | 115 | 115 | 13 | 4 | 13 | 0 | 0 | 0 | 0 |
| Vegetable Shortening | 1 cup | 1812 | 1844 | 205 | 51 | 0 | 8 | 0 | 0 | 0 |
| **MARGARINES & MARGARINE SUBSTITUTES** | | | | | | | | | | |
| Butter-Margarine Blend, Stick, without Salt | 1 tbsp | 101 | 102 | 11 | 4 | 12 | 4 | 0 | 0 | 0 |
| Margarine-Like Spread with Yogurt | 1 tbsp | 88 | 88 | 10 | 2 | 0 | 83 | 0 | 0 | 0 |
| Margarine-Like Spread with Yogurt, Light | 1 tbsp | 46 | 44 | 5 | 1 | 0 | 88 | 0 | 0 | 0 |
| Margarine-Like, Vegetable Oil Spread, Fat-Free, Tub | 1 tbsp | 6 | 4 | 0 | 0 | 0 | 85 | 1 | 0 | 0 |
| Margarine-Like, Vegetable Oil Spread, Light, with Salt | 1 tbsp | 26 | 26 | 3 | 0 | 0 | 110 | 0 | 0 | 0 |
| Margarine-Like, Vegetable Oil Spread, Light, without Salt | 1 tbsp | 22 | 22 | 2 | 0 | 0 | 0 | 0 | 0 | 0 |
| Margarine-Like, Vegetable Oil Spread, Stick/Tub/Bottle, with Salt | 1 tbsp | 75 | 76 | 8 | 1 | 0 | 112 | 0 | 0 | 0 |
| Regular Margarine, Stick, with Salt | 1 tbsp | 100 | 102 | 11 | 2 | 0 | 132 | 0 | 0 | 0 |

| | SERVING SIZE | CAL | CAL FAT | TOT FAT (G) | SAT FAT (G) | CHOL (MG) | SOD (MG) | CARB (G) | FIBER (G) | PROT (G) |
|---|---|---|---|---|---|---|---|---|---|---|
| Stick Margarine, without Salt | 1 tbsp | 102 | 103 | 11 | 2 | 0 | 0 | 0 | 0 | 0 |
| Tub Margarine, Light | 1 tbsp | 59 | 60 | 7 | 1 | 0 | 90 | 0 | 0 | 0 |
| Tub Margarine, with Salt | 1 tbsp | 101 | 102 | 11 | 2 | 0 | 93 | 0 | 0 | 0 |
| Tub Margarine, without Salt | 1 tbsp | 101 | 102 | 11 | 2 | 0 | 4 | 0 | 0 | 0 |
| **MAYONNAISES** | | | | | | | | | | |
| Low-Sodium Mayonnaise, Low Calorie | 1 tbsp | 32 | 24 | 3 | 0 | 3 | 15 | 2 | 0 | 0 |
| Mayonnaise | 1 tbsp | 57 | 45 | 5 | 1 | 4 | 105 | 4 | 0 | 0 |
| Mayonnaise Made with Tofu | 1 tbsp | 48 | 43 | 5 | 0 | 0 | 116 | 0 | 0 | 1 |
| No Cholesterol Mayonnaise | 1 tbsp | 103 | 105 | 12 | 2 | 0 | 73 | 0 | 0 | 0 |
| Reduced-Calorie, Cholesterol-Free Mayonnaise | 1 tbsp | 49 | 44 | 5 | 1 | 0 | 107 | 1 | 0 | 0 |
| **OILS** | | | | | | | | | | |
| Almond Oil | 1 tbsp | 120 | 122 | 14 | 1 | 0 | 0 | 0 | 0 | 0 |
| Avocado Oil | 1 tbsp | 124 | 126 | 14 | 2 | 0 | 0 | 0 | 0 | 0 |
| Canola Oil | 1 tbsp | 124 | 126 | 14 | 1 | 0 | 0 | 0 | 0 | 0 |
| Cocoa Butter Oil | 1 tbsp | 120 | 122 | 14 | 8 | 0 | 0 | 0 | 0 | 0 |
| Coconut Oil | 1 tbsp | 117 | 122 | 14 | 12 | 0 | 0 | 0 | 0 | 0 |
| Corn and Canola Oil | 1 tbsp | 124 | 126 | 14 | 1 | 0 | 0 | 0 | 0 | 0 |
| Cottonseed, Salad or Cooking Oil | 1 tbsp | 120 | 122 | 14 | 4 | 0 | 0 | 0 | 0 | 0 |
| Fish Oil, Cod Liver | 1 tbsp | 123 | 122 | 14 | 3 | 78 | 0 | 0 | 0 | 0 |
| Fish Oil, Herring | 1 tbsp | 123 | 122 | 14 | 3 | 104 | 0 | 0 | 0 | 0 |
| Fish Oil, Menhaden | 1 tbsp | 123 | 122 | 14 | 4 | 71 | 0 | 0 | 0 | 0 |
| Fish Oil, Menhaden, Fully Hydrogenated | 1 tbsp | 113 | 113 | 13 | 12 | 63 | 0 | 0 | 0 | 0 |
| Fish Oil, Salmon | 1 tbsp | 123 | 122 | 14 | 3 | 66 | 0 | 0 | 0 | 0 |
| Fish Oil, Sardine | 1 tbsp | 123 | 122 | 14 | 4 | 97 | 0 | 0 | 0 | 0 |
| Flaxseed Oil | 1 tbsp | 120 | 122 | 14 | 1 | 0 | 0 | 0 | 0 | 0 |
| Grapeseed Oil | 1 tbsp | 120 | 122 | 14 | 1 | 0 | 0 | 0 | 0 | 0 |
| Hazelnut Oil | 1 tbsp | 120 | 122 | 14 | 1 | 0 | 0 | 0 | 0 | 0 |
| Olive, Salad or Cooking Oil | 1 tbsp | 119 | 122 | 14 | 2 | 0 | 0 | 0 | 0 | 0 |
| Palm Oil | 1 tbsp | 120 | 122 | 14 | 7 | 0 | 0 | 0 | 0 | 0 |
| Peanut and Olive Oil | 1 tbsp | 124 | 126 | 14 | 2 | 0 | 0 | 0 | 0 | 0 |
| Sesame, Salad or Cooking Oil | 1 tbsp | 120 | 122 | 14 | 2 | 0 | 0 | 0 | 0 | 0 |
| Soybean, Salad or Cooking Oil | 1 tbsp | 120 | 122 | 14 | 2 | 0 | 0 | 0 | 0 | 0 |
| Sunflower Oil | 1 tbsp | 120 | 122 | 14 | 1 | 0 | 0 | 0 | 0 | 0 |
| Vegetable Oil | 1 tbsp | 124 | 126 | 14 | 1 | 0 | 0 | 0 | 0 | 0 |
| Walnut Oil | 1 tbsp | 120 | 122 | 14 | 1 | 0 | 0 | 0 | 0 | 0 |
| Wheat Germ Oil | 1 tbsp | 120 | 122 | 14 | 3 | 0 | 0 | 0 | 0 | 0 |

# common foods

## Fish & Other Seafoods
### FISH

| | SERVING SIZE | CAL | CAL FAT | TOT FAT (G) | SAT FAT (G) | CHOL (MG) | SOD (MG) | CARB (G) | FIBER (G) | PROT (G) |
|---|---|---|---|---|---|---|---|---|---|---|
| **Anchovy**, Canned, in Oil, Boneless | 1 oz | 60 | 25 | 3 | 1 | 24 | 1040 | 0 | 0 | 8 |
| **Bass**, Freshwater, Cooked | 3 oz | 124 | 36 | 4 | 1 | 74 | 77 | 0 | 0 | 21 |
| Bass, Striped, Cooked | 3 oz | 105 | 23 | 3 | 1 | 88 | 75 | 0 | 0 | 19 |
| **Blackfish**, Whole | 3 oz | 82 | 16 | 2 | 0 | 0 | 0 | 0 | 0 | 16 |
| **Bluefish**, Cooked | 3 oz | 135 | 42 | 5 | 1 | 65 | 65 | 0 | 0 | 22 |
| **Carp**, Cooked | 3 oz | 138 | 55 | 6 | 1 | 71 | 54 | 0 | 0 | 19 |
| **Catfish**, Channel, Breaded & Fried | 3 oz | 195 | 102 | 11 | 3 | 69 | 238 | 7 | 1 | 15 |
| Catfish, Channel, Farmed, Cooked | 3 oz | 129 | 61 | 7 | 2 | 54 | 68 | 0 | 0 | 16 |
| Catfish, Channel, Wild, Cooked | 3 oz | 89 | 22 | 2 | 1 | 61 | 43 | 0 | 0 | 16 |
| **Cod**, Atlantic, Canned | 3 oz | 89 | 7 | 1 | 0 | 47 | 185 | 0 | 0 | 19 |
| Cod, Atlantic, Cooked | 3 oz | 89 | 7 | 1 | 0 | 47 | 66 | 0 | 0 | 19 |
| Cod, Pacific, Cooked | 3 oz | 89 | 6 | 1 | 0 | 40 | 316 | 0 | 0 | 20 |
| **Fish Portions & Steaks**, Frozen, Preheated | 1 stick | 70 | 33 | 4 | 1 | 9 | 118 | 6 | 0 | 3 |
| **Fish Sticks**, Meatless | 1 stick | 81 | 45 | 5 | 1 | 0 | 137 | 3 | 2 | 6 |
| **Flatfish** (Flounder & Sole), Cooked | 3 oz | 99 | 12 | 1 | 0 | 48 | 309 | 0 | 0 | 21 |
| **Grouper**, Cooked | 3 oz | 100 | 10 | 1 | 0 | 40 | 45 | 0 | 0 | 21 |
| **Haddock**, Cooked | 3 oz | 95 | 7 | 1 | 0 | 63 | 222 | 0 | 0 | 21 |
| Haddock, Smoked, Boneless | 1 oz | 33 | 2 | 0 | 0 | 22 | 216 | 0 | 0 | 7 |
| **Halibut**, Atlantic & Pacific, Cooked | 3 oz | 119 | 22 | 2 | 0 | 35 | 59 | 0 | 0 | 23 |
| Halibut, Cooked, with Skin | 3 oz | 113 | 25 | 3 | 0 | 75 | 86 | 0 | 0 | 22 |
| Halibut, Greenland, Cooked | 3 oz | 203 | 136 | 15 | 3 | 50 | 88 | 0 | 0 | 16 |
| **Herring**, Atlantic, Cooked | 3 oz | 173 | 89 | 10 | 2 | 65 | 98 | 0 | 0 | 20 |
| Herring, Atlantic, Kippered, Boneless | 1 oz | 62 | 32 | 4 | 1 | 23 | 260 | 0 | 0 | 7 |
| Herring, Atlantic, Pickled, Boneless | 1 oz | 74 | 46 | 5 | 1 | 4 | 247 | 3 | 0 | 4 |
| Herring, Pacific, Cooked | 3 oz | 213 | 136 | 15 | 4 | 84 | 81 | 0 | 0 | 18 |
| **Mackerel**, Atlantic, Cooked | 3 oz | 223 | 136 | 15 | 4 | 64 | 71 | 0 | 0 | 20 |
| Mackerel, Jack, Canned, Boneless | 1 oz | 44 | 16 | 2 | 1 | 22 | 107 | 0 | 0 | 7 |
| Mackerel, King, Cooked | 3 oz | 114 | 20 | 2 | 0 | 58 | 173 | 0 | 0 | 22 |
| Mackerel, Pacific & Jack, Cooked, Boneless | 1 oz | 57 | 26 | 3 | 1 | 17 | 31 | 0 | 0 | 7 |
| Mackerel, Salted, Cooked | 1 cup | 415 | 307 | 34 | 10 | 129 | 6052 | 0 | 0 | 25 |
| Mackerel, Spanish, Cooked | 3 oz | 134 | 48 | 5 | 2 | 62 | 56 | 0 | 0 | 20 |
| **Monkfish**, Cooked | 3 oz | 82 | 15 | 2 | 0 | 27 | 20 | 0 | 0 | 16 |
| **Mullet**, Striped, Cooked | 3 oz | 128 | 37 | 4 | 1 | 54 | 60 | 0 | 0 | 21 |
| **Ocean Perch**, Atlantic, Cooked | 3 oz | 103 | 16 | 2 | 0 | 46 | 295 | 0 | 0 | 20 |
| **Orange Roughy**, Cooked | 3 oz | 89 | 7 | 1 | 0 | 68 | 59 | 0 | 0 | 19 |

| | SERVING SIZE | CAL | CAL FAT | TOT FAT (G) | SAT FAT (G) | CHOL (MG) | SOD (MG) | CARB (G) | FIBER (G) | PROT (G) |
|---|---|---|---|---|---|---|---|---|---|---|
| **Perch**, Cooked | 3 oz | 99 | 9 | 1 | 0 | 98 | 67 | 0 | 0 | 21 |
| **Pike**, Cooked | 3 oz | 101 | 12 | 1 | 0 | 94 | 55 | 0 | 0 | 21 |
| **Pollock**, Cooked | 3 oz | 100 | 10 | 1 | 0 | 77 | 94 | 0 | 0 | 21 |
| **Pout**, Ocean, Cooked | 3 oz | 87 | 9 | 1 | 0 | 57 | 66 | 0 | 0 | 18 |
| **Rockfish**, Pacific, Cooked | 3 oz | 103 | 15 | 2 | 0 | 37 | 65 | 0 | 0 | 20 |
| **Sablefish**, Cooked | 3 oz | 213 | 150 | 17 | 3 | 54 | 61 | 0 | 0 | 15 |
| Sablefish, Smoked | 3 oz | 218 | 154 | 17 | 4 | 54 | 626 | 0 | 0 | 15 |
| **Salmon**, Atlantic, Farmed, Cooked | 3 oz | 175 | 94 | 10 | 2 | 54 | 52 | 0 | 0 | 19 |
| Salmon, Atlantic, Wild, Cooked | 3 oz | 155 | 62 | 7 | 1 | 60 | 48 | 0 | 0 | 22 |
| Salmon, Red (Sockeye), Filets with Skin, Smoked | 3 oz | 345 | 99 | 11 | 2.5 | 155 | 51 | 0 | 0 | 61 |
| Salmon, Red, (Sockeye), Canned, Smoked | 3 oz | 206 | 65 | 7 | 1 | 93 | 600 | 0 | 0 | 35 |
| Salmon, Red, (Sockeye), Kippered | 3 oz | 141 | 43 | 5 | 1 | 68 | 460 | 0 | 0 | 25 |
| Salmon, Red (Sockeye), Canned, No Bones | 3 oz | 161 | 52 | 6 | 1 | 69 | 390 | 0 | 0 | 27 |
| Salmon, Smoked, (Lox) | 1 oz | 33 | 11 | 1 | 0 | 7 | 567 | 0 | 0 | 5 |
| Salmon, Sockeye, Canned, with Bone | 3 oz | 141 | 56 | 6 | 1 | 37 | 306 | 0 | 0 | 20 |
| Salmon, Sockeye, Canned, without Salt, with Bone | 3 oz | 130 | 56 | 6 | 1 | 37 | 64 | 0 | 0 | 17 |
| Salmon, Sockeye, Cooked | 3 oz | 184 | 84 | 9 | 2 | 74 | 56 | 0 | 0 | 23 |
| **Sardine**, Atlantic, Canned in Oil, Drained, with Solids and Bone | 1 oz | 59 | 29 | 3 | 0 | 40 | 143 | 0 | 0 | 7 |
| **Sardine**, Pacific, Canned in Tomato Sauce, with Bone | 1 cup | 165 | 84 | 9 | 2 | 54 | 368 | 0 | 0 | 19 |
| **Sea Bass**, Cooked | 3 oz | 105 | 20 | 2 | 1 | 45 | 74 | 0 | 0 | 20 |
| **Sea Trout**, Cooked | 3 oz | 113 | 35 | 4 | 1 | 90 | 63 | 0 | 0 | 18 |
| **Snapper**, Cooked | 3 oz | 109 | 13 | 1 | 0 | 40 | 48 | 0 | 0 | 22 |
| **Sturgeon**, Cooked, Boneless | 1 oz | 38 | 13 | 1 | 0 | 22 | 20 | 0 | 0 | 6 |
| Sturgeon, Smoked | 3 oz | 147 | 34 | 4 | 1 | 68 | 628 | 0 | 0 | 27 |
| **Swordfish**, Cooked | 3 oz | 132 | 39 | 4 | 1 | 43 | 98 | 0 | 0 | 22 |
| **Tilapia**, Cooked | 3 oz | 128 | 24 | 3 | 1 | 57 | 56 | 0 | 0 | 26 |
| **Tilefish**, Cooked | 3 oz | 125 | 36 | 4 | 1 | 54 | 50 | 0 | 0 | 21 |
| **Trout**, Cooked | 3 oz | 162 | 65 | 7 | 1 | 63 | 57 | 0 | 0 | 23 |
| Trout, Rainbow, Farmed, Cooked | 3 oz | 144 | 55 | 6 | 2 | 58 | 36 | 0 | 0 | 21 |
| Trout, Rainbow, Wild, Cooked | 3 oz | 128 | 45 | 5 | 1 | 59 | 48 | 0 | 0 | 19 |
| **Tuna**, Fresh, Blue Fin, Cooked | 3 oz | 156 | 48 | 5 | 1 | 42 | 43 | 0 | 0 | 25 |
| Tuna, Light, Canned, in Oil | 3 oz | 168 | 63 | 7 | 1 | 15 | 301 | 0 | 0 | 25 |
| Tuna, Light, Canned, in Water | 3 oz | 99 | 6 | 1 | 0 | 26 | 287 | 0 | 0 | 22 |

| | SERVING SIZE | CAL | CAL FAT | TOT FAT (G) | SAT FAT (G) | CHOL (MG) | SOD (MG) | CARB (G) | FIBER (G) | PROT (G) |
|---|---|---|---|---|---|---|---|---|---|---|
| Tuna, Skipjack, Fresh, Cooked | 3 oz | 112 | 10 | 1 | 0 | 51 | 40 | 0 | 0 | 24 |
| Tuna, White, Canned in Oil | 3 oz | 158 | 62 | 7 | 1 | 26 | 337 | 0 | 0 | 23 |
| Tuna, White, Canned in Water | 3 oz | 109 | 23 | 3 | 1 | 36 | 320 | 0 | 0 | 20 |
| Tuna, Yellow Fin, Fresh, Cooked | 3 oz | 118 | 9 | 1 | 0 | 49 | 40 | 0 | 0 | 25 |
| **Turbot**, European, Cooked | 3 oz | 104 | 29 | 3 | 0 | 53 | 163 | 0 | 0 | 17 |
| **Whitefish**, Cooked | 3 oz | 146 | 57 | 6 | 1 | 65 | 55 | 0 | 0 | 21 |
| Whitefish, Smoked, Boneless | 1 oz | 31 | 2 | 0 | 0 | 9 | 289 | 0 | 0 | 7 |
| Whiting, Cooked | 3 oz | 99 | 13 | 1 | 0 | 71 | 112 | 0 | 0 | 20 |
| **Yellowtail**, Cooked | 3 oz | 159 | 51 | 6 | 0 | 60 | 43 | 0 | 0 | 25 |
| **FISH JERKY** | | | | | | | | | | |
| Cod, Atlantic, Dried & Salted | 1 oz | 82 | 6 | 1 | 0 | 43 | 1992 | 0 | 0 | 18 |
| Whitefish, Dried | 3 oz | 371 | 121 | 13 | 3 | 266 | 200 | 0 | 0 | 62 |
| **OTHER SEAFOOD** | | | | | | | | | | |
| Caviar, Black & Red, Granular | 1 oz | 71 | 46 | 5 | 1 | 167 | 425 | 1 | 0 | 7 |
| Devilfish, Meat | 3 oz | 97 | 48 | 5 | 0 | 0 | 0 | 0 | 0 | 12 |
| Eel, Cooked, Boneless | 1 oz | 67 | 38 | 4 | 1 | 46 | 18 | 0 | 0 | 7 |
| Eel, Cooked with Bone | 1 oz | 52 | 30 | 3 | 1 | 35 | 14 | 0 | 0 | 5 |
| Octopus, Cooked | 3 oz | 139 | 16 | 2 | 0 | 82 | 391 | 4 | 0 | 25 |
| Squid, Cooked, Fried | 3 oz | 149 | 57 | 6 | 2 | 221 | 260 | 7 | 0 | 15 |
| **SHELLFISH & MOLLUSKS** | | | | | | | | | | |
| **Abalone**, Breaded & Fried | 3 oz | 161 | 52 | 6 | 1 | 80 | 502 | 9 | 0 | 17 |
| **Clam**, Breaded & Fried | 3 oz | 172 | 85 | 9 | 2 | 52 | 309 | 9 | 0 | 12 |
| Clam, Canned | 3 oz | 126 | 15 | 2 | 0 | 57 | 95 | 4 | 0 | 22 |
| Clam, Cooked | 3 oz | 126 | 15 | 2 | 0 | 57 | 95 | 4 | 0 | 22 |
| Clam, Raw | 1 large | 15 | 2 | 0 | 0 | 7 | 120 | 1 | 0 | 3 |
| **Crab**, Alaska King, Cooked | 3 oz | 82 | 12 | 1 | 0 | 45 | 911 | 0 | 0 | 16 |
| Crab, Alaska King, Imitation, Made from Surimi | 3 oz | 81 | 4 | 0 | 0 | 17 | 715 | 13 | 0 | 6 |
| Crab, Blue, Canned | 1 oz | 28 | 3 | 0 | 0 | 25 | 94 | 0 | 0 | 6 |
| Crab, Blue, Cooked, Flaked & Pieces | 1 cup | 120 | 19 | 2 | 0 | 118 | 466 | 0 | 0 | 24 |
| Crab, Blue, Cooked (not packed) | 1 cup | 138 | 22 | 2 | 0 | 135 | 533 | 0 | 0 | 27 |
| Crab, Blue, Crab Cakes | 1 cake | 93 | 41 | 5 | 1 | 90 | 198 | 0 | 0 | 12 |
| Crab, Dungeness, Cooked | 3 oz | 94 | 9 | 1 | 0 | 65 | 321 | 1 | 0 | 19 |
| Crab, Queen, Cooked | 3 oz | 98 | 12 | 1 | 0 | 60 | 587 | 0 | 0 | 20 |
| **Crayfish**, Farmed, Cooked, | 3 oz | 74 | 10 | 1 | 0 | 116 | 82 | 0 | 0 | 15 |
| Crayfish, Wild, Cooked | 3 oz | 70 | 9 | 1 | 0 | 113 | 80 | 0 | 0 | 14 |
| **Lobster**, Northern, Cooked | 3 oz | 83 | 5 | 1 | 0 | 124 | 413 | 1 | 0 | 17 |

| | SERVING SIZE | CAL | CAL FAT | TOT FAT (G) | SAT FAT (G) | CHOL (MG) | SOD (MG) | CARB (G) | FIBER (G) | PROT (G) |
|---|---|---|---|---|---|---|---|---|---|---|
| Lobster, Spiny, Cooked | 3 oz | 122 | 15 | 2 | 0 | 77 | 193 | 3 | 0 | 22 |
| **Mussel,** Blue, Cooked | 3 oz | 146 | 34 | 4 | 1 | 48 | 314 | 6 | 0 | 20 |
| **Oyster,** Eastern, Canned & Drained | 1 cup | 112 | 36 | 4 | 1 | 89 | 181 | 6 | 0 | 11 |
| Oyster, Eastern, Cooked, Breaded & Fried | 3 oz | 167 | 96 | 11 | 3 | 69 | 354 | 10 | 0 | 7 |
| Oyster, Eastern, Farmed, Cooked | 3 oz | 67 | 16 | 2 | 1 | 32 | 139 | 6 | 0 | 6 |
| Oyster, Eastern, Farmed, Raw | 6 med | 50 | 12 | 1 | 0 | 21 | 150 | 5 | 0 | 4 |
| Oyster, Eastern, Wild, Cooked, Dry Heat | 3 oz | 67 | 20 | 2 | .6 | 53 | 112 | 4 | 0 | 8 |
| Oyster, Eastern, Wild, Cooked, Moist Heat | 3 oz | 87 | 26 | 3 | 1 | 67 | 141 | 5 | 0 | 10 |
| Oyster, Eastern, Wild, Raw | 6 med | 57 | 19 | 2 | 1 | 45 | 71 | 3 | 0 | 6 |
| Oyster, Pacific, Cooked | 3 oz | 139 | 35 | 4 | 1 | 85 | 180 | 8 | 0 | 16 |
| Oyster, Pacific, Raw | 1 med | 41 | 10 | 1 | 0 | 25 | 53 | 2 | 0 | 5 |
| **Scallop,** Bay & Sea, Cooked | 3 oz | 111 | 0 | 1 | 0 | 41 | 667 | 5 | 0 | 20 |
| Scallop, Cooked, Breaded & Fried | 2 large | 67 | 31 | 3 | 1 | 19 | 144 | 3 | 0 | 6 |
| Scallop, Imitation, Made from Surimi | 3 oz | 84 | 3 | 0 | 0 | 19 | 676 | 9 | 0 | 11 |
| **Shrimp,** Breaded & Fried | 3 oz | 206 | 94 | 10 | 2 | 150 | 292 | 10 | 0 | 18 |
| Shrimp, Canned | 1 oz | 28 | 3 | 0 | 0 | 71 | 220 | 0 | 0 | 6 |
| Shrimp, Cooked | 3 oz | 84 | 8 | 1 | 0 | 166 | 805 | 0 | 0 | 18 |
| Shrimp, Imitation, Made from Surimi | 3 oz | 86 | 11 | 1 | 0 | 31 | 599 | 8 | 0 | 11 |
| **Fruits** | | | | | | | | | | |
| **Apples,** Canned, Sweetened, Slices | 1 cup | 137 | 8 | 1 | 0 | 0 | 6 | 34 | 4 | 0 |
| Apples, Dehydrated (Low-Moisture), Sulfured, Stewed | 1 cup | 143 | 2 | 0 | 0 | 0 | 50 | 38 | 5 | 1 |
| Apples, Dehydrated (Low-Moisture), Sulfured, Uncooked | 1 cup | 208 | 3 | 0 | 0 | 0 | 74 | 56 | 7 | 1 |
| Apples, Dried, Sulfured, Stewed, with Sugar | 1 cup | 232 | 2 | 0 | 0 | 0 | 53 | 58 | 5 | 1 |
| Apples, Dried, Sulfured, Stewed, without Sugar | 1 cup | 145 | 2 | 0 | 0 | 0 | 51 | 39 | 5 | 1 |
| Apples, Dried, Sulfured, Uncooked | 1 cup | 209 | 2 | 0 | 0 | 0 | 75 | 57 | 7 | 1 |
| Apples, Frozen, Unsweetened, Heated, Slices | 1 cup | 97 | 6 | 1 | 0 | 0 | 6 | 25 | 4 | 1 |
| Apples, Frozen, Unsweetened, Unheated, Slices | 1 cup | 83 | 5 | 1 | 0 | 0 | 5 | 21 | 3 | 0 |
| Apple, with Skin | 1 medium | 95 | 0 | 0 | 0 | 0 | 2 | 25 | 4 | 0 |
| Apples, with Skin, Quartered or Chopped | 1 cup | 65 | 2 | 0 | 0 | 0 | 1 | 17 | 3 | 0 |
| Apples, without Skin | 1 large | 104 | 3 | 0 | 0 | 0 | 0 | 28 | 3 | 1 |
| Apples, without Skin, Cooked, Slices | 1 cup | 91 | 6 | 1 | 0 | 0 | 2 | 23 | 4 | 0 |
| Applesauce, Sweetened | 1 cup | 194 | 4 | 0 | 0 | 0 | 71 | 51 | 3 | 0 |

# common foods

| | SERVING SIZE | CAL | CAL FAT | TOT FAT (G) | SAT FAT (G) | CHOL (MG) | SOD (MG) | CARB (G) | FIBER (G) | PROT (G) |
|---|---|---|---|---|---|---|---|---|---|---|
| Applesauce, Unsweetened | 1 cup | 102 | 2 | 0 | 0 | 0 | 5 | 27 | 3 | 0 |
| **Apricots**, Canned, Extra Light Syrup, Halves | 1 cup | 121 | 2 | 0 | 0 | 0 | 5 | 31 | 4 | 1 |
| Apricots, Canned, Heavy Syrup, Drained, Halves | 1 cup | 182 | 2 | 0 | 0 | 0 | 9 | 47 | 6 | 1 |
| Apricots, Canned, Heavy Syrup, Halves | 1 cup | 214 | 2 | 0 | 0 | 0 | 10 | 55 | 4 | 1 |
| Apricots, Canned, Juice, Halves | 1 cup | 117 | 1 | 0 | 0 | 0 | 10 | 30 | 4 | 2 |
| Apricots, Canned, Light Syrup, Halves | 1 cup | 159 | 1 | 0 | 0 | 0 | 10 | 42 | 4 | 1 |
| Apricots, Canned, Water, Halves | 1 cup | 66 | 3 | 0 | 0 | 0 | 7 | 16 | 4 | 2 |
| Apricots, Dehydrated (Low-Moisture), Sulfured, Stewed | 1 cup | 314 | 5 | 1 | 0 | 0 | 12 | 81 | 0 | 5 |
| Apricots, Dehydrated (Low-Moisture), Sulfured, Uncooked | 1 cup | 381 | 7 | 1 | 0 | 0 | 15 | 99 | 0 | 6 |
| Apricots, Dried, Sulfured, Stewed with Sugar, Halved | 1 cup | 305 | 4 | 0 | 0 | 0 | 8 | 79 | 11 | 3 |
| Apricots, Dried, Sulfured, Stewed without Sugar, Halved | 1 cup | 213 | 4 | 0 | 0 | 0 | 10 | 55 | 7 | 3 |
| Apricots, Dried, Sulfured, Uncooked, Halved | 1 cup | 313 | 6 | 1 | 0 | 0 | 13 | 81 | 9 | 4 |
| Apricots, Frozen, Sweetened | 1 cup | 237 | 2 | 0 | 0 | 0 | 10 | 61 | 5 | 2 |
| Apricots, Halves | 1 cup | 74 | 5 | 1 | 0 | 0 | 2 | 17 | 3 | 2 |
| **Bananas** | small | 88 | 0 | 0 | 0 | 0 | 1 | 27 | 3 | 1 |
| Banana Chips | 1 oz | 147 | 86 | 10 | 8 | 0 | 2 | 17 | 2 | 1 |
| Bananas, Sliced | 1 cup | 134 | 4 | 0 | 0 | 0 | 2 | 34 | 4 | 2 |
| **Blackberries** | 1 cup | 62 | 6 | 1 | 0 | 0 | 1 | 14 | 8 | 2 |
| Blackberries, Canned, Heavy Syrup | 1 cup | 236 | 3 | 0 | 0 | 0 | 8 | 59 | 9 | 3 |
| Blackberries, Frozen, Unsweetened | 1 cup | 97 | 6 | 1 | 0 | 0 | 2 | 24 | 8 | 2 |
| **Blueberries** | 1 cup | 84 | 4 | 0 | 0 | 0 | 1 | 21 | 4 | 1 |
| Blueberries, Canned, Heavy Syrup | 1 cup | 225 | 8 | 1 | 0 | 0 | 8 | 56 | 4 | 2 |
| Blueberries, Canned, Light Syrup, Drained | 1 cup | 214 | 9 | 1 | 0 | 0 | 7 | 55 | 6 | 3 |
| Blueberries, Frozen then Thawed, Sweetened | 1 cup | 186 | 3 | 0 | 0 | 0 | 2 | 50 | 5 | 1 |
| Blueberries, Frozen, Unsweetened | 1 cup | 79 | 9 | 1 | 0 | 0 | 2 | 19 | 4 | 1 |
| Blueberries, Wild, Canned, Heavy Syrup, Drained | 1 cup | 341 | 10 | 1 | 0 | 0 | 3 | 90 | 16 | 2 |
| Blueberries, Wild, Frozen | 1 cup | 71 | 2 | 0 | 0 | 0 | 4 | 19 | 6 | 0 |
| **Boysenberries**, Canned, Heavy Syrup | 1 cup | 225 | 3 | 0 | 0 | 0 | 8 | 57 | 7 | 3 |
| Boysenberries, Frozen, Unsweetened | 1 cup | 66 | 3 | 0 | 0 | 0 | 1 | 16 | 7 | 1 |
| **Cantaloupe**, Diced | 1 cup | 54 | 3 | 0 | 0 | 0 | 26 | 13 | 1 | 1 |

| | SERVING SIZE | CAL | CAL FAT | TOT FAT (G) | SAT FAT (G) | CHOL (MG) | SOD (MG) | CARB (G) | FIBER (G) | PROT (G) |
|---|---|---|---|---|---|---|---|---|---|---|
| **Carambola**, (Star Fruit), Sliced | 1 cup | 33 | 3 | 0 | 0 | 0 | 2 | 7 | 3 | 1 |
| **Casaba Melon**, Cubed | 1 cup | 48 | 2 | 0 | 0 | 0 | 15 | 11 | 2 | 2 |
| **Cherries**, Maraschino, Canned, Drained | 1 cherry | 8 | 0 | 0 | 0 | 0 | 0 | 2 | 0 | 0 |
| Cherries, Pie | 1 cup | 52 | 3 | 0 | 0 | 0 | 3 | 13 | 2 | 1 |
| Cherries, Pie, Canned, Heavy Syrup | 1 cup | 233 | 2 | 0 | 0 | 0 | 18 | 60 | 3 | 2 |
| Cherries, Pie, Canned, Light Syrup | 1 cup | 189 | 2 | 0 | 0 | 0 | 18 | 49 | 2 | 2 |
| Cherries, Pie, Frozen, Unsweetened | 1 cup | 71 | 6 | 1 | 0 | 0 | 2 | 17 | 2 | 1 |
| Cherries, Sweet | 1 cup | 87 | 2 | 0 | 0 | 0 | 0 | 22 | 3 | 1 |
| Cherries, Sweet, Canned, Juice, Pitted | 1 cup | 135 | 0 | 0 | 0 | 0 | 8 | 35 | 4 | 2 |
| Cherries, Sweet, Canned, Light Syrup, Pitted | 1 cup | 169 | 3 | 0 | 0 | 0 | 8 | 44 | 4 | 2 |
| Cherries, Sweet, Canned, Pitted, Heavy Syrup | 1 cup | 210 | 3 | 0 | 0 | 0 | 8 | 54 | 4 | 2 |
| Cherries, Sweet, Canned, Pitted, Heavy Syrup, Drained | 1 cup | 149 | 3 | 0 | 0 | 0 | 5 | 38 | 4 | 1 |
| Cherries, Sweet, Canned, Water, Pitted | 1 cup | 114 | 3 | 0 | 0 | 0 | 2 | 29 | 4 | 2 |
| Cherries, Sweet, Frozen then Thawed, Sweetened | 1 cup | 231 | 3 | 0 | 0 | 0 | 3 | 58 | 5 | 3 |
| **Clementines** | 1 fruit | 35 | 1 | 0 | 0 | 0 | 1 | 9 | 1 | 1 |
| **Coconut Meat**, Shredded | 1 cup | 283 | 241 | 27 | 24 | 0 | 16 | 12 | 7 | 3 |
| Coconut Meat, Dried (Desiccated), Sweetened, Shredded | 1 cup | 466 | 297 | 33 | 29 | 0 | 244 | 44 | 4 | 3 |
| Coconut Meat, Dried (Desiccated), Toasted | 1 oz | 168 | 120 | 13 | 12 | 0 | 10 | 13 | 0 | 2 |
| **Crabapples**, Slices | 1 cup | 84 | 3 | 0 | 0 | 0 | 1 | 22 | n/a | 0 |
| **Cranberries** | 1 cup | 46 | 1 | 0 | 0 | 0 | 2 | 12 | 5 | 0 |
| **Cranberries**, Dried, Sweetened | 1/3 cup | 123 | 5 | 1 | 0 | 0 | 1 | 33 | 2 | 0 |
| **Dates**, Pitted | 1 date | 20 | 0 | 0 | 0 | 0 | 0 | 5 | 1 | 0 |
| **Elderberries** | 1 cup | 106 | 7 | 1 | 0 | 0 | 9 | 27 | 10 | 1 |
| **Figs**, Medium | 1 fig | 37 | 1 | 0 | 0 | 0 | 1 | 10 | 1 | 0 |
| Figs, Large | 1 fig | 47 | 2 | 0 | 0 | 0 | 1 | 12 | 2 | 0 |
| Figs, Dried, Stewed | 1 cup | 277 | 9 | 1 | 0 | 0 | 10 | 71 | 11 | 4 |
| Figs, Dried, Uncooked | 1 cup | 371 | 12 | 1 | 0 | 0 | 15 | 95 | 15 | 5 |
| Figs, Dried, Uncooked | 1 fig | 21 | 1 | 0 | 0 | 0 | 1 | 5 | 1 | 0 |
| **Gooseberries** | 1 cup | 66 | 8 | 1 | 0 | 0 | 2 | 15 | 6 | 1 |
| **Grapefruit**, Pink, Red, White | 1/2 large | 53 | 1 | 0 | 0 | 0 | 0 | 13 | 2 | 1 |
| Grapefruit, Sections, Canned, Juice | 1 cup | 92 | 2 | 0 | 0 | 0 | 17 | 23 | 1 | 2 |
| Grapefruit, Sections, Canned, Light Syrup | 1 cup | 152 | 2 | 0 | 0 | 0 | 5 | 39 | 1 | 1 |

| | SERVING SIZE | CAL | CAL FAT | TOT FAT (G) | SAT FAT (G) | CHOL (MG) | SOD (MG) | CARB (G) | FIBER (G) | PROT (G) |
|---|---|---|---|---|---|---|---|---|---|---|
| Grapefruit, Sections, Canned, Water | 1 cup | 88 | 2 | 0 | 0 | 0 | 5 | 22 | 1 | 1 |
| **Grapes**, Canned, Seedless, Heavy Syrup | 1 cup | 195 | 2 | 0 | 0 | 0 | 13 | 50 | 2 | 1 |
| Grapes, Canned, Seedless, Water | 1 cup | 98 | 2 | 0 | 0 | 0 | 15 | 25 | 1 | 1 |
| Grapes, Red or Green | 1 cup | 104 | 2 | 0 | 0 | 0 | 3 | 27 | 1 | 1 |
| **Ground Cherries** (Husk Tomatoes) | 1 cup | 74 | 9 | 1 | 0 | 0 | 0 | 16 | 0 | 3 |
| **Guavas** | 1 cup | 112 | 14 | 2 | 0 | 0 | 3 | 24 | 9 | 4 |
| Guavas | 1 fruit | 37 | 5 | 1 | 0 | 0 | 1 | 8 | 3 | 1 |
| **Honeydew**, Diced | 1 cup | 64 | 2 | 0 | 0 | 0 | 32 | 16 | 1 | 1 |
| **Kiwi** | 1 fruit | 42 | 3 | 0 | 0 | 0 | 2 | 10 | 2 | 1 |
| **Kumquats** | 1 fruit | 13 | 1 | 0 | 0 | 0 | 2 | 3 | 1 | 0 |
| **Lemons** with Peel | 1 fruit | 22 | 3 | 0 | 0 | 0 | 3 | 12 | 5 | 1 |
| **Limes** | 1 fruit | 20 | 1 | 0 | 0 | 0 | 1 | 7 | 2 | 0 |
| **Loganberries**, Frozen | 1 cup | 81 | 4 | 0 | 0 | 0 | 1 | 19 | 8 | 2 |
| **Mandarin Oranges**, Canned, Juice | 1 cup | 92 | 1 | 0 | 0 | 0 | 12 | 24 | 2 | 2 |
| Mandarin Oranges, Canned, Juice, Drained | 1 cup | 72 | 1 | 0 | 0 | 0 | 9 | 18 | 2 | 1 |
| Mandarin Oranges, Canned, Light Syrup | 1 cup | 154 | 2 | 0 | 0 | 0 | 15 | 41 | 2 | 1 |
| **Mangoes** | 1 fruit | 202 | 11 | 1 | 0 | 0 | 4 | 50 | 4 | 3 |
| Mangoes, Sliced | 1 cup | 107 | 4 | 0 | 0 | 0 | 3 | 28 | 3 | 1 |
| **Melon Balls**, Frozen | 1 cup | 57 | 4 | 0 | 0 | 0 | 54 | 14 | 1 | 1 |
| **Mulberries** | 1 cup | 60 | 5 | 1 | 0 | 0 | 14 | 14 | 2 | 2 |
| **Nectarines** | 1 small | 57 | 4 | 0 | 0 | 0 | 0 | 14 | 2 | 1 |
| **Oranges** | 1 large | 86 | 2 | 0 | 0 | 0 | 0 | 22 | 4 | 2 |
| **Papayas**, Cubes | 1 cup | 55 | 2 | 0 | 0 | 0 | 4 | 14 | 3 | 1 |
| **Passion-Fruit**, (Granadilla), Purple | 1 fruit | 17 | 1 | 0 | 0 | 0 | 5 | 4 | 2 | 0 |
| **Peaches** | 1 small | 51 | 3 | 0 | 0 | 0 | 0 | 12 | 2 | 1 |
| Peaches, Canned, Extra Light Syrup, Halves or Slices | 1 cup | 104 | 2 | 0 | 0 | 0 | 12 | 27 | 2 | 1 |
| Peaches, Canned, Heavy Syrup | 1 cup | 194 | 2 | 0 | 0 | 0 | 16 | 52 | 3 | 1 |
| Peaches, Canned, Heavy Syrup, Drained | 1 cup | 171 | 3 | 0 | 0 | 0 | 13 | 44 | 5 | 1 |
| Peaches, Canned, Juice, Halves or Slices | 1 cup | 109 | 1 | 0 | 0 | 0 | 10 | 29 | 3 | 2 |
| Peaches, Canned, Light Syrup, Halves or Slices | 1 cup | 136 | 1 | 0 | 0 | 0 | 13 | 37 | 3 | 1 |
| Peaches, Canned, Water, Halves or Slices | 1 cup | 59 | 1 | 0 | 0 | 0 | 7 | 15 | 3 | 1 |
| Peaches, Dehydrated (Low-Moisture), Sulfured, Stewed | 1 cup | 322 | 9 | 1 | 0 | 0 | 10 | 83 | 0 | 5 |
| Peaches, Dehydrated (Low-Moisture), Sulfured, Uncooked | 1 cup | 377 | 11 | 1 | 0 | 0 | 12 | 96 | 0 | 6 |

| | SERVING SIZE | CAL | CAL FAT | TOT FAT (G) | SAT FAT (G) | CHOL (MG) | SOD (MG) | CARB (G) | FIBER (G) | PROT (G) |
|---|---|---|---|---|---|---|---|---|---|---|
| Peaches, Dried, Sulfured, Stewed, with Sugar | 1 cup | 278 | 5 | 1 | 0 | 0 | 5 | 72 | 6 | 3 |
| Peaches, Dried, Sulfured, Stewed, without Sugar | 1 cup | 199 | 6 | 1 | 0 | 0 | 5 | 51 | 7 | 3 |
| Peaches, Dried, Sulfured, Uncooked, Halved | 1 cup | 382 | 11 | 1 | 0 | 0 | 11 | 98 | 13 | 6 |
| Peaches, Frozen then Thawed, Sliced, Sweetened | 1 cup | 235 | 3 | 0 | 0 | 0 | 15 | 60 | 5 | 2 |
| Peaches, Spiced, Canned, Heavy Syrup, Whole | 1 cup | 182 | 2 | 0 | 0 | 0 | 10 | 49 | 3 | 1 |
| **Pears** | 1 small | 86 | 2 | 0 | 0 | 0 | 1 | 23 | 5 | 1 |
| Pears | 1 medium | 103 | 2 | 0 | 0 | 0 | 2 | 28 | 6 | 1 |
| Pears, Asian, Small | 1 fruit | 51 | 3 | 0 | 0 | 0 | 0 | 13 | 4 | 1 |
| Pears, Asian, Medium | 1 fruit | 116 | 6 | 1 | 0 | 0 | 0 | 29 | 10 | 1 |
| Pears, Canned, Extra Light Syrup, Halves | 1 cup | 116 | 2 | 0 | 0 | 0 | 5 | 30 | 4 | 1 |
| Pears, Canned, Heavy Syrup | 1 cup | 197 | 3 | 0 | 0 | 0 | 13 | 51 | 4 | 1 |
| Pears, Canned, Heavy Syrup, Drained | 1 cup | 149 | 3 | 0 | 0 | 0 | 10 | 38 | 5 | 0 |
| Pears, Canned, Juice, Halves | 1 cup | 124 | 2 | 0 | 0 | 0 | 10 | 32 | 4 | 1 |
| Pears, Canned, Light Syrup, Halves | 1 cup | 143 | 1 | 0 | 0 | 0 | 13 | 38 | 4 | 0 |
| Pears, Canned, Water, Halves | 1 cup | 71 | 1 | 0 | 0 | 0 | 5 | 19 | 4 | 0 |
| Pears, Dried, Sulfured, Stewed, with Sugar, Halved | 1 cup | 392 | 7 | 1 | 0 | 0 | 8 | 104 | 16 | 2 |
| Pears, Dried, Sulfured, Stewed, without Sugar, Halved | 1 cup | 324 | 7 | 1 | 0 | 0 | 8 | 86 | 16 | 2 |
| Pears, Dried, Sulfured, Uncooked, Halved | 1 cup | 472 | 10 | 1 | 0 | 0 | 11 | 125 | 14 | 3 |
| **Persimmons**, Japanese | 1 fruit | 118 | 3 | 0 | 0 | 0 | 2 | 31 | 6 | 1 |
| Persimmons, Japanese, Dried | 1 fruit | 93 | 2 | 0 | 0 | 0 | 1 | 25 | 5 | 0 |
| Persimmons, Native | 1 fruit | 32 | 1 | 0 | 0 | 0 | 0 | 8 | 0 | 0 |
| **Pineapple** | 1 cup | 82 | 2 | 0 | 0 | 0 | 2 | 22 | 2 | 1 |
| Pineapple, Canned, Heavy Syrup, Chunks | 1 cup | 198 | 3 | 0 | 0 | 0 | 3 | 51 | 2 | 1 |
| Pineapple, Canned, Juice, Crushed, Sliced, or Chunks | 1 cup | 149 | 2 | 0 | 0 | 0 | 2 | 39 | 2 | 1 |
| Pineapple, Canned, Juice, Drained, Chunks | 1 cup | 109 | 2 | 0 | 0 | 0 | 2 | 28 | 2 | 1 |
| Pineapple, Canned, Juice, Drained, Crushed | 1 cup | 117 | 2 | 0 | 0 | 0 | 2 | 30 | 3 | 1 |
| Pineapple, Canned, Light Syrup, Crushed, Sliced, or Chunks | 1 cup | 131 | 3 | 0 | 0 | 0 | 3 | 34 | 2 | 1 |
| Pineapple, Canned, Water, Crushed, Sliced, or Chunks | 1 cup | 79 | 2 | 0 | 0 | 0 | 2 | 20 | 2 | 1 |

# common foods

| | SERVING SIZE | CAL | CAL FAT | TOT FAT (G) | SAT FAT (G) | CHOL (MG) | SOD (MG) | CARB (G) | FIBER (G) | PROT (G) |
|---|---|---|---|---|---|---|---|---|---|---|
| Pineapple, Frozen, Chunks, Sweetened | 1 cup | 211 | 2 | 0 | 0 | 0 | 5 | 54 | 3 | 1 |
| **Plantains** | 1 medium | 218 | 6 | 1 | 0 | 0 | 7 | 57 | 4 | 2 |
| Plantains, Cooked, Mashed | 1 cup | 232 | 3 | 0 | 0 | 0 | 10 | 62 | 5 | 2 |
| Plantains, Green, Fried | 1 cup | 364 | 125 | 14 | 4 | 0 | 2 | 58 | 4 | 2 |
| Plantains, Yellow, Fried | 1 cup | 399 | 114 | 13 | 3 | 0 | 10 | 69 | 5 | 2 |
| **Plums** | 1 fruit | 30 | 2 | 0 | 0 | 0 | 0 | 8 | 1 | 0 |
| Plums, Canned, Heavy Syrup, Drained | 1 cup | 163 | 2 | 0 | 0 | 0 | 35 | 42 | 3 | 1 |
| Plums, Canned, Purple, Heavy Syrup, Pitted | 1 cup | 230 | 2 | 0 | 0 | 0 | 49 | 60 | 2 | 1 |
| Plums, Canned, Purple, Juice, Pitted | 1 cup | 146 | 0 | 0 | 0 | 0 | 3 | 38 | 2 | 1 |
| Plums, Canned, Purple, Light Syrup, Pitted | 1 cup | 159 | 2 | 0 | 0 | 0 | 50 | 41 | 2 | 1 |
| Plums, Canned, Purple, Water, Pitted | 1 cup | 102 | 0 | 0 | 0 | 0 | 2 | 27 | 2 | 1 |
| Plums, Dried (Prunes), Stewed, with Added Sugar, Pitted | 1 cup | 308 | 5 | 1 | 0 | 0 | 5 | 82 | 9 | 3 |
| Plums, Dried (Prunes), Stewed, without Added Sugar, Pitted | 1 cup | 265 | 4 | 0 | 0 | 0 | 2 | 70 | 8 | 2 |
| Plums, Dried (Prunes), Uncooked, Pitted | 1 prune | 23 | 0 | 0 | 0 | 0 | 0 | 6 | 1 | 0 |
| **Pomegranates** | 1/2 cup | 72 | 9 | 1 | 0 | 0 | 3 | 16 | 3 | 1 |
| **Prunes**, Canned, Heavy Syrup | 1 cup | 246 | 4 | 0 | 0 | 0 | 7 | 65 | 9 | 2 |
| Prunes, Dehydrated (Low-Moisture), Stewed | 1 cup | 316 | 6 | 1 | 0 | 0 | 6 | 83 | 0 | 3 |
| Prunes, Dehydrated (Low-Moisture), Uncooked | 1 cup | 447 | 9 | 1 | 0 | 0 | 7 | 118 | 0 | 5 |
| **Quinces** | 1 fruit | 52 | 1 | 0 | 0 | 0 | 4 | 14 | 2 | 0 |
| **Raisins** (All Varieties) | 1 cup | 438 | 6 | 1 | 0 | 0 | 17 | 115 | 6 | 5 |
| **Raspberries** | 1 cup | 64 | 7 | 1 | 0 | 0 | 1 | 15 | 8 | 1 |
| Raspberries, Canned, Red, Heavy Syrup | 1 cup | 233 | 3 | 0 | 0 | 0 | 8 | 60 | 8 | 2 |
| Raspberries, Frozen, Red, Sweetened | 1 cup | 258 | 4 | 0 | 0 | 0 | 3 | 65 | 11 | 2 |
| **Strawberries**, Halved | 1 cup | 49 | 4 | 0 | 0 | 0 | 2 | 12 | 3 | 1 |
| Strawberries, Frozen then Thawed, Sweetened, Sliced | 1 cup | 245 | 3 | 0 | 0 | 0 | 8 | 66 | 5 | 1 |
| Strawberries, Frozen then Thawed, Sweetened, Whole | 1 cup | 199 | 3 | 0 | 0 | 0 | 3 | 54 | 5 | 1 |
| Strawberries, Frozen then Thawed, Unsweetened | 1 cup | 77 | 2 | 0 | 0 | 0 | 4 | 20 | 5 | 1 |
| Strawberries, Frozen, Unsweetened | 1 cup | 52 | 1 | 0 | 0 | 0 | 3 | 14 | 3 | 1 |
| **Tangerines** | 1 small | 40 | 2 | 0 | 0 | 0 | 2 | 10 | 1 | 1 |
| **Watermelon**, Diced | 1 cup | 46 | 2 | 0 | 0 | 0 | 2 | 12 | 1 | 1 |

## Grains

### FLOURS

| | SERVING SIZE | CAL | CAL FAT | TOT FAT (G) | SAT FAT (G) | CHOL (MG) | SOD (MG) | CARB (G) | FIBER (G) | PROT (G) |
|---|---|---|---|---|---|---|---|---|---|---|
| Arrowroot Flour | 1 cup | 457 | 1 | 0 | 0 | 0 | 3 | 113 | 4 | 0 |
| Barley Flour or Meal | 1 cup | 511 | 21 | 2 | 0 | 0 | 6 | 110 | 15 | 16 |
| Barley Malt Flour | 1 cup | 585 | 27 | 3 | 1 | 0 | 18 | 127 | 12 | 17 |
| Buckwheat Flour, Whole-Groat | 1 cup | 402 | 33 | 4 | 1 | 0 | 13 | 85 | 12 | 15 |
| Rice Flour, Brown | 1 cup | 574 | 40 | 4 | 1 | 0 | 13 | 121 | 7 | 11 |
| Rice Flour, White | 1 cup | 578 | 20 | 2 | 1 | 0 | 0 | 127 | 4 | 9 |
| Rye Flour, Dark | 1 cup | 416 | 26 | 3 | 0 | 0 | 3 | 88 | 30 | 20 |
| Rye Flour, Light | 1 cup | 364 | 12 | 1 | 0 | 0 | 2 | 78 | 8 | 10 |
| Rye Flour, Medium | 1 cup | 356 | 14 | 2 | 0 | 0 | 2 | 77 | 12 | 11 |
| Semolina | 1 cup | 601 | 16 | 2 | 0 | 0 | 2 | 122 | 7 | 21 |
| Sesame Flour, High-Fat | 1 oz | 149 | 95 | 11 | 1 | 0 | 12 | 8 | 0 | 9 |
| Sesame Flour, Low-Fat | 1 oz | 94 | 4 | 0 | 0 | 0 | 11 | 10 | 0 | 14 |
| Sesame Flour, Partially Defatted | 1 oz | 108 | 30 | 3 | 0 | 0 | 12 | 10 | 0 | 11 |
| Sesame Meal, Partially Defatted | 1 oz | 161 | 122 | 14 | 2 | 0 | 11 | 7 | 0 | 5 |
| Soy Flour, Defatted | 1 cup | 348 | 12 | 1 | 0 | 0 | 21 | 40 | 18 | 50 |
| Soy Flour, Full-Fat | 1 cup | 366 | 156 | 17 | 3 | 0 | 11 | 30 | 8 | 29 |
| Soy Flour, Low-Fat | 1 cup | 330 | 70 | 8 | 1 | 0 | 8 | 31 | 14 | 40 |
| Soy Meal, Defatted | 1 cup | 414 | 26 | 3 | 0 | 0 | 4 | 49 | 0 | 55 |
| Wheat Flour, Bread | 1 cup | 495 | 20 | 2 | 0 | 0 | 3 | 99 | 3 | 16 |
| Wheat Flour, White, All-Purpose | 1 cup | 455 | 11 | 1 | 0 | 0 | 3 | 95 | 3 | 13 |
| Wheat Flour, White, Bread | 1 cup | 495 | 20 | 2 | 0 | 0 | 3 | 99 | 3 | 16 |
| Wheat Flour, White, Cake | 1 cup | 496 | 11 | 1 | 0 | 0 | 3 | 107 | 2 | 11 |
| Wheat Flour, Whole-Grain | 1 cup | 407 | 20 | 2 | 0 | 0 | 6 | 87 | 15 | 16 |

### GRAINS

| | SERVING SIZE | CAL | CAL FAT | TOT FAT (G) | SAT FAT (G) | CHOL (MG) | SOD (MG) | CARB (G) | FIBER (G) | PROT (G) |
|---|---|---|---|---|---|---|---|---|---|---|
| Barley, Hulled | 1 cup | 651 | 38 | 4 | 1 | 0 | 22 | 135 | 32 | 23 |
| Barley, Pearled, Cooked | 1 cup | 193 | 6 | 1 | 0 | 0 | 5 | 44 | 6 | 4 |
| Barley, Pearled, Dry | 1 cup | 704 | 21 | 2 | 0 | 0 | 18 | 155 | 31 | 20 |
| Buckwheat | 1 cup | 583 | 52 | 6 | 1 | 0 | 2 | 122 | 17 | 23 |
| Buckwheat Groats, Roasted, Cooked | 1 cup | 155 | 9 | 1 | 0 | 0 | 7 | 33 | 5 | 6 |
| Buckwheat Groats, Roasted, Dry | 1 cup | 567 | 40 | 4 | 1 | 0 | 18 | 123 | 17 | 19 |
| Bulgur, Cooked | 1 cup | 151 | 4 | 0 | 0 | 0 | 9 | 34 | 8 | 6 |
| Bulgur, Dry | 1 cup | 479 | 17 | 2 | 0 | 0 | 24 | 106 | 26 | 17 |
| Millet, Cooked | 1 cup | 207 | 16 | 2 | 0 | 0 | 3 | 41 | 2 | 6 |
| Millet, Puffed | 1 cup | 74 | 6 | 1 | 0 | 0 | 1 | 17 | 1 | 3 |
| Millet, Raw | 1 cup | 756 | 76 | 8 | 1 | 0 | 10 | 146 | 17 | 22 |

# common foods

| | SERVING SIZE | CAL | CAL FAT | TOT FAT (G) | SAT FAT (G) | CHOL (MG) | SOD (MG) | CARB (G) | FIBER (G) | PROT (G) |
|---|---|---|---|---|---|---|---|---|---|---|
| Oat Bran, Cooked | 1 cup | 88 | 17 | 2 | 0 | 0 | 2 | 25 | 6 | 7 |
| Oat Bran, Raw | 1 cup | 231 | 59 | 7 | 1 | 0 | 4 | 62 | 14 | 16 |
| Oats | 1 cup | 607 | 97 | 11 | 2 | 0 | 3 | 103 | 17 | 26 |
| Quinoa, Cooked | 1 cup | 222 | 32 | 4 | 0 | 0 | 13 | 39 | 5 | 8 |
| Quinoa, Raw | 1 cup | 626 | 93 | 10 | 1 | 0 | 9 | 109 | 12 | 24 |
| Rye | 1 cup | 571 | 25 | 3 | 0 | 0 | 3 | 128 | 26 | 17 |
| Spelt, Cooked | 1 cup | 246 | 15 | 2 | 0 | 0 | 10 | 51 | 8 | 11 |
| Spelt, Dry | 1 cup | 587 | 38 | 4 | 1 | 0 | 14 | 122 | 19 | 25 |
| Wheat Bran, Crude | 1 cup | 125 | 22 | 2 | 0 | 0 | 1 | 37 | 25 | 9 |
| Wheat Germ, Crude | 1 cup | 414 | 101 | 11 | 2 | 0 | 14 | 60 | 15 | 27 |
| Wheat, Durum | 1 cup | 651 | 43 | 5 | 1 | 0 | 4 | 137 | 0 | 26 |
| Wheat, Hard Red Spring | 1 cup | 632 | 33 | 4 | 1 | 0 | 4 | 131 | 23 | 30 |
| Wheat, Hard Red Winter | 1 cup | 628 | 27 | 3 | 1 | 0 | 4 | 137 | 23 | 24 |
| Wheat, Hard White | 1 cup | 657 | 30 | 3 | 1 | 0 | 4 | 146 | 23 | 22 |
| Wheat, Soft Red Winter | 1 cup | 556 | 24 | 3 | 0 | 0 | 3 | 125 | 21 | 17 |
| Wheat, Soft White | 1 cup | 571 | 30 | 3 | 1 | 0 | 3 | 127 | 21 | 18 |
| Wheat, Sprouted | 1 cup | 214 | 12 | 1 | 0 | 0 | 17 | 46 | 1 | 8 |
| **RICES** | | | | | | | | | | |
| Brown, Long-Grain, Cooked | 1 cup | 216 | 16 | 2 | 0 | 0 | 10 | 45 | 4 | 5 |
| Brown, Long-Grain, Raw | 1 cup | 685 | 49 | 5 | 1 | 0 | 13 | 143 | 6 | 15 |
| Brown, Medium-Grain, Cooked | 1 cup | 218 | 15 | 2 | 0 | 0 | 2 | 46 | 4 | 5 |
| Brown, Medium-Grain, Raw | 1 cup | 688 | 46 | 5 | 1 | 0 | 8 | 145 | 6 | 14 |
| White, Glutinous, Cooked | 1 cup | 169 | 3 | 0 | 0 | 0 | 9 | 37 | 2 | 4 |
| White, Glutinous, Raw | 1 cup | 685 | 9 | 1 | 0 | 0 | 13 | 151 | 5 | 13 |
| White, Long-Grain, Cooked | 1 cup | 205 | 4 | 0 | 0 | 0 | 2 | 45 | 1 | 4 |
| White, Long-Grain, Dry | 1 cup | 675 | 11 | 1 | 0 | 0 | 9 | 148 | 2 | 13 |
| White, Long-Grain, Instant, Dry | 1 cup | 361 | 8 | 1 | 0 | 0 | 10 | 78 | 2 | 7 |
| White, Long-Grain, Instant, Prepared | 1 cup | 193 | 7 | 1 | 0 | 0 | 7 | 41 | 1 | 4 |
| White, Long-Grain, Parboiled, Cooked | 1 cup | 195 | 5 | 1 | 0 | 0 | 3 | 41 | 1 | 5 |
| White, Long-Grain, Parboiled, Dry | 1 cup | 698 | 17 | 2 | 1 | 0 | 6 | 150 | 4 | 15 |
| White, Medium-Grain, Cooked | 1 cup | 242 | 4 | 0 | 0 | 0 | 0 | 53 | 1 | 4 |
| White, Medium-Grain, Dry | 1 cup | 702 | 10 | 1 | 0 | 0 | 2 | 155 | 3 | 13 |
| White, Short-Grain, Cooked | 1 cup | 242 | 3 | 0 | 0 | 0 | 0 | 53 | 0 | 4 |
| White, Short-Grain, Dry | 1 cup | 716 | 9 | 1 | 0 | 0 | 2 | 158 | 6 | 13 |
| White, Steamed, Chinese Restaurant | 1 cup | 200 | 3 | 0 | 0 | 0 | 7 | 45 | 1 | 4 |
| Wild Rice, Cooked | 1 cup | 166 | 5 | 1 | 0 | 0 | 5 | 35 | 3 | 7 |
| Wild Rice, Raw | 1 cup | 571 | 16 | 2 | 0 | 0 | 11 | 120 | 10 | 24 |

| | SERVING SIZE | CAL | CAL FAT | TOT FAT (G) | SAT FAT (G) | CHOL (MG) | SOD (MG) | CARB (G) | FIBER (G) | PROT (G) |
|---|---|---|---|---|---|---|---|---|---|---|
| **Herbs & Spices** | | | | | | | | | | |
| Allspice, Ground | 1 tbsp | 16 | 5 | 1 | 0 | 0 | 5 | 4 | 1 | 0 |
| Basil, Dried | 1 tbsp | 5 | 1 | 0 | 0 | 0 | 1 | 1 | 1 | 0 |
| Bay Leaf, Crumbled | 1 tbsp | 6 | 1 | 0 | 0 | 0 | 0 | 1 | 0 | 0 |
| Cardamom, Ground | 1 tbsp | 18 | 3 | 0 | 0 | 0 | 1 | 4 | 2 | 1 |
| Chili Powder | 1 tbsp | 24 | 11 | 1 | 0 | 0 | 76 | 4 | 3 | 1 |
| Cinnamon, Ground | 1 tbsp | 19 | 1 | 0 | 0 | 0 | 1 | 6 | 4 | 0 |
| Curry Powder | 1 tbsp | 20 | 8 | 1 | 0 | 0 | 3 | 4 | 2 | 1 |
| Garlic Powder | 1 tbsp | 32 | 1 | 0 | 0 | 0 | 6 | 7 | 1 | 2 |
| Mustard, Ground | 1 tbsp | 32 | 21 | 2 | 0 | 0 | 1 | 2 | 1 | 2 |
| Nutmeg, Ground | 1 tbsp | 37 | 23 | 3 | 2 | 0 | 1 | 3 | 1 | 0 |
| Onion Powder | 1 tbsp | 24 | 1 | 0 | 0 | 0 | 5 | 5 | 1 | 1 |
| Oregano, Dried | 1 tsp | 3 | 0 | 0 | 0 | 0 | 0 | 1 | 0 | 0 |
| Parsley, Dried | 1 tbsp | 5 | 1 | 0 | 0 | 0 | 7 | 1 | 0 | 0 |
| Parsley, Fresh | 1 tbsp | 1 | 0 | 0 | 0 | 0 | 2 | 0 | 0 | 0 |
| Pepper, Black | 1 tbsp | 16 | 2 | 0 | 0 | 0 | 3 | 4 | 2 | 1 |
| Pepper, Red or Cayenne | 1 tbsp | 17 | 8 | 1 | 0 | 0 | 2 | 3 | 1 | 1 |
| Pepper, White, Ground | 1 tbsp | 21 | 1 | 0 | 0 | 0 | 0 | 5 | 2 | 1 |
| Pumpkin Pie Spice | 1 tbsp | 19 | 6 | 1 | 0 | 0 | 3 | 4 | 1 | 0 |
| Rosemary, Dried | 1 tbsp | 11 | 5 | 1 | 0 | 0 | 2 | 2 | 1 | 0 |
| Rosemary, Fresh | 1 tbsp | 2 | 1 | 0 | 0 | 0 | 0 | 0 | 0 | 0 |
| Saffron | 1 tbsp | 7 | 1 | 0 | 0 | 0 | 3 | 1 | 0 | 0 |
| Sage, Ground | 1 tbsp | 6 | 2 | 0 | 0 | 0 | 0 | 1 | 1 | 0 |
| Salt, Table | 1 tbsp | 0 | 0 | 0 | 0 | 0 | 6976 | 0 | 0 | 0 |
| Spearmint, Dried | 1 tbsp | 5 | 1 | 0 | 0 | 0 | 6 | 1 | 0 | 0 |
| Spearmint, Fresh | 2 tbsp | 5 | 1 | 0 | 0 | 0 | 3 | 1 | 1 | 0 |
| Tarragon, Dried | 1 tbsp | 5 | 1 | 0 | 0 | 0 | 1 | 1 | 0 | 0 |
| Thyme, Dried | 1 tbsp | 7 | 2 | 0 | 0 | 0 | 1 | 2 | 1 | 0 |
| Thyme, Fresh | 1 tsp | 1 | 0 | 0 | 0 | 0 | 0 | 0 | 0 | 0 |
| Turmeric, Ground | 1 tbsp | 24 | 6 | 1 | 0 | 0 | 3 | 4 | 1 | 1 |
| **Meats** | | | | | | | | | | |
| **BEEF** | | | | | | | | | | |
| *Cured Meats* | | | | | | | | | | |
| Corned Beef, Brisket, Cooked | 3 oz | 213 | 145 | 16 | 5 | 83 | 964 | 0 | 0 | 15 |
| Dried | 10 slices | 43 | 5 | 1 | 0 | 22 | 781 | 1 | 0 | 9 |
| Sausage, Cooked, Smoked | 1 oz | 88 | 69 | 8 | 3 | 19 | 321 | 1 | 0 | 4 |
| Smoked, Chopped Beef | 1 oz | 38 | 11 | 1 | 1 | 13 | 357 | 1 | 0 | 6 |

| | SERVING SIZE | CAL | CAL FAT | TOT FAT (G) | SAT FAT (G) | CHOL (MG) | SOD (MG) | CARB (G) | FIBER (G) | PROT (G) |
|---|---|---|---|---|---|---|---|---|---|---|
| *Ground Beef* | | | | | | | | | | |
| Ground, 70% Lean Meat / 30% Fat, Crumbles, Cooked, Pan-Browned | 3 oz | 230 | 137 | 15 | 6 | 75 | 82 | 0 | 0 | 22 |
| Ground, 70% Lean Meat / 30% Fat, Patty, Cooked, Broiled | 3 oz | 232 | 139 | 15 | 6 | 70 | 69 | 0 | 0 | 22 |
| Ground, 70% Lean Meat / 30% Fat, Patty Cooked, Pan-Broiled | 3 oz | 202 | 119 | 13 | 5 | 66 | 78 | 0 | 0 | 19 |
| Ground, 75% Lean Meat / 25% Fat, Crumbles, Cooked, Pan-Browned | 3 oz | 235 | 139 | 15 | 6 | 76 | 79 | 0 | 0 | 22 |
| Ground, 75% Lean Meat / 25% Fat, Patty, Cooked, Broiled | 3 oz | 236 | 143 | 16 | 6 | 76 | 66 | 0 | 0 | 22 |
| Ground, 75% Lean Meat / 25% Fat, Patty, Cooked, Pan-Broiled | 3 oz | 211 | 126 | 14 | 5 | 71 | 74 | 0 | 0 | 20 |
| Ground, 80% Lean Meat / 20% Fat, Crumbles, Cooked, Pan-Browned | 3 oz | 231 | 133 | 15 | 6 | 76 | 77 | 0 | 0 | 23 |
| Ground, 80% Lean Meat / 20% Fat, Patty, Cooked, Broiled | 3 oz | 230 | 136 | 15 | 6 | 77 | 64 | 0 | 0 | 22 |
| Ground, 80% Lean Meat / 20% Fat, Patty, Cooked, Pan-Broiled | 3 oz | 209 | 122 | 14 | 5 | 73 | 71 | 0 | 0 | 20 |
| Ground, 85% Lean Meat / 15% Fat, Crumbles, Cooked, Pan-Browned | 3 oz | 218 | 117 | 13 | 5 | 77 | 76 | 0 | 0 | 24 |
| Ground, 85% Lean Meat / 15% Fat, Patty, Cooked, Pan-Broiled | 3 oz | 197 | 107 | 12 | 5 | 73 | 67 | 0 | 0 | 21 |
| Ground, 90% Lean Meat / 10% Fat, Crumbles, Cooked, Pan-Browned | 3 oz | 196 | 92 | 10 | 4 | 76 | 74 | 0 | 0 | 24 |
| Ground, 90% Lean Meat / 10% Fat, Patty, Cooked, Broiled | 3 oz | 184 | 90 | 10 | 4 | 72 | 58 | 0 | 0 | 22 |
| Ground, 90% Lean Meat / 10% Fat, Patty, Cooked, Pan-Broiled | 3 oz | 173 | 82 | 9 | 4 | 70 | 64 | 0 | 0 | 21 |
| Ground, 95% Lean Meat / 5% Fat, Crumbles, Cooked, Pan-Browned | 3 oz | 164 | 58 | 6 | 3 | 76 | 72 | 0 | 0 | 25 |
| Ground, 95% Lean Meat / 5% Fat, Patty, Cooked, Broiled | 3 oz | 145 | 50 | 6 | 3 | 65 | 55 | 0 | 0 | 22 |
| Ground, 95% Lean Meat / 5% Fat, Patty, Cooked, Pan-Broiled | 3 oz | 139 | 45 | 5 | 2 | 65 | 60 | 0 | 0 | 22 |
| *Roasts* | | | | | | | | | | |
| Brisket, Flat Half, 1/8" Fat, Cooked | 3 oz | 246 | 141 | 16 | 6 | 65 | 41 | 0 | 0 | 24 |

| | SERVING SIZE | CAL | CAL FAT | TOT FAT (G) | SAT FAT (G) | CHOL (MG) | SOD (MG) | CARB (G) | FIBER (G) | PROT (G) |
|---|---|---|---|---|---|---|---|---|---|---|
| Brisket, Whole, 1/8" Fat, Cooked | 3 oz | 281 | 187 | 21 | 8 | 79 | 54 | 0 | 0 | 22 |
| Chuck, (Blade) Roast, 1/8" Fat, Cooked | 3 oz | 290 | 192 | 21 | 9 | 88 | 55 | 0 | 0 | 23 |
| Chuck, Pot Roast, 1/8" Fat, Cooked | 3 oz | 257 | 147 | 16 | 6 | 67 | 43 | 0 | 0 | 26 |
| Rib, Large End, 1/8" Fat, Broiled | 3 oz | 287 | 208 | 23 | 9 | 68 | 54 | 0 | 0 | 18 |
| Rib, Large End, 1/8" Fat, Roasted | 3 oz | 302 | 218 | 24 | 10 | 72 | 54 | 0 | 0 | 20 |
| Rib, Short Ribs, Cooked | 3 oz | 400 | 321 | 36 | 15 | 80 | 43 | 0 | 0 | 18 |
| Rib, Small End, 1/8" Fat, Broiled | 3 oz | 247 | 153 | 17 | 7 | 89 | 45 | 0 | 0 | 22 |
| Rib, Small End, 1/8" Fat, Roasted | 3 oz | 290 | 208 | 23 | 9 | 71 | 54 | 0 | 0 | 19 |
| Rib, Whole, 1/8" Fat, Broiled | 3 oz | 286 | 205 | 23 | 9 | 70 | 54 | 0 | 0 | 19 |
| Rib, Whole, 1/8" Fat, Roasted | 3 oz | 298 | 215 | 24 | 10 | 71 | 54 | 0 | 0 | 19 |
| Round, Bottom Round, Roast, 1/8" Fat, Cooked | 3 oz | 185 | 90 | 10 | 4 | 72 | 30 | 0 | 0 | 22 |
| Round, Eye of Round, Roast, 1/8" Fat, Cooked | 3 oz | 177 | 74 | 8 | 3 | 53 | 31 | 0 | 0 | 24 |
| Round, Full Cut, 1/8" Fat, Cooked | 3 oz | 200 | 99 | 11 | 4 | 67 | 53 | 0 | 0 | 23 |
| Round, Tip Round, Roast, 1/8" Fat, Cooked | 3 oz | 186 | 87 | 10 | 4 | 70 | 54 | 0 | 0 | 23 |
| Round, Top Round, 1/8" Fat, Cooked | 3 oz | 202 | 77 | 9 | 3 | 77 | 38 | 0 | 0 | 29 |
| Tenderloin, 1/8" Fat, Cooked | 3 oz | 275 | 188 | 21 | 8 | 72 | 48 | 0 | 0 | 20 |
| Top Sirloin, 1/8" Fat, Cooked | 3 oz | 207 | 109 | 12 | 5 | 64 | 48 | 0 | 0 | 23 |
| Top Sirloin, 1/8" Fat, Cooked, Pan-Fried | 3 oz | 266 | 161 | 18 | 7 | 83 | 60 | 0 | 0 | 24 |
| *Steaks* | | | | | | | | | | |
| Filet, 1/8" Fat, Cooked | 3 oz | 227 | 131 | 15 | 6 | 71 | 46 | 0 | 0 | 22 |
| Flank, Cooked | 3 oz | 201 | 99 | 11 | 5 | 60 | 61 | 0 | 0 | 24 |
| NY Strip/ Club Top Loin, 1/8" Fat, Cooked | 3 oz | 224 | 128 | 14 | 6 | 75 | 46 | 0 | 0 | 22 |
| Plate, Skirt Steak, Cooked | 3 oz | 187 | 92 | 10 | 4 | 51 | 64 | 0 | 0 | 22 |
| Porterhouse Steak, 1/8" Fat, Cooked | 3 oz | 252 | 167 | 19 | 7 | 60 | 54 | 0 | 0 | 20 |
| Rib Eye, Small End, Cooked | 3 oz | 249 | 135 | 15 | 6 | 89 | 56 | 0 | 0 | 27 |
| Rib, Small End, 1/8" Fat, Cooked | 3 oz | 258 | 169 | 19 | 7 | 99 | 42 | 0 | 0 | 21 |
| Sirloin, 1/8" Fat, Cooked | 3 oz | 218 | 120 | 13 | 5 | 71 | 46 | 0 | 0 | 23 |
| T-Bone Steak, 1/8" Fat, Cooked | 3 oz | 238 | 149 | 17 | 6 | 53 | 56 | 0 | 0 | 21 |
| **DELI MEAT** | | | | | | | | | | |
| Beef, Thin Sliced | 1 oz | 50 | 10 | 1 | 0 | 12 | 408 | 2 | 0 | 8 |
| Bologna, Pork & Turkey, Light | 2 oz | 118 | 81 | 9 | 3 | 44 | 401 | 2 | 0 | 7 |
| Bologna, Turkey | 1 oz | 59 | 40 | 4 | 1 | 21 | 351 | 1 | 0 | 3 |
| Bologna, Lebanon, Beef | 2 oz | 98 | 54 | 6 | 2 | 31 | 783 | 0 | 0 | 11 |
| Bologna, Pork Turkey & Beef | 1 oz | 95 | 75 | 8 | 3 | 21 | 299 | 2 | 0 | 3 |
| Bologna, Beef | 3 oz | 311 | 252 | 28 | 11 | 56 | 1080 | 4 | 0 | 10 |
| Bologna, Beef & Pork | 3 oz | 308 | 221 | 25 | 9 | 60 | 736 | 5 | 0 | 15 |

# common foods

| | SERVING SIZE | CAL | CAL FAT | TOT FAT (G) | SAT FAT (G) | CHOL (MG) | SOD (MG) | CARB (G) | FIBER (G) | PROT (G) |
|---|---|---|---|---|---|---|---|---|---|---|
| Bologna, Beef & Pork, Low Fat | 3 oz | 230 | 171 | 19 | 7 | 39 | 1108 | 3 | 0 | 12 |
| Bologna, Beef, Low Fat | 3 oz | 204 | 135 | 15 | 5 | 44 | 1180 | 5 | 0 | 12 |
| Bologna, Pork | 1 oz | 70 | 51 | 6 | 2 | 17 | 336 | 0 | 0 | 4 |
| Ham, Sliced, Extra Lean | 3 oz | 107 | 27 | 3 | 1 | 45 | 1060 | 1 | 0 | 19 |
| Ham, Sliced, Regular (11% Fat) | 3 oz | 163 | 81 | 9 | 3 | 57 | 1304 | 4 | 1 | 17 |
| Headcheese, Pork | 1 oz | 45 | 28 | 3 | 1 | 20 | 235 | 0 | 0 | 4 |
| Pastrami, Beef 98% Fat Free | 3 oz | 95 | 9 | 1 | 0 | 47 | 1010 | 2 | 0 | 20 |
| Pastrami, Cured | 3 oz | 147 | 54 | 6 | 3 | 68 | 885 | 0 | 0 | 22 |
| Salami, Cooked Beef | 3 oz | 261 | 198 | 22 | 10 | 71 | 1140 | 2 | 0 | 13 |
| Salami, Italian Pork | 1 oz | 119 | 93 | 10 | 4 | 22 | 529 | 0 | 0 | 6 |
| Salami, Italian, Pork & Beef, Dry, Sliced, 50% Less Salt | 3 oz | 350 | 234 | 26 | 10 | 89 | 936 | 6 | 0 | 22 |
| Salami, Pork Beef Low Salt | 3 oz | 396 | 275 | 31 | 11 | 90 | 623 | 15 | 0 | 15 |
| Salami, Cooked, Beef & Pork | 3 oz | 336 | 234 | 26 | 9 | 89 | 1449 | 2 | 0 | 22 |
| Salami, Dry or Hard, Pork | 3 oz | 407 | 306 | 34 | 12 | 79 | 2260 | 2 | 0 | 23 |
| Salami, Dry or Hard, Pork, Beef | 3 oz | 385 | 270 | 30 | 11 | 100 | 2010 | 4 | 0 | 23 |
| **FAKE MEAT & SOY MEAT ANALOGUES** | | | | | | | | | | |
| Bacon, Cooked | 1 oz | 50 | 43 | 5 | 1 | 0 | 234 | 1 | 0 | 2 |
| Bacon Bits | 1 tbsp | 33 | 16 | 2 | 0 | 0 | 124 | 2 | 1 | 2 |
| Chicken | 1 cup | 376 | 192 | 21 | 3 | 0 | 1191 | 6 | 6 | 40 |
| Chicken, Breaded, Fried | 3 oz | 234 | 117 | 13 | 1 | 0 | 400 | 9 | 4 | 21 |
| Frankfurter, Meatless, Sliced | 1 cup | 326 | 173 | 19 | 3 | 0 | 659 | 11 | 5 | 27 |
| Meatballs, Imitation | 1 cup | 284 | 117 | 13 | 2 | 0 | 792 | 12 | 7 | 30 |
| Sausage, Meatless | 1 link | 64 | 41 | 5 | 1 | 0 | 222 | 2 | 1 | 5 |
| **GAME MEAT** | | | | | | | | | | |
| Bear, cooked | 3 oz | 220 | 102 | 12 | 3 | 83 | 60 | 0 | 0 | 28 |
| Bison, Chuck, Shoulder Clod, 3-5 LB Roast, Cooked | 3 oz | 164 | 42 | 5 | 2 | 94 | 48 | 0 | 0 | 29 |
| Bison, Cooked | 3 oz | 122 | 19 | 2 | 1 | 70 | 48 | 0 | 0 | 24 |
| Bison, Ground, Cooked | 3 oz | 202 | 116 | 13 | 0 | 71 | 62 | 0 | 0 | 20 |
| Bison, Ground, Grass-Fed, Cooked | 3 oz | 152 | 66 | 7 | 3 | 60 | 65 | 0 | 0 | 22 |
| Bison, Rib Eye, 1" Steak, Cooked | 3 oz | 150 | 43 | 5 | 2 | 67 | 44 | 0 | 0 | 25 |
| Bison, Top Round, 1" Steak, Cooked | 3 oz | 148 | 38 | 4 | 2 | 72 | 35 | 0 | 0 | 26 |
| Bison, Top Sirloin, 1" Steak, Cooked | 3 oz | 145 | 43 | 5 | 2 | 73 | 45 | 0 | 0 | 24 |
| Buffalo, Free Range, Top Round Steak, Cooked (Shoshone Bannock) | 3 oz | 146 | 18 | 2 | 1 | 82 | 41 | 0 | 0 | 33 |

| | SERVING SIZE | CAL | CAL FAT | TOT FAT (G) | SAT FAT (G) | CHOL (MG) | SOD (MG) | CARB (G) | FIBER (G) | PROT (G) |
|---|---|---|---|---|---|---|---|---|---|---|
| Deer, Cooked | 3 oz | 134 | 24 | 3 | 1 | 95 | 46 | 0 | 0 | 26 |
| Deer, Ground, Cooked | 3 oz | 159 | 63 | 7 | 3 | 83 | 66 | 0 | 0 | 22 |
| Deer, Loin, 1" Steak, Cooked | 3 oz | 128 | 18 | 2 | 1 | 67 | 48 | 0 | 0 | 26 |
| Deer, Shoulder Clod, 3-5 LB Roast, Cooked | 3 oz | 162 | 30 | 3 | 2 | 96 | 44 | 0 | 0 | 31 |
| Deer, Tenderloin, 0.5-1 LB Roast, Cooked | 3 oz | 127 | 18 | 2 | 1 | 75 | 48 | 0 | 0 | 25 |
| Deer, Top Round, 1" Steak, Cooked | 3 oz | 129 | 15 | 2 | 1 | 72 | 38 | 0 | 0 | 27 |
| Goat, Cooked | 3 oz | 122 | 23 | 3 | 1 | 64 | 73 | 0 | 0 | 23 |
| Moose, Cooked | 3 oz | 114 | 7 | 1 | 0 | 66 | 59 | 0 | 0 | 25 |
| **LAMB** | | | | | | | | | | |
| Cubed For Stew (Leg & Shoulder), 1/4" Fat, Cooked | 3 oz | 190 | 67 | 7 | 3 | 92 | 60 | 0 | 0 | 29 |
| Foreshank, 1/8" Fat, Cooked | 3 oz | 207 | 103 | 11 | 5 | 90 | 61 | 0 | 0 | 24 |
| Ground, Cooked | 3 oz | 241 | 150 | 17 | 7 | 82 | 69 | 0 | 0 | 21 |
| Lamb, Leg, Center Slice, Bone-in, Broiled | 3 oz | 183 | 90 | 10 | 5 | 72 | 55 | 0 | 0 | 22 |
| Lamb, Sirlion Chops, without Bones, Broiled | 3 oz | 200 | 106 | 11.5 | 5 | 72 | 54 | 0 | 0 | 22 |
| Lamb, Steak, Boneless | 3 oz | 105 | 32 | 4 | 1 | 39 | 1080 | 0 | 0 | 17 |
| Leg, Shank Half, 1/8" Fat, Cooked | 3 oz | 184 | 87 | 10 | 4 | 77 | 55 | 0 | 0 | 23 |
| Leg, Sirloin Half, 1/8" Fat, Cooked | 3 oz | 241 | 150 | 17 | 7 | 82 | 58 | 0 | 0 | 21 |
| Leg, Whole (Shank & Sirloin), 1/8" Fat, Cooked | 3 oz | 206 | 110 | 12 | 5 | 78 | 57 | 0 | 0 | 22 |
| Loin, 1/8" Fat, Cooked | 3 oz | 252 | 158 | 18 | 7 | 84 | 66 | 0 | 0 | 22 |
| Rib, 1/8" Fat, Cooked | 3 oz | 290 | 211 | 23 | 10 | 82 | 63 | 0 | 0 | 19 |
| Shoulder, Arm, 1/8" Fat, Cooked | 3 oz | 286 | 173 | 19 | 8 | 102 | 61 | 0 | 0 | 26 |
| Shoulder, Blade, 1/8" Fat, Cooked | 3 oz | 288 | 183 | 20 | 8 | 99 | 64 | 0 | 0 | 25 |
| Shoulder, Whole (Arm & Blade), 1/8" Fat, Cooked | 3 oz | 287 | 180 | 20 | 8 | 99 | 63 | 0 | 0 | 25 |
| **PORK** | | | | | | | | | | |
| *Cured* | | | | | | | | | | |
| Bacon, Cooked | 1 slice | 43 | 30 | 3 | 1 | 9 | 185 | 0 | 0 | 3 |
| Canadian-Style Bacon, Grilled | 2 slices | 86 | 35 | 4 | 1 | 27 | 719 | 1 | 0 | 11 |
| Ham, Boneless, Regular (Approx 11% Fat), Roasted | 3 oz | 151 | 69 | 8 | 3 | 50 | 1275 | 0 | 0 | 19 |
| Ham, Center Slice, Unheated | 1 oz | 58 | 33 | 4 | 1 | 15 | 393 | 0 | 0 | 6 |
| Ham, Low Salt, Cooked | 1 oz | 49 | 21 | 2 | 1 | 16 | 275 | 0 | 0 | 6 |

# common foods

| | SERVING SIZE | CAL | CAL FAT | TOT FAT (G) | SAT FAT (G) | CHOL (MG) | SOD (MG) | CARB (G) | FIBER (G) | PROT (G) |
|---|---|---|---|---|---|---|---|---|---|---|
| Ham, Patties, Grilled | 1 patty | 203 | 165 | 18 | 7 | 43 | 632 | 1 | 0 | 8 |
| Ham, Regular (Approx 13% Fat), Canned, Roasted | 3 oz | 192 | 116 | 13 | 4 | 53 | 800 | 0 | 0 | 17 |
| Ham, Rump, Bone-In, Roasted | 3 oz | 150 | 68 | 8 | 2 | 60 | 702 | 0 | 0 | 20 |
| Ham, Shank, Bone-In, Roasted | 3 oz | 156 | 72 | 8 | 2 | 60 | 689 | 0 | 0 | 21 |
| Ham, Slice, Boneless, Pan-Broiled | 3 oz | 106 | 39 | 4 | 1 | 46 | 1030 | 1 | 0 | 16 |
| Ham, Slice, Bone-In, Pan-Broiled | 3 oz | 153 | 65 | 7 | 1 | 62 | 724 | 0 | 0 | 22 |
| Ham, Whole, Boneless, Roasted | 3 oz | 107 | 42 | 5 | 2 | 46 | 1004 | 1 | 0 | 15 |
| Ham, Whole, Roasted | 3 oz | 207 | 128 | 14 | 5 | 53 | 1009 | 0 | 0 | 18 |
| Picnic (Shoulder), Roasted | 3 oz | 238 | 163 | 18 | 7 | 49 | 911 | 0 | 0 | 17 |
| Shoulder, Blade Roll, Roasted | 3 oz | 244 | 180 | 20 | 7 | 57 | 827 | 0 | 0 | 15 |
| *Fresh Chops* | | | | | | | | | | |
| Blade (Loin), Bone-In, Cooked | 3 oz | 275 | 195 | 22 | 8 | 72 | 47 | 0 | 0 | 19 |
| Blade (Loin), Bone-In, Cooked, Pan-Fried | 3 oz | 291 | 212 | 24 | 9 | 72 | 57 | 0 | 0 | 18 |
| Center Loin, Bone-In, Cooked | 3 oz | 210 | 108 | 12 | 5 | 73 | 50 | 0 | 0 | 24 |
| Center Loin, Bone-In, Cooked, Pan-Fried | 3 oz | 235 | 127 | 14 | 5 | 78 | 68 | 0 | 0 | 25 |
| Loin, Center Rib, Bone-In, Cooked | 3 oz | 213 | 115 | 13 | 5 | 62 | 34 | 0 | 0 | 23 |
| Loin, Center Rib, Bone-In, Cooked, Pan-Fried | 3 oz | 225 | 130 | 14 | 5 | 62 | 43 | 0 | 0 | 22 |
| Loin, Center Rib, Boneless, Cooked | 3 oz | 217 | 121 | 13 | 5 | 62 | 34 | 0 | 0 | 22 |
| Loin, Center Rib, Boneless, Cooked, Pan-Fried | 3 oz | 232 | 138 | 15 | 6 | 62 | 43 | 0 | 0 | 22 |
| Sirloin, Bone-In, Cooked | 3 oz | 208 | 116 | 13 | 5 | 70 | 43 | 0 | 0 | 22 |
| Sirloin, Boneless, Cooked | 3 oz | 161 | 64 | 7 | 3 | 69 | 39 | 0 | 0 | 23 |
| Top Loin, Boneless, Cooked | 3 oz | 198 | 97 | 11 | 4 | 64 | 36 | 0 | 0 | 24 |
| Top Loin, Boneless, Cooked, Pan-Fried | 3 oz | 218 | 113 | 13 | 5 | 66 | 47 | 0 | 0 | 25 |
| *Fresh Ribs* | | | | | | | | | | |
| Back Ribs, Cooked | 3 oz | 315 | 226 | 25 | 9 | 100 | 86 | 0 | 0 | 21 |
| Loin, Country-Style Ribs, Cooked, Braised | 3 oz | 232 | 135 | 15 | 5 | 88 | 49 | 0 | 0 | 23 |
| Spareribs, Cooked, Braised | 3 oz | 337 | 232 | 26 | 9 | 103 | 79 | 0 | 0 | 25 |
| *Fresh Roasts* | | | | | | | | | | |
| Boston Butt (Shoulder), Cooked | 3 oz | 227 | 135 | 15 | 6 | 83 | 49 | 0 | 0 | 21 |
| Center Loin (Roasts), Bone-In, Cooked | 3 oz | 199 | 103 | 11 | 4 | 68 | 54 | 0 | 0 | 22 |
| Leg Sirloin, Tip Roast, Boneless, Cooked | 3 oz | 156 | 27 | 3 | 1 | 84 | 43 | 0 | 0 | 31 |
| Loin, Blade (Roasts), Bone-In, Cooked | 3 oz | 275 | 188 | 21 | 8 | 79 | 26 | 0 | 0 | 20 |
| Loin, Center Rib (Roasts), Bone-In, Cooked | 3 oz | 217 | 117 | 13 | 5 | 62 | 39 | 0 | 0 | 23 |
| Loin, Center Rib (Roasts), Boneless, Cooked | 3 oz | 214 | 116 | 13 | 5 | 69 | 41 | 0 | 0 | 23 |

| | SERVING SIZE | CAL | CAL FAT | TOT FAT (G) | SAT FAT (G) | CHOL (MG) | SOD (MG) | CARB (G) | FIBER (G) | PROT (G) |
|---|---|---|---|---|---|---|---|---|---|---|
| Loin, Whole, Cooked | 3 oz | 203 | 104 | 12 | 4 | 68 | 41 | 0 | 0 | 23 |
| Picnic (Shoulder), Cooked | 3 oz | 280 | 178 | 20 | 7 | 93 | 75 | 0 | 0 | 24 |
| Shoulder, Blade, Boston (Roasts), Cooked | 3 oz | 229 | 144 | 16 | 6 | 73 | 57 | 0 | 0 | 20 |
| Shoulder, Whole, Cooked | 3 oz | 248 | 164 | 18 | 7 | 77 | 58 | 0 | 0 | 20 |
| Sirloin (Roasts), Bone-In, Cooked | 3 oz | 196 | 98 | 11 | 3 | 76 | 48 | 0 | 0 | 23 |
| Sirloin (Roasts), Boneless, Cooked | 3 oz | 176 | 72 | 8 | 3 | 73 | 48 | 0 | 0 | 24 |
| Tenderloin, Cooked | 3 oz | 171 | 62 | 7 | 2 | 80 | 54 | 0 | 0 | 25 |
| Top Loin (Roasts), Boneless, Cooked | 3 oz | 163 | 67 | 7 | 2 | 68 | 39 | 0 | 0 | 22 |
| *Ground* | | | | | | | | | | |
| Fresh, Ground, Cooked | 3 oz | 252 | 159 | 18 | 7 | 80 | 62 | 0 | 0 | 22 |
| Ground, 72% Lean / 28% Fat, Cooked, Crumbles | 3 oz | 393 | 297 | 33 | 11 | 100 | 94 | 1 | 0 | 23 |
| Ground, 72% Lean / 28% Fat, Cooked, Pan-Broiled | 3 oz | 377 | 279 | 31 | 11 | 99 | 91 | 1 | 0 | 23 |
| Ground, 84% Lean / 16% Fat, Cooked, Crumbles | 3 oz | 289 | 180 | 20 | 7 | 89 | 89 | 1 | 0 | 27 |
| Ground, 84% Lean / 16% Fat, Cooked, Pan-Broiled | 3 oz | 301 | 193 | 21 | 7 | 97 | 89 | 0 | 0 | 27 |
| Ground, 96% Lean / 4% Fat, Cooked, Crumbles | 3 oz | 187 | 63 | 7 | 2 | 78 | 84 | 0 | 0 | 31 |
| Ground, 96% Lean / 4% Fat, Cooked, Pan-Broiled | 3 oz | 185 | 45 | 6 | 2 | 85 | 88 | 1 | 0 | 32 |
| *Ham* | | | | | | | | | | |
| Fresh, Leg (Ham), Rump Half, Cooked | 3 oz | 214 | 109 | 12 | 4 | 82 | 53 | 0 | 0 | 25 |
| Fresh, Leg (Ham), Shank Half, Cooked | 3 oz | 246 | 153 | 17 | 6 | 78 | 50 | 0 | 0 | 22 |
| Fresh, Leg (Ham), Whole, Cooked | 3 oz | 232 | 135 | 15 | 5 | 80 | 51 | 0 | 0 | 23 |
| Ham Steak, Boneless, Cooked | 1 piece | 307 | 77 | 9 | 3 | 157 | 148 | 0 | 0 | 54 |
| *Other Pork Products* | | | | | | | | | | |
| Bacon & Beef Sticks | 1 oz | 145 | 111 | 12 | 4 | 29 | 398 | 0 | 0 | 8 |
| Feet, Pickled | 1 oz | 40 | 26 | 3 | 1 | 24 | 159 | 0 | 0 | 3 |
| **SAUSAGE** | | | | | | | | | | |
| Berliner Sausage, Pork & Beef | 1 oz | 65 | 44 | 5 | 2 | 13 | 368 | 1 | 0 | 4 |
| Breakfast Sausage Links, Turkey, Mild | 2 oz | 132 | 91 | 10 | 2 | 90 | 328 | 1 | 0 | 9 |
| Blood Sausage | 3 oz | 379 | 311 | 35 | 13 | 120 | 680 | 1 | 0 | 15 |
| Bratwurst, Beef & Pork, Smoked | 3 oz | 297 | 234 | 26 | 6 | 78 | 848 | 2 | 0 | 12 |
| Bratwurst, Pork Beef & Turkey Light Smoked | 3 oz | 186 | 126 | 14 | 0 | 56 | 982 | 2 | 0 | 14 |

# common foods

| | SERVING SIZE | CAL | CAL FAT | TOT FAT (G) | SAT FAT (G) | CHOL (MG) | SOD (MG) | CARB (G) | FIBER (G) | PROT (G) |
|---|---|---|---|---|---|---|---|---|---|---|
| Bratwurst, Pork, Cooked | 3 oz | 333 | 261 | 29 | 10 | 74 | 846 | 3 | 0 | 14 |
| Bratwurst, Veal, Cooked | 3 oz | 341 | 288 | 32 | 15 | 79 | 60 | 0 | 0 | 14 |
| Brotwurst, Pork, Beef | 3 oz | 323 | 252 | 28 | 10 | 63 | 1112 | 3 | 0 | 14 |
| Chorizo, Pork & Beef | 1 oz | 129 | 98 | 11 | 4 | 25 | 350 | 1 | 0 | 7 |
| Frankfurter, Beef | 2 oz | 170 | 135 | 15 | 6 | 29 | 600 | 2 | 0 | 6 |
| Frankfurter, Beef & Pork | 1 frank | 137 | 112 | 12 | 5 | 23 | 504 | 1 | 0 | 5 |
| Frankfurter, Beef & Pork, Low-Fat | 2 oz | 87 | 54 | 6 | 2 | 25 | 716 | 3 | 0 | 6 |
| Frankfurter, Beef, Low-Fat | 2 oz | 131 | 99 | 11 | 5 | 23 | 593 | 1 | 0 | 7 |
| Frankfurter, Beef, Pork, & Turkey, Fat-Free | 3-1/2 oz | 109 | 18 | 2 | 1 | 41 | 798 | 11 | 0 | 13 |
| Frankfurter, Meat & Poultry, Low-Fat | 3-1/2 oz | 121 | 27 | 3 | 1 | 44 | 983 | 8 | 0 | 16 |
| Frankfurter, Pork | 1 link | 204 | 162 | 18 | 7 | 50 | 620 | 0 | 0 | 10 |
| Fresh Sausage, Cooked | 3 oz | 196 | 90 | 10 | 2 | 92 | 665 | 0 | 0 | 24 |
| Italian Sausage, Pork, Cooked | 3 oz | 344 | 243 | 27 | 10 | 57 | 1207 | 4 | 0 | 19 |
| Italian Sausage, Sweet Links | 3 oz | 125 | 64 | 7 | 3 | 25 | 479 | 2 | 0 | 14 |
| Kielbasa, Kolbassy, Pork, Beef, Nonfat Dry Milk | 1 link | 232 | 184 | 20 | 7 | 50 | 678 | 2 | 0 | 9 |
| Kielbasa, Polish, Turkey & Beef, Smoked | 2 oz | 127 | 89 | 10 | 3 | 39 | 672 | 2 | 0 | 7 |
| Knackwurst, Knockwurst, Pork & Beef | 1 oz | 87 | 71 | 8 | 3 | 17 | 264 | 1 | 0 | 3 |
| Liverwurst Spread | 1/4 cup | 168 | 126 | 14 | 5 | 65 | 385 | 3 | 1 | 7 |
| Polish Sausage, Beef with Chicken, Hot | 3 oz | 259 | 171 | 19 | 8 | 66 | 1540 | 4 | 0 | 18 |
| Polish Sausage, Pork | 1 oz | 92 | 73 | 8 | 3 | 20 | 248 | 0 | 0 | 4 |
| Polish Sausage, Pork & Beef, Smoked | 3 oz | 228 | 181 | 20 | 7 | 54 | 641 | 1 | 0 | 9 |
| Pork & Beef with Cheddar Cheese Sausage, Smoked | 3 oz | 227 | 178 | 20 | 7 | 48 | 649 | 2 | 0 | 10 |
| Pork & Beef Sausage, Fresh, Cooked | 4" link | 51 | 42 | 5 | 2 | 9 | 105 | 0 | 0 | 2 |
| Pork & Rice Sausage Links, Brown & Serve, Cooked | 3 oz | 407 | 342 | 38 | 7 | 66 | 689 | 2 | 0 | 14 |
| Pork & Turkey Sausage, Pre-Cooked | 3 oz | 342 | 279 | 31 | 10 | 72 | 876 | 4 | 0 | 12 |
| Pork Sausage, Fresh, Cooked | 3 oz | 339 | 252 | 28 | 9 | 84 | 749 | 0 | 0 | 19 |
| Pork Sausage, Pre-Cooked | 3 oz | 378 | 315 | 35 | 12 | 74 | 752 | 0 | 0 | 14 |
| Smoked Sausage Link, Pork | 3 oz | 307 | 252 | 28 | 9 | 61 | 827 | 0 | 0 | 12 |
| Smoked Sausage Link, Pork & Beef | 16 oz | 1452 | 1173 | 130 | 44 | 263 | 4132 | 11 | 0 | 54 |
| Smoked Sausage Link, Pork & Beef, Flour & Nonfat Dry Milk | 2 oz | 152 | 109 | 12 | 4 | 37 | 721 | 2 | 0 | 8 |
| Smoked Sausage Link, Pork & Beef, Nonfat Dry Milk | 2 oz | 153 | 108 | 12 | 4 | 37 | 725 | 2 | 0 | 8 |

| | SERVING SIZE | CAL | CAL FAT | TOT FAT (G) | SAT FAT (G) | CHOL (MG) | SOD (MG) | CARB (G) | FIBER (G) | PROT (G) |
|---|---|---|---|---|---|---|---|---|---|---|
| Summer Sausage, Pork & Beef Steaks with Cheddar Cheese | 1 oz | 121 | 97 | 11 | 3 | 25 | 420 | 1 | 0 | 6 |
| Vienna Sausage, Canned, Chicken, Beef, Pork | 3 oz | 230 | 171 | 19 | 7 | 87 | 969 | 3 | 0 | 11 |

## Nuts, Nut Butters, and Seeds

### NUTS

| | SERVING SIZE | CAL | CAL FAT | TOT FAT (G) | SAT FAT (G) | CHOL (MG) | SOD (MG) | CARB (G) | FIBER (G) | PROT (G) |
|---|---|---|---|---|---|---|---|---|---|---|
| **Almonds**, Sliced | 1 cup | 528 | 408 | 45 | 3 | 0 | 1 | 20 | 11 | 19 |
| Almonds, Dry Roasted, with Salt | 1 oz | 169 | 135 | 15 | 1 | 0 | 96 | 5 | 3 | 6 |
| Almonds, Dry Roasted, without Salt | 1 oz | 169 | 135 | 15 | 1 | 0 | 0 | 5 | 3 | 6 |
| Almonds, Honey Roasted, Unblanched | 1 oz | 168 | 127 | 14 | 1 | 0 | 37 | 8 | 4 | 5 |
| Almonds, Oil Roasted, with Salt | 1 oz | 172 | 141 | 16 | 1 | 0 | 96 | 5 | 3 | 6 |
| Almonds, Oil Roasted, without Salt | 1 oz | 172 | 141 | 16 | 1 | 0 | 0 | 5 | 3 | 6 |
| **Cashews**, Dry Roasted, with Salt | 1 cup | 786 | 571 | 63 | 13 | 0 | 877 | 45 | 4 | 21 |
| Cashews, Dry Roasted, without Salt | 1 cup | 786 | 571 | 63 | 13 | 0 | 22 | 45 | 4 | 21 |
| Cashews, Oil Roasted, with Salt | 1 cup | 750 | 555 | 62 | 11 | 0 | 398 | 39 | 4 | 22 |
| Cashews, Oil Roasted, without Salt | 1 cup | 749 | 555 | 62 | 11 | 0 | 17 | 39 | 4 | 22 |
| Cashews, Raw | 1 oz | 157 | 112 | 12 | 2 | 0 | 3 | 9 | 1 | 5 |
| **Chestnuts**, European, Boiled & Steamed | 1 oz | 37 | 4 | 0 | 0 | 0 | 8 | 8 | 0 | 1 |
| Chestnuts, European, Dried, Peeled | 1 oz | 105 | 10 | 1 | 0 | 0 | 10 | 22 | 0 | 1 |
| Chestnuts, European, Dried, Unpeeled | 1 oz | 106 | 11 | 1 | 0 | 0 | 10 | 22 | 3 | 2 |
| Chestnuts, European, Raw, Peeled | 1 oz | 56 | 3 | 0 | 0 | 0 | 1 | 13 | 0 | 0 |
| Chestnuts, European, Raw, Unpeeled | 1 oz | 60 | 6 | 1 | 0 | 0 | 1 | 13 | 2 | 1 |
| Chestnuts, European, Roasted | 1 oz | 69 | 6 | 1 | 0 | 0 | 1 | 15 | 1 | 1 |
| **Hazelnuts** or Filberts, Chopped | 1 cup | 722 | 629 | 70 | 5 | 0 | 0 | 19 | 11 | 17 |
| Hazelnuts or Filberts, Dry Roasted, without Salt | 1 oz | 183 | 159 | 18 | 1 | 0 | 0 | 5 | 3 | 4 |
| **Macadamias**, Dry Roasted, with Salt | 1 oz | 203 | 194 | 22 | 3 | 0 | 75 | 4 | 2 | 2 |
| Macadamias, Dry Roasted, without Salt | 1 oz | 204 | 194 | 22 | 3 | 0 | 1 | 4 | 2 | 2 |
| Macadamias, Raw | 1 oz | 204 | 193 | 21 | 3 | 0 | 1 | 4 | 2 | 2 |
| **Mixed**, Dry Roasted, with Peanuts & Salt | 1 oz | 168 | 131 | 15 | 2 | 0 | 190 | 7 | 3 | 5 |
| Mixed, Dry Roasted, with Peanuts, without Salt | 1 oz | 168 | 131 | 15 | 2 | 0 | 3 | 7 | 3 | 5 |
| Mixed, Oil Roasted, with Peanuts, without Salt | 1 tbsp | 55 | 45 | 5 | 1 | 0 | 1 | 2 | 1 | 1 |
| Mixed, Oil Roasted, without Peanuts, without Salt | 1 oz | 174 | 143 | 16 | 3 | 0 | 3 | 6 | 2 | 4 |

| | SERVING SIZE | CAL | CAL FAT | TOT FAT (G) | SAT FAT (G) | CHOL (MG) | SOD (MG) | CARB (G) | FIBER (G) | PROT (G) |
|---|---|---|---|---|---|---|---|---|---|---|
| Mixed, with Peanuts, Oil Roasted, with Salt | 1 oz | 175 | 144 | 16 | 2 | 0 | 119 | 6 | 3 | 5 |
| Mixed, without Peanuts, Oil Roasted, with Salt | 1 oz | 174 | 143 | 16 | 3 | 0 | 87 | 6 | 2 | 4 |
| **Peanuts**, Dry-Roasted, with Salt | 1 oz | 166 | 127 | 14 | 2 | 0 | 230 | 6 | 2 | 7 |
| Peanuts, Dry-Roasted, without Salt | 1 oz | 166 | 127 | 14 | 2 | 0 | 2 | 6 | 2 | 7 |
| Peanuts, Oil Roasted, with Salt | 1 cup | 863 | 680 | 76 | 13 | 0 | 461 | 22 | 14 | 40 |
| Peanuts, Oil Roasted, without Salt, Shelled | 1 oz | 165 | 126 | 14 | 2 | 0 | 2 | 5 | 2 | 7 |
| Peanuts, Raw | 1 oz | 161 | 126 | 14 | 2 | 0 | 5 | 5 | 2 | 7 |
| **Pecans**, Chopped | 1 cup | 756 | 709 | 79 | 7 | 0 | 0 | 15 | 11 | 10 |
| Pecans, Halved | 1 cup | 685 | 642 | 71 | 6 | 0 | 0 | 14 | 10 | 9 |
| Pecans, Dry Roasted, with Salt | 1 oz | 201 | 189 | 21 | 2 | 0 | 109 | 4 | 3 | 3 |
| Pecans, Dry Roasted, without Salt | 1 oz | 201 | 189 | 21 | 2 | 0 | 0 | 4 | 3 | 3 |
| Pecans, Oil Roasted, with Salt | 1 oz | 203 | 192 | 21 | 2 | 0 | 111 | 4 | 3 | 3 |
| Pecans, Oil Roasted, without Salt | 1 oz | 203 | 192 | 21 | 2 | 0 | 0 | 4 | 3 | 3 |
| **Pilinuts**, Dried | 1 oz | 204 | 203 | 23 | 9 | 0 | 1 | 1 | 0 | 3 |
| **Pine Nuts**, Pinyon, Dried | 1 oz | 178 | 156 | 17 | 3 | 0 | 20 | 5 | 3 | 3 |
| **Pistachios**, Dry Roasted, with Salt | 1 oz | 161 | 117 | 13 | 2 | 0 | 115 | 8 | 3 | 6 |
| Pistachios, Dry Roasted, without Salt | 1 oz | 162 | 117 | 13 | 2 | 0 | 3 | 8 | 3 | 6 |
| Pistachios, Raw | 1 oz | 159 | 116 | 13 | 2 | 0 | 0 | 8 | 3 | 6 |
| **Walnuts**, Black, Dried, Chopped | 1 cup | 773 | 664 | 74 | 4 | 0 | 3 | 12 | 9 | 30 |
| Walnuts, English, Chopped | 1 cup | 766 | 687 | 76 | 7 | 0 | 2 | 16 | 8 | 18 |
| **NUT BUTTERS** | | | | | | | | | | |
| **Almond**, Plain, with Salt | 1 tbsp | 101 | 85 | 9 | 1 | 0 | 72 | 3 | 1 | 2 |
| Almond, Plain, without Salt | 1 tbsp | 101 | 85 | 9 | 1 | 0 | 2 | 3 | 1 | 2 |
| **Cashew**, Plain, with Salt | 1 tbsp | 94 | 71 | 8 | 2 | 0 | 98 | 4 | 0 | 3 |
| Cashew, Plain, without Salt | 1 tbsp | 94 | 71 | 8 | 2 | 0 | 2 | 4 | 0 | 3 |
| **Peanut** with Omega-3, Creamy | 1 tbsp | 99 | 79 | 9 | 2 | 0 | 58 | 3 | 1 | 4 |
| Peanut, Chunky, with Salt | 2 tbsp | 188 | 144 | 16 | 3 | 0 | 156 | 7 | 3 | 8 |
| Peanut, Chunky, without Salt | 2 tbsp | 188 | 144 | 16 | 3 | 0 | 5 | 7 | 3 | 8 |
| Peanut, Chunky, Vitamin & Mineral Fortified | 2 tbsp | 190 | 148 | 16 | 3 | 0 | 117 | 6 | 2 | 8 |
| Peanut, Smooth Style, with Salt | 2 tbsp | 188 | 145 | 16 | 3 | 0 | 147 | 6 | 2 | 8 |
| Peanut, Smooth Style, without Salt | 2 tbsp | 188 | 145 | 16 | 3 | 0 | 5 | 6 | 2 | 8 |
| Peanut, Smooth Style, Vitamin & Mineral Fortified | 2 tbsp | 189 | 146 | 16 | 3 | 0 | 134 | 6 | 2 | 8 |
| **Sesame**, Paste | 1 tbsp | 94 | 73 | 8 | 1 | 0 | 2 | 4 | 1 | 3 |
| Sesame, Tahini | 1 tbsp | 89 | 72 | 8 | 1 | 0 | 5 | 3 | 1 | 3 |

| | SERVING SIZE | CAL | CAL FAT | TOT FAT (G) | SAT FAT (G) | CHOL (MG) | SOD (MG) | CARB (G) | FIBER (G) | PROT (G) |
|---|---|---|---|---|---|---|---|---|---|---|
| **Sunflower**, with Salt | 1 tbsp | 93 | 69 | 8 | 1 | 0 | 83 | 4 | 0 | 3 |
| Sunflower, without Salt | 1 tbsp | 93 | 69 | 8 | 1 | 0 | 0 | 4 | 0 | 3 |
| **SEEDS** | | | | | | | | | | |
| **Flax** | 1 tbsp | 55 | 39 | 4 | 0 | 0 | 3 | 3 | 3 | 2 |
| **Pumpkin** & Squash Seeds, Roasted, with Salt | 1 cup | 285 | 112 | 12 | 2 | 0 | 1626 | 34 | 12 | 12 |
| **Sesame**, Whole, Dried | 1 tbsp | 52 | 40 | 4 | 1 | 0 | 1 | 2 | 1 | 2 |
| Sesame, Whole, Roasted & Toasted | 1 oz | 160 | 122 | 14 | 2 | 0 | 3 | 7 | 4 | 5 |
| **Sunflower**, Dried, with Hulls | 1 cup | 269 | 213 | 24 | 2 | 0 | 4 | 9 | 4 | 10 |
| Sunflower, Dried | 1 cup | 816 | 647 | 72 | 6 | 0 | 13 | 28 | 12 | 29 |
| Sunflower, Dry Roasted with Salt | 1 oz | 165 | 127 | 14 | 1 | 0 | 116 | 7 | 3 | 5 |
| Sunflower, Dry Roasted without Salt | 1 oz | 165 | 127 | 14 | 1 | 0 | 1 | 7 | 3 | 5 |
| Sunflower, Oil Roasted with Salt | 1 oz | 168 | 131 | 15 | 2 | 0 | 116 | 6 | 3 | 6 |
| Sunflower, Oil Roasted without Salt | 1 oz | 168 | 131 | 15 | 2 | 0 | 1 | 6 | 3 | 6 |
| Sunflower, Toasted with Salt | 1 oz | 175 | 145 | 16 | 2 | 0 | 174 | 6 | 3 | 5 |
| Sunflower, Toasted without Salt | 1 oz | 175 | 145 | 16 | 2 | 0 | 1 | 6 | 3 | 5 |
| **Pasta** | | | | | | | | | | |
| Couscous, Cooked | 1 cup | 176 | 2 | 0 | 0 | 0 | 8 | 36 | 2 | 6 |
| Couscous, Dry | 1 cup | 650 | 10 | 1 | 0 | 0 | 17 | 134 | 9 | 22 |
| Macaroni, Cooked, Elbow Shaped | 1 cup | 221 | 12 | 1 | 0 | 0 | 1 | 43 | 3 | 8 |
| Macaroni, Dry, Elbow Shaped | 1 cup | 390 | 14 | 2 | 0 | 0 | 6 | 78 | 3 | 14 |
| Macaroni, Dry, Spiral Shaped | 1 cup | 312 | 11 | 1 | 0 | 0 | 5 | 63 | 3 | 11 |
| Macaroni, Whole-Wheat, Cooked, Elbow Shaped | 1 cup | 174 | 7 | 1 | 0 | 0 | 4 | 37 | 4 | 7 |
| Macaroni, Whole-Wheat, Dry, Elbow Shape | 1 cup | 365 | 13 | 1 | 0 | 0 | 8 | 79 | 9 | 15 |
| Noodles, Chinese, Cellophane or Long Rice (Mung Beans), Dehydrated | 1 cup | 491 | 1 | 0 | 0 | 0 | 14 | 121 | 1 | 0 |
| Noodles, Chinese, Chow Mein | 1 cup | 237 | 125 | 14 | 2 | 0 | 198 | 26 | 2 | 4 |
| Noodles, Egg, Cooked | 1 cup | 221 | 30 | 3 | 1 | 46 | 8 | 40 | 2 | 7 |
| Noodles, Egg, Dry | 1 cup | 146 | 15 | 2 | 0 | 32 | 8 | 27 | 1 | 5 |
| Noodles, Flat, Crunchy, Chinese Restaurant | 1 cup | 234 | 128 | 14 | 2 | 0 | 170 | 23 | 1 | 5 |
| Noodles, Japanese, Soba, Cooked | 1 cup | 113 | 1 | 0 | 0 | 0 | 68 | 24 | 0 | 6 |
| Noodles, Japanese, Soba, Dry | 2 oz | 192 | 4 | 0 | 0 | 0 | 451 | 43 | 0 | 8 |
| Noodles, Japanese, Somen, Cooked | 1 cup | 231 | 3 | 0 | 0 | 0 | 283 | 48 | 0 | 7 |
| Noodles, Japanese, Somen, Dry | 2 oz | 203 | 4 | 0 | 0 | 0 | 1049 | 42 | 2 | 6 |
| Pasta with Meatballs in Tomato Sauce, Canned | 1 cup | 273 | 117 | 13 | 5 | 23 | 742 | 28 | 7 | 11 |

# common foods

| | SERVING SIZE | CAL | CAL FAT | TOT FAT (G) | SAT FAT (G) | CHOL (MG) | SOD (MG) | CARB (G) | FIBER (G) | PROT (G) |
|---|---|---|---|---|---|---|---|---|---|---|
| Pasta with Sliced Franks in Tomato Sauce, Canned | 1 cup | 227 | 54 | 6 | 2.5 | 23 | 600 | 32 | 4 | 11 |
| Pasta with Tomato Sauce, Canned | 1 cup | 189 | 17 | 2 | 1 | 3 | 867 | 37 | 3 | 6 |
| Pasta, Corn, Cooked | 1 cup | 176 | 9 | 1 | 0 | 0 | 0 | 39 | 7 | 4 |
| Pasta, Corn, Dry | 1 cup | 375 | 20 | 2 | 0 | 0 | 3 | 83 | 12 | 8 |
| Pasta, Fresh-Refrigerated | 4-1/2 oz | 369 | 26 | 3 | 0 | 93 | 33 | 70 | 0 | 14 |
| Pasta, Fresh-Refrigerated, Cooked | 2 oz | 75 | 5 | 1 | 0 | 19 | 3 | 14 | 0 | 3 |
| Pasta, Fresh-Refrigerated, Spinach | 4-1/2 oz | 370 | 24 | 3 | 1 | 93 | 35 | 71 | 0 | 14 |
| Pasta, Fresh-Refrigerated, Spinach, Cooked | 2 oz | 74 | 5 | 1 | 0 | 19 | 3 | 14 | 0 | 3 |
| Pasta, Homemade, with Egg, Cooked | 2 oz | 74 | 9 | 1 | 0 | 23 | 47 | 13 | 0 | 3 |
| Pasta, Homemade, without Egg, Cooked | 2 oz | 71 | 5 | 1 | 0 | 0 | 42 | 14 | 0 | 2 |
| Rice Noodles, Cooked | 1 cup | 192 | 3 | 0 | 0 | 0 | 33 | 44 | 2 | 2 |
| Rice Noodles, Dry | 2 oz | 206 | 3 | 0 | 0 | 0 | 103 | 47 | 1 | 2 |
| Spaghetti, Cooked with Salt | 1 cup | 220 | 12 | 1 | 0 | 0 | 183 | 43 | 3 | 8 |
| Spaghetti, Dry | 2 oz | 211 | 8 | 1 | 0 | 0 | 3 | 43 | 2 | 7 |
| Spaghetti, Spinach, Cooked | 1 cup | 182 | 8 | 1 | 0 | 0 | 20 | 37 | 0 | 6 |
| Spaghetti, Spinach, Dry | 2 oz | 212 | 8 | 1 | 0 | 0 | 21 | 43 | 6 | 8 |
| Spaghetti, Whole-Wheat, Cooked | 1 cup | 174 | 7 | 1 | 0 | 0 | 4 | 37 | 6 | 7 |
| Spaghetti, Whole-Wheat, Dry | 2 oz | 198 | 7 | 1 | 0 | 0 | 5 | 43 | 0 | 8 |
| Tortellini, Pasta with Cheese Filling | 3/4 cup | 249 | 53 | 6 | 3 | 34 | 499 | 38 | 2 | 11 |
| **Pizza** | | | | | | | | | | |
| Pizza, Cheese Topping, Frozen, Cooked | 24-oz pizza | 1947 | 803 | 89 | 31 | 102 | 3248 | 211 | 16 | 75 |
| Pizza, Cheese Topping, Rising Crust, Frozen, Cooked | 30-oz pizza | 2170 | 659 | 73 | 32 | 134 | 4639 | 275 | 21 | 103 |
| Pizza, Meat & Vegetable Topping, Frozen, Cooked | 24-oz pizza | 1969 | 927 | 103 | 36 | 114 | 3960 | 179 | 16 | 80 |
| Pizza, Meat & Vegetable Topping, Rising Crust, Frozen, Cooked | 35-oz pizza | 2766 | 1079 | 120 | 47 | 194 | 6531 | 294 | 23 | 129 |
| **Poultry** | | | | | | | | | | |
| **CHICKEN** | | | | | | | | | | |
| *Average of All Dark Meat* | | | | | | | | | | |
| Meat, Fried | 1 cup | 335 | 146 | 16 | 4 | 134 | 136 | 4 | 0 | 41 |
| Meat, Roasted, Chopped or Diced | 1 cup | 287 | 123 | 14 | 4 | 130 | 130 | 0 | 0 | 38 |
| Meat, Stewed, Chopped or Diced | 1 cup | 269 | 113 | 13 | 3 | 123 | 104 | 0 | 0 | 36 |
| Meat & Skin, Fried, Batter | 3-1/2 oz | 298 | 171 | 19 | 5 | 89 | 295 | 9 | 0 | 22 |
| Meat & Skin, Fried, Flour | 3-1/2 oz | 285 | 153 | 17 | 5 | 92 | 89 | 4 | 0 | 27 |

| | SERVING SIZE | CAL | CAL FAT | TOT FAT (G) | SAT FAT (G) | CHOL (MG) | SOD (MG) | CARB (G) | FIBER (G) | PROT (G) |
|---|---|---|---|---|---|---|---|---|---|---|
| Meat & Skin, Roasted | 3-1/2 oz | 253 | 144 | 16 | 4 | 91 | 87 | 0 | 0 | 26 |
| Meat & Skin, Stewed | 3-1/2 oz | 233 | 135 | 15 | 4 | 82 | 70 | 0 | 0 | 24 |
| *Average of All Light Meat* | | | | | | | | | | |
| Meat, Fried | 1 cup | 269 | 70 | 8 | 2 | 126 | 113 | 1 | 0 | 46 |
| Meat, Roasted, Chopped or Diced | 1 cup | 242 | 57 | 6 | 2 | 119 | 108 | 0 | 0 | 43 |
| Meat, Stewed, Chopped or Diced | 1 cup | 223 | 50 | 6 | 2 | 108 | 91 | 0 | 0 | 40 |
| Meat & Skin, Cooked, Stewed, Bone Removed | 1/2 bird | 302 | 135 | 15 | 4 | 111 | 95 | 0 | 0 | 39 |
| Meat & Skin, Fried, Batter, Bone Removed | 1/2 bird | 521 | 261 | 29 | 8 | 158 | 540 | 18 | 0 | 44 |
| Meat & Skin, Fried, Flour, Bone Removed | 1/2 bird | 320 | 141 | 16 | 4 | 113 | 100 | 2 | 0 | 40 |
| Meat & Skin, Roasted, Bone Removed | 1/2 bird | 293 | 129 | 14 | 4 | 111 | 99 | 0 | 0 | 38 |
| *Breast* | | | | | | | | | | |
| Meat, Fried; Breast, Bone, and Skin Removed | 1/2 breast | 161 | 36 | 4 | 1 | 78 | 68 | 0 | 0 | 29 |
| Meat, Roasted, Chopped or Diced | 1 cup | 231 | 45 | 5 | 1 | 119 | 104 | 0 | 0 | 43 |
| Meat, Rotisserie | 3-1/2 oz | 148 | 27 | 3 | 1 | 89 | 341 | 0 | 0 | 29 |
| Meat, Stewed, Chopped or Diced | 1 cup | 211 | 38 | 4 | 1 | 108 | 88 | 0 | 0 | 41 |
| Meat & Skin, Fried, Batter, Bone Removed | 1/2 breast | 364 | 166 | 18 | 5 | 119 | 385 | 13 | 0 | 35 |
| Meat & Skin, Fried, Flour, Bone Removed | 1/2 breast | 218 | 78 | 9 | 2 | 87 | 74 | 2 | n/a | 31 |
| Meat & Skin, Roasted, Chopped or Diced | 1 cup | 276 | 98 | 11 | 3 | 118 | 99 | 0 | 0 | 42 |
| Meat & Skin, Rotisserie | 3-1/2 oz | 184 | 72 | 8 | 2 | 96 | 347 | 0 | 0 | 27 |
| Meat & Skin, Stewed, Chopped or Diced | 1 cup | 258 | 93 | 10 | 3 | 105 | 87 | 0 | 0 | 38 |
| *Chicken Offal* | | | | | | | | | | |
| Giblets, Fried, Chopped or Diced | 1 cup | 402 | 176 | 20 | 6 | 647 | 164 | 6 | 0 | 47 |
| Giblets, Simmered, Chopped or Diced | 1 cup | 228 | 59 | 7 | 2 | 641 | 97 | 0 | 0 | 39 |
| *Chicken Products* | | | | | | | | | | |
| Chicken Breast Tenders, Cooked, Conventional Oven | 3-1/2 oz | 293 | 162 | 18 | 4 | 44 | 457 | 17 | 1 | 16 |
| Chicken Nuggets, Frozen, Cooked | 3-1/2 oz | 296 | 180 | 20 | 4 | 43 | 557 | 14 | 2 | 15 |
| Chicken Patty, Frozen, Cooked | 3-1/2 oz | 287 | 180 | 20 | 4 | 43 | 532 | 13 | 0 | 15 |
| Chicken Spread | 1 serving | 88 | 89 | 10 | 2 | 31 | 404 | 2 | 0 | 10 |
| Wing, Frozen, Glazed, Barbecue Flavor, Heated | 3-1/2 oz | 242 | 135 | 15 | 4 | 136 | 559 | 3 | 0 | 22 |
| *Drumstick* | | | | | | | | | | |
| Meat, Fried, Bone & Skin Removed | 1 drumstick | 82 | 31 | 3 | 1 | 39 | 40 | 0 | 0 | 12 |

| | SERVING SIZE | CAL | CAL FAT | TOT FAT (G) | SAT FAT (G) | CHOL (MG) | SOD (MG) | CARB (G) | FIBER (G) | PROT (G) |
|---|---|---|---|---|---|---|---|---|---|---|
| Meat, Roasted, Chopped or Diced | 1 cup | 241 | 71 | 8 | 2 | 130 | 133 | 0 | 0 | 40 |
| Meat, Rotisserie | 3-1/2 oz | 176 | 63 | 7 | 2 | 160 | 417 | 0 | 0 | 29 |
| Meat, Stewed, Chopped or Diced | 1 cup | 270 | 82 | 9 | 2 | 141 | 128 | 0 | 0 | 44 |
| Meat & Skin, Fried, Batter, Bone Removed | 1 drumstick | 193 | 102 | 11 | 3 | 62 | 194 | 6 | 0 | 16 |
| Meat & Skin, Fried, Flour, Bone Removed | 1 drumstick | 120 | 61 | 7 | 2 | 44 | 44 | 1 | 0 | 13 |
| Meat & Skin, Roasted, Chopped or Diced | 1 cup | 302 | 140 | 16 | 4 | 127 | 126 | 0 | 0 | 38 |
| Meat & Skin, Rotisserie | 3-1/2 oz | 215 | 108 | 12 | 3 | 156 | 411 | 0 | 0 | 27 |
| Meat & Skin, Stewed, Chopped or Diced | 1 cup | 286 | 134 | 15 | 4 | 116 | 106 | 0 | 0 | 35 |
| *Game Hens* | | | | | | | | | | |
| Cornish Game Hens, Meat Only, Cooked, Roasted | 1/2 bird | 147 | 38 | 4 | 1 | 117 | 69 | 0 | 0 | 26 |
| Cornish Game Hens, Meat & Skin, Cooked, Roasted | 1/2 bird | 334 | 211 | 23 | 7 | 169 | 83 | 0 | 0 | 29 |
| *Leg* | | | | | | | | | | |
| Meat, Fried, Bone & Skin Removed | 1 leg | 196 | 79 | 9 | 2 | 93 | 90 | 1 | 0 | 27 |
| Meat, Roasted, Chopped or Diced | 1 cup | 267 | 106 | 12 | 3 | 132 | 127 | 0 | 0 | 38 |
| Meat, Stewed, Chopped or Diced | 1 cup | 296 | 116 | 13 | 4 | 142 | 125 | 0 | 0 | 42 |
| Meat & Skin, Fried, Batter, Bone Removed | 1 leg | 431 | 230 | 26 | 7 | 142 | 441 | 14 | 0 | 34 |
| Meat & Skin, Fried, Flour, Bone Removed | 1 leg | 284 | 145 | 16 | 4 | 105 | 99 | 3 | 0 | 30 |
| Meat & Skin, Roasted, Chopped or Diced | 1 cup | 325 | 170 | 19 | 5 | 129 | 122 | 0 | 0 | 36 |
| Meat & Skin, Stewed, Chopped or Diced | 1 cup | 308 | 163 | 18 | 5 | 118 | 102 | 0 | 0 | 34 |
| *Other* | | | | | | | | | | |
| Canned, No Broth | 1 cup | 379 | 149 | 17 | 5 | 103 | 277 | 2 | 0 | 52 |
| Canned, Meat Only, with Broth | 5 oz | 234 | 102 | 11 | 3 | 88 | 714 | 0 | 0 | 31 |
| Ground, Crumbles, Cooked, Pan-Browned, Crumbled | 3 oz | 161 | 84 | 9 | 3 | 91 | 64 | 0 | 0 | 20 |
| *Stewing Chicken* | | | | | | | | | | |
| Dark Meat, Cooked, Chopped or Diced | 1 cup | 361 | 193 | 21 | 6 | 133 | 133 | 0 | 0 | 39 |
| Giblets, Simmered, Chopped or Diced | 1 cup | 281 | 121 | 13 | 4 | 515 | 81 | 0 | 0 | 37 |
| Light Meat, Cooked, Chopped or Diced | 1 cup | 298 | 101 | 11 | 3 | 98 | 81 | 0 | 0 | 46 |
| *Thigh* | | | | | | | | | | |
| Meat & Skin, Rotisserie | 3-1/2 oz | 233 | 144 | 16 | 4 | 132 | 345 | 0 | 0 | 23 |
| Meat, Fried, Bone & Skin Removed | 1 thigh | 113 | 48 | 5 | 1 | 53 | 49 | 1 | 0 | 15 |
| Meat, Roasted, Chopped or Diced | 1 cup | 293 | 137 | 15 | 4 | 133 | 123 | 0 | 0 | 36 |
| Meat, Rotisserie | 3-1/2 oz | 196 | 99 | 11 | 3 | 130 | 337 | 0 | 0 | 24 |
| Meat, Stewed, Chopped or Diced | 1 cup | 273 | 123 | 14 | 4 | 126 | 105 | 0 | 0 | 35 |

| | SERVING SIZE | CAL | CAL FAT | TOT FAT (G) | SAT FAT (G) | CHOL (MG) | SOD (MG) | CARB (G) | FIBER (G) | PROT (G) |
|---|---|---|---|---|---|---|---|---|---|---|
| Meat & Skin, Fried, Batter, Bone Removed | 1 thigh | 238 | 128 | 14 | 4 | 80 | 248 | 8 | 0 | 19 |
| Meat & Skin, Fried, Flour, Bone Removed | 1 thigh | 162 | 84 | 9 | 3 | 60 | 55 | 2 | 0 | 17 |
| Meat & Skin, Roasted, Chopped or Diced | 1 cup | 346 | 195 | 22 | 6 | 130 | 118 | 0 | 0 | 35 |
| Meat & Skin, Stewed, Bone Removed | 1 thigh | 158 | 90 | 10 | 3 | 57 | 48 | 0 | 0 | 16 |
| *Wing* | | | | | | | | | | |
| Meat, Fried, Bone & Skin Removed | 1 wing | 42 | 16 | 2 | 1 | 17 | 18 | 0 | 0 | 6 |
| Meat, Roasted, Bone & Skin Removed | 1 wing | 43 | 15 | 2 | 0 | 18 | 19 | 0 | 0 | 6 |
| Meat, Rotisserie | 3-1/2 oz | 197 | 90 | 10 | 2 | 140 | 725 | 0 | 0 | 28 |
| Meat, Stewed, Chopped or Diced | 1 cup | 253 | 90 | 10 | 3 | 104 | 102 | 0 | 0 | 38 |
| Meat & Skin, Fried, Batter, Bone Removed | 1 wing | 159 | 96 | 11 | 3 | 39 | 157 | 5 | 0 | 10 |
| Meat & Skin, Fried, Flour, Bone Removed | 1 wing | 103 | 64 | 7 | 2 | 26 | 25 | 1 | 0 | 8 |
| Meat & Skin, Roasted, Chopped or Diced | 1 cup | 406 | 245 | 27 | 8 | 118 | 115 | 0 | 0 | 38 |
| Meat & Skin, Rotisserie | 3-1/2 oz | 266 | 171 | 19 | 5 | 140 | 610 | 0 | 0 | 24 |
| Meat & Skin, Stewed, Chopped or Diced | 1 cup | 349 | 212 | 24 | 7 | 98 | 94 | 0 | 0 | 32 |
| *Roasting Chicken* | | | | | | | | | | |
| Dark Meat, Cooked, Chopped or Diced | 1 cup | 249 | 110 | 12 | 3 | 105 | 133 | 0 | 0 | 33 |
| Giblets, Simmered, Chopped or Diced | 1 cup | 239 | 68 | 8 | 2 | 518 | 87 | 1 | 0 | 39 |
| Light Meat, Cooked, Chopped or Diced | 1 cup | 214 | 51 | 6 | 2 | 105 | 71 | 0 | 0 | 38 |
| **DELI MEATS** | | | | | | | | | | |
| Bologna, Chicken, Pork | 3-1/2 oz | 336 | 279 | 31 | 10 | 87 | 1240 | 4 | 0 | 10 |
| Bologna, Chicken, Pork, Beef | 3-1/2 oz | 272 | 207 | 23 | 7 | 83 | 1120 | 6 | 0 | 11 |
| Bologna, Chicken, Turkey, Pork | 3-1/2 oz | 298 | 234 | 26 | 8 | 80 | 922 | 6 | 0 | 10 |
| Chicken Breast, Fat Free, Mesquite Flavor, Sliced | 3-1/2 oz | 80 | 0 | 0 | 0 | 36 | 1040 | 2 | 0 | 17 |
| Chicken Breast, Oven Roasted, Fat Free, Sliced | 3-1/2 oz | 79 | 0 | 0 | 0 | 36 | 1087 | 2 | 0 | 17 |
| Chicken Roll, Light Meat | 3-1/2 oz | 110 | 27 | 3 | 1 | 45 | 1059 | 5 | 0 | 17 |
| Pastrami, Turkey | 3-1/2 oz | 133 | 54 | 6 | 2 | 68 | 981 | 2 | 0 | 16 |
| Salami, Cooked, Turkey | 3-1/2 oz | 172 | 81 | 9 | 3 | 76 | 1004 | 2 | 0 | 19 |
| Turkey Breast | 3-1/2 oz | 104 | 18 | 2 | 0 | 43 | 1015 | 4 | 1 | 17 |
| Turkey Breast, Low Salt | 3-1/2 oz | 99 | 0 | 1 | 0 | 44 | 772 | 0 | 1 | 23 |
| Turkey Breast, Smoked, Lemon Pepper Flavor, 97% Fat Free | 3-1/2 oz | 95 | 9 | 1 | 0 | 48 | 1160 | 1 | 0 | 21 |
| Turkey, White, Rotisserie | 3-1/2 oz | 112 | 27 | 3 | 0 | 55 | 1200 | 8 | 0 | 14 |
| Turkey Ham, Sliced, Extra Lean | 3-1/2 oz | 124 | 36 | 4 | 1 | 67 | 1038 | 3 | 0 | 20 |
| Turkey Roll, Light Meat | 3-1/2 oz | 98 | 18 | 2 | 0 | 34 | 1042 | 5 | 0 | 15 |
| Turkey Roll, Light & Dark Meat | 1 oz | 42 | 18 | 2 | 1 | 16 | 166 | 1 | 0 | 5 |

# common foods

| | SERVING SIZE | CAL | CAL FAT | TOT FAT (G) | SAT FAT (G) | CHOL (MG) | SOD (MG) | CARB (G) | FIBER (G) | PROT (G) |
|---|---|---|---|---|---|---|---|---|---|---|
| **GAME POULTRY** | | | | | | | | | | |
| Duck, Domesticated, Meat & Skin, Cooked | 3-1/2 oz | 337 | 252 | 28 | 10 | 84 | 59 | 0 | 0 | 19 |
| Duck, Domesticated, Meat, Cooked | 3-1/2 oz | 201 | 99 | 11 | 4 | 89 | 65 | 0 | 0 | 23 |
| Duck, Whole Pekin, Breast, Meat & Skin, Boneless, Cooked | 3-1/2 oz | 172 | 83 | 9 | 2 | 116 | 71 | 0 | 0 | 21 |
| Duck, Whole Pekin, Breast, Meat, Boneless, Cooked without Skin | 3-1/2 oz | 140 | 27 | 3 | 1 | 143 | 105 | 0 | 0 | 28 |
| Duck, Whole Pekin, Leg, Meat & Skin, Bone In, Cooked | 3-1/2 oz | 217 | 99 | 11 | 3 | 114 | 110 | 0 | 0 | 27 |
| Duck, Whole Pekin, Leg, Meat, Bone In, Cooked without Skin | 3-1/2 oz | 178 | 54 | 6 | 1 | 105 | 108 | 0 | 0 | 29 |
| Emu, Fan Fillet, Cooked | 3 oz | 131 | 18 | 2 | 0 | 70 | 45 | 0 | 0 | 27 |
| Emu, Full Rump, Cooked | 3 oz | 143 | 21 | 2 | 1 | 110 | 94 | 0 | 0 | 29 |
| Emu, Ground, Cooked | 3 oz | 139 | 36 | 4 | 1 | 74 | 55 | 0 | 0 | 24 |
| Emu, Inside Drums, Cooked | 3 oz | 133 | 15 | 2 | 1 | 77 | 100 | 0 | 0 | 28 |
| Emu, Top Loin, Cooked | 3 oz | 129 | 24 | 3 | 1 | 75 | 49 | 0 | 0 | 25 |
| Pheasant, Cooked | 3-1/2 oz | 239 | 108 | 12 | 4 | 89 | 43 | 0 | 0 | 32 |
| Quail, Cooked | 3-1/2 oz | 227 | 126 | 14 | 4 | 86 | 52 | 0 | 0 | 25 |
| **SAUSAGE** | | | | | | | | | | |
| Bratwurst, Chicken, Cooked | 3-1/2 oz | 176 | 90 | 10 | 0 | 71 | 72 | 0 | 0 | 19 |
| Chicken & Beef Sausage, Smoked | 3-1/2 oz | 295 | 216 | 24 | 7 | 70 | 1020 | 0 | 0 | 19 |
| Chicken, Beef, & Pork Sausage, Skinless, Smoked | 1 link | 181 | 108 | 12 | 4 | 101 | 869 | 7 | 0 | 11 |
| Frankfurter, Chicken | 1 link | 101 | 66 | 7 | 2 | 43 | 382 | 1 | 0 | 7 |
| Frankfurter, Turkey | 1 frank | 100 | 72 | 8 | 2 | 35 | 485 | 2 | 0 | 6 |
| Italian Sausage, Turkey, Smoked | 2 oz | 88 | 44 | 5 | 0 | 30 | 520 | 3 | 1 | 8 |
| Turkey & Pork, Patty or Link, Cooked | 1 oz | 86 | 58 | 6 | 2 | 24 | 246 | 0 | 0 | 6 |
| Turkey Sausage, Hot, Smoked | 2 oz | 88 | 44 | 5 | 2 | 30 | 520 | 3 | 1 | 8 |
| **TURKEY** | | | | | | | | | | |
| *Average for All Dark Meat* | | | | | | | | | | |
| Meat & Skin, Fryer-Roaster (Young Turkey) | 3-1/2 oz | 182 | 63 | 7 | 2 | 117 | 76 | 0 | 0 | 28 |
| Meat & Skin, Roasted | 3-1/2 oz | 221 | 108 | 12 | 3 | 89 | 76 | 0 | 0 | 27 |
| Meat, Fryer-Roaster (Young Turkey) | 3-1/2 oz | 162 | 36 | 4 | 1 | 112 | 79 | 0 | 0 | 29 |
| Meat, Roasted | 3-1/2 oz | 188 | 63 | 7 | 2 | 85 | 79 | 0 | 0 | 29 |
| *Average for All Light Meat* | | | | | | | | | | |
| Meat & Skin, Fryer-Roaster (Young Turkey) | 3-1/2 oz | 164 | 45 | 5 | 1 | 95 | 57 | 0 | 0 | 29 |

| | SERVING SIZE | CAL | CAL FAT | TOT FAT (G) | SAT FAT (G) | CHOL (MG) | SOD (MG) | CARB (G) | FIBER (G) | PROT (G) |
|---|---|---|---|---|---|---|---|---|---|---|
| Meat & Skin, Roasted | 3-1/2 oz | 208 | 90 | 10 | 3 | 82 | 68 | 0 | 0 | 28 |
| Meat, Fryer-Roaster (Young Turkey) | 3-1/2 oz | 140 | 9 | 1 | 0 | 86 | 56 | 0 | 0 | 30 |
| Meat, Roasted | 3-1/2 oz | 170 | 45 | 5 | 1 | 76 | 70 | 0 | 0 | 29 |
| *Breast* | | | | | | | | | | |
| Meat & Skin, Fryer-Roaster (Young Turkey) | 3-1/2 oz | 153 | 27 | 3 | 1 | 90 | 53 | 0 | 0 | 22 |
| Meat & Skin, Pre-Basted, Roasted | 3-1/2 oz | 126 | 27 | 3 | 1 | 42 | 397 | 0 | 0 | 29 |
| Meat & Skin, Roasted | 3-1/2 oz | 189 | 63 | 7 | 2 | 74 | 63 | 0 | 0 | 29 |
| Meat, Fryer-Roaster (Young Turkey) | 3-1/2 oz | 135 | 9 | 1 | 0 | 83 | 52 | 0 | 0 | 30 |
| *Drumstick* | | | | | | | | | | |
| Smoked, with Skin, Bone Removed | 1 oz | 42 | 19 | 2 | 1 | 18 | 209 | 0 | 0 | 6 |
| *Leg* | | | | | | | | | | |
| Meat & Skin, Fryer-Roaster (Young Turkey) | 3-1/2 oz | 170 | 45 | 5 | 2 | 70 | 80 | 0 | 0 | 28 |
| Meat & Skin, Roasted | 3-1/2 oz | 208 | 90 | 10 | 3 | 85 | 77 | 0 | 0 | 28 |
| Meat, Fryer-Roaster (Young Turkey) | 3-1/2 oz | 159 | 36 | 4 | 1 | 119 | 81 | 0 | 0 | 29 |
| *Offal* | | | | | | | | | | |
| Giblets, Cooked, Simmered, some Giblet Fat, Chopped or Diced | 1 cup | 289 | 155 | 17 | 6 | 419 | 93 | 1 | 0 | 30 |
| Neck, Meat, Cooked, Simmered, Bone & Skin Removed | 1 neck | 274 | 99 | 11 | 3 | 185 | 85 | 0 | 0 | 41 |
| *Other* | | | | | | | | | | |
| Bacon, Cooked | 1 oz | 107 | 70 | 8 | 2 | 27 | 640 | 1 | 0 | 8 |
| Canned, Meat Only, with Broth | 1 cup | 228 | 83 | 9 | 3 | 89 | 630 | 2 | 0 | 32 |
| Patties, Breaded, Battered, Fried | 3 oz | 266 | 153 | 17 | 4 | 70 | 752 | 15 | 1 | 13 |
| Turkey Ham, Cured Thigh Meat | 1 oz | 35 | 12 | 1 | 0 | 20 | 312 | 1 | 0 | 5 |
| *Thigh* | | | | | | | | | | |
| Meat & Skin, Pre-Basted, Roasted | 3-1/2 oz | 157 | 63 | 9 | 3 | 62 | 437 | 0 | 0 | 19 |
| *Wing* | | | | | | | | | | |
| Meat & Skin, Fryer-Roaster (Young Turkey) | 3-1/2 oz | 207 | 90 | 10 | 3 | 115 | 73 | 0 | 0 | 28 |
| Meat & Skin, Roasted | 3-1/2 oz | 229 | 108 | 12 | 3 | 81 | 61 | 0 | 0 | 27 |
| Meat, Fryer-Roaster (Young Turkey) | 3-1/2 oz | 163 | 27 | 3 | 1 | 102 | 78 | 0 | 0 | 31 |
| **Snacks** | | | | | | | | | | |
| **Beef Sticks**, Smoked | 1 stick | 109 | 88 | 10 | 4 | 26 | 293 | 1 | 0 | 4 |
| **Granola Bars**, Soft, Almond, Confectioners Coating | 1 bar | 159 | 63 | 7 | 2 | 1 | 170 | 21 | 2 | 3 |
| **Plantain Chips**, Salted | 1 oz | 151 | 75 | 8 | 2 | 0 | 57 | 18 | 1 | 1 |

# common foods

| | SERVING SIZE | CAL | CAL FAT | TOT FAT (G) | SAT FAT (G) | CHOL (MG) | SOD (MG) | CARB (G) | FIBER (G) | PROT (G) |
|---|---|---|---|---|---|---|---|---|---|---|
| **POPCORN** | | | | | | | | | | |
| Popcorn, Air-Popped | 1 cup | 31 | 3 | 0 | 0 | 0 | 1 | 6 | 1 | 1 |
| Popcorn, Cakes | 1 cake | 38 | 3 | 0 | 0 | 0 | 29 | 8 | 0 | 1 |
| Popcorn, Cheese Flavor | 1 cup | 58 | 33 | 4 | 1 | 1 | 98 | 6 | 1 | 1 |
| Popcorn, Microwave, Butter Flavor | 1 oz | 149 | 76 | 8 | 2 | 1 | 219 | 16 | 3 | 2 |
| Popcorn, Oil-Popped | 1 cup | 64 | 43 | 5 | 1 | 0 | 116 | 5 | 1 | 1 |
| **Pork Skins**, Barbecue Flavor | 1 oz | 153 | 81 | 9 | 3 | 33 | 756 | 0 | 0 | 16 |
| Pork Skins, Plain | 1 oz | 154 | 80 | 9 | 3 | 27 | 521 | 0 | 0 | 17 |
| **POTATO CHIPS** | | | | | | | | | | |
| Potato Chips, Barbecue Flavor | 1 oz | 139 | 83 | 9 | 2 | 0 | 213 | 15 | 1 | 2 |
| Potato Chips, Cheese Flavor | 1 oz | 141 | 69 | 8 | 2 | 1 | 225 | 16 | 1 | 2 |
| Potato Chips, Fat Free, Salted | 1 oz | 107 | 2 | 0 | 0 | 0 | 182 | 24 | 2 | 3 |
| Potato Chips, Light | 1 oz | 134 | 53 | 6 | 1 | 0 | 139 | 19 | 2 | 2 |
| Potato Chips, Plain, Salted | 1 oz | 154 | 93 | 10 | 1 | 0 | 149 | 14 | 1 | 2 |
| Potato Chips, Plain, Unsalted | 1 oz | 152 | 88 | 10 | 3 | 0 | 2 | 15 | 1 | 2 |
| Potato Chips, Sour Cream & Onion Flavor | 1 oz | 155 | 94 | 10 | 3 | 1 | 204 | 15 | 0 | 2 |
| **PRETZELS** | | | | | | | | | | |
| Pretzels, Hard, Plain, Salted | 1 oz | 108 | 7 | 1 | 0 | 0 | 385 | 23 | 1 | 3 |
| Pretzels, Hard, Whole-Wheat | 1 oz | 103 | 7 | 1 | 0 | 0 | 58 | 23 | 2 | 3 |
| Pretzels, Soft | 1 large | 483 | 40 | 4 | 1 | 4 | 1151 | 99 | 2 | 12 |
| **Soy Chips** or Crisps, Salted | 1 oz | 109 | 19 | 2 | 0 | 0 | 239 | 15 | 1 | 8 |
| **Sweet Potato Chips** | 1 oz | 141 | 63 | 7 | 1 | 0 | 10 | 18 | 1 | 1 |
| **TORTILLA CHIPS** | | | | | | | | | | |
| Tortilla Chips, Light | 10 chips | 74 | 22 | 2 | 0 | 0 | 160 | 12 | 1 | 1 |
| Tortilla Chips, Low Fat, Baked | 1 oz | 118 | 15 | 2 | 0 | 0 | 119 | 23 | 2 | 3 |
| Tortilla Chips, Nacho Cheese | 1 oz | 146 | 67 | 7 | 1 | 0 | 174 | 18 | 1 | 2 |
| Tortilla Chips, Ranch Flavor | 1 oz | 142 | 63 | 7 | n/a | 0 | 147 | 18 | 1 | 2 |
| Tortilla Chips, Taco Flavor | 1 oz | 136 | 62 | 7 | 1 | 1 | 223 | 18 | 2 | 2 |
| Tortilla Chips, Unsalted, White Corn | 1 cup | 131 | 55 | 6 | 1 | 0 | 4 | 17 | 1 | 2 |
| **TRAIL MIXES** | | | | | | | | | | |
| Trail Mix, Regular | 1 cup | 693 | 397 | 44 | 8 | 0 | 344 | 67 | 0 | 21 |
| Tropical | 1 cup | 570 | 215 | 24 | 12 | 0 | 14 | 92 | 0 | 9 |
| With Chocolate Chips, Salted Nuts & Seeds | 1 cup | 707 | 419 | 47 | 9 | 6 | 177 | 66 | 0 | 21 |

## Soups
### BEAN

| | SERVING SIZE | CAL | CAL FAT | TOT FAT (G) | SAT FAT (G) | CHOL (MG) | SOD (MG) | CARB (G) | FIBER (G) | PROT (G) |
|---|---|---|---|---|---|---|---|---|---|---|
| Bean with Ham, Canned, Chunky, Ready-to-Serve | 1 cup | 231 | 77 | 9 | 3 | 22 | 972 | 27 | 11 | 13 |

| | SERVING SIZE | CAL | CAL FAT | TOT FAT (G) | SAT FAT (G) | CHOL (MG) | SOD (MG) | CARB (G) | FIBER (G) | PROT (G) |
|---|---|---|---|---|---|---|---|---|---|---|
| Bean with Pork, Canned, Prepared with Water | 1 cup | 168 | 52 | 6 | 1 | 3 | 930 | 22 | 8 | 8 |
| Black Bean, Canned, Prepared with Water | 1 cup | 114 | 15 | 2 | 0 | 0 | 1203 | 19 | 8 | 6 |
| **BEEF** | | | | | | | | | | |
| Beef Broth or Bouillon, Canned, Ready-to-Serve | 1 cup | 17 | 5 | 1 | 0 | 0 | 893 | 0 | 0 | 3 |
| Beef Broth, Cubed, Dry | 1 cube | 6 | 1 | 0 | 0 | 0 | 864 | 1 | 0 | 1 |
| Beef Broth, Cubed, Prepared with Water | 1 cup | 7 | 2 | 0 | 0 | 0 | 623 | 1 | 0 | 1 |
| Beef Chili, Canned, Prepared with Water | 1 cup | 149 | 29 | 3 | 2 | 13 | 1011 | 24 | 3 | 6 |
| Beef Mushroom, Canned, Prepared with Water | 1 cup | 73 | 27 | 3 | 1 | 7 | 942 | 6 | 0 | 6 |
| Beef Noodle, Canned, Prepared with Water | 1 cup | 83 | 27 | 3 | 1 | 5 | 930 | 9 | 1 | 5 |
| Beef Stock, Home-Prepared | 1 cup | 31 | 2 | 0 | 0 | 0 | 475 | 3 | 0 | 5 |
| **CHICKEN** | | | | | | | | | | |
| Chicken Broth Cubes, Dry | 1 cube | 10 | 2 | 0 | 0 | 1 | 1152 | 1 | 0 | 1 |
| Chicken Broth or Bouillon, Prepared with Water | 1 cup | 10 | 5 | 1 | 0 | 0 | 753 | 1 | 0 | 1 |
| Chicken Gumbo, Canned, Prepared with Water | 1 cup | 56 | 13 | 1 | 0 | 5 | 954 | 8 | 2 | 3 |
| Chicken Mushroom, Canned, Prepared with Water | 1 cup | 132 | 82 | 9 | 2 | 10 | 798 | 9 | 0 | 4 |
| Chicken Noodle, Canned, Prepared with Water | 1 cup | 62 | 21 | 2 | 1 | 12 | 866 | 7 | 0 | 3 |
| Chicken Noodle, Dry, Mix, Prepared with Water | 1 cup | 56 | 12 | 1 | 0 | 10 | 561 | 9 | 0 | 2 |
| Chicken Rice, Canned, Chunky, Ready-to-Serve | 1 cup | 127 | 29 | 3 | 1 | 12 | 888 | 13 | 1 | 12 |
| Chicken Stock, Home-Prepared | 1 cup | 86 | 26 | 3 | 1 | 7 | 343 | 8 | 0 | 6 |
| Chicken Vegetable, Canned, Chunky, Ready-to-Serve | 1 cup | 166 | 43 | 5 | 1 | 17 | 833 | 19 | 0 | 12 |
| Chicken Vegetable, Canned, Prepared with Water | 1 cup | 77 | 26 | 3 | 1 | 10 | 972 | 9 | 1 | 4 |
| Chicken with Dumplings, Canned, Prepared with Water | 1 cup | 96 | 50 | 6 | 1 | 34 | 735 | 6 | 0 | 6 |
| Chicken with Rice, Canned, Prepared with Water | 1 cup | 58 | 17 | 2 | 0 | 7 | 578 | 7 | 1 | 4 |

# common foods

| | SERVING SIZE | CAL | CAL. FAT | TOT. FAT (G) | SAT FAT (G) | CHOL (MG) | SOD (MG) | CARB (G) | FIBER (G) | PROT (G) |
|---|---|---|---|---|---|---|---|---|---|---|
| Cream of Chicken, Canned, Prepared with Milk | 1 cup | 191 | 103 | 11 | 5 | 27 | 898 | 15 | 0 | 7 |
| Cream of Chicken, Canned, Prepared with Water | 1 cup | 117 | 66 | 7 | 2 | 10 | 847 | 9 | 0 | 3 |
| **CLAM CHOWDER** | | | | | | | | | | |
| Clam Chowder, Manhattan, Canned, Prepared with Water | 1 cup | 75 | 19 | 2 | 0 | 2 | 563 | 12 | 1 | 2 |
| Clam Chowder, Manhattan Style, Canned, Chunky, Ready-to-Serve | 1 cup | 134 | 30 | 3 | 2 | 14 | 1001 | 19 | 3 | 7 |
| Clam Chowder, New England, Canned, Prepared with 2% Milk | 1 cup | 154 | 46 | 5 | 3 | 18 | 688 | 19 | 1 | 8 |
| Clam Chowder, New England, Canned, Prepared with Water | 1 cup | 87 | 23 | 3 | 1 | 7 | 630 | 13 | 1 | 4 |
| **Fish Stock**, Home-Prepared | 1 cup | 40 | 17 | 2 | 0 | 2 | 363 | 0 | 0 | 5 |
| **Gazpacho**, Canned, Ready-to-Serve | 1 cup | 46 | 2 | 0 | 0 | 0 | 739 | 4 | 0 | 7 |
| **Hot & Sour**, Chinese Restaurant | 1 cup | 91 | 25 | 3 | 1 | 49 | 877 | 10 | 1 | 6 |
| **Lentil** with Ham, Canned, Ready-to-Serve | 1 cup | 139 | 25 | 3 | 1 | 7 | 1319 | 20 | 0 | 9 |
| **Minestrone**, Canned, Ready-to-Serve | 1 cup | 127 | 25 | 3 | 1 | 5 | 691 | 21 | 6 | 5 |
| **MUSHROOM** | | | | | | | | | | |
| Cream of Mushroom, Canned, Prepared with 2% Milk | 1 cup | 169 | 88 | 10 | 3 | 10 | 844 | 14 | 0 | 6 |
| Cream of Mushroom, Canned, Prepared with Water | 1 cup | 104 | 64 | 7 | 2 | 0 | 789 | 8 | 0 | 2 |
| Mushroom Barley, Canned, Prepared with Water | 1 cup | 73 | 20 | 2 | 0 | 0 | 891 | 12 | 1 | 2 |
| Mushroom with Beef Stock, Canned, Prepared with Water | 1 cup | 85 | 36 | 4 | 2 | 7 | 969 | 9 | 1 | 3 |
| **Ramen** Noodle, Any Flavor, Dry | 1 package | 371 | 120 | 13 | 6 | 0 | 1731 | 54 | 2 | 9 |
| **SPLIT PEA** | | | | | | | | | | |
| Split Pea, with Ham, Canned, Prepared with Water | 1 cup | 190 | 40 | 4 | 2 | 8 | 1007 | 28 | 2 | 10 |
| Split Pea, with Ham, Canned, Chunky, Ready-to-Serve | 1 cup | 185 | 36 | 4 | 2 | 7 | 722 | 27 | 4 | 11 |
| **TOMATO** | | | | | | | | | | |
| Tomato Bisque, Canned, Prepared with Milk | 1 cup | 198 | 59 | 7 | 3 | 23 | 1109 | 29 | 1 | 6 |
| Tomato Bisque, Canned, Prepared with Water | 1 cup | 124 | 23 | 3 | 1 | 5 | 1047 | 24 | 0 | 2 |

| | SERVING SIZE | CAL | CAL FAT | TOT FAT (G) | SAT FAT (G) | CHOL. (MG) | SOD (MG) | CARB (G) | FIBER (G) | PROT (G) |
|---|---|---|---|---|---|---|---|---|---|---|
| Tomato Rice, Canned, Prepared with Water | 1 cup | 116 | 24 | 3 | 0 | 2 | 788 | 21 | 2 | 2 |
| Tomato, Canned, Prepared with 2% Milk | 1 cup | 139 | 29 | 3 | 2 | 10 | 529 | 23 | 2 | 6 |
| Tomato, Canned, Prepared with Water | 1 cup | 74 | 6 | 1 | 0 | 0 | 471 | 16 | 2 | 2 |
| **TURKEY** | | | | | | | | | | |
| Turkey, Canned, Chunky, Ready-to-Serve | 1 cup | 135 | 40 | 4 | 1 | 9 | 923 | n/a | 0 | 10 |
| Turkey Noodle, Canned, Prepared with Water | 1 cup | 68 | 18 | 2 | 1 | 5 | 815 | 9 | 1 | 4 |
| Turkey Vegetable, Canned, Prepared with Water | 1 cup | 72 | 27 | 3 | 1 | 2 | 906 | 9 | 0 | 3 |
| **VEGETABLE** | | | | | | | | | | |
| Vegetable Beef, Canned, Prepared with Water | 1 cup | 76 | 17 | 2 | 1 | 5 | 852 | 10 | 2 | 5 |
| Vegetable, Canned, Chunky, Ready-to-Serve | 1 cup | 125 | 34 | 4 | 1 | 0 | 880 | 19 | 1 | 4 |
| Vegetarian Vegetable, Canned, Prepared with Water | 1 cup | 67 | 17 | 2 | 0 | 0 | 815 | 12 | 1 | 2 |
| **Wonton**, Chinese Restaurant | 1 cup | 71 | 5 | 1 | 0 | 9 | 905 | 12 | 0 | 5 |
| **Sugars** | | | | | | | | | | |
| Brown Sugar, Packed | 1 cup | 836 | 0 | 0 | 0 | 0 | 62 | 216 | 0 | 0 |
| Granulated Sugar | 1 tsp | 16 | 0 | 0 | 0 | 0 | 0 | 4 | 0 | 0 |
| Powdered Sugar, Unsifted | 1 cup | 467 | 0 | 0 | 0 | 0 | 2 | 120 | 0 | 0 |
| **Syrups** | | | | | | | | | | |
| Chocolate Syrup, Fudge-Type | 2 tbsp | 133 | 30 | 3 | 2 | 0 | 131 | 24 | 1 | 2 |
| Corn Syrup, Dark | 1 tbsp | 57 | 0 | 0 | 0 | 0 | 31 | 16 | 0 | 0 |
| Corn Syrup, High-Fructose | 1 tbsp | 53 | 0 | 0 | 0 | 0 | 0 | 14 | 0 | 0 |
| Corn Syrup, Light | 1 tbsp | 62 | 0 | 0 | 0 | 0 | 14 | 17 | 0 | 0 |
| Grenadine | 1 tbsp | 54 | 0 | 0 | 0 | 0 | 5 | 13 | 0 | 0 |
| Malt Syrup | 1 tbsp | 76 | 0 | 0 | 0 | 0 | 8 | 17 | 0 | 1 |
| Maple Syrup | 1 tbsp | 52 | 0 | 0 | 0 | 0 | 2 | 13 | 0 | 0 |
| Sorghum Syrup | 1 tbsp | 61 | 0 | 0 | 0 | 0 | 2 | 16 | 0 | 0 |
| Pancake Syrup | 1 tbsp | 47 | 0 | 0 | 0 | 0 | 16 | 12 | 0 | 0 |
| Pancake Syrup, Reduced-Calorie | 1 tbsp | 25 | 0 | 0 | 0 | 0 | 27 | 7 | 0 | 0 |
| Pancake Syrup, with 2% Maple | 1 tbsp | 53 | 0 | 0 | 0 | 0 | 12 | 14 | 0 | 0 |
| Pancake Syrup, with Butter | 1 tbsp | 59 | 3 | 0 | 0 | 1 | 20 | 15 | 0 | 0 |
| **Tempeh and Tofu** | | | | | | | | | | |
| Tempeh | 1 cup | 320 | 161 | 18 | 4 | 0 | 15 | 16 | 0 | 31 |
| Tofu, Extra Firm, Nigari | 1/5 block | 83 | 48 | 5 | 0 | 0 | 7 | 2 | 0 | 9 |

# common foods

| | SERVING SIZE | CAL | CAL FAT | TOT FAT (G) | SAT FAT (G) | CHOL (MG) | SOD (MG) | CARB (G) | FIBER (G) | PROT (G) |
|---|---|---|---|---|---|---|---|---|---|---|
| Tofu, Firm, Nigari | 1/2 cup | 88 | 47 | 5 | 1 | 0 | 15 | 2 | 1 | 10 |
| Tofu, Fried | 1 oz | 77 | 51 | 6 | 1 | 0 | 5 | 3 | 1 | 5 |
| **Vegetables** | | | | | | | | | | |
| **Artichokes** | 1 medium | 60 | 2 | 0 | 0 | 0 | 120 | 13 | 7 | 4 |
| Artichokes, Cooked with Salt | 1 medium | 64 | 4 | 0 | 0 | 0 | 72 | 14 | 10 | 3 |
| Artichokes, Frozen | 9 oz | 97 | 10 | 1 | 0 | 0 | 120 | 20 | 10 | 7 |
| Artichokes, Frozen, Cooked with Salt | 1 cup | 76 | 8 | 1 | 0 | 0 | 486 | 15 | 8 | 5 |
| **Arugula** | 1/2 cup | 2 | 1 | 0 | 0 | 0 | 3 | 0 | 0 | 0 |
| **Asparagus** | 1 cup | 27 | 1 | 0 | 0 | 0 | 3 | 5 | 3 | 3 |
| Asparagus, Canned | 1 cup | 46 | 14 | 2 | 0 | 0 | 695 | 6 | 4 | 5 |
| Asparagus, Cooked | 4 spears | 13 | 1 | 0 | 0 | 0 | 8 | 2 | 1 | 1 |
| Asparagus, Frozen | 4 spears | 14 | 1 | 0 | 0 | 0 | 5 | 2 | 1 | 2 |
| Asparagus, Frozen, Cooked, with Salt | 1 cup | 32 | 7 | 1 | 0 | 0 | 432 | 3 | 3 | 5 |
| **Avocados**, California | 1 fruit | 227 | 188 | 21 | 3 | 0 | 11 | 12 | 9 | 3 |
| Avocados, Florida | 1 fruit | 365 | 275 | 31 | 6 | 0 | 6 | 24 | 17 | 7 |
| **Bamboo Shoots** | 1 cup | 41 | 4 | 0 | 0 | 0 | 6 | 8 | 3 | 4 |
| Bamboo Shoots, Canned | 1 cup | 25 | 5 | 1 | 0 | 0 | 9 | 4 | 2 | 2 |
| Bamboo Shoots, Cooked with Salt | 1 cup | 13 | 2 | 0 | 0 | 0 | 288 | 2 | 1 | 2 |
| **BEANS** | | | | | | | | | | |
| **Baked**, Canned, Plain or Vegetarian | 1 cup | 239 | 8 | 1 | 0 | 0 | 871 | 54 | 10 | 12 |
| Baked, Canned, with Beef | 1 cup | 322 | 83 | 9 | 4 | 59 | 1264 | 45 | 0 | 17 |
| Baked, Canned, with Franks | 1 cup | 368 | 153 | 17 | 6 | 16 | 1114 | 40 | 18 | 17 |
| Baked, Canned, with Pork | 1 cup | 268 | 35 | 4 | 2 | 18 | 1047 | 51 | 14 | 13 |
| Baked, Canned, with Pork & Sweet Sauce | 1 cup | 283 | 33 | 4 | 1 | 18 | 845 | 53 | 11 | 13 |
| Baked, Canned, with Pork & Tomato Sauce | 1 cup | 231 | 21 | 2 | 1 | 17 | 1075 | 46 | 10 | 13 |
| Baked, Home Prepared | 1 cup | 392 | 117 | 13 | 5 | 13 | 1068 | 55 | 14 | 14 |
| **Black**, Mature Seeds, Cooked, Boiled, with Salt | 1 cup | 227 | 8 | 1 | 0 | 0 | 408 | 41 | 15 | 15 |
| Black, Mature Seeds, Raw | 1 cup | 662 | 25 | 3 | 1 | 0 | 10 | 121 | 30 | 42 |
| **Black Turtle Soup**, Mature Seeds, Canned | 1 cup | 218 | 6 | 1 | 0 | 0 | 922 | 40 | 17 | 14 |
| Black Turtle Soup, Mature Seeds, Cooked, Boiled, with Salt | 1 cup | 240 | 6 | 1 | 0 | 0 | 442 | 45 | 10 | 15 |
| Black Turtle Soup, Mature Seeds, Raw | 1 cup | 624 | 15 | 2 | 0 | 0 | 17 | 116 | 46 | 39 |
| **Broadbeans** (Fava Beans), Mature Seeds, Canned | 1 cup | 182 | 5 | 1 | 0 | 0 | 1160 | 32 | 9 | 14 |
| Broadbeans (Fava Beans), Mature Seeds, Cooked, Boiled, with Salt | 1 cup | 187 | 6 | 1 | 0 | 0 | 410 | 33 | 9 | 13 |

| | SERVING SIZE | CAL | CAL FAT | TOT FAT (G) | SAT FAT (G) | CHOL (MG) | SOD (MG) | CARB (G) | FIBER (G) | PROT (G) |
|---|---|---|---|---|---|---|---|---|---|---|
| Broadbeans (Fava Beans), Mature Seeds, Raw | 1 cup | 512 | 21 | 2 | 0 | 0 | 20 | 87 | 38 | 39 |
| Broadbeans, Immature Seeds, Raw | 1 cup | 78 | 6 | 1 | 0 | 0 | 54 | 13 | 5 | 6 |
| **Chickpeas** (Garbanzo Beans), Mature Seeds, Canned | 1 cup | 286 | 25 | 3 | 0 | 0 | 718 | 54 | 11 | 12 |
| Chickpeas, Mature Seeds, Cooked, Boiled, with Salt | 1 cup | 269 | 38 | 4 | 0 | 0 | 399 | 45 | 13 | 15 |
| Chickpeas, Mature Seeds, Raw | 1 cup | 728 | 109 | 12 | 1 | 0 | 48 | 121 | 35 | 39 |
| **Chili**, Barbecue, Ranch Style, Cooked | 1 cup | 245 | 23 | 3 | 0 | 0 | 1834 | 43 | 11 | 13 |
| **Cowpeas**, Common (Blackeyes, Crowder, Southern), Mature Seeds, Boiled, w/o Salt | 1 cup | 198 | 8 | 1 | 0 | 0 | 7 | 36 | 11 | 13 |
| Cowpeas, Common (Blackeyes, Crowder, Southern), Mature Seeds, Raw | 1 cup | 561 | 19 | 2 | 1 | 0 | 27 | 100 | 18 | 39 |
| Cowpeas, Common, Mature Seeds, Canned, Plain | 1 cup | 185 | 12 | 1 | 0 | 0 | 718 | 33 | 8 | 11 |
| Cowpeas, Common, Mature Seeds, Canned with Pork | 1 cup | 199 | 35 | 4 | 1 | 17 | 840 | 40 | 8 | 7 |
| Cowpeas, Common, Mature Seeds, Cooked, Boiled, with Salt | 1 cup | 198 | 8 | 1 | 0 | 0 | 410 | 35 | 11 | 13 |
| **Cranberry** (Roman), Mature Seeds, Canned | 1 cup | 216 | 7 | 1 | 0 | 0 | 863 | 39 | 16 | 14 |
| Cranberry (Roman), Mature Seeds, Cooked, Boiled, with Salt | 1 cup | 241 | 7 | 1 | 0 | 0 | 419 | 43 | 18 | 17 |
| Cranberry (Roman), Mature Seeds, Raw | 1 cup | 653 | 22 | 2 | 1 | 0 | 12 | 117 | 48 | 45 |
| **Edamame**, Frozen, Prepared | 1 cup | 189 | 73 | 8 | 1 | 0 | 9 | 15 | 8 | 17 |
| Edamame, Frozen, Unprepared | 1 cup | 130 | 50 | 6 | 0 | 0 | 7 | 10 | 6 | 12 |
| **French**, Mature Seeds, Cooked, Boiled, with Salt | 1 cup | 228 | 12 | 1 | 0 | 0 | 428 | 43 | 17 | 12 |
| French, Mature Seeds, Raw | 1 cup | 631 | 33 | 4 | 0 | 0 | 33 | 118 | 46 | 35 |
| **Great Northern**, Mature Seeds, Canned | 1 cup | 299 | 9 | 1 | 0 | 0 | 10 | 55 | 13 | 19 |
| Great Northern, Mature Seeds, Cooked, Boiled, with Salt | 1 cup | 209 | 7 | 1 | 0 | 0 | 421 | 37 | 12 | 15 |
| Great Northern, Mature Seeds, Raw | 1 cup | 620 | 19 | 2 | 1 | 0 | 26 | 114 | 37 | 40 |
| **Hummus**, Commercial | 1 cup | 408 | 213 | 24 | 4 | 0 | 932 | 35 | 15 | 19 |
| Hummus, Commercial | 1 tbsp | 25 | 13 | 1 | 0 | 0 | 57 | 2 | 1 | 1 |
| Hummus, Home Prepared | 1 cup | 435 | 190 | 21 | 3 | 0 | 595 | 50 | 10 | 12 |
| Hummus, Home Prepared | 1 tbsp | 27 | 12 | 1 | 0 | 0 | 36 | 3 | 1 | 1 |
| **Kidney**, All Types, Mature Seeds, Canned | 1 cup | 215 | 14 | 2 | 0 | 0 | 758 | 37 | 14 | 13 |

# common foods

| | SERVING SIZE | CAL | CAL FAT | TOT FAT (G) | SAT FAT (G) | CHOL (MG) | SOD (MG) | CARB (G) | FIBER (G) | PROT (G) |
|---|---|---|---|---|---|---|---|---|---|---|
| Kidney, All Types, Mature Seeds, Cooked, Boiled, with Salt | 1 cup | 225 | 8 | 1 | 0 | 0 | 421 | 40 | 11 | 15 |
| Kidney, All Types, Mature Seeds, Raw | 1 cup | 613 | 14 | 2 | 0 | 0 | 44 | 110 | 46 | 43 |
| **Lentils**, Mature Seeds, Cooked, Boiled, with Salt | 1 cup | 226 | 7 | 1 | 0 | 0 | 471 | 39 | 16 | 18 |
| Lentils, Pink, Raw | 1 cup | 662 | 37 | 4 | 1 | 0 | 13 | 114 | 21 | 48 |
| Lentils, Raw | 1 cup | 678 | 18 | 2 | 0 | 0 | 12 | 115 | 59 | 50 |
| **Lima Beans**, Immature Seeds, Canned, No Salt | 1/2 cup | 88 | 3 | 0 | 0 | 0 | 5 | 17 | 5 | 5 |
| Lima Beans, Immature Seeds, Canned, Regular | 1/2 cup | 88 | 3 | 0 | 0 | 0 | 312 | 17 | 5 | 5 |
| Lima Beans, Immature Seeds, Cooked, Boiled, Drained, with Salt | 1 cup | 209 | 5 | 1 | 0 | 0 | 430 | 40 | 9 | 12 |
| Lima Beans, Immature Seeds, Frozen, Cooked, Boiled, Drained, with Salt | 1/2 cup | 94 | 2 | 0 | 0 | 0 | 238 | 18 | 5 | 6 |
| Lima Beans, Immature Seeds, Frozen, Unprepared | 1/2 cup | 108 | 3 | 0 | 0 | 0 | 43 | 21 | 5 | 6 |
| Lima Beans, Immature Seeds, Raw | 1 cup | 176 | 12 | 1 | 0 | 0 | 12 | 31 | 8 | 11 |
| Lima Beans, Large, Mature Seeds, Canned | 1 cup | 190 | 4 | 0 | 0 | 0 | 810 | 36 | 12 | 12 |
| Lima Beans, Large, Mature Seeds, Cooked, Boiled, with Salt | 1 cup | 216 | 6 | 1 | 0 | 0 | 447 | 39 | 13 | 15 |
| Lima Beans, Large, Mature Seeds, Raw | 1 cup | 602 | 11 | 1 | 0 | 0 | 32 | 113 | 34 | 38 |
| **Mung Beans**, Mature Seeds, Cooked, Boiled, with Salt | 1 cup | 212 | 7 | 1 | 0 | 0 | 481 | 39 | 15 | 14 |
| Mung Beans, Mature Seeds, Raw | 1 cup | 718 | 21 | 2 | 1 | 0 | 31 | 130 | 34 | 49 |
| **Mungo Beans**, Mature Seeds, Cooked, Boiled, with Salt | 1 cup | 189 | 9 | 1 | 0 | 0 | 437 | 33 | 12 | 14 |
| Mungo Beans, Mature Seeds, Raw | 1 cup | 706 | 31 | 3 | 0 | 0 | 79 | 122 | 38 | 52 |
| **Navy**, Mature Seeds, Canned | 1 cup | 296 | 10 | 1 | 0 | 0 | 1174 | 54 | 13 | 20 |
| Navy, Mature Seeds, Cooked, Boiled, with Salt | 1 cup | 255 | 10 | 1 | 0 | 0 | 431 | 47 | 19 | 15 |
| Navy, Mature Seeds, Raw | 1 cup | 701 | 28 | 3 | 0 | 0 | 10 | 126 | 51 | 46 |
| **Pigeon Peas** (Red Gram), Immature Seeds, Cooked, Boiled, Drained, with Salt | 1 cup | 170 | 19 | 2 | 0 | 0 | 367 | 30 | 9 | 9 |
| Pigeon Peas, Immature Seeds, Raw | 1 cup | 209 | 23 | 3 | 1 | 0 | 8 | 37 | 8 | 11 |
| Pigeon Peas, Mature Seeds, Cooked, Boiled, with Salt | 1 cup | 203 | 6 | 1 | 0 | 0 | 405 | 39 | 11 | 11 |

| | SERVING SIZE | CAL | CAL FAT | TOT FAT (G) | SAT FAT (G) | CHOL (MG) | SOD (MG) | CARB (G) | FIBER (G) | PROT (G) |
|---|---|---|---|---|---|---|---|---|---|---|
| Pigeon Peas, Mature Seeds, Raw | 1 cup | 703 | 27 | 3 | 1 | 0 | 35 | 129 | 31 | 44 |
| **Pink**, Mature Seeds, Cooked, Boiled, with Salt | 1 cup | 252 | 7 | 1 | 0 | 0 | 402 | 47 | 9 | 15 |
| Pink, Mature Seeds, Raw | 1 cup | 720 | 21 | 2 | 1 | 0 | 17 | 135 | 27 | 44 |
| **Pinto**, Mature Seeds, Canned | 1 cup | 206 | 17 | 2 | 0 | 0 | 706 | 37 | 11 | 12 |
| Pinto, Mature Seeds, Cooked, Boiled, with Salt | 1 cup | 245 | 10 | 1 | 0 | 0 | 407 | 45 | 15 | 15 |
| Pinto, Mature Seeds, Raw | 1 cup | 670 | 21 | 2 | 0 | 0 | 23 | 121 | 30 | 41 |
| **Refried Beans**, Canned, Fat-Free | 1 cup | 182 | 9 | 1 | 0 | 0 | 1069 | 31 | 11 | 12 |
| Refried Beans, Canned, Traditional Style | 1 cup | 217 | 25 | 3 | 1 | 0 | 1041 | 36 | 12 | 13 |
| Refried Beans, Canned, Vegetarian | 1 cup | 201 | 19 | 2 | 0 | 0 | 1041 | 33 | 11 | 13 |
| **Snap Beans, Green** | 1 cup | 31 | 2 | 0 | 0 | 0 | 6 | 7 | 3 | 2 |
| Snap Beans, Green, Canned | 1 cup | 35 | 2 | 0 | 0 | 0 | 402 | 7 | 4 | 2 |
| Snap Beans, Green, Cooked, with Salt | 1 cup | 44 | 3 | 0 | 0 | 0 | 299 | 10 | 4 | 2 |
| Snap Beans, Green, Frozen | 1 cup | 47 | 2 | 0 | 0 | 0 | 4 | 9 | 3 | 2 |
| Snap Beans, Green, Frozen, Cooked, Salted | 1 cup | 35 | 2 | 0 | 0 | 0 | 331 | 8 | 4 | 2 |
| **Snap Beans, Yellow** | 1 cup | 31 | 1 | 0 | 0 | 0 | 6 | 7 | 3 | 2 |
| Snap Beans, Yellow, Canned | 1 cup | 31 | 1 | 0 | 0 | 0 | 384 | 7 | 2 | 2 |
| Snap Beans, Yellow, Cooked, with Salt | 1 cup | 44 | 3 | 0 | 0 | 0 | 299 | 10 | 4 | 2 |
| Snap Beans, Yellow, Frozen | 1 cup | 40 | 2 | 0 | 0 | 0 | 4 | 9 | 3 | 2 |
| Snap Beans, Yellow, Frozen, Cooked, with Salt | 1 cup | 35 | 2 | 0 | 0 | 0 | 331 | 8 | 4 | 2 |
| **Soybeans**, Green, Cooked, Boiled, Drained, with Salt | 1 cup | 254 | 104 | 12 | 1 | 0 | 450 | 20 | 8 | 22 |
| Soybeans, Green, Raw | 1 cup | 376 | 157 | 17 | 2 | 0 | 38 | 28 | 11 | 33 |
| Soybeans, Mature Seeds, Cooked, Boiled, with Salt | 1 cup | 298 | 139 | 15 | 2 | 0 | 408 | 17 | 10 | 29 |
| Soybeans, Mature Seeds, Dry Roasted | 1 cup | 776 | 335 | 37 | 5 | 0 | 3 | 56 | 14 | 68 |
| Soybeans, Mature Seeds, Raw | 1 cup | 830 | 334 | 37 | 5 | 0 | 4 | 56 | 17 | 68 |
| Soybeans, Mature Seeds, Roasted, Salted | 1 cup | 810 | 393 | 44 | 6 | 0 | 280 | 58 | 30 | 61 |
| **Split Peas**, Mature Seeds, Cooked, Boiled, with Salt | 1 cup | 227 | 7 | 1 | 0 | 0 | 466 | 40 | 16 | 16 |
| **Yellow Beans**, Mature Seeds | 1 cup | 676 | 46 | 5 | 1 | 0 | 24 | 119 | 49 | 43 |
| Yellow Beans, Mature Seeds, Cooked, with Salt | 1 cup | 255 | 17 | 2 | 0 | 0 | 427 | 45 | 18 | 16 |
| **Beet Greens** | 1 cup | 8 | 0 | 0 | 0 | 0 | 86 | 2 | 1 | 1 |
| Beet Greens, Cooked, with Salt | 1 cup | 39 | 3 | 0 | 0 | 0 | 687 | 8 | 4 | 4 |

| common foods | SERVING SIZE | CAL | CAL FAT | TOT FAT (G) | SAT FAT (G) | CHOL (MG) | SOD (MG) | CARB (G) | FIBER (G) | PROT (G) |
|---|---|---|---|---|---|---|---|---|---|---|
| **Beets** | 1 cup | 58 | 2 | 0 | 0 | 0 | 106 | 13 | 4 | 2 |
| Beets, Canned | 1 cup | 74 | 2 | 0 | 0 | 0 | 352 | 18 | 3 | 2 |
| Beets, Harvard, Canned, Slices | 1 cup | 180 | 1 | 0 | 0 | 0 | 399 | 45 | 6 | 2 |
| Beets, Pickled, Slices | 1 cup | 148 | 2 | 0 | 0 | 0 | 599 | 37 | 6 | 2 |
| **Bok Choi**, Cooked, with Salt, Shredded | 1 cup | 20 | 2 | 0 | 0 | 0 | 631 | 3 | 2 | 3 |
| Bok Choi, Shredded | 1 cup | 9 | 1 | 0 | 0 | 0 | 46 | 2 | 1 | 1 |
| **Broccoli** | 1 cup | 31 | 3 | 0 | 0 | 0 | 30 | 6 | 2 | 3 |
| Broccoli, Chinese, Cooked | 1 cup | 19 | 6 | 1 | 0 | 0 | 6 | 3 | 2 | 1 |
| Broccoli, Cooked, with Salt, Medium | 1 stalk | 63 | 7 | 1 | 0 | 0 | 472 | 13 | 6 | 4 |
| Broccoli, Flower Clusters | 1 cup | 20 | 2 | 0 | 0 | 0 | 19 | 4 | 0 | 2 |
| Broccoli, Frozen, Chopped | 1 cup | 41 | 4 | 0 | 0 | 0 | 37 | 7 | 5 | 4 |
| Broccoli, Frozen, Chopped, Cooked, with Salt | 1 cup | 52 | 2 | 0 | 0 | 0 | 478 | 10 | 6 | 6 |
| Broccoli, Frozen, Spears | 10 oz | 82 | 9 | 1 | 0 | 0 | 48 | 15 | 9 | 9 |
| Broccoli, Frozen, Spears, Cooked, with Salt | 1/2 cup | 26 | 1 | 0 | 0 | 0 | 239 | 5 | 3 | 3 |
| Broccoli, Stalks | 1 stalk | 32 | 4 | 0 | 0 | 0 | 31 | 6 | 0 | 3 |
| **Broccoli Rabe**, Chopped | 1 cup | 9 | 2 | 0 | 0 | 0 | 13 | 1 | 1 | 1 |
| Broccoli Rabe, Cooked | 1 bunch | 144 | 20 | 2 | 0 | 0 | 245 | 14 | 12 | 17 |
| **Brussels Sprouts** | 1 cup | 38 | 2 | 0 | 0 | 0 | 22 | 8 | 3 | 3 |
| Brussels Sprouts, Cooked, with Salt | 1/2 cup | 28 | 4 | 0 | 0 | 0 | 200 | 6 | 2 | 2 |
| Brussels Sprouts, Frozen | 10 oz | 116 | 10 | 1 | 0 | 0 | 28 | 22 | 11 | 11 |
| Brussels Sprouts, Frozen, Cooked, with Salt | 1 cup | 65 | 5 | 1 | 0 | 0 | 401 | 13 | 6 | 6 |
| **Cabbage**, Common (Danish, Domestic, and Pointed Types), Shredded | 1/2 cup | 8 | 1 | 0 | 0 | 0 | 6 | 2 | 1 | 0 |
| Cabbage, Common, Cooked, with Salt, Shredded | 1/2 cup | 17 | 0 | 0 | 0 | 0 | 191 | 4 | 1 | 1 |
| Cabbage, Japanese Style, Pickled | 1 cup | 45 | 1 | 0 | 0 | 0 | 416 | 9 | 5 | 2 |
| Cabbage, Mustard, with Salt | 1 cup | 36 | 1 | 0 | 0 | 0 | 918 | 7 | 4 | 1 |
| Cabbage, Nappa, Cooked | 1 cup | 13 | 2 | 0 | 0 | 0 | 12 | 2 | 0 | 1 |
| Cabbage, Red, Cooked, with Salt, Shredded | 1/2 cup | 22 | 1 | 0 | 0 | 0 | 183 | 5 | 2 | 1 |
| Cabbage, Red, Shredded | 1 cup | 22 | 1 | 0 | 0 | 0 | 19 | 5 | 2 | 1 |
| Cabbage, Savoy, Cooked, with Salt, Shredded | 1 cup | 35 | 1 | 0 | 0 | 0 | 377 | 8 | 4 | 3 |
| Cabbage, Savoy, Shredded | 1 cup | 19 | 1 | 0 | 0 | 0 | 20 | 4 | 2 | 1 |
| Cabbage, Shredded | 1 cup | 18 | 1 | 0 | 0 | 0 | 13 | 4 | 2 | 1 |
| **Carrots**, Baby | 1 carrot | 4 | 0 | 0 | 0 | 0 | 8 | 1 | 0 | 0 |
| Carrots, Canned, Sliced | 1 cup | 36 | 3 | 0 | 0 | 0 | 353 | 8 | 2 | 1 |
| Carrots, Chopped | 1 cup | 52 | 3 | 0 | 0 | 0 | 88 | 12 | 4 | 1 |

| | SERVING SIZE | CAL | CAL FAT | TOT FAT (G) | SAT FAT (G) | CHOL (MG) | SOD (MG) | CARB (G) | FIBER (G) | PROT (G) |
|---|---|---|---|---|---|---|---|---|---|---|
| Carrots, Cooked, with Salt, Sliced | 1/2 cup | 27 | 1 | 0 | 0 | 0 | 236 | 6 | 2 | 1 |
| Carrots, Frozen, Cooked, with Salt, Sliced | 1 cup | 54 | 9 | 1 | 0 | 0 | 431 | 11 | 5 | 1 |
| Carrots, Frozen, Sliced | 1/2 cup | 23 | 3 | 0 | 0 | 0 | 44 | 5 | 2 | 0 |
| **Cassava** | 1 cup | 330 | 5 | 1 | 0 | 0 | 29 | 78 | 4 | 3 |
| **Cauliflower**, Chopped | 1 cup | 27 | 3 | 0 | 0 | 0 | 32 | 5 | 2 | 2 |
| Cauliflower, Cooked, with Salt | 1/2 cup | 14 | 3 | 0 | 0 | 0 | 150 | 3 | 1 | 1 |
| Cauliflower, Frozen | 1/2 cup | 16 | 2 | 0 | 0 | 0 | 16 | 3 | 2 | 1 |
| Cauliflower, Frozen, Cooked, with Salt | 1 cup | 31 | 4 | 0 | 0 | 0 | 457 | 6 | 5 | 3 |
| Cauliflower, Green | 1 cup | 20 | 2 | 0 | 0 | 0 | 15 | 4 | 2 | 2 |
| Cauliflower, Green, Cooked, with Salt | 1/2 cup | 20 | 2 | 0 | 0 | 0 | 161 | 4 | 2 | 2 |
| **Celeriac** | 1 cup | 66 | 4 | 0 | 0 | 0 | 156 | 14 | 3 | 2 |
| Celeriac, Cooked, with Salt, Pieces | 1 cup | 42 | 3 | 0 | 0 | 0 | 460 | 9 | 0 | 1 |
| **Celery**, Chopped | 1 cup | 16 | 2 | 0 | 0 | 0 | 81 | 3 | 2 | 1 |
| Celery, Cooked, with Salt, Diced | 1 cup | 27 | 2 | 0 | 0 | 0 | 490 | 6 | 2 | 1 |
| **Chard, Swiss** | 1 cup | 7 | 1 | 0 | 0 | 0 | 77 | 1 | 1 | 1 |
| Chard, Swiss, Cooked, with Salt, Chopped | 1 cup | 35 | 1 | 0 | 0 | 0 | 726 | 7 | 4 | 3 |
| **Collards**, Chopped | 1 cup | 11 | 1 | 0 | 0 | 0 | 7 | 2 | 1 | 1 |
| Collards, Cooked, with Salt, Chopped | 1 cup | 49 | 6 | 1 | 0 | 0 | 479 | 9 | 5 | 4 |
| Collards, Frozen, Chopped | 10 oz | 94 | 9 | 1 | 0 | 0 | 136 | 18 | 10 | 8 |
| Collards , Frozen, Chopped, Cooked, Salted | 1 cup | 61 | 6 | 1 | 0 | 0 | 486 | 12 | 5 | 5 |
| **Corn, Sweet, White** | 1 med ear | 77 | 10 | 1 | 0 | 0 | 14 | 17 | 2 | 3 |
| Corn, Sweet, White, Canned, Cream Style | 1 cup | 184 | 10 | 1 | 0 | 0 | 730 | 46 | 3 | 4 |
| Corn, Sweet, White, Canned, Whole Kernel | 1 cup | 133 | 15 | 2 | 0 | 0 | 530 | 30 | 3 | 4 |
| Corn, Sweet, White, Cooked, with Salt | 1 med ear | 100 | 13 | 1 | 0 | 0 | 261 | 22 | 3 | 3 |
| Corn, Sweet, White, Frozen, Kernels | 1/2 cup | 73 | 6 | 1 | 0 | 0 | 2 | 17 | 2 | 2 |
| Corn, Sweet, White, Frozen, Kernels on Cob | 1 ear | 122 | 9 | 1 | 0 | 0 | 6 | 29 | 4 | 4 |
| Corn, Sweet, White, Frozen, Kernels on Cob, Cooked, with Salt | 1 ear | 59 | 4 | 0 | 0 | 0 | 151 | 14 | 2 | 2 |
| Corn, Sweet, White, Frozen, Kernels, with Salt | 1/2 cup | 66 | 3 | 0 | 0 | 0 | 201 | 16 | 2 | 2 |
| **Corn, Sweet, Yellow** | 1 lg ear | 123 | 15 | 2 | 0 | 0 | 21 | 27 | 3 | 5 |
| Corn, Sweet, Yellow, Canned, Cream Style | 1 cup | 184 | 10 | 1 | 0 | 0 | 730 | 46 | 3 | 4 |
| Corn, Sweet, Yellow, Canned, Whole Kernel | 1 cup | 133 | 14 | 2 | 0 | 0 | 489 | 31 | 3 | 4 |
| Corn, Sweet, Yellow, Cooked, with Salt | 1 med ear | 99 | 14 | 2 | 0 | 0 | 261 | 22 | 2 | 4 |
| Corn, Sweet, Yellow, Frozen, Kernels | 1 cup | 120 | 10 | 1 | 0 | 0 | 4 | 28 | 3 | 4 |
| Corn, Sweet, Yellow, Frozen, Kernels on Cob, Cooked, with Salt | 1 ear | 59 | 4 | 0 | 0 | 0 | 151 | 14 | 2 | 2 |

# common foods

| | SERVING SIZE | CAL | CAL FAT | TOT FAT (G) | SAT FAT (G) | CHOL (MG) | SOD (MG) | CARB (G) | FIBER (G) | PROT (G) |
|---|---|---|---|---|---|---|---|---|---|---|
| Corn, Sweet, Yellow, Frozen, Kernels on Cob | 1 ear | 122 | 9 | 1 | 0 | 0 | 6 | 29 | 4 | 4 |
| Corn, Sweet, Yellow, Frozen, Kernels, Cooked, with Salt | 1/2 cup | 65 | 5 | 1 | 0 | 0 | 201 | 15 | 2 | 2 |
| **Cucumber** | 1 cucumber | 45 | 3 | 0 | 0 | 0 | 6 | 11 | 2 | 2 |
| Cucumber, Peeled, Sliced | 1 cup | 14 | 2 | 0 | 0 | 0 | 2 | 3 | 1 | 1 |
| **Dandelion Greens**, Chopped | 1 cup | 25 | 3 | 0 | 0 | 0 | 42 | 5 | 2 | 1 |
| Dandelion Greens, Cooked, with Salt, Chopped | 1 cup | 35 | 6 | 1 | 0 | 0 | 294 | 7 | 3 | 2 |
| **Eggplant**, Cooked, with Salt | 1 cup | 33 | 2 | 0 | 0 | 0 | 237 | 8 | 3 | 1 |
| Eggplant, Cubed | 1 cup | 20 | 1 | 0 | 0 | 0 | 2 | 5 | 3 | 1 |
| Eggplant, Pickled | 1 cup | 67 | 9 | 1 | 0 | 0 | 2277 | 13 | 3 | 1 |
| **Endive**, Chopped | 1/2 cup | 4 | 0 | 0 | 0 | 0 | 6 | 1 | 1 | 0 |
| **Fennel, Bulb**, Sliced | 1 cup | 27 | 2 | 0 | 0 | 0 | 45 | 6 | 3 | 1 |
| **Garlic** | 1 tsp | 4 | 0 | 0 | 0 | 0 | 0 | 0 | 0 | 0 |
| **Grape Leaves** | 1 leaf | 3 | 1 | 0 | 0 | 0 | 0 | 1 | 0 | 0 |
| Grape Leaves, Canned | 1 leaf | 3 | 1 | 0 | 0 | 0 | 114 | 0 | 0 | 0 |
| **Hearts Of Palm**, Canned | 1 cup | 41 | 8 | 1 | 0 | 0 | 622 | 7 | 4 | 4 |
| **Jerusalem Artichokes**, Sliced | 1 cup | 110 | 0 | 0 | 0 | 0 | 6 | 26 | 2 | 3 |
| **Kale**, Chopped | 1 cup | 34 | 4 | 0 | 0 | 0 | 29 | 7 | 1 | 2 |
| Kale, Cooked, with Salt, Chopped | 1 cup | 36 | 5 | 1 | 0 | 0 | 337 | 7 | 3 | 2 |
| Kale, Frozen | 10 oz | 80 | 12 | 1 | 0 | 0 | 43 | 14 | 6 | 8 |
| Kale, Frozen, Cooked, with Salt, Chopped | 1 cup | 39 | 6 | 1 | 0 | 0 | 326 | 7 | 3 | 4 |
| **Kohlrabi** | 1 cup | 36 | 1 | 0 | 0 | 0 | 27 | 8 | 5 | 2 |
| Kohlrabi, Cooked, with Salt, Sliced | 1 cup | 48 | 2 | 0 | 0 | 0 | 424 | 11 | 2 | 3 |
| **Leeks** | 1 cup | 54 | 2 | 0 | 0 | 0 | 18 | 13 | 2 | 1 |
| Leeks, Cooked, with Salt, Chopped | 1/4 cup | 8 | 0 | 0 | 0 | 0 | 64 | 2 | 0 | 0 |
| **LETTUCE** | | | | | | | | | | |
| Butterhead/ Boston/Bibb, Shredded or Chopped | 1 cup | 7 | 1 | 0 | 0 | 0 | 3 | 1 | 1 | 1 |
| Green Leaf, Shredded | 1 cup | 5 | 0 | 0 | 0 | 0 | 10 | 1 | 0 | 0 |
| Iceberg/Crisphead, Shredded | 1 cup | 10 | 1 | 0 | 0 | 0 | 7 | 2 | 1 | 1 |
| Red Leaf, Shredded | 1 cup | 4 | 1 | 0 | 0 | 0 | 7 | 1 | 0 | 0 |
| Romaine, Shredded | 1 cup | 8 | 1 | 0 | 0 | 0 | 4 | 2 | 1 | 1 |
| **MUSHROOMS** | | | | | | | | | | |
| Brown/Italian/Crimini | 1 cup | 19 | 1 | 0 | 0 | 0 | 5 | 4 | 1 | 2 |
| Canned | 1 cup | 39 | 4 | 0 | 0 | 0 | 663 | 8 | 4 | 3 |
| Chanterelle | 1 cup | 21 | 3 | 0 | 0 | 0 | 5 | 4 | 2 | 1 |

| | SERVING SIZE | CAL | CAL FAT | TOT FAT (G) | SAT FAT (G) | CHOL (MG) | SOD (MG) | CARB (G) | FIBER (G) | PROT (G) |
|---|---|---|---|---|---|---|---|---|---|---|
| Enoki | 1 medium | 1 | 0 | 0 | 0 | 0 | 0 | 0 | 0 | 0 |
| Maitake, Diced | 1 cup | 22 | 1 | 0 | 0 | 0 | 1 | 5 | 2 | 1 |
| Morel | 1 cup | 20 | 3 | 0 | 0 | 0 | 14 | 3 | 2 | 2 |
| Oyster | 1 small | 5 | 1 | 0 | 0 | 0 | 3 | 1 | 0 | 0 |
| Portabella | 1 piece | 18 | 3 | 0 | 0 | 0 | 8 | 3 | 1 | 2 |
| Portabella, Grilled, Sliced | 1 cup | 35 | 6 | 1 | 0 | 0 | 13 | 5 | 3 | 4 |
| Shiitake | 1 piece | 6 | 1 | 0 | 0 | 0 | 2 | 1 | 0 | 0 |
| Shiitake, Cooked, with Salt, Pieces | 1 cup | 81 | 3 | 0 | 0 | 0 | 348 | 21 | 3 | 2 |
| Shiitake, Dried | 1 medium | 11 | 0 | 0 | 0 | 0 | 0 | 3 | 0 | 0 |
| Shiitake, Stir-Fried, Sliced | 1 cup | 38 | 3 | 0 | 0 | 0 | 5 | 7 | 4 | 3 |
| Straw, Canned | 1 cup | 58 | 11 | 1 | 0 | 0 | 699 | 8 | 5 | 7 |
| White | 1 cup | 21 | 3 | 0 | 0 | 0 | 5 | 3 | 1 | 3 |
| White, Cooked, with Salt, Pieces | 1 cup | 44 | 7 | 1 | 0 | 0 | 371 | 8 | 3 | 3 |
| White, Stir-Fried, Sliced | 1 cup | 28 | 3 | 0 | 0 | 0 | 13 | 4 | 2 | 4 |
| **Mustard Greens**, Chopped | 1 cup | 15 | 1 | 0 | 0 | 0 | 14 | 3 | 2 | 2 |
| Mustard Greens, Cooked, with Salt, Chopped | 1 cup | 21 | 3 | 0 | 0 | 0 | 353 | 3 | 3 | 3 |
| Mustard Greens, Frozen, Chopped | 1 cup | 29 | 4 | 0 | 0 | 0 | 42 | 5 | 5 | 4 |
| Mustard Greens, Frozen, Cooked, with Salt, Chopped or Diced | 1/2 cup | 14 | 2 | 0 | 0 | 0 | 196 | 2 | 2 | 2 |
| **Mustard Spinach**, (Tendergreen), Chopped | 1 cup | 33 | 4 | 0 | 0 | 0 | 32 | 6 | 4 | 3 |
| Mustard Spinach, (Tendergreen), Cooked, with Salt, Chopped | 1 cup | 29 | 3 | 0 | 0 | 0 | 450 | 5 | 4 | 3 |
| **Okra** | 1 cup | 31 | 1 | 0 | 0 | 0 | 8 | 7 | 3 | 2 |
| Okra, Cooked, with Salt, Sliced | 1/2 cup | 18 | 2 | 0 | 0 | 0 | 193 | 4 | 2 | 1 |
| Okra, Frozen | 10 oz | 85 | 6 | 1 | 0 | 0 | 9 | 19 | 6 | 5 |
| Okra, Frozen, Cooked, with Salt, Sliced | 1/2 cup | 31 | 2 | 0 | 0 | 0 | 220 | 6 | 2 | 2 |
| **Onions**, Canned, Chopped or Diced | 1/2 cup | 21 | 1 | 0 | 0 | 0 | 416 | 5 | 1 | 1 |
| Onions, Chopped | 1 cup | 64 | 1 | 0 | 0 | 0 | 6 | 15 | 3 | 2 |
| Onions, Cooked, with Salt | 1 cup | 88 | 4 | 0 | 0 | 0 | 502 | 20 | 3 | 3 |
| Onions, Frozen, Chopped | 10 oz | 82 | 3 | 0 | 0 | 0 | 34 | 19 | 5 | 2 |
| Onions, Frozen, Cooked, with Salt | 1 cup | 55 | 1 | 0 | 0 | 0 | 521 | 13 | 4 | 2 |
| Onions, Frozen, Cooked, with Salt, Chopped or Diced | 1/2 cup | 27 | 0 | 0 | 0 | 0 | 256 | 6 | 2 | 1 |
| Onions, Frozen, Whole | 10 oz | 99 | 2 | 0 | 0 | 0 | 28 | 24 | 5 | 3 |
| Onions, Spring or Scallions, Chopped | 1 cup | 32 | 2 | 0 | 0 | 0 | 16 | 7 | 3 | 2 |
| Onions, Sweet | 1 onion | 106 | 2 | 0 | 0 | 0 | 26 | 25 | 3 | 3 |

# common foods

| | SERVING SIZE | CAL | CAL FAT | TOT FAT (G) | SAT FAT (G) | CHOL (MG) | SOD (MG) | CARB (G) | FIBER (G) | PROT (G) |
|---|---|---|---|---|---|---|---|---|---|---|
| Onions, Yellow, Sautéed, Chopped | 1 cup | 115 | 84 | 9 | 0 | 0 | 10 | 7 | 2 | 1 |
| **Parsnips**, Cooked, with Salt, Sliced | 1/2 cup | 55 | 2 | 0 | 0 | 0 | 192 | 13 | 3 | 1 |
| **Peapods** | 1 cup | 26 | 1 | 0 | 0 | 0 | 3 | 5 | 2 | 2 |
| Peapods, Cooked, with Salt | 1 cup | 64 | 3 | 0 | 0 | 0 | 384 | 10 | 4 | 5 |
| Peapods, Frozen | 1/2 cup | 30 | 2 | 0 | 0 | 0 | 3 | 5 | 2 | 2 |
| Peapods, Frozen, Cooked, with Salt | 1 cup | 80 | 5 | 1 | 0 | 0 | 386 | 13 | 5 | 6 |
| **Peas**, Green | 1 cup | 117 | 5 | 1 | 0 | 0 | 7 | 21 | 7 | 8 |
| Peas, Green, Canned | 1/2 cup | 66 | 3 | 0 | 0 | 0 | 310 | 12 | 4 | 4 |
| Peas, Green, Cooked, with Salt | 1 cup | 134 | 3 | 0 | 0 | 0 | 382 | 25 | 9 | 9 |
| Peas, Green, Frozen | 1 cup | 103 | 5 | 1 | 0 | 0 | 145 | 18 | 6 | 7 |
| Peas, Green, Frozen, Cooked, with Salt | 1/2 cup | 62 | 2 | 0 | 0 | 0 | 258 | 11 | 4 | 4 |
| **PEPPERS** | | | | | | | | | | |
| Banana, Small | 1 sm pepper | 9 | 1 | 0 | 0 | 0 | 4 | 2 | 1 | 1 |
| Hot Chili, Green | 1 pepper | 18 | 1 | 0 | 0 | 0 | 3 | 4 | 1 | 1 |
| Hot Chili, Red | 1 pepper | 18 | 2 | 0 | 0 | 0 | 4 | 4 | 1 | 1 |
| Hot Chili, Red, Canned, Chopped or Diced | 1/2 cup | 14 | 1 | 0 | 0 | 0 | 798 | 3 | 1 | 1 |
| Hungarian | 1 pepper | 8 | 1 | 0 | 0 | 0 | 0 | 2 | 0 | 0 |
| Jalapeño | 1 pepper | 4 | 0 | 0 | 0 | 0 | 0 | 1 | 0 | 0 |
| Jalapeño, Canned, Chopped | 1 cup | 37 | 12 | 1 | 0 | 0 | 2273 | 6 | 4 | 1 |
| Pasilla, Dried | 1 pepper | 24 | 10 | 1 | 0 | 0 | 6 | 4 | 2 | 1 |
| Sweet, Green, Canned, Halved | 1 cup | 25 | 4 | 0 | 0 | 0 | 1917 | 5 | 2 | 1 |
| Sweet, Green, Chopped | 1 cup | 30 | 2 | 0 | 0 | 0 | 4 | 7 | 3 | 1 |
| Sweet, Green, Cooked, with Salt | 1 pepper | 19 | 1 | 0 | 0 | 0 | 174 | 4 | 1 | 1 |
| Sweet, Green, Frozen, Cooked, with Salt, Chopped or Strips | 1 cup | 22 | 2 | 0 | 0 | 0 | 324 | 4 | 0 | 1 |
| Sweet, Green, Frozen, Chopped | 10 oz | 57 | 5 | 1 | 0 | 0 | 14 | 13 | 5 | 3 |
| Sweet, Red, Chopped | 1 cup | 46 | 4 | 0 | 0 | 0 | 6 | 9 | 3 | 1 |
| Sweet, Red, Cooked, with Salt | 1 pepper | 19 | 1 | 0 | 0 | 0 | 174 | 4 | 1 | 1 |
| Sweet, Red, Frozen, Chopped | 10 oz | 57 | 5 | 1 | 0 | 0 | 14 | 13 | 5 | 3 |
| Sweet, Red, Frozen, Cooked, with Salt, Chopped or Strips | 1 cup | 22 | 2 | 0 | 0 | 0 | 324 | 4 | 0 | 1 |
| Sweet, Yellow, Large | 1 pepper | 50 | 4 | 0 | 0 | 0 | 4 | 12 | 2 | 2 |
| **PICKLES** | | | | | | | | | | |
| Cucumber, Dill or Kosher Dill, Sliced | 1 cup | 19 | 2 | 0 | 0 | 0 | 1356 | 4 | 2 | 1 |
| Cucumber, Sour, Sliced | 1 cup | 17 | 3 | 0 | 0 | 0 | 1872 | 6 | 2 | 1 |
| Cucumber, Sweet (Includes Bread & Butter Pickles) | 1 cup | 146 | 6 | 1 | 0 | 0 | 699 | 32 | 2 | 1 |

| | SERVING SIZE | CAL | CAL FAT | TOT FAT (G) | SAT FAT (G) | CHOL (MG) | SOD (MG) | CARB (G) | FIBER (G) | PROT (G) |
|---|---|---|---|---|---|---|---|---|---|---|
| **POTATOES** | | | | | | | | | | |
| Au Gratin, Home-Prepared from Recipe Using Butter | 1 cup | 323 | 167 | 19 | 12 | 56 | 1061 | 28 | 4 | 12 |
| Au Gratin, Home-Prepared from Recipe Using Margarine | 1 cup | 323 | 167 | 19 | 9 | 37 | 1061 | 28 | 4 | 12 |
| Baked, Flesh & Skin, with Salt, Medium | 1 potato | 161 | 2 | 0 | 0 | 0 | 421 | 37 | 4 | 4 |
| Baked, Flesh, with Salt, Medium | 1 potato | 145 | 1 | 0 | 0 | 0 | 376 | 34 | 2 | 3 |
| Baked Skin, with Salt | 1 skin | 115 | 1 | 0 | 0 | 0 | 149 | 27 | 5 | 2 |
| Boiled, Cooked with Skin, Flesh Only, with Salt | 1 potato | 118 | 1 | 0 | 0 | 0 | 326 | 27 | 3 | 3 |
| Boiled, Cooked without Skin, Flesh Only, with Salt, Medium | 1 potato | 144 | 2 | 0 | 0 | 0 | 402 | 33 | 3 | 3 |
| Canned | 1 cup | 108 | 3 | 0 | 0 | 0 | 394 | 25 | 4 | 3 |
| Hashed Brown, Home-Prepared | 1 cup | 413 | 176 | 20 | 3 | 0 | 534 | 55 | 5 | 5 |
| Mashed, Home-Prepared, Whole Milk & Butter Added | 1 cup | 237 | 80 | 9 | 5 | 23 | 666 | 35 | 3 | 4 |
| Mashed, Home-Prepared, Whole Milk & Margarine Added | 1 cup | 233 | 79 | 9 | 2 | 2 | 699 | 36 | 3 | 4 |
| Mashed, Home-Prepared, Whole Milk Added | 1 cup | 174 | 11 | 1 | 1 | 4 | 634 | 37 | 3 | 4 |
| Mashed, Prepared from Flakes, Whole Milk & Margarine | 1 cup | 237 | 106 | 12 | 3 | 8 | 697 | 32 | 5 | 4 |
| Mashed, Prepared from Granules, Whole Milk & Margarine | 1 cup | 227 | 93 | 10 | 3 | 6 | 552 | 30 | 5 | 4 |
| Red, Flesh & Skin, Baked, Medium | 1 potato | 154 | 2 | 0 | 0 | 0 | 21 | 34 | 3 | 4 |
| Russet, Flesh & Skin, Baked, Medium | 1 potato | 168 | 2 | 0 | 0 | 0 | 24 | 37 | 4 | 5 |
| Scalloped, Home-Prepared | 1 cup | 216 | 81 | 9 | 3 | 15 | 821 | 26 | 5 | 7 |
| Scalloped, Home-Prepared with Butter | 1 cup | 216 | 81 | 9 | 6 | 29 | 821 | 26 | 5 | 7 |
| White, Flesh & Skin, Baked, Medium | 1 potato | 130 | 2 | 0 | 0 | 0 | 10 | 29 | 3 | 3 |
| **Pumpkin**, Canned, with Salt | 1 cup | 83 | 6 | 1 | 0 | 0 | 590 | 20 | 7 | 3 |
| Pumpkin, Cooked, with Salt, Mashed | 1 cup | 49 | 2 | 0 | 0 | 0 | 581 | 12 | 3 | 2 |
| Pumpkin, Flowers, Cooked, with Salt | 1 cup | 20 | 1 | 0 | 0 | 0 | 324 | 4 | 1 | 1 |
| **Radicchio**, Shredded | 1 cup | 9 | 1 | 0 | 0 | 0 | 9 | 2 | 0 | 1 |
| **Radishes**, Large | 1 radish | 1 | 0 | 0 | 0 | 0 | 4 | 0 | 0 | 0 |
| Radish Seeds, Sprouted | 1 cup | 16 | 9 | 1 | 0 | 0 | 2 | 1 | 0 | 1 |
| Radishes, Hawaiian Style, Pickled | 1 cup | 42 | 4 | 0 | 0 | 0 | 1184 | 8 | 3 | 2 |
| Radishes, Oriental, Cooked, with Salt, Sliced | 1 cup | 25 | 3 | 0 | 0 | 0 | 366 | 5 | 2 | 1 |

| | SERVING SIZE | CAL | CAL FAT | TOT FAT (G) | SAT FAT (G) | CHOL (MG) | SOD (MG) | CARB (G) | FIBER (G) | PROT (G) |
|---|---|---|---|---|---|---|---|---|---|---|
| Radishes, Oriental | 1 radish | 61 | 3 | 0 | 0 | 0 | 71 | 14 | 5 | 2 |
| Radishes, Oriental, Dried | 1 cup | 314 | 8 | 1 | 0 | 0 | 322 | 74 | 0 | 9 |
| Radishes, White Icicle | 1 radish | 2 | 0 | 0 | 0 | 0 | 3 | 0 | 0 | 0 |
| **Rhubarb**, Diced | 1 cup | 26 | 2 | 0 | 0 | 0 | 5 | 6 | 2 | 1 |
| Rhubarb, Frozen, Diced | 1 cup | 29 | 1 | 0 | 0 | 0 | 3 | 7 | 2 | 1 |
| **Rutabagas**, Cooked, with Salt, Mashed | 1/2 cup | 47 | 2 | 0 | 0 | 0 | 305 | 10 | 0 | 2 |
| **SEAWEED** | | | | | | | | | | |
| Seaweed, Agar | 2 tbsp | 3 | 0 | 0 | 0 | 0 | 1 | 1 | 0 | 0 |
| Seaweed, Irish Moss | 2 tbsp | 5 | 0 | 0 | 0 | 0 | 7 | 1 | 0 | 0 |
| Seaweed, Kelp | 2 tbsp | 4 | 1 | 0 | 0 | 0 | 23 | 1 | 0 | 0 |
| Seaweed, Laver | 10 sheets | 9 | 1 | 0 | 0 | 0 | 12 | 1 | 0 | 2 |
| Seaweed, Spirulina, Dried | 1 tbsp | 20 | 5 | 1 | 0 | 0 | 73 | 2 | 0 | 4 |
| Seaweed, Wakame | 2 tbsp | 5 | 1 | 0 | 0 | 0 | 87 | 1 | 0 | 0 |
| **Shallots**, Chopped | 1 tbsp | 7 | 0 | 0 | 0 | 0 | 1 | 2 | 0 | 0 |
| **Spinach** | 1 cup | 7 | 1 | 0 | 0 | 0 | 24 | 1 | 1 | 1 |
| Spinach, Canned | 1 cup | 49 | 10 | 1 | 0 | 0 | 689 | 7 | 5 | 6 |
| Spinach, Cooked, with Salt | 1 cup | 41 | 4 | 0 | 0 | 0 | 551 | 7 | 4 | 5 |
| Spinach, Frozen, Chopped | 1 cup | 45 | 8 | 1 | 0 | 0 | 115 | 7 | 5 | 6 |
| Spinach, Frozen, Chopped, Cooked, with Salt | 1/2 cup | 32 | 7 | 1 | 0 | 0 | 306 | 5 | 4 | 4 |
| **SPROUTS** | | | | | | | | | | |
| Mung Beans, Mature Seeds, Canned, Drained Solids | 1 cup | 15 | 1 | 0 | 0 | 0 | 175 | 3 | 1 | 2 |
| Mung Beans, Mature Seeds, Cooked, Boiled, Drained, with Salt | 1 cup | 24 | 1 | 0 | 0 | 0 | 305 | 4 | 1 | 3 |
| Mung Beans, Mature Seeds, Cooked, Stir-Fried | 1 cup | 62 | 2 | 0 | 0 | 0 | 11 | 13 | 2 | 5 |
| Mung Beans, Mature Seeds, Raw | 1 cup | 31 | 2 | 0 | 0 | 0 | 6 | 6 | 2 | 3 |
| Navy, Mature Seeds, Raw | 1 cup | 70 | 7 | 1 | 0 | 0 | 14 | 14 | 0 | 6 |
| Peas, Mature Seeds, Sprouted, Raw | 1 cup | 149 | 7 | 1 | 0 | 0 | 24 | 33 | 0 | 11 |
| Soybeans, Mature Seeds, Cooked, Steamed | 1 cup | 76 | 38 | 4 | 1 | 0 | 9 | 6 | 1 | 8 |
| Soybeans, Mature Seeds, Cooked, Steamed, with Salt | 1 cup | 76 | 38 | 4 | 1 | 0 | 231 | 6 | 1 | 8 |
| Soybeans, Mature Seeds, Raw | 1/2 cup | 43 | 21 | 2 | 0 | 0 | 5 | 3 | 0 | 5 |
| **Sweet Potato** | 1, 5" long | 112 | 1 | 0 | 0 | 0 | 72 | 26 | 4 | 2 |
| Sweet Potato, Canned, Mashed | 1 cup | 258 | 5 | 1 | 0 | 0 | 191 | 59 | 4 | 5 |
| Sweet Potato, Canned, Syrup | 1 cup | 212 | 6 | 1 | 0 | 0 | 76 | 50 | 6 | 3 |

| | SERVING SIZE | CAL | CAL FAT | TOT FAT (G) | SAT FAT (G) | CHOL (MG) | SOD (MG) | CARB (G) | FIBER (G) | PROT (G) |
|---|---|---|---|---|---|---|---|---|---|---|
| Sweet Potato, Cooked, Baked in Skin, with Salt | 1 medium | 105 | 2 | 0 | 0 | 0 | 280 | 24 | 4 | 2 |
| Sweet Potato, Cooked, Boiled, without Skin | 1 medium | 115 | 2 | 0 | 0 | 0 | 41 | 27 | 4 | 2 |
| Sweet Potato, Frozen, Cooked, with Salt, Cubed | 1 cup | 176 | 2 | 0 | 0 | 0 | 429 | 41 | 3 | 3 |
| Sweet Potato, Frozen, Cubed | 1 cup | 169 | 3 | 0 | 0 | 0 | 11 | 39 | 3 | 3 |
| **TOMATOES** | | | | | | | | | | |
| Tomato Products, Canned, Paste, with Salt | 1/2 cup | 107 | 6 | 1 | 0 | 0 | 1035 | 25 | 5 | 6 |
| Tomato Products, Canned, Puree, with Salt | 1 cup | 95 | 5 | 1 | 0 | 0 | 998 | 22 | 5 | 4 |
| Tomato Products, Canned, Sauce | 1 cup | 59 | 4 | 0 | 0 | 0 | 1284 | 13 | 4 | 3 |
| Tomatoes, Cherry | 1 cup | 27 | 3 | 0 | 0 | 0 | 7 | 6 | 2 | 1 |
| Tomatoes, Green | 1 tomato | 42 | 3 | 0 | 0 | 0 | 24 | 9 | 2 | 2 |
| Tomatoes, Orange | 1 tomato | 18 | 2 | 0 | 0 | 0 | 47 | 4 | 1 | 1 |
| Tomatoes, Red, Canned, Stewed | 1 cup | 66 | 4 | 0 | 0 | 0 | 564 | 16 | 3 | 2 |
| Tomatoes, Red, Cooked | 1 cup | 43 | 2 | 0 | 0 | 0 | 26 | 10 | 2 | 2 |
| Tomatoes, Sun-Dried | 1 cup | 139 | 14 | 2 | 0 | 0 | 1131 | 30 | 7 | 8 |
| Tomatoes, Sun-Dried, Packed in Oil, Drained | 1 cup | 234 | 139 | 15 | 2 | 0 | 293 | 26 | 6 | 6 |
| Tomatoes, Yellow | 1 tomato | 32 | 5 | 1 | 0 | 0 | 49 | 6 | 2 | 2 |
| **Turnip Greens**, Canned | 1/2 cup | 16 | 3 | 0 | 0 | 0 | 324 | 3 | 2 | 2 |
| Turnip Greens, Chopped | 1 cup | 18 | 2 | 0 | 0 | 0 | 22 | 4 | 2 | 1 |
| Turnip Greens, Cooked, with Salt, Chopped | 1 cup | 29 | 3 | 0 | 0 | 0 | 382 | 6 | 5 | 2 |
| Turnip Greens, Frozen, Chopped or Diced | 1/2 cup | 18 | 2 | 0 | 0 | 0 | 10 | 3 | 2 | 2 |
| Turnip Greens, Frozen, Cooked, with Salt | 1/2 cup | 29 | 3 | 0 | 0 | 0 | 219 | 4 | 3 | 3 |
| **Turnips**, Cubed | 1 cup | 36 | 1 | 0 | 0 | 0 | 87 | 8 | 2 | 1 |
| Turnips & Greens, Frozen | 10 oz | 60 | 5 | 1 | 0 | 0 | 51 | 10 | 7 | 7 |
| Turnips & Greens, Frozen, Cooked, with Salt | 1 cup | 55 | 6 | 1 | 0 | 0 | 416 | 8 | 5 | 5 |
| Turnips, Cooked, with Salt, Cubed | 1 cup | 34 | 1 | 0 | 0 | 0 | 446 | 8 | 3 | 1 |
| Turnips, Frozen, Mashed | 10 oz | 45 | 4 | 0 | 0 | 0 | 71 | 8 | 5 | 3 |
| Turnips, Frozen, Cooked, with Salt | 1 cup | 33 | 3 | 0 | 0 | 0 | 424 | 6 | 3 | 2 |
| **Vegetables, Mixed**, Canned | 1 cup | 80 | 4 | 0 | 0 | 0 | 243 | 15 | 5 | 4 |
| Vegetables, Mixed, Frozen | 10 oz | 182 | 13 | 1 | 0 | 0 | 133 | 38 | 11 | 9 |
| Vegetables, Mixed, Frozen, Cooked, with Salt | 1/2 cup | 55 | 1 | 0 | 0 | 0 | 247 | 12 | 4 | 3 |
| **Water Chestnuts**, Chinese, (Matai), Sliced | 1/2 cup | 60 | 1 | 0 | 0 | 0 | 9 | 15 | 2 | 1 |
| Water Chestnuts, Chinese, Canned, Sliced | 1/2 cup | 35 | 0 | 0 | 0 | 0 | 6 | 9 | 2 | 1 |
| **Watercress**, Chopped | 1 cup | 4 | 0 | 0 | 0 | 0 | 14 | 0 | 0 | 1 |

# common foods

| | SERVING SIZE | CAL | CAL FAT (G) | TOT FAT (G) | SAT FAT (G) | CHOL (MG) | SOD (MG) | CARB (G) | FIBER (G) | PROT (G) |
|---|---|---|---|---|---|---|---|---|---|---|
| **WINTER SQUASH** | | | | | | | | | | |
| Acorn, Cooked, with Salt, Cubed | 1 cup | 115 | 3 | 0 | 0 | 0 | 492 | 30 | 9 | 2 |
| Acorn, Cooked, with Salt, Mashed | 1 cup | 83 | 2 | 0 | 0 | 0 | 586 | 22 | 6 | 2 |
| Butternut, Cooked, with Salt, Cubed | 1 cup | 82 | 2 | 0 | 0 | 0 | 492 | 22 | 7 | 2 |
| Butternut, Frozen, Cooked, with Salt, Mashed | 1 cup | 94 | 2 | 0 | 0 | 0 | 571 | 24 | 0 | 3 |
| Hubbard, Cooked, with Salt, Cubed | 1 cup | 102 | 11 | 1 | 0 | 0 | 500 | 22 | 0 | 5 |
| Hubbard, Cooked, with Salt, Mashed | 1 cup | 71 | 8 | 1 | 0 | 0 | 569 | 15 | 7 | 3 |
| Spaghetti, Cooked, with Salt | 1 cup | 42 | 4 | 0 | 0 | 0 | 394 | 10 | 2 | 1 |
| **Yam**, Cooked or Baked, with Salt, Cubed | 1 cup | 155 | 2 | 0 | 0 | 0 | 332 | 37 | 5 | 2 |
| **Zucchini**, Baby | 1 medium | 2 | 0 | 0 | 0 | 0 | 0 | 0 | 0 | 0 |
| Zucchini, Includes Skin, Chopped | 1 cup | 21 | 4 | 0 | 0 | 0 | 10 | 4 | 1 | 2 |
| Zucchini, Includes Skin, Cooked, with Salt, Sliced | 1/2 cup | 14 | 3 | 0 | 0 | 0 | 215 | 3 | 1 | 1 |
| Zucchini, Includes Skin, Frozen | 10 oz | 48 | 3 | 0 | 0 | 0 | 6 | 10 | 4 | 3 |

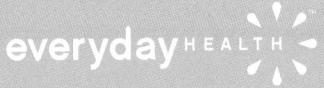

# store brands

# store brands

| | SERVING SIZE | CAL | CAL FAT | TOT FAT (G) | SAT FAT (G) | CHOL (MG) | SOD (MG) | CARB (G) | FIBER (G) | PROT (G) |
|---|---|---|---|---|---|---|---|---|---|---|
| **A.1. Steak Sauce** | | | | | | | | | | |
| Original | 1 tbsp | 15 | 0 | 0 | 0 | 0 | 280 | 3 | 0 | 0 |
| Steak House Cracked Peppercorn | 1 tbsp | 15 | 0 | 0 | 0 | 0 | 230 | 0 | 0 | 0 |
| Thick & Hearty | 1 tbsp | 25 | 0 | 0 | 0 | 0 | 290 | 6 | 0 | 0 |
| **A&W Soft Drinks** | | | | | | | | | | |
| Cream Soda | 8 fl oz | 120 | 0 | 0 | 0 | n/a | 30 | 31 | 0 | 0 |
| Root Beer | 8 fl oz | 120 | 0 | 0 | 0 | n/a | 30 | 31 | 0 | 0 |
| **Act II Popcorn** | | | | | | | | | | |
| 94% Fat Free Butter | 7 cups | 130 | 20 | 2.5 | 1 | 0 | 220 | 28 | 5 | 4 |
| Butter | 4-1/2 cups | 160 | 80 | 9 | 4 | 0 | 310 | 18 | 3 | 3 |
| HomePop Classic | 4 cups | 150 | 90 | 10 | 5 | 0 | 210 | 16 | 3 | 2 |
| Kettle Corn | 4-1/2 cups | 160 | 90 | 10 | 4.5 | 0 | 150 | 18 | 3 | 3 |
| **Activia (Dannon)** | | | | | | | | | | |
| **FIBER YOGURT** | | | | | | | | | | |
| Peach | 4 oz | 110 | 15 | 2 | 1 | 5 | 60 | 20 | 3 | 3 |
| Strawberry | 4 oz | 110 | 15 | 2 | 1 | 5 | 60 | 20 | 3 | 3 |
| Vanilla | 4 oz | 110 | 15 | 2 | 1 | 5 | 60 | 19 | 3 | 3 |
| **LIGHT YOGURT** | | | | | | | | | | |
| Blueberry | 4 oz | 70 | 0 | 0 | 0 | <5 | 65 | 13 | 2 | 4 |
| Peach | 4 oz | 70 | 0 | 0 | 0 | <5 | 65 | 12 | 2 | 4 |
| Raspberry | 4 oz | 70 | 0 | 0 | 0 | <5 | 75 | 13 | 2 | 4 |
| Strawberry | 4 oz | 70 | 0 | 0 | 0 | <5 | 70 | 13 | 2 | 4 |
| Vanilla | 4 oz | 70 | 0 | 0 | 0 | <5 | 70 | 14 | 3 | 5 |
| **YOGURT** | | | | | | | | | | |
| Blueberry | 4 oz | 110 | 15 | 2 | 1 | 5 | 65 | 20 | 0 | 4 |
| Cherry | 4 oz | 110 | 15 | 2 | 1 | 10 | 70 | 19 | 0 | 5 |
| Mixed Berry | 4 oz | 110 | 20 | 2 | 1 | 10 | 65 | 19 | 0 | 5 |
| Peach | 4 oz | 120 | 20 | 2 | 1 | 10 | 65 | 19 | 0 | 5 |
| Plain | 8 oz | 170 | 40 | 4.5 | 3 | 15 | 170 | 20 | 0 | 11 |
| Strawberry | 4 oz | 110 | 15 | 2 | 1 | 5 | 75 | 19 | 0 | 4 |
| **Alexia** | | | | | | | | | | |
| **APPETIZERS** | | | | | | | | | | |
| Chicken Nuggets with Broccoli & Cheddar Cheese | 6 nuggets | 200 | 110 | 12 | 3.5 | 30 | 420 | 13 | <1 | 11 |
| Mozzarella Stix, Italian Herbs & Olive Oil | 2 stix | 120 | 60 | 6 | 2.5 | 10 | 230 | 10 | 1 | 5 |
| Mushroom Bites Roasted Garlic & Olive Oil | 2 oz | 110 | 40 | 4.5 | .5 | 0 | 290 | 14 | 2 | 3 |
| Onion Rings with Sea Salt | 6 rings | 240 | 120 | 13 | 2 | 0 | 150 | 27 | 2 | 4 |

| | SERVING SIZE | CAL | CAL FAT | TOT FAT (G) | SAT FAT (G) | CHOL (MG) | SOD (MG) | CARB (G) | FIBER (G) | PROT (G) |
|---|---|---|---|---|---|---|---|---|---|---|
| **ARTISAN BREADS** | | | | | | | | | | |
| Biscuits | 1-3/4 oz | 170 | 80 | 9 | 5 | 0 | 450 | 20 | 1 | 3 |
| Ciabatta Rolls with Rosemary & Olive Oil | 1 roll | 100 | 15 | 1.5 | 0 | 0 | 220 | 19 | 1 | 3 |
| Focaccia Rolls, Asiago & Parmesan Cheeses | 1 roll | 120 | 20 | 2 | .5 | 0 | 230 | 21 | 1 | 4 |
| French Rolls | 1 roll | 100 | 0 | 0 | 0 | 0 | 230 | 21 | 1 | 4 |
| Garlic Baguette | 2 pieces | 130 | 45 | 5 | 3.5 | 15 | 260 | 18 | 1 | 3 |
| Whole Grain Rolls with Whole Wheat & Flaxseed | 1 roll | 90 | 10 | 1 | 0 | 0 | 200 | 18 | 1 | 4 |
| **CRUNCHY SNACKS** | | | | | | | | | | |
| Aged Cheddar Cheese Waffle Fries | 1 oz | 140 | 60 | 7 | .5 | 0 | 200 | 18 | 1 | 1 |
| Bold & Spicy BBQ Waffle Fries | 1 oz | 140 | 60 | 7 | .5 | 0 | 200 | 18 | 1 | 1 |
| Classic Ranch Waffle Fries | 1 oz | 140 | 60 | 7 | .5 | 0 | 200 | 18 | 1 | 1 |
| Hot Pepper Waffle Fries | 1 oz | 140 | 60 | 7 | .5 | 0 | 200 | 18 | 1 | 1 |
| Jalapeno Onion Strips | 1 oz | 150 | 70 | 8 | .5 | 0 | 200 | 18 | 1 | 2 |
| Savory Seasoned Onion Strips | 1 oz | 150 | 70 | 8 | .5 | 0 | 200 | 18 | 1 | 2 |
| **JULIENNE FRIES** | | | | | | | | | | |
| Spicy Sweet Potato | 3 oz | 130 | 35 | 4 | 0 | 0 | 250 | 23 | 3 | 1 |
| Sweet Potato | 3 oz | 140 | 45 | 5 | 0 | 0 | 140 | 24 | 3 | 1 |
| Yukon Gold with Sea Salt | 3 oz | 130 | 30 | 3.5 | 0 | 0 | 180 | 22 | 2 | 2 |
| **OVEN FRIES & OVEN REDS** | | | | | | | | | | |
| Oven Fries with Olive Oil & Sea Salt | 3 oz | 90 | 20 | 2 | 0 | 0 | 230 | 16 | 2 | 2 |
| Oven Fries with Olive Oil, Rosemary & Garlic | 3 oz | 130 | 30 | 3.5 | 0 | 0 | 240 | 22 | 2 | 2 |
| Oven Reds with Olive Oil, Parmesan & Roasted Garlic | 3 oz | 120 | 30 | 3.5 | .5 | 0 | 270 | 19 | 2 | 3 |
| Potato Nuggets with Seasoned Salt | 3 oz | 150 | 60 | 7 | .5 | 0 | 440 | 19 | 3 | 2 |
| Waffle Fries with Seasoned Salt | 1 cup | 160 | 60 | 7 | .5 | 0 | 330 | 21 | 2 | 2 |
| **Almond Joy** | | | | | | | | | | |
| Bar | 1 item | 220 | 110 | 13 | 8 | 0 | 50 | 26 | 2 | 2 |
| **Amy's Kitchen** | | | | | | | | | | |
| **BEANS & CHILI** | | | | | | | | | | |
| Organic Medium Chili with Vegetables | 1 cup | 190 | 50 | 6 | .5 | 0 | 590 | 29 | 8 | 7 |
| Organic Traditional Refried Beans, Light in Sodium | 1/2 cup | 140 | 30 | 3 | 0 | 0 | 190 | 22 | 6 | 7 |
| Southwestern Black Bean Chili | 1 cup | 240 | 35 | 4 | .5 | 0 | 680 | 40 | 10 | 12 |
| **BOWLS** | | | | | | | | | | |
| Brown Rice & Vegetables Bowl | 1 item | 260 | 80 | 9 | 1 | 0 | 550 | 36 | 5 | 9 |
| Santa Fe Enchilada Bowl | 1 item | 350 | 100 | 11 | 2 | 5 | 780 | 47 | 9 | 16 |

## store brands

| | SERVING SIZE | CAL | CAL FAT | TOT FAT (G) | SAT FAT (G) | CHOL (MG) | SOD (MG) | CARB (G) | FIBER (G) | PROT (G) |
|---|---|---|---|---|---|---|---|---|---|---|
| Stuffed Pasta Shells Bowl | 1 item | 310 | 120 | 13 | 7 | 30 | 740 | 30 | 5 | 19 |
| **BREAKFAST** | | | | | | | | | | |
| Breakfast Scramble Wrap | 1 item | 380 | 180 | 19 | 4.5 | 10 | 490 | 30 | 4 | 21 |
| Multi-Grain Hot Cereal Bowl | 1 item | 190 | 10 | 1.5 | 0 | 0 | 300 | 40 | 5 | 4 |
| Steel-Cut Oats Hot Cereal Bowl | 1 item | 220 | 30 | 3.5 | .5 | 0 | 190 | 42 | 5 | 6 |
| **BURRITOS & WRAPS** | | | | | | | | | | |
| Bean & Cheese Burrito, Light in Sodium | 1 item | 330 | 80 | 9 | 2.5 | 10 | 290 | 51 | 7 | 12 |
| Bean & Rice Burrito (Dairy Free), Light in Sodium | 1 item | 320 | 70 | 8 | 1 | 0 | 290 | 52 | 8 | 10 |
| **DESSERT** | | | | | | | | | | |
| Gluten Free Chocolate Cake | 1 slice | 180 | 60 | 7 | 1 | 0 | 200 | 27 | 2 | 3 |
| **ENTRÉES** | | | | | | | | | | |
| Black Bean Tamale Verde | 1 item | 330 | 90 | 10 | 1 | 0 | 780 | 55 | 8 | 7 |
| Cheese Lasagna | 1 item | 380 | 130 | 14 | 8 | 45 | 680 | 44 | 4 | 20 |
| Chili & Cornbread Whole Meal | 1 item | 340 | 60 | 6 | 2.5 | 10 | 680 | 59 | 10 | 11 |
| Enchilada Verde Whole Meal | 1 item | 390 | 120 | 13 | 6 | 30 | 690 | 54 | 8 | 15 |
| Macaroni & Cheese, Light in Sodium | 1 item | 400 | 140 | 16 | 10 | 40 | 290 | 47 | 3 | 16 |
| Veggie Loaf Whole Meal | 1 item | 290 | 70 | 8 | 1 | 0 | 690 | 47 | 10 | 9 |
| **PIZZA** | | | | | | | | | | |
| Broccoli & Spinach White Pizza | 1/3 item | 290 | 130 | 14 | 6 | 25 | 570 | 31 | 2 | 10 |
| Cheese Pizza | 1/3 item | 290 | 110 | 12 | 5 | 15 | 590 | 33 | 2 | 12 |
| Single Serve Mushroom & Olive Pizza | 1 item | 450 | 170 | 19 | 6 | 20 | 780 | 56 | 3 | 18 |
| Single Serve Non-Dairy Rice Crust Cheeze Pizza | 1 item | 460 | 250 | 28 | 3 | 20 | 640 | 46 | 4 | 10 |
| **SNACKS** | | | | | | | | | | |
| Cheese Pizza Snacks | 5–6 pieces | 210 | 80 | 9 | 4.5 | 20 | 440 | 25 | 2 | 9 |
| Nacho Snacks | 5–6 pieces | 220 | 80 | 9 | 5 | 25 | 420 | 25 | 2 | 9 |
| **SOUPS** | | | | | | | | | | |
| No Chicken Noodle Soup | 1 cup | 100 | 30 | 3 | 0 | 0 | 540 | 13 | 2 | 5 |
| Organic Black Bean Vegetable Soup | 1 cup | 140 | 15 | 1.5 | 0 | 0 | 620 | 26 | 5 | 6 |
| Organic Chunky Tomato Bisque | 1 cup | 130 | 30 | 3.5 | 2 | 10 | 680 | 21 | 3 | 3 |
| Organic Fire Roasted Southwestern Vegetable Soup | 1 cup | 140 | 40 | 4 | .5 | 0 | 680 | 21 | 4 | 4 |
| Organic Lentil Soup | 1 cup | 180 | 45 | 5 | 1 | 0 | 590 | 25 | 6 | 8 |
| Organic Vegetable Barley Soup | 1 cup | 70 | 10 | 1 | 0 | 0 | 580 | 13 | 3 | 2 |
| **VEGGIE BURGERS** | | | | | | | | | | |
| Bistro Burger | 1 item | 110 | 20 | 2.5 | 0 | 0 | 370 | 16 | 2 | 5 |

| | SERVING SIZE | CAL | CAL FAT | TOT FAT (G) | SAT FAT (G) | CHOL (MG) | SOD (MG) | CARB (G) | FIBER (G) | PROT (G) |
|---|---|---|---|---|---|---|---|---|---|---|
| California Veggie Burger, Light in Sodium | 1 item | 110 | 35 | 4 | 0 | 0 | 250 | 16 | 3 | 5 |

## Applegate Farms

### BACON

| | | | | | | | | | | |
|---|---|---|---|---|---|---|---|---|---|---|
| Natural Canadian Bacon | 2 slices | 90 | 35 | 4 | 1.5 | 35 | 500 | 1 | 0 | 12 |
| Natural Dry Cured | 2 slices | 60 | 45 | 5 | 2 | 10 | 290 | 0 | 0 | 4 |
| Natural Peppered | 2 slices | 60 | 45 | 5 | 2 | 10 | 290 | 0 | 0 | 4 |
| Natural Turkey | 1 slice | 35 | 15 | 1.5 | 0 | 25 | 200 | 0 | 0 | 6 |
| Organic Turkey | 1 slice | 35 | 15 | 1.5 | 0 | 25 | 200 | 0 | 0 | 6 |

### HOT DOGS

| | | | | | | | | | | |
|---|---|---|---|---|---|---|---|---|---|---|
| The Great Organic | 1 hot dog | 110 | 80 | 8 | 3 | 30 | 330 | 0 | 0 | 7 |
| The Greatest Little Organic Smokey Pork Cocktail Franks | 7 franks | 120 | 90 | 9 | 3.5 | 35 | 390 | 1 | 0 | 8 |
| Natural Beef | 1 hot dog | 70 | 50 | 6 | 2 | 20 | 330 | 0 | 0 | 6 |
| Natural Big Apple | 1 hot dog | 110 | 80 | 9 | 3 | 20 | 360 | 1 | 0 | 7 |
| Natural Chicken | 1 hot dog | 60 | 30 | 3 | 1 | 35 | 370 | 0 | 0 | 7 |
| Natural Turkey | 1 hot dog | 40 | 20 | 3.5 | 1 | 25 | 260 | 0 | 0 | 5 |
| Organic Beef | 1 hot dog | 90 | 60 | 6 | 2.5 | 25 | 380 | 0 | 0 | 6 |
| Organic Chicken | 1 hot dog | 70 | 30 | 3.5 | 1 | 35 | 420 | 0 | 0 | 8 |
| Organic Stadium-Style | 1 hot dog | 110 | 80 | 8 | 3 | 30 | 330 | 0 | 0 | 7 |
| Organic Stadium-Style Ballpark | 1 hot dog | 70 | 40 | 4.5 | 1 | 30 | 430 | 0 | 0 | 7 |
| Organic Turkey | 1 hot dog | 60 | 30 | 3.5 | 1 | 25 | 370 | 0 | 0 | 7 |

### SAUSAGES

| | | | | | | | | | | |
|---|---|---|---|---|---|---|---|---|---|---|
| Organic Andouille | 1 sausage | 140 | 60 | 6 | 2 | 60 | 620 | 3 | 1 | 13 |
| Organic Chicken & Apple | 1 sausage | 140 | 60 | 7 | 1.5 | 65 | 500 | 6 | 1 | 14 |
| Organic Fire Roasted Red Pepper | 1 sausage | 120 | 60 | 6 | 1.5 | 65 | 500 | 2 | 1 | 14 |
| Organic Pork Bratwurst | 1 link | 170 | 110 | 12 | 4 | 45 | 660 | 2 | 0 | 12 |
| Organic Pork Kielbasa | 1 sausage | 190 | 130 | 14 | 5 | 50 | 600 | 2 | 0 | 12 |
| Organic Port Bratwurst | 1 slice | 35 | 15 | 1.5 | 0 | 25 | 200 | 0 | 0 | 6 |
| Organic Spinach & Feta | 1 sausage | 120 | 60 | 7 | 2.5 | 60 | 470 | 2 | 0 | 13 |
| Organic Sweet Italian | 1 sausage | 130 | 60 | 7 | 2 | 70 | 500 | 2 | 1 | 15 |

## AriZona Beverage Co.

| | | | | | | | | | | |
|---|---|---|---|---|---|---|---|---|---|---|
| Asia Plum Green Tea | 8 fl oz | 70 | n/a | 0 | 0 | 0 | 20 | 18 | 0 | 0 |
| Black Tea with Ginseng | 8 fl oz | 60 | 0 | 0 | 0 | 0 | 20 | 15 | 0 | 0 |
| Green Tea with Ginseng & Honey | 8 fl oz | 70 | 0 | 0 | 0 | 0 | 20 | 18 | 0 | 0 |
| Mandarin Orange Green Tea | 8 fl oz | 70 | n/a | 0 | 0 | 0 | 20 | 19 | 0 | 0 |
| Organic Green Tea | 8 fl oz | 20 | 0 | 0 | 0 | 0 | 0 | 6 | 0 | 0 |
| Pomegranate Green Tea | 8 fl oz | 70 | n/a | 0 | 0 | 0 | 10 | 19 | 0 | 0 |

# store brands

## Arnold Bread

| | SERVING SIZE | CAL | CAL FAT | TOT FAT (G) | SAT FAT (G) | CHOL (MG) | SOD (MG) | CARB (G) | FIBER (G) | PROT (G) |
|---|---|---|---|---|---|---|---|---|---|---|
| **ROLLS** | | | | | | | | | | |
| 100% Whole Wheat Sandwich | 1 item | 160 | 20 | 2 | .5 | 0 | 310 | 26 | 4 | 8 |
| Dinner | 1 item | 110 | 15 | 1.5 | 0 | 0 | 200 | 21 | <1 | 3 |
| White Hamburger | 1 item | 150 | 20 | 2 | .5 | 0 | 350 | 30 | 1 | 5 |
| White Hot Dog | 1 item | 130 | 20 | 2 | .5 | 0 | 310 | 26 | 1 | 4 |
| **SLICED BREAD** | | | | | | | | | | |
| 100% Whole Wheat | 1 slice | 110 | 10 | 1 | 0 | 0 | 170 | 20 | 3 | 5 |
| 12 Grain | 1 slice | 110 | 15 | 1.5 | 0 | 0 | 170 | 21 | 3 | 5 |
| 7 Grain | 1 slice | 110 | 15 | 1.5 | 0 | 0 | 170 | 21 | 3 | 4 |
| Bakery Carb Counting, Multi-Grain | 1 slice | 60 | 15 | 1.5 | 0 | 0 | 120 | 9 | 3 | 5 |
| Bakery Light, 100 % Whole Wheat | 2 slices | 80 | 5 | .5 | 0 | 0 | 170 | 18 | 5 | 5 |
| Brick Oven, Premium White | 1 slice | 90 | 15 | 1.5 | 0 | 0 | 190 | 17 | <1 | 3 |
| Country Oat Bran | 1 slice | 110 | 15 | 1.5 | 0 | 0 | 180 | 21 | 1 | 4 |
| Country Wheat | 1 slice | 120 | 15 | 1.5 | 0 | 0 | 170 | 22 | 2 | 4 |
| Country White | 1 slice | 120 | 15 | 1.5 | 0 | 0 | 180 | 22 | 1 | 3 |
| Country Whole Grain White | 1 slice | 100 | 10 | 1 | 0 | 0 | 170 | 20 | 3 | 5 |
| Double Fiber | 1 slice | 100 | 15 | 1.5 | 0 | 0 | 170 | 21 | 6 | 4 |
| Double Protein | 1 slice | 110 | 15 | 1.5 | 0 | 0 | 170 | 18 | 3 | 7 |
| German Dark Wheat | 1 slice | 110 | 20 | 2 | 0 | 0 | 170 | 20 | 3 | 5 |
| Grain Lover's | 1 slice | 120 | 25 | 2.5 | 0 | 0 | 170 | 21 | 3 | 5 |
| Health Nut | 1 slice | 120 | 20 | 2 | 0 | 0 | 170 | 21 | 2 | 5 |
| Healthful 10 Grain | 1 slice | 80 | 10 | 1 | 0 | 0 | 160 | 16 | 4 | 5 |
| Healthy Multi-Grain | 1 slice | 110 | 15 | 1.5 | 0 | 0 | 160 | 20 | 4 | 5 |
| Honey Whole Wheat | 1 slice | 110 | 10 | 1 | 0 | 0 | 170 | 20 | 3 | 5 |
| Oatnut | 1 slice | 120 | 25 | 2.5 | 0 | 0 | 170 | 22 | 2 | 4 |
| Premium Italian | 1 slice | 90 | 15 | 1.5 | 0 | 0 | 180 | 16 | <1 | 2 |
| Real Jewish Marble Rye | 1 slice | 80 | 10 | 1 | 0 | 0 | 210 | 14 | <1 | 2 |
| Real Jewish Seedless Rye | 2 slices | 110 | 15 | 1.5 | 0 | 0 | 290 | 20 | <1 | 3 |
| Stone Ground—100 % Whole Wheat | 2 slices | 130 | 20 | 2 | 0 | 0 | 260 | 22 | 3 | 6 |
| **SANDWICH THINS** | | | | | | | | | | |
| 100% Whole Wheat | 1 item | 100 | 10 | 1 | 0 | 0 | 230 | 21 | 5 | 5 |
| Honey Wheat | 1 item | 100 | 10 | 1 | 0 | 0 | 220 | 22 | 5 | 5 |
| Multi-Grain | 1 item | 100 | 10 | 1 | 0 | 0 | 230 | 22 | 5 | 5 |
| Seedless Rye | 1 item | 100 | 10 | 1 | 0 | 0 | 210 | 23 | 5 | 4 |
| Whole Grain White | 1 item | 100 | 10 | 1 | 0 | 0 | 230 | 22 | 5 | 4 |

| | SERVING SIZE | CAL | CAL FAT | TOT FAT (G) | SAT FAT (G) | CHOL (MG) | SOD (MG) | CARB (G) | FIBER (G) | PROT (G) |
|---|---|---|---|---|---|---|---|---|---|---|
| **Athenos** | | | | | | | | | | |
| Reduced Fat Crumbled Feta Cheese | 1/4 cup | 70 | 40 | 4 | 2.5 | 10 | 470 | 1 | 0 | 7 |
| Traditional Crumbled Feta Cheese | 1/4 cup | 90 | 60 | 7 | 4 | 25 | 390 | 2 | 1 | 7 |
| **Aunt Jemima** | | | | | | | | | | |
| Lite Syrup | 1/4 cup | 100 | 0 | 0 | 0 | 0 | 190 | 26 | 1 | 0 |
| Original Syrup | 1/4 cup | 210 | 0 | 0 | 0 | 0 | 120 | 52 | n/a | 0 |
| **Balance Bar** | | | | | | | | | | |
| Bare, Sweet & Salty Peanut Butter | 1 bar | 210 | 80 | 9 | 3 | 0 | 290 | 23 | 3 | 13 |
| Bare, Trail Mix Chocolate Chip | 1 bar | 200 | 60 | 7 | 3 | 0 | 310 | 22 | 3 | 14 |
| Carb Well, Caramel 'n Chocolate | 1 bar | 190 | 60 | 7 | 4 | 5 | 190 | 23 | 1 | 14 |
| Original, Chocolate Craze | 1 bar | 200 | 60 | 7 | 4 | 0 | 160 | 21 | 2 | 14 |
| **Banquet** | | | | | | | | | | |
| **ENTRÉES** | | | | | | | | | | |
| Cheesy Smothered Meat Patty Dinner | 1 item | 310 | 150 | 16 | 7 | 35 | 1160 | 30 | 3 | 13 |
| Crock-Pot Classics Beef Pot Roast | 2/3 cup | 150 | 35 | 3.5 | 2 | 20 | 660 | 18 | 3 | 11 |
| Crock-Pot Classics Chicken & Dumplings | 2/3 cup | 200 | 70 | 8 | 2 | 35 | 940 | 21 | 6 | 10 |
| Crock-Pot Classics Hearty Beef & Vegetables | 1 serving | 140 | 30 | 6 | 2 | 35 | 620 | 15 | 4 | 12 |
| Family Entrée—Salisbury Steak with Gravy | 1 steak | 180 | 120 | 13 | 5 | 25 | 710 | 9 | 2 | 9 |
| Family Entrée—Homestyle Gravy & Sliced Turkey Meal | 2 slices | 90 | 45 | 5 | 1 | 20 | 710 | 6 | <1 | 5 |
| Family Entrée—Broccoli, Chicken, & Cheese | 1 cup | 200 | 70 | 7 | 2.5 | 30 | 940 | 210 | 24 | 1 |
| Fettucini Alfredo Dinner | 1 item | 280 | 100 | 11 | 4.5 | 20 | 700 | 35 | 3 | 10 |
| Fried Chicken Classics Original Drumsticks | 9 oz | 400 | 180 | 20 | 4.5 | 90 | 910 | 30 | 5 | 24 |
| Homestyle Grilled Meat Patty Dinner | 1 item | 280 | 150 | 15 | 6 | 35 | 860 | 23 | 2 | 12 |
| Macaroni & Beef Dinner | 1 item | 210 | 40 | 4.5 | 1.5 | 10 | 820 | 32 | 4 | 9 |
| Macaroni & Cheese | 1 meal | 260 | 60 | 6 | 3 | 15 | 770 | 40 | 4 | 11 |
| Mexican Style Chicken Enchilada | 1 item | 280 | 80 | 9 | 3 | 10 | 870 | 44 | 5 | 7 |
| Mozzarella Cheese Nuggets | 7 pieces | 290 | 160 | 18 | 8 | 15 | 330 | 22 | 3 | 10 |
| Pot Pie, Beef | 1 item | 300 | 200 | 22 | 9 | 22 | 1010 | 36 | 3 | 12 |
| Pot Pie, Chicken with Broccoli | 1 item | 360 | 180 | 20 | 8 | 30 | 930 | 34 | 3 | 9 |
| Pot Pie, Turkey | 1 item | 370 | 190 | 21 | 8 | 30 | 980 | 35 | 3 | 10 |
| Salisbury Steak Dinner | 1 item | 290 | 150 | 16 | 7 | 30 | 1100 | 25 | 4 | 11 |
| Select Recipes—Classic Fried Chicken | 1 item | 350 | 160 | 17 | 4 | 35 | 930 | 35 | 5 | 12 |
| Select Recipes—Classic Fried Chicken Premium Meal | 1 item | 440 | 240 | 26 | 6 | 80 | 1140 | 30 | 4 | 22 |

# store brands

| | SERVING SIZE | CAL | CAL FAT | TOT FAT (G) | SAT FAT (G) | CHOL (MG) | SOD (MG) | CARB (G) | FIBER (G) | PROT (G) |
|---|---|---|---|---|---|---|---|---|---|---|
| Select Recipes—Corn Dog Meal | 1 item | 460 | 150 | 16 | 3.5 | 45 | 750 | 68 | 6 | 10 |
| Select Recipes—Enchilada Combo Meal | 1 item | 310 | 90 | 10 | 3.5 | 10 | 930 | 44 | 11 | 10 |
| Select Recipes—Herb Grilled Chicken | 1 item | 270 | 90 | 10 | 3.5 | 35 | 750 | 29 | 4 | 15 |
| Select Recipes—Homestyle Pot Roast | 1 item | 170 | 45 | 5 | 2 | 20 | 860 | 19 | 5 | 13 |
| Select Recipes—Slow Cooked Beef | 1 item | 220 | 60 | 6 | 2 | 40 | 680 | 27 | 5 | 16 |
| Select Recipes—Smothered Burritos | 1 item | 500 | 180 | 20 | 8 | 25 | 1200 | 65 | 11 | 16 |
| Spaghetti & Meatballs Dinner | 1 item | 330 | 130 | 14 | 5 | 20 | 650 | 35 | 5 | 15 |
| Zesty Smothered Meat Patty Dinner | 1 item | 300 | 130 | 15 | 5 | 25 | 860 | 30 | 4 | 11 |
| **MEATS** | | | | | | | | | | |
| Boneless Buffalo Chicken Tender | 5 pieces | 220 | 120 | 13 | 2.5 | 15 | 330 | 15 | 2 | 12 |
| Boneless Chicken Breast Nuggets | 6 pieces | 240 | 120 | 11 | 2.5 | 15 | 400 | 17 | 3 | 12 |
| Boneless Chicken Breast Patty | 1 item | 160 | 80 | 9 | 1.5 | 15 | 340 | 11 | 1 | 10 |
| Boneless Chicken Breast Strips | 2 pieces | 190 | 90 | 10 | 1.5 | 15 | 500 | 14 | 2 | 12 |
| Boneless Chicken Breast Tender | 5 pieces | 220 | 130 | 14 | 2 | 15 | 470 | 12 | <1 | 11 |
| Boneless Fun Chicken Nuggets | 4 pieces | 200 | 100 | 11 | 0 | 15 | 430 | 13 | 0 | 13 |
| Boneless Original Chicken Nuggets | 5 pieces | 270 | 170 | 19 | 4 | 15 | 480 | 15 | 2 | 11 |
| Boneless Original Chicken Patty | 1 item | 220 | 120 | 13 | 2.5 | 15 | 340 | 11 | 1 | 9 |
| Boneless Southern Chicken Tender | 5 pieces | 220 | 110 | 12 | 2 | 15 | 360 | 15 | 0 | 12 |
| Brown 'N Serve Beef Link | 3 items | 190 | 160 | 17 | 8 | 15 | 420 | 1 | 0 | 7 |
| Brown 'N Serve Beef Sausage Patties | 2 pieces | 160 | 130 | 14 | 6 | 15 | 350 | 1 | 0 | 6 |
| Brown 'N Serve Country Recipe Link | 3 items | 200 | 160 | 18 | 6 | 30 | 510 | 3 | 1 | 7 |
| Brown 'N Serve Lite Maple Link | 3 pieces | 130 | 80 | 9 | 3 | 35 | 450 | 4 | 0 | 9 |
| Brown 'N Serve Lite Original Link | 3 items | 120 | 80 | 9 | 3 | 25 | 430 | 2 | 0 | 9 |
| Brown 'N Serve Maple Link | 3 items | 210 | 170 | 19 | 6 | 25 | 520 | 2 | 0 | 8 |
| Brown 'N Serve Original Link | 3 items | 200 | 160 | 18 | 6 | 30 | 490 | 2 | 1 | 8 |
| Brown 'N Serve Original Patty | 2 items | 170 | 130 | 15 | 5 | 25 | 410 | 2 | <1 | 6 |
| Brown 'N Serve Turkey Link | 3 items | 110 | 60 | 7 | 2 | 40 | 390 | 2 | 0 | 9 |
| Brown 'N Serve Turkey Sausage Patty | 2 pieces | 90 | 50 | 6 | 2 | 35 | 320 | 2 | 0 | 8 |
| Country Fried Chicken | 1 item | 350 | 210 | 24 | 5 | 70 | 1180 | 11 | 1 | 24 |
| Crispy Chicken | 1 piece | 330 | 190 | 21 | 5 | 75 | 890 | 12 | <1 | 24 |
| Patty Fritters Popcorn Chicken | 10 pieces | 220 | 90 | 10 | 1.5 | 10 | 140 | 23 | 0 | 10 |
| Skinless Crispy Chicken | 1 piece | 360 | 210 | 23 | 5 | 65 | 720 | 13 | 1 | 25 |
| Southern Crispy Chicken | 1 piece | 360 | 220 | 24 | 6 | 65 | 1050 | 14 | 2 | 22 |
| Sweet & Sour Chicken | 1 item | 390 | 120 | 14 | 2.5 | 15 | 570 | 56 | 3 | 10 |
| Wings, Honey BBQ | 3 oz | 270 | 160 | 18 | 4.5 | 50 | 540 | 11 | 1 | 16 |
| Wings, Hot & Spicy | 3 oz | 270 | 160 | 18 | 4.5 | 55 | 470 | 11 | 1 | 15 |

| | SERVING SIZE | CAL | CAL FAT | TOT FAT (G) | SAT FAT (G) | CHOL (MG) | SOD (MG) | CARB (G) | FIBER (G) | PROT (G) |
|---|---|---|---|---|---|---|---|---|---|---|
| **Barq's** | | | | | | | | | | |
| Root Beer | 12 fl oz | 160 | 0 | 0 | 0 | 0 | 70 | 45 | 0 | 0 |
| **Ben & Jerry's** | | | | | | | | | | |
| **ICE CREAM** | | | | | | | | | | |
| Cherry Garcia | 1/2 cup | 240 | 120 | 13 | 9 | 60 | 35 | 28 | <1 | 4 |
| Chocolate | 1/2 cup | 250 | 130 | 14 | 10 | 40 | 50 | 25 | 2 | 4 |
| Chocolate Chip Cookie Dough | 1/2 cup | 270 | 130 | 14 | 8 | 65 | 60 | 33 | 0 | 4 |
| Chubby Hubby | 1/2 cup | 340 | 180 | 20 | 10 | 55 | 140 | 33 | 1 | 7 |
| Chunky Monkey | 1/2 cup | 290 | 160 | 18 | 10 | 65 | 35 | 29 | 1 | 4 |
| Half Baked | 1/2 cup | 270 | 120 | 13 | 7 | 55 | 70 | 35 | 1 | 4 |
| Phish Food | 1/2 cup | 280 | 120 | 13 | 8 | 35 | 80 | 39 | 2 | 4 |
| Turtle Soup | 1/2 cup | 280 | 140 | 16 | 10 | 60 | 100 | 30 | 1 | 4 |
| Vanilla | 1/2 cup | 200 | 110 | 12 | 7 | 65 | 35 | 20 | 0 | 4 |
| **ICE CREAM BARS** | | | | | | | | | | |
| Cherry Garcia | 1 item | 260 | 140 | 16 | 11 | 40 | 40 | 23 | 1 | 8 |
| Half Baked | 1 item | 360 | 200 | 22 | 13 | 45 | 100 | 37 | 1 | 4 |
| Vanilla | 1 item | 300 | 180 | 20 | 13 | 50 | 40 | 25 | 1 | 3 |
| **Bertolli** | | | | | | | | | | |
| **FROZEN ENTRÉES** | | | | | | | | | | |
| Chianti Braised Beef & Rigatoni | 1/2 entrée | 350 | 110 | 12 | 2 | 70 | 890 | 41 | 5 | 17 |
| Chicken Alfredo & Fettuccine | 1/2 entrée | 630 | 290 | 32 | 17 | 125 | 1200 | 50 | 4 | n/a |
| Chicken Alla Vodka & Farfalle | 1/2 entrée | 500 | 230 | 25 | 11 | 125 | 1360 | 40 | 3 | 21 |
| Chicken Florentine & Farfalle | 1/2 entrée | 570 | 260 | 31 | 17 | 175 | 1040 | 40 | 3 | 25 |
| Chicken Marsala & Roasted Redskin Potatoes | 1/2 entrée | 390 | 120 | 13 | 5 | 55 | 920 | 35 | 3 | 19 |
| Chicken Parmigiana & Penne | 1/2 entrée | 490 | 200 | 22 | 6 | 40 | 1330 | 52 | 5 | 23 |
| Chicken, Rigatoni & Broccoli | 1/2 entrée | 390 | 150 | 15 | 4 | 40 | 970 | 37 | 4 | 22 |
| Garlic Shrimp, Penne & Cherry Tomatoes | 1/2 entrée | 340 | 100 | 11 | 1 | 40 | 740 | 42 | 5 | 13 |
| Grilled Chicken & Roasted Vegetables | 1/2 entrée | 400 | 160 | 18 | 2.5 | 65 | 950 | 33 | 4 | 22 |
| Italian Sausage & Rigatoni | 1/2 entrée | 500 | 230 | 26 | 8 | 50 | 1120 | 46 | 4 | 18 |
| Italian Sausage Stuffed Shells | 1/2 entrée | 480 | 230 | 26 | 9 | 55 | 1160 | 41 | 4 | 20 |
| Lemon Herb Shrimp & Penne | 1/2 entrée | 410 | 150 | 17 | 3.5 | 95 | 910 | 44 | 4 | 18 |
| Meat Lasagna Rustica | 1/2 entrée | 520 | 340 | 31 | 13 | 60 | 1110 | 36 | 4 | 25 |
| Mushroom Lasagna Al Forno | 1/2 entrée | 480 | 240 | 27 | 14 | 70 | 1210 | 41 | 5 | 18 |
| Roasted Chicken & Linguine | 1/2 entrée | 390 | 150 | 17 | 5 | 70 | 1350 | 36 | 5 | 24 |
| Roasted Chicken Cannelloni | 1/2 entrée | 490 | 250 | 28 | 11 | 100 | 1030 | 37 | 2 | 23 |

# store brands

| | SERVING SIZE | CAL | CAL FAT | TOT FAT (G) | SAT FAT (G) | CHOL (MG) | SOD (MG) | CARB (G) | FIBER (G) | PROT (G) |
|---|---|---|---|---|---|---|---|---|---|---|
| Rosemary Chicken, Linguine & Cherry Tomatoes | 1/2 entrée | 380 | 130 | 14 | 3 | 60 | 800 | 38 | 4 | 20 |
| Shrimp Asparagus & Penne | 1/2 entrée | 420 | 140 | 16 | 8 | 80 | 990 | 50 | 3 | 18 |
| Shrimp Scampi & Linguine | 1/2 entrée | 550 | 220 | 24 | 11 | 130 | 990 | 58 | 3 | 19 |
| Steak, Rigatoni & Portobello Mushrooms | 1/2 entrée | 390 | 150 | 17 | 4.5 | 30 | 890 | 38 | 4 | 19 |
| Stuffed Shells in Scampi Sauce | 1/2 entrée | 600 | 310 | 34 | 19 | 120 | 1200 | 41 | 2 | 21 |
| Tri-Color Four Cheese Ravioli | 1/2 entrée | 620 | 290 | 32 | 19 | 115 | 1150 | 52 | 3 | 26 |
| Tuscan-Style Braised Beef, with Gold Potatoes | 1/2 entrée | 310 | 100 | 11 | 2.5 | 25 | 920 | 35 | 3 | 16 |
| **SAUCES** | | | | | | | | | | |
| Alfredo Sauce | 1/4 cup | 110 | 90 | 10 | 5 | 40 | 410 | 2 | 0 | 2 |
| Arrabbiata Sauce | 1/2 cup | 60 | 15 | 1.5 | 0 | 0 | 450 | 11 | 2 | 1 |
| Organic Traditional Tomato & Basil Sauce | 1/2 cup | 90 | 40 | 7.5 | .5 | 0 | 510 | 11 | 2 | 2 |
| Tomato & Basil Sauce | 1/2 cup | 70 | 20 | 2 | 0 | 0 | 460 | 13 | 3 | 3 |
| Vodka Sauce | 1/2 cup | 150 | 80 | 9 | 4.5 | 25 | 700 | 11 | 2 | 3 |
| **Betty Crocker** | | | | | | | | | | |
| **FROSTING** | | | | | | | | | | |
| Mix Home Style Fluffy White | 3 tbsp | 100 | 0 | 0 | 0 | 0 | 55 | 24 | 0 | <1 |
| Rich & Creamy Chocolate | 2 tbsp | 130 | 45 | 5 | 1.5 | 0 | 95 | 21 | <1 | 0 |
| Whipped Butter Cream | 2 tbsp | 100 | 45 | 5 | 1.5 | 0 | 25 | 15 | 0 | 0 |
| Whipped Chocolate (made with Hershey's) | 2 tbsp | 90 | 40 | 4.5 | 1.5 | 0 | 60 | 14 | <1 | <1 |
| Whipped Vanilla | 2 tbsp | 100 | 45 | 5 | 1.5 | 0 | 25 | 15 | 0 | 0 |
| **POTATOES** | | | | | | | | | | |
| Casserole Au Gratin | 1/2 cup | 90 | 0 | 0 | 0 | 0 | 590 | 22 | 1 | 2 |
| Casserole Cheddar and Bacon | 1/2 cup | 100 | 5 | .5 | 0 | 0 | 640 | 22 | 1 | 2 |
| Casserole Cheesy Scalloped | 2/3 cup | 90 | 0 | 0 | 0 | 0 | 650 | 21 | 2 | 2 |
| Casserole Julienne | 1/3 cup | 80 | 0 | 0 | 0 | 0 | 620 | 20 | 1 | 1 |
| Casserole Loaded Baked | 2/3 cup | 90 | 0 | 0 | 0 | 0 | 590 | 21 | 1 | 2 |
| Casserole Roasted Garlic | 2/3 cup | 90 | 10 | 1 | 0 | 0 | 500 | 21 | 1 | 2 |
| Casserole Scalloped | 1/2 cup | 90 | 0 | 0 | 0 | 0 | 600 | 21 | 1 | 2 |
| Casserole Sour Cream and Chives | 2/3 cup | 90 | 5 | .5 | 0 | 0 | 710 | 21 | 1 | 1 |
| Casserole Three Cheese | 2/3 cup | 100 | 5 | .5 | 0 | 0 | 610 | 22 | 1 | 2 |
| Deluxe, Cheesy Cheddar Au Gratin | 2/3 cup | 120 | 30 | 3.5 | .5 | 0 | 650 | 22 | 1 | 2 |
| Deluxe, Loaded Au Gratin | 2/3 cup | 130 | 30 | 3.5 | 1 | 0 | 650 | 22 | 1 | 2 |
| Deluxe, Three Cheese Mashed Potato Bake | 1/2 cup | 150 | 40 | 4.5 | 1 | <5 | 740 | 25 | 1 | 3 |
| Flavored Mashed, Butter and Herb | 1/3 cup | 80 | 5 | .5 | 0 | 0 | 410 | 17 | 1 | 2 |
| Flavored Mashed, Four Cheese | 1/3 cup | 80 | 0 | 0 | 0 | 0 | 440 | 17 | 1 | 2 |

| | SERVING SIZE | CAL | CAL FAT | TOT FAT (G) | SAT FAT (G) | CHOL (MG) | SOD (MG) | CARB (G) | FIBER (G) | PROT (G) |
|---|---|---|---|---|---|---|---|---|---|---|
| Flavored Mashed, Homestyle Creamy Butter | 1/3 cup | 80 | 5 | .5 | 0 | 0 | 390 | 17 | 1 | 2 |
| Flavored Mashed, Loaded | 1/2 cup | 80 | 0 | 0 | 0 | 0 | 460 | 17 | 1 | 2 |
| Flavored Mashed, Roasted Garlic | 1/3 cup | 80 | 0 | 0 | 0 | 0 | 400 | 17 | 1 | 2 |
| Flavored Mashed, Roasted Garlic & Cheddar | 1/3 cup | 80 | 0 | 0 | 0 | 0 | 430 | 17 | 1 | 2 |
| Flavored Mashed, Sour Cream and Chives | 1/3 cup | 80 | 0 | 0 | 0 | 0 | 400 | 17 | 1 | 2 |
| Flavored Mashed, Sweet | 1/3 cup | 120 | 5 | 1 | .5 | 0 | 310 | 26 | 1 | 2 |
| Flavored Mashed, Yukon Gold | 1/3 cup | 90 | 5 | 1 | .5 | 0 | 390 | 18 | 1 | 2 |
| Potato Buds | 1/3 cup | 90 | 0 | 0 | 0 | 0 | 25 | 19 | 1 | 2 |
| Pouch, Cheddar and Sour Cream Mashed | 1/3 cup | 80 | 5 | 1 | 0 | 0 | 470 | 18 | 3 | 2 |
| Pouch, Creamy Butter | 1/3 cup | 80 | 10 | 1 | .5 | <5 | 460 | 17 | 3 | 2 |
| Pouch, Homestyle Reds | 1/3 cup | 80 | 10 | 1.5 | 1 | <5 | 480 | 17 | 3 | 2 |
| Pouch, Loaded Mashed | 1/3 cup | 80 | 10 | 1 | .5 | 5 | 480 | 17 | 3 | 2 |
| Pouch, Roasted Garlic Mashed | 1/3 cup | 80 | 10 | 1 | .5 | <5 | 420 | 17 | 3 | 2 |
| Seasoned Skillets, Hash Brown | 1/3 cup | 80 | 5 | .5 | 0 | 0 | 410 | 18 | 2 | 2 |
| Seasoned Skillets, Roasted Garlic and Herb | 3/4 cup | 90 | 5 | .5 | 0 | 0 | 410 | 21 | 2 | 2 |
| Seasoned Skillets, Traditional Recipe | 3/4 cup | 90 | 5 | .5 | 0 | 0 | 490 | 22 | 2 | 2 |
| **SUPER MOIST CAKE MIX** | | | | | | | | | | |
| Butter Pecan | 1/12 pckg | 160 | 15 | 1.5 | 1 | 0 | 280 | 35 | n/a | 1 |
| Butter Recipe Chocolate | 1/12 pckg | 160 | 15 | 2 | 1 | 0 | 380 | 35 | 1 | 2 |
| Butter Recipe Yellow | 1/12 pckg | 160 | 15 | 1.5 | .5 | 0 | 280 | 35 | n/a | 1 |
| Cake Mix Lemon | 1/12 pckg | 160 | 15 | 1.5 | 1 | 0 | 280 | 35 | n/a | 1 |
| Carrot | 1/12 pckg | 160 | 15 | 1.5 | .5 | 0 | 270 | 35 | n/a | 1 |
| Cherry Chip | 1/12 pckg | 160 | 15 | 1.5 | 1 | 0 | 300 | 35 | <1 | 2 |
| Chocolate Fudge | 1/12 pckg | 160 | 15 | 2 | 1 | 0 | 360 | 35 | 1 | 2 |
| Dark Chocolate | 1/12 pckg | 170 | 15 | 2 | 1 | 0 | 410 | 37 | 1 | 2 |
| Devil's Food | 1/12 pckg | 160 | 15 | 2 | 1 | 0 | 370 | 35 | 1 | 2 |
| French Vanilla | 1/12 pckg | 160 | 15 | 1.5 | 1 | 0 | 280 | 35 | n/a | 1 |
| German Chocolate | 1/12 pckg | 160 | 15 | 1.5 | 1 | 0 | 350 | 35 | <1 | 2 |
| Golden Vanilla | 1/12 pckg | 160 | 15 | 1.5 | 1 | 0 | 280 | 35 | n/a | 1 |
| Milk Chocolate | 1/12 pckg | 160 | 15 | 2 | 1 | 0 | 280 | 35 | <1 | 2 |
| Party Rainbow Chip | 1/12 pckg | 160 | 15 | 1.5 | 1 | 0 | 300 | 35 | n/a | 2 |
| Spice | 1/12 pckg | 160 | 20 | 2.5 | 1.5 | 0 | 370 | 34 | 1 | 2 |
| Strawberry | 1/12 pckg | 170 | 25 | 3 | 1 | 0 | 280 | 34 | n/a | 2 |
| Triple Chocolate Fudge | 1/12 pckg | 160 | 20 | 2.5 | 1.5 | 0 | 370 | 34 | 1 | 2 |
| Vanilla | 1/12 pckg | 160 | 15 | 1.5 | 1 | 0 | 300 | 35 | n/a | 2 |
| White | 1/12 pckg | 160 | 15 | 1.5 | 1 | 0 | 300 | 35 | n/a | 2 |
| Yellow | 1/12 pckg | 160 | 15 | 1.5 | 1 | 0 | 280 | 35 | n/a | 1 |

| Boar's Head | SERVING SIZE | CAL | CAL FAT | TOT FAT (G) | SAT FAT (G) | CHOL (MG) | SOD (MG) | CARB (G) | FIBER (G) | PROT (G) |
|---|---|---|---|---|---|---|---|---|---|---|
| **DELI MEATS** | | | | | | | | | | |
| All Natural Oven Roasted Beef | 2 oz | 80 | 20 | 2 | 1 | 35 | 140 | 0 | 0 | 14 |
| All Natural Roasted Turkey Breast | 2 oz | 60 | 10 | 1 | 0 | 30 | 330 | 1 | 0 | 13 |
| All Natural Uncured Ham | 2 oz | 70 | 10 | 1 | 0 | 35 | 340 | 1 | 0 | 12 |
| Bologna (Pork & Beef) | 2 oz | 150 | 120 | 13 | 4.5 | 35 | 530 | 1 | 0 | 7 |
| Classic Oven Roasted Chicken Breast | 2 oz | 50 | 5 | 1 | 0 | 35 | 440 | 0 | 0 | 13 |
| Cooked Salami | 2 oz | 130 | 100 | 11 | 5 | 40 | 590 | 0 | 0 | 8 |
| Genoa Salami | 2 oz | 190 | 130 | 15 | 5 | 50 | 920 | 1 | 0 | 12 |
| Sandwich Style Pepperoni | 1 oz | 130 | 100 | 11 | 4.5 | 25 | 480 | 1 | 0 | 6 |
| **Boca** | | | | | | | | | | |
| **MEATLESS BURGERS** | | | | | | | | | | |
| Cheeseburger | 1 burger | 100 | 40 | 4.5 | 1.5 | 10 | 320 | 6 | 4 | 13 |
| Grilled Vegetable | 1 burger | 80 | 10 | 1 | 0 | 0 | 300 | 7 | 4 | 12 |
| Original | 1 burger | 100 | 5 | 1 | 0 | 0 | 520 | 8 | 6 | 19 |
| Vegan (Made with Non-GMO Soy) | 1 burger | 100 | 20 | 2.5 | 0 | 0 | 470 | 9 | 4 | 13 |
| **MEATLESS CHICK'N** | | | | | | | | | | |
| Original Nuggets | 3 oz | 180 | 60 | 7 | .5 | 0 | 500 | 17 | 3 | 14 |
| Original Patty | 1 patty | 160 | 50 | 6 | 1 | 0 | 430 | 15 | 2 | 11 |
| **MEATLESS CRUMBLES, LINKS & ENTRÉES** | | | | | | | | | | |
| Breakfast Links | 1-1/2 oz | 70 | 30 | 3 | 1 | 0 | 330 | 5 | 2 | 8 |
| Ground Crumbles | 2 oz | 60 | 0 | .5 | 0 | 0 | 270 | 6 | 3 | 13 |
| **Bolthouse Farms** | | | | | | | | | | |
| **BEVERAGES** | | | | | | | | | | |
| 100% Carrot Juice | 8 fl oz | 70 | 0 | 0 | 0 | 0 | 150 | 14 | <1 | 2 |
| 100% Pomegranate Juice | 8 fl oz | 150 | 0 | 0 | 0 | 0 | 20 | 38 | 0 | 0 |
| 50/50 Berry Juice | 8 fl oz | 140 | 0 | 0 | 0 | 0 | 80 | 32 | 1 | 1 |
| Açai Blueberry | 8 fl oz | 140 | 0 | 0 | 0 | 0 | 25 | 39 | 1 | 0 |
| Açai Pomegranate | 8 fl oz | 160 | 5 | .5 | 0 | 0 | 25 | 39 | 0 | 0 |
| Berry Boost Smoothie | 8 fl oz | 130 | 10 | 1 | 0 | 0 | 20 | 30 | 4 | 0 |
| C-Boost | 8 fl oz | 152 | 0 | 0 | 0 | 0 | 15 | 36 | <1 | 1 |
| Green Tea with Açai | 8 fl oz | 70 | 0 | 0 | 0 | 0 | 10 | 16 | 0 | 0 |
| Mango Lemonade | 8 fl oz | 120 | 0 | 0 | 0 | 0 | 0 | 30 | <1 | <1 |
| Perfectly Protein Hazelnut Latte | 8 fl oz | 199 | 23 | 2.5 | 1.5 | 13 | 115 | 34 | 0 | 10 |
| Perfectly Protein Mocha Cappuccino | 8 fl oz | 180 | 20 | 2.5 | 1.5 | 13 | 106 | 29 | 0 | 10 |
| Perfectly Protein Vanilla Chai Tea | 8 fl oz | 160 | 28 | 3 | 1 | 0 | 60 | 25 | 0 | 10 |

| | SERVING SIZE | CAL | CAL FAT | TOT FAT (G) | SAT FAT (G) | CHOL (MG) | SOD (MG) | CARB (G) | FIBER (G) | PROT (G) |
|---|---|---|---|---|---|---|---|---|---|---|
| **SALAD DRESSINGS** | | | | | | | | | | |
| Olive Oil Vinaigrette Chunky Blue Cheese | 2 tbsp | 60 | 45 | 5 | 1 | 5 | 150 | 4 | 0 | 1 |
| Olive Oil Vinaigrette Classic Balsamic Vinaigrette | 2 tbsp | 30 | 0 | 0 | 0 | 0 | 150 | 6 | 0 | 0 |
| Yogurt Dressing Chunky Blue Cheese | 2 tbsp | 50 | 40 | 4.5 | 1.5 | 10 | 140 | 1 | 0 | 1 |
| Yogurt Dressing Classic Ranch | 2 tbsp | 70 | 60 | 6 | 1.5 | 5 | 280 | 2 | 0 | 1 |
| Yogurt Dressing Creamy Italian | 2 tbsp | 70 | 60 | 7 | 1.5 | 10 | 105 | 2 | 0 | 1 |
| Yogurt Dressing Honey Mustard | 2 tbsp | 45 | 15 | 2 | .5 | 5 | 80 | 7 | 0 | 1 |
| Yogurt Dressing Thousand Island | 2 tbsp | 70 | 50 | 5.5 | 1 | 5 | 180 | 4 | <1 | 1 |
| **VEGETABLES** | | | | | | | | | | |
| Snack Packs Baby Cut Carrots | 3 oz | 35 | 0 | 0 | 0 | 0 | 65 | 8 | 2 | 1 |
| *Buitoni* | | | | | | | | | | |
| **FROZEN MEALS** | | | | | | | | | | |
| Braised Beef & Sausage Ravioli, Creamy Marinara Sauce | 1/2 item | 590 | 170 | 19 | 9 | 120 | 1200 | 72 | 5 | 33 |
| Chicken & Mushroom Ravioli, Marsala Wine Sauce | 1/2 item | 530 | 180 | 20 | 11 | 110 | 1140 | 59 | 5 | 29 |
| Five Cheese Cannelloni, Tomato Basil Sauce | 1/2 item | 560 | 240 | 27 | 15 | 115 | 1560 | 52 | 5 | 27 |
| Four Cheese Spinach Ravioli, Tomato Basil Sauce | 1/2 item | 550 | 190 | 21 | 12 | 100 | 1270 | 55 | 7 | 24 |
| Maine Lobster Ravioli, White Wine Butter | 1/4 item | 430 | 180 | 20 | 12 | 105 | 890 | 106 | 2 | 14 |
| **PASTA** | | | | | | | | | | |
| Cheese & Roasted Garlic Tortelloni | 3 oz | 270 | 70 | 8 | 4 | 35 | 360 | 37 | 2 | 12 |
| Chicken & Four Cheese Ravioli | 1 cup | 300 | 100 | 11 | 6 | 85 | 793 | 35 | 2 | 16 |
| Quattro Formaggi Agnolotti | 1 cup | 360 | 150 | 17 | 9 | 90 | 698 | 35 | 2 | 17 |
| Three Cheese Ravioletti | 3 oz | 270 | 45 | 5 | 2.5 | 30 | 340 | 43 | 2 | 12 |
| Whole Wheat Three Cheese Tortellini | 4 oz | 330 | 90 | 10 | 3 | 60 | 500 | 45 | 6 | 16 |
| Wild Mushroom Agnolotti | 1 cup | 320 | 110 | 13 | 6 | 75 | 796 | 39 | 3 | 14 |
| **SAUCES** | | | | | | | | | | |
| Alfredo | 2 oz | 140 | 110 | 12 | 7 | 30 | 350 | 4 | 0 | 4 |
| Marinara | 4 oz | 70 | 25 | 3 | 0 | 0 | 540 | 10 | 2 | 0 |
| Pesto with Basil | 2 oz | 270 | 200 | 23 | 3.5 | 10 | 450 | 6 | 1 | 6 |
| Vodka | 4 oz | 90 | 50 | 6 | 4 | 15 | 550 | 5 | 1 | 3 |
| *Bull's Eye* | | | | | | | | | | |
| Hickory Smoke BBQ Sauce | 2 tbsp | 60 | 0 | 0 | 0 | 0 | 360 | 14 | 0 | 0 |
| Original BBQ Sauce | 2 tbsp | 60 | 0 | 0 | 0 | 0 | 370 | 14 | 0 | 0 |
| Sauce Sweet & Tangy BBQ Sauce | 2 tbsp | 60 | 0 | 0 | 0 | 0 | 310 | 13 | 0 | 0 |

# store brands

| | SERVING SIZE | CAL | CAL FAT | TOT FAT (G) | SAT FAT (G) | CHOL (MG) | SOD (MG) | CARB (G) | FIBER (G) | PROT (G) |
|---|---|---|---|---|---|---|---|---|---|---|
| **Bumble Bee** | | | | | | | | | | |
| **CLAMS** | | | | | | | | | | |
| Chopped | 2 oz | 25 | 0 | 0 | 0 | 5 | 350 | 3 | 0 | 3 |
| Fancy Whole Baby | 2 oz | 45 | 10 | 1 | .5 | 70 | 290 | 2 | 0 | 9 |
| **CRABMEAT** | | | | | | | | | | |
| Lump | 2 oz | 40 | 5 | .5 | 0 | 60 | 260 | 0 | 0 | 9 |
| Pink | 2 oz | 40 | 5 | .5 | 0 | 60 | 260 | 0 | 0 | 9 |
| White | 2 oz | 40 | 5 | .5 | 0 | 60 | 260 | 0 | 0 | 9 |
| **SALMON** | | | | | | | | | | |
| Pink | 2-1/5 oz | 80 | 30 | 3 | 1 | 50 | 270 | 0 | 0 | 12 |
| Premium Wild Pink Skinless & Boneless | 2 oz | 60 | 10 | 1.5 | .5 | 30 | 180 | 0 | 0 | 12 |
| **SARDINES** | | | | | | | | | | |
| In Oil | 1 can | 190 | 110 | 13 | 3 | 110 | 230 | 0 | 0 | 20 |
| In Water | 1 can | 140 | 70 | 7.5 | 1.5 | 100 | 270 | 0 | 0 | 19 |
| **SHRIMP** | | | | | | | | | | |
| Deveined Large | 2 oz | 40 | 0 | 0 | 0 | 115 | 430 | 0 | 0 | 10 |
| Deveined Medium | 2 oz | 70 | 5 | 1 | 0 | 130 | 250 | 0 | 0 | 15 |
| Deveined Small | 2 oz | 40 | 0 | 0 | 0 | 115 | 430 | 0 | 0 | 10 |
| Tiny | 2 oz | 70 | 5 | 1 | 0 | 130 | 250 | 0 | 0 | 15 |
| **TUNA** | | | | | | | | | | |
| Chunk Light in Oil | 2 oz | 70 | 25 | 3 | .5 | 25 | 180 | 0 | 0 | 13 |
| Chunk Light in Water | 2 oz | 50 | 5 | .5 | 0 | 30 | 180 | 0 | 0 | 13 |
| Chunk White Albacore in Oil | 2 oz | 80 | 30 | 3 | .5 | 25 | 140 | 0 | 0 | 12 |
| Chunk White Albacore in Water | 2 oz | 60 | 10 | 1 | 0 | 25 | 140 | 0 | 0 | 12 |
| Sensations Seasoned Medley Bowl, Lemon & Pepper | 3 oz | 110 | 30 | 3 | .5 | 25 | 350 | 2 | 0 | 18 |
| Solid White Albacore in Oil | 2 oz | 80 | 25 | 3 | .5 | 25 | 140 | 0 | 0 | 14 |
| Solid White Albacore in Water | 2 oz | 60 | 10 | 1 | 0 | 25 | 140 | 0 | 0 | 13 |
| **Bush's Best** | | | | | | | | | | |
| Baked Beans, Bold & Spicy | 1/2 cup | 110 | 10 | 1 | 0 | 0 | 560 | 24 | 5 | 6 |
| Boston Recipe Baked Beans | 1/2 cup | 150 | 10 | 1 | 0 | 0 | 440 | 31 | 5 | 6 |
| Country Style Baked Beans | 1/2 cup | 160 | 10 | 1 | 0 | 0 | 680 | 33 | 5 | 6 |
| Homestyle Baked Beans | 1/2 cup | 140 | 10 | 1 | 0 | 0 | 550 | 29 | 5 | 6 |
| Honey Baked Beans | 1/2 cup | 160 | 10 | 1 | 0 | 0 | 540 | 32 | 6 | 6 |
| Hot Chili | 1 cup | 250 | 90 | 10 | 4 | 15 | 1260 | 26 | 7 | 14 |
| Maple Cured Bacon Baked Beans | 1/2 cup | 140 | 10 | 1 | 0 | 0 | 620 | 28 | 5 | 6 |
| No Bean Chili | 1 cup | 240 | 120 | 14 | 5 | 25 | 1380 | 16 | 3 | 13 |

| | SERVING SIZE | CAL | CAL FAT | TOT FAT (G) | SAT FAT (G) | CHOL (MG) | SOD (MG) | CARB (G) | FIBER (G) | PROT (G) |
|---|---|---|---|---|---|---|---|---|---|---|
| Original Baked Beans | 1/2 cup | 140 | 10 | 1 | 0 | 0 | 550 | 29 | 5 | 6 |
| Original Chili | 1 cup | 250 | 90 | 10 | 4 | 15 | 1250 | 26 | 7 | 14 |
| Refried Beans, Fat Free | 1/2 cup | 130 | 0 | 0 | 0 | 0 | 490 | 24 | 7 | 9 |
| Refried Beans, Traditional | 1/2 cup | 150 | 25 | 3 | 1 | 0 | 490 | 24 | 7 | 9 |

## Cabot
### CHEDDAR

| | | | | | | | | | | |
|---|---|---|---|---|---|---|---|---|---|---|
| 50% Reduced Fat | 1 oz | 70 | 40 | 4.5 | 3 | 15 | 170 | <1 | 0 | 8 |
| 50% Reduced Fat Pepper Jack | 1 oz | 70 | 40 | 4.5 | 3 | 15 | 170 | <1 | 0 | 8 |
| 75% Reduced Fat | 1 oz | 60 | 20 | 2.5 | 1.5 | 10 | 200 | <1 | 0 | 9 |
| Chipotle | 1 oz | 110 | 80 | 9 | 6 | 30 | 180 | <1 | 0 | 7 |
| Classic Vermont Sharp Cheddar | 1 oz | 110 | 80 | 9 | 6 | 30 | 180 | <1 | 0 | 7 |
| Extra Sharp | 1 oz | 110 | 80 | 9 | 6 | 30 | 180 | <1 | 0 | 7 |
| Horseradish | 1 oz | 110 | 80 | 9 | 5 | 30 | 270 | 1 | 0 | 6 |
| Mild | 1 oz | 110 | 80 | 9 | 6 | 30 | 180 | 0 | 0 | 7 |
| New York Extra Sharp | 1 oz | 110 | 80 | 9 | 6 | 30 | 180 | <1 | 0 | 7 |
| Seriously Sharp | 1 oz | 110 | 80 | 9 | 6 | 30 | 180 | <1 | 0 | 7 |
| Sharp | 1 oz | 110 | 80 | 9 | 6 | 30 | 180 | <1 | 0 | 7 |

### OTHER CHEESES

| | | | | | | | | | | |
|---|---|---|---|---|---|---|---|---|---|---|
| American, White Slices | 1 slice | 70 | 45 | 5 | 3.5 | 10 | 260 | 2 | 0 | 4 |
| Colby Jack | 1 oz | 110 | 80 | 9 | 5 | 30 | 180 | 1 | 0 | 7 |
| Fancy Blend Shredded | 1/4 cup | 100 | 60 | 7 | 4 | 20 | 180 | 1 | 0 | 7 |
| Monterey Jack | 1 oz | 110 | 80 | 9 | 6 | 30 | 170 | <1 | 0 | 7 |
| Mozzarella, Shredded | 1/4 cup | 80 | 50 | 6 | 3.5 | 15 | 170 | 1 | 0 | 8 |
| Pepper Jack | 1 oz | 110 | 80 | 9 | 6 | 30 | 170 | <1 | 0 | 7 |
| Swiss, Slices | 1 oz | 110 | 70 | 8 | 4.5 | 25 | 60 | 1 | 0 | 8 |

## Campbell's
### CHUNKY SOUP

| | | | | | | | | | | |
|---|---|---|---|---|---|---|---|---|---|---|
| Baked Potato with Cheddar & Bacon Bits | 1 cup | 190 | 81 | 9 | 3 | 10 | 790 | 23 | 2 | 5 |
| Baked Potato with Steak & Cheese | 1 cup | 200 | 81 | 9 | 2.5 | 15 | 840 | 21 | 3 | 8 |
| Beef & Dumplings, Hearty Vegetables | 1 cup | 130 | 14 | 1.5 | .5 | 25 | 800 | 20 | 3 | 8 |
| Beef Rib Roast with Potatoes & Herbs | 1 cup | 110 | 9 | 1 | 1 | 10 | 890 | 17 | 2 | 7 |
| Beef with Country Vegetables | 1 cup | 130 | 27 | 3 | 1 | 15 | 920 | 18 | 3 | 8 |
| Beef with White & Wild Rice | 1 cup | 140 | 14 | 1.5 | .5 | 10 | 890 | 24 | 2 | 8 |
| Chicken & Dumplings Microwavable Bowls | 1 cup | 190 | 81 | 9 | 2 | 30 | 890 | 18 | 3 | 8 |
| Chicken Broccoli Cheese & Potato | 1 cup | 210 | 99 | 11 | 4 | 20 | 880 | 20 | 3 | 7 |
| Chicken Corn Chowder | 1 cup | 200 | 90 | 10 | 3 | 15 | 860 | 20 | 2 | 7 |
| Chicken Noodle Microwavable Bowls | 1 cup | 110 | 27 | 3 | 1 | 25 | 790 | 14 | 2 | 6 |

# store brands

| | SERVING SIZE | CAL | CAL FAT | TOT FAT (G) | SAT FAT (G) | CHOL (MG) | SOD (MG) | CARB (G) | FIBER (G) | PROT (G) |
|---|---|---|---|---|---|---|---|---|---|---|
| Classic Chicken Noodle | 1 cup | 120 | 28 | 3 | 1 | 25 | 790 | 14 | 2 | 8 |
| Creamy Chicken & Dumplings | 1 cup | 180 | 72 | 8 | 2 | 30 | 890 | 19 | 3 | 8 |
| Fajita Chicken with Rice and Beans | 1 cup | 130 | 14 | 1.5 | .5 | 15 | 850 | 23 | 2 | 7 |
| Grilled Chicken & Sausage Gumbo | 1 cup | 140 | 27 | 3 | 1.5 | 20 | 850 | 21 | 2 | 7 |
| Grilled Chicken with Vegetables & Pasta | 1 cup | 100 | 23 | 2.5 | .5 | 15 | 880 | 14 | 2 | 6 |
| Grilled Sirloin Steak with Hearty Vegetables | 1 cup | 130 | 18 | 2 | 1 | 10 | 890 | 19 | 3 | 8 |
| Grilled Steak Chili with Beans | 1 cup | 200 | 27 | 3 | 1 | 20 | 870 | 27 | 7 | 16 |
| Hearty Bean 'N' Ham | 1 cup | 170 | 14 | 1.5 | .5 | 10 | 780 | 28 | 8 | 10 |
| Hearty Beef Barley | 1 cup | 160 | 18 | 2 | .5 | 10 | 790 | 26 | 4 | 9 |
| Hearty Beef Noodle | 1 cup | 100 | 9 | 1 | .5 | 20 | 650 | 15 | 2 | 7 |
| Hearty Chicken with Vegetables | 1 cup | 110 | 18 | 2 | .5 | 15 | 710 | 17 | 3 | 6 |
| Hearty Italian Style Wedding | 1 cup | 160 | 27 | 3 | 1 | 15 | 650 | 24 | 3 | 8 |
| Hearty Tomato with Pasta | 1 cup | 140 | 9 | 1 | .5 | 5 | 650 | 28 | 3 | 5 |
| Manhattan Clam Chowder | 1 cup | 130 | 32 | 3.5 | 1 | 5 | 830 | 19 | 3 | 5 |
| New England Clam Chowder | 1 cup | 230 | 117 | 13 | 2 | 10 | 890 | 20 | 3 | 7 |
| Old Fashioned Potato Ham Chowder | 1 cup | 190 | 99 | 11 | 4 | 20 | 800 | 17 | 3 | 6 |
| Old Fashioned Vegetable Beef | 1 cup | 120 | 23 | 2.5 | 1 | 15 | 890 | 17 | 3 | 8 |
| Roasted Beef Tips with Vegetables | 1 cup | 130 | 14 | 1.5 | .5 | 15 | 800 | 20 | 2 | 8 |
| Salisbury Steak Mushrooms & Onions | 1 cup | 140 | 41 | 4.5 | 2.5 | 15 | 800 | 19 | 2 | 7 |
| Savory Chicken with White & Wild Rice | 1 cup | 110 | 18 | 2 | .5 | 10 | 810 | 18 | 2 | 6 |
| Savory Pot Roast | 1 cup | 120 | 9 | 1 | .5 | 10 | 790 | 20 | 2 | 7 |
| Savory Vegetable | 1 cup | 110 | 9 | 1 | .5 | 0 | 770 | 22 | 4 | 3 |
| Sirloin Burger with Country Vegetables | 1 cup | 130 | 23 | 2.5 | 1 | 15 | 800 | 18 | 3 | 8 |
| Slow Roasted Beef with Mushrooms | 1 cup | 120 | 14 | 1.5 | 1 | 15 | 830 | 18 | 3 | 8 |
| Split Pea 'N' Ham | 1 cup | 190 | 23 | 2.5 | 1 | 10 | 780 | 30 | 5 | 12 |
| Steak 'N' Potato | 1 cup | 120 | 18 | 2 | .5 | 15 | 920 | 18 | 3 | 8 |
| **CONDENSED SOUP** | | | | | | | | | | |
| Chicken & Stars | 1/2 cup | 70 | 18 | 2 | .5 | 5 | 480 | 11 | 1 | 3 |
| Chicken Noodle | 1/2 cup | 60 | 18 | 2 | .5 | 15 | 890 | 8 | 1 | 3 |
| Chicken Vegetable | 1/2 cup | 80 | 9 | 1 | .5 | 5 | 890 | 15 | 2 | 3 |
| Chicken with Rice | 1/2 cup | 70 | 14 | 1.5 | .5 | 5 | 610 | 13 | 1 | 2 |
| Cream of Broccoli | 1/2 cup | 90 | 45 | 5 | 1.5 | 5 | 750 | 12 | 1 | 2 |
| Cream of Chicken | 1/2 cup | 120 | 72 | 8 | 2.5 | 10 | 870 | 10 | 2 | 2 |
| Cream of Mushroom | 1/2 cup | 100 | 54 | 6 | 1 | 5 | 870 | 9 | 2 | 1 |
| Green Pea | 1/2 cup | 180 | 27 | 3 | 1 | 0 | 870 | 28 | 4 | 9 |
| Minestrone | 1/2 cup | 90 | 9 | 1 | .5 | 5 | 650 | 17 | 3 | 4 |
| New England Clam Chowder | 1/2 cup | 90 | 23 | 2.5 | .5 | 5 | 650 | 13 | 1 | 4 |

| | SERVING SIZE | CAL | CAL FAT | TOT FAT (G) | SAT FAT (G) | CHOL (MG) | SOD (MG) | CARB (G) | FIBER (G) | PROT (G) |
|---|---|---|---|---|---|---|---|---|---|---|
| Split Pea with Ham & Bacon | 1/2 cup | 180 | 18 | 2 | .5 | 5 | 850 | 30 | 4 | 10 |
| Tomato | 1/2 cup | 90 | 0 | 0 | 0 | 0 | 480 | 20 | 1 | 2 |
| Vegetable | 1/2 cup | 100 | 5 | .5 | .5 | 5 | 650 | 21 | 3 | 4 |
| Vegetable Beef | 1/2 cup | 90 | 9 | 1 | .5 | 5 | 890 | 15 | 3 | 5 |
| **HEALTHY REQUEST** | | | | | | | | | | |
| Chicken Noodle | 1/2 cup | 60 | 18 | 2 | .5 | 10 | 410 | 8 | 1 | 3 |
| Chicken Rice | 1/2 cup | 70 | 14 | 1.5 | .5 | 5 | 410 | 13 | 1 | 2 |
| Cream of Celery | 1/2 cup | 70 | 18 | 2 | .5 | <5 | 410 | 12 | 1 | 1 |
| Cream of Chicken | 1/2 cup | 80 | 23 | 2.5 | 1 | 5 | 410 | 12 | 1 | 2 |
| Cream of Mushroom | 1/2 cup | 70 | 18 | 2 | .5 | 5 | 410 | 10 | 1 | 2 |
| Homestyle Chicken Noodle | 1/2 cup | 60 | 14 | 1.5 | .5 | 10 | 410 | 10 | 1 | 3 |
| Minestrone | 1/2 cup | 80 | 5 | .5 | 0 | 0 | 410 | 15 | 3 | 3 |
| Tomato | 1/2 cup | 90 | 14 | 1.5 | .5 | 0 | 410 | 17 | 1 | 2 |
| Vegetable | 1/2 cup | 100 | 9 | 1 | 0 | 0 | 410 | 20 | 3 | 4 |
| Vegetable Beef | 1/2 cup | 90 | 9 | 1 | .5 | 5 | 410 | 15 | 3 | 5 |
| **Canada Dry** | | | | | | | | | | |
| Ginger Ale | 8 fl oz | 90 | 0 | 0 | 0 | 0 | 35 | 25 | 0 | 0 |
| **Cascadian Farm** | | | | | | | | | | |
| **CEREALS** | | | | | | | | | | |
| Multi Grain Squares | 3/4 cup | 110 | 5 | 1 | 0 | 0 | 115 | 25 | 2 | 3 |
| Oats & Honey Granola | 2/3 cup | 230 | 50 | 6 | 1 | 0 | 120 | 42 | 3 | 5 |
| Purely O's | 1 cup | 110 | 10 | 1 | 0 | 0 | 200 | 24 | 3 | 3 |
| Raisin Bran | 1 cup | 180 | 10 | 1 | 0 | 0 | 340 | 43 | 6 | 5 |
| **GRANOLA BARS** | | | | | | | | | | |
| Chewy Chocolate Chip | 1 bar | 140 | 30 | 4 | 1 | 0 | 100 | 25 | 1 | 2 |
| Chewy Dark Chocolate Almond | 1 bar | 130 | 35 | 4 | 1 | 0 | 100 | 25 | 5 | 2 |
| Chewy Sweet & Salty Mixed Nut | 1 bar | 160 | 70 | 8 | 3 | 0 | 125 | 20 | 1 | 3 |
| Chewy Fruit & Nut | 1 bar | 140 | 35 | 4 | 1 | 0 | 100 | 24 | 1 | 2 |
| **Cheerios** | | | | | | | | | | |
| Apple Cinnamon | 3/4 cup | 120 | 15 | 1.5 | 0 | 0 | 135 | 24 | 2 | 2 |
| Honey Nut | 3/4 cup | 110 | 10 | 1.5 | 0 | 0 | 160 | 22 | 2 | 2 |
| MultiGrain | 1 cup | 110 | 10 | 1 | 0 | 0 | 160 | 23 | 3 | 2 |
| Original | 1 cup | 110 | 15 | 2 | 0 | 0 | 160 | 20 | 3 | 3 |
| **Cheetos** | | | | | | | | | | |
| **CRUNCHY SNACKS** | | | | | | | | | | |
| Baked Flamin' Cheese | 1 oz | 130 | 45 | 5 | .5 | 0 | 240 | 19 | <1 | 3 |
| Cheese, Baked | 1 oz | 130 | 45 | 5 | 1 | 0 | 240 | 19 | 0 | 2 |

# store brands

| | SERVING SIZE | CAL | CAL FAT | TOT FAT (G) | SAT FAT (G) | CHOL (MG) | SOD (MG) | CARB (G) | FIBER (G) | PROT (G) |
|---|---|---|---|---|---|---|---|---|---|---|
| Puffs Cheese | 1 oz | 160 | 90 | 10 | 1.5 | 0 | 370 | 15 | <1 | 2 |
| Twisted Cheese | 1 oz | 160 | 90 | 10 | 1.5 | 0 | 350 | 13 | 0 | 2 |
| **Cheez Whiz** | | | | | | | | | | |
| Light | 1 oz | 80 | 30 | 3.5 | 2 | 20 | 500 | 6 | 0 | 6 |
| Original | 1 oz | 90 | 60 | 7 | 1.5 | 5 | 440 | 4 | 0 | 3 |
| **Chef Boyardee** | | | | | | | | | | |
| **BEEFARONI** | | | | | | | | | | |
| Big | 1 cup | 260 | 80 | 9 | 3.5 | 20 | 860 | 32 | 4 | 12 |
| Original | 1 cup | 240 | 80 | 9 | 3.5 | 15 | 720 | 30 | 3 | 9 |
| Whole Grain | 1 cup | 240 | 80 | 9 | 3.5 | 20 | 750 | 31 | 3 | 9 |
| **LASAGNA** | | | | | | | | | | |
| Original | 1 cup | 270 | 90 | 10 | 5 | 25 | 830 | 36 | 2 | 9 |
| Whole Grain | 1 cup | 270 | 90 | 10 | 4.5 | 15 | 670 | 35 | 4 | 9 |
| **PASTA** | | | | | | | | | | |
| Cheesy Burger Macaroni | 1 cup | 200 | 45 | 5 | 2.5 | 15 | 820 | 30 | 3 | 9 |
| Chili Mac | 1 cup | 260 | 120 | 13 | 5 | 20 | 940 | 26 | 3 | 9 |
| Spaghetti & Meatballs | 1 cup | 260 | 100 | 11 | 4 | 15 | 750 | 30 | 4 | 10 |
| **RAVIOLI** | | | | | | | | | | |
| 99% Fat Free Beef | 1 cup | 170 | 15 | 1.5 | .5 | 10 | 880 | 33 | 2 | 7 |
| Beef | 1 cup | 230 | 70 | 8 | 3 | 15 | 750 | 31 | 3 | 8 |
| Big Italian Sausage | 1 cup | 240 | 40 | 4.5 | 1.5 | 15 | 990 | 40 | 4 | 9 |
| **Chex** | | | | | | | | | | |
| **CEREAL** | | | | | | | | | | |
| Chocolate | 3/4 cup | 130 | 25 | 2.5 | 0 | 0 | 240 | 26 | <1 | 2 |
| Corn | 1 cup | 120 | 5 | .5 | 0 | 0 | 240 | 26 | 2 | 2 |
| Multi-Bran | 3/4 cup | 160 | 15 | 1.5 | 0 | 0 | 270 | 39 | 6 | 4 |
| Rice | 1 cup | 100 | 0 | 0 | 0 | 0 | 240 | 23 | 1 | 2 |
| Wheat | 3/4 cup | 160 | 10 | 1 | 0 | 0 | 300 | 39 | 5 | 5 |
| **CHEX MIX** | | | | | | | | | | |
| Cheddar | 1/2 cup | 130 | 35 | 4 | .5 | 0 | 220 | 21 | 1 | 2 |
| Bold Party Blend | 1/2 cup | 120 | 35 | 4 | 1 | 0 | 190 | 20 | 1 | 2 |
| Peanut Lovers | 1/2 cup | 140 | 50 | 6 | 1 | 0 | 200 | 19 | 1 | 3 |
| Select, Sweet 'n Salty Trail Mix | 1/2 cup | 150 | 45 | 5 | 1.5 | 0 | 95 | 24 | 1 | 3 |
| Traditional | 1/2 cup | 120 | 35 | 4 | 1 | 0 | 210 | 20 | 1 | 2 |
| **Chobani** | | | | | | | | | | |
| **LOWFAT GREEK YOGURT** | | | | | | | | | | |
| Pineapple | 6 oz | 160 | 25 | 2.5 | 2 | 5 | 65 | 21 | 0 | 13 |

| | SERVING SIZE | CAL | CAL FAT | TOT FAT (G) | SAT FAT (G) | CHOL (MG) | SOD (MG) | CARB (G) | FIBER (G) | PROT (G) |
|---|---|---|---|---|---|---|---|---|---|---|
| Plain | 6 oz | 130 | 30 | 3.5 | 2 | 10 | 70 | 7 | 0 | 17 |
| Strawberry Banana | 6 oz | 160 | 25 | 3 | 2 | 5 | 65 | 19 | 1 | 14 |
| **NONFAT GREEK YOGURT** | | | | | | | | | | |
| Blueberry | 6 oz | 140 | 0 | 0 | 0 | 0 | 65 | 20 | 1 | 14 |
| Honey | 6 oz | 150 | 0 | 0 | 0 | 0 | 75 | 20 | 0 | 16 |
| Peach | 6 oz | 140 | 0 | 0 | 0 | 0 | 65 | 20 | 1 | 14 |
| Plain | 6 oz | 100 | 0 | 0 | 0 | 0 | 80 | 7 | 0 | 18 |
| Pomegranate | 6 oz | 140 | 0 | 0 | 0 | 0 | 75 | 21 | 0 | 14 |
| Raspberry | 6 oz | 140 | 0 | 0 | 0 | 0 | 65 | 22 | 1 | 14 |
| Strawberry | 6 oz | 140 | 0 | 0 | 0 | 0 | 65 | 20 | 1 | 14 |
| Vanilla | 6 oz | 120 | 0 | 0 | 0 | 0 | 75 | 13 | 0 | 16 |
| **Claussen Pickles** | | | | | | | | | | |
| Bread 'n Butter Chips | 1 oz | 20 | 0 | 0 | 0 | 0 | 180 | 4 | 0 | 0 |
| Bread 'n Butter Sandwich Slices | 2 pieces | 25 | 0 | 0 | 0 | 0 | 210 | 5 | 0 | 0 |
| Deli Style Kosher Dill Spears | 2 pieces | 5 | 0 | 0 | 0 | 0 | 310 | 1 | 0 | 0 |
| Deli Style Kosher Dill, Halves | 1-1/2 oz | 5 | 0 | 0 | 0 | 0 | 450 | 1 | 0 | 0 |
| Half Sours, New York Deli Style, Wholes | 1 oz | 5 | 0 | 0 | 0 | 0 | 270 | 1 | 0 | 0 |
| Hearty Garlic Deli Style Wholes | 1 oz | 5 | 0 | 0 | 0 | 0 | 270 | 1 | 0 | 0 |
| Kosher Dill Burger Slices | 1 oz | 5 | 0 | 0 | 0 | 0 | 300 | 1 | 0 | 0 |
| Kosher Dill Halves | 1 oz | 5 | 0 | 0 | 0 | 0 | 270 | 1 | 0 | 0 |
| Kosher Dill Minis | 2 pieces | 5 | 0 | 0 | 0 | 0 | 290 | 1 | 0 | 0 |
| Kosher Dill Sandwich Slices | 2 pieces | 5 | 0 | 0 | 0 | 0 | 420 | 1 | 0 | 0 |
| Pickle Relish, Sweet Squeeze | 1-1/2 oz | 10 | 0 | 0 | 0 | 0 | 85 | 3 | 0 | 0 |
| Sauerkraut, Crisp | 1 oz | 5 | 0 | 0 | 0 | 0 | 220 | 1 | 1 | 0 |
| **Clif Bar** | | | | | | | | | | |
| Apricot | 1 bar | 230 | 30 | 3 | .5 | 0 | 125 | 45 | 5 | 10 |
| Banana Nut Bread | 1 bar | 240 | 50 | 6 | 1 | 0 | 120 | 42 | 4 | 9 |
| Black Cherry Almond | 1 bar | 250 | 45 | 5 | 1.5 | 0 | 110 | 44 | 5 | 10 |
| Blueberry Crisp | 1 bar | 240 | 50 | 5 | .5 | 0 | 150 | 43 | 5 | 9 |
| Cool Mint Chocolate | 1 bar | 250 | 50 | 5 | 1.5 | 0 | 140 | 43 | 5 | 10 |
| Cranberry Orange Nut Bread | 1 bar | 240 | 50 | 6 | 1 | 0 | 130 | 43 | 5 | 9 |
| Iced Gingerbread | 1 bar | 250 | 60 | 6 | 1.5 | 0 | 170 | 43 | 4 | 9 |
| Maple Nut | 1 bar | 240 | 50 | 5 | 1 | 0 | 220 | 42 | 5 | 10 |
| Oatmeal Raisin Walnut | 1 bar | 240 | 45 | 5 | 1 | 0 | 130 | 43 | 5 | 10 |
| Peanut Toffee Buzz | 1 bar | 250 | 50 | 6 | 2 | 0 | 200 | 42 | 5 | 11 |
| Spiced Pumpkin Pie | 1 bar | 240 | 40 | 4.5 | 1 | 0 | 170 | 45 | 4 | 9 |
| White Chocolate Macadamia Nut | 1 bar | 240 | 60 | 7 | 1.5 | 0 | 160 | 41 | 4 | 9 |

| | SERVING SIZE | CAL | CAL FAT | TOT FAT (G) | SAT FAT (G) | CHOL (MG) | SOD (MG) | CARB (G) | FIBER (G) | PROT (G) |
|---|---|---|---|---|---|---|---|---|---|---|
| **Coca-Cola** | | | | | | | | | | |
| **SOFT DRINKS** | | | | | | | | | | |
| Cherry | 12 fl oz | 150 | 0 | 0 | 0 | 0 | 35 | 42 | 0 | 0 |
| Classic | 12 fl oz | 140 | 0 | 0 | 0 | 0 | 45 | 39 | 0 | 0 |
| Vanilla | 12 fl oz | 150 | 0 | 0 | 0 | 0 | 35 | 42 | 0 | 0 |
| **Coffee-Mate** | | | | | | | | | | |
| **LIQUID CREAMER** | | | | | | | | | | |
| Fat Free Cinnamon Vanilla Crème | 1 tbsp | 25 | 0 | 0 | 0 | 0 | 25 | 5 | n/a | 0 |
| Fat Free French Vanilla | 1 tbsp | 25 | 0 | 0 | 0 | 0 | 25 | 5 | n/a | 0 |
| Fat Free Hazelnut | 1 tbsp | 25 | 0 | 0 | 0 | 0 | 25 | 5 | n/a | 0 |
| Fat Free Original | 1 tbsp | 10 | 0 | 0 | 0 | 0 | 0 | 1 | n/a | 0 |
| Fat Free Vanilla Caramel | 1 tbsp | 25 | 0 | 0 | 0 | 0 | 25 | 5 | n/a | 0 |
| French Vanilla | 1 tbsp | 35 | 15 | 1.5 | 0 | 0 | 30 | 5 | n/a | 0 |
| Hazelnut | 1 tbsp | 35 | 15 | 1.5 | 0 | 0 | 0 | 5 | n/a | 0 |
| Low Fat Original | 1 tbsp | 10 | 5 | .5 | 0 | 0 | 5 | 2 | n/a | 0 |
| Original | 1 tbsp | 20 | 10 | 1 | 0 | 0 | 0 | 2 | n/a | 0 |
| Sugar Free French Vanilla | 1 tbsp | 15 | 10 | 1 | 0 | 0 | 0 | 2 | n/a | 0 |
| Sugar Free Hazelnut | 1 tbsp | 15 | 10 | 1 | 0 | 0 | 5 | 2 | n/a | 0 |
| Sugar Free Vanilla Caramel | 1 tbsp | 15 | 10 | 1 | 0 | 0 | 0 | 2 | n/a | 0 |
| **POWDER CREAMER** | | | | | | | | | | |
| Fat Free French Vanilla | 4 tsp | 50 | 0 | 0 | 0 | 0 | 15 | 11 | n/a | 0 |
| Fat Free Original | 1 tsp | 10 | 0 | 0 | 0 | 0 | 0 | 2 | n/a | 0 |
| French Vanilla | 4 tsp | 60 | 25 | 2.5 | 2 | 0 | 15 | 9 | n/a | 0 |
| Hazelnut | 4 tsp | 60 | 25 | 3 | 2.5 | 0 | 15 | 9 | n/a | 0 |
| Original | 2 tsp | 10 | 5 | .5 | .5 | 0 | 0 | 1 | n/a | 0 |
| Sugar Free French Vanilla | 1 tbsp | 30 | 25 | 2.5 | 2 | 0 | 15 | 2 | n/a | 0 |
| Sugar Free Hazelnut | 3 tsp | 30 | 25 | 2.5 | 2 | 0 | 15 | 2 | n/a | 0 |
| **Combos** | | | | | | | | | | |
| Cheddar Cheese Cracker | 1 oz | 140 | 60 | 6 | 3 | 0 | 290 | 18 | 0 | 2 |
| Cheddar Cheese Pretzel | 1 oz | 130 | 40 | 4.5 | 3 | 0 | 440 | 19 | 0 | 3 |
| Nacho Cheese Pretzel | 1 oz | 130 | 40 | 4.5 | 3 | 0 | 460 | 19 | 1 | 3 |
| Pepperoni Pizza Cracker | 1 oz | 140 | 60 | 6 | 3 | 0 | 280 | 18 | 0 | 2 |
| Pizzeria Pretzel | 1 oz | 130 | 40 | 4.5 | 2.5 | 0 | 450 | 19 | 1 | 2 |
| **Comet Cups** | | | | | | | | | | |
| Ice Cream Cup | 1 cone | 20 | 0 | 0 | 0 | 0 | 10 | 4 | 0 | 0 |
| Ice Cream Cup, Rainbow | 1 cone | 20 | 0 | 0 | 0 | 1 | 10 | 4 | 1 | 0 |
| Sugar Cone | 1 cone | 50 | 0 | 0 | 0 | 0 | 20 | 11 | 0 | 1 |

| | SERVING SIZE | CAL | CAL FAT | TOT FAT (G) | SAT FAT (G) | CHOL (MG) | SOD (MG) | CARB (G) | FIBER (G) | PROT (G) |
|---|---|---|---|---|---|---|---|---|---|---|
| **Cool Whip** | | | | | | | | | | |
| Extra Creamy | 1/3 oz | 20 | 15 | 2 | 1.5 | 0 | 5 | 2 | 0 | 0 |
| Lite | 1/3 oz | 20 | 10 | 1 | 1 | 0 | 0 | 3 | 1 | 0 |
| Original | 1/3 oz | 25 | 15 | 1.5 | 1.5 | 0 | 0 | 2 | 0 | 0 |
| **Country Time** | | | | | | | | | | |
| Lemonade | 8 fl oz | 60 | n/a | 0 | n/a | n/a | 25 | 16 | n/a | 0 |
| Lemonade Iced Tea | 8 fl oz | 90 | n/a | 0 | n/a | n/a | 10 | 22 | n/a | 0 |
| Lite Lemonade | 8 fl oz | 35 | n/a | 0 | n/a | n/a | 10 | 8 | n/a | 0 |
| Lite Pink Lemonade | 8 fl oz | 35 | n/a | 0 | n/a | n/a | 10 | 8 | n/a | 0 |
| Pink Lemonade | 8 fl oz | 60 | n/a | 0 | n/a | n/a | 25 | 16 | n/a | 0 |
| Raspberry Lemonade | 8 fl oz | 80 | n/a | 0 | n/a | n/a | 0 | 19 | n/a | 0 |
| Strawberry Lemonade | 8 fl oz | 80 | n/a | 0 | n/a | n/a | 0 | 20 | n/a | 0 |
| **Cracker Barrel** | | | | | | | | | | |
| **CHEDDAR, EXTRA SHARP** | | | | | | | | | | |
| 2% Milk, Reduced Fat | 1 oz | 90 | 50 | 6 | 3.5 | 20 | 240 | 1 | 0 | 7 |
| 2% Reduced Fat, Shredded | 1 oz | 80 | 50 | 6 | 3.5 | 20 | 240 | 1 | 0 | 7 |
| Cheddar | 1 oz | 120 | 90 | 10 | 7 | 30 | 180 | 0 | 0 | 6 |
| Vermont Sharp White | 1 oz | 110 | 80 | 9 | 6 | 30 | 180 | 1 | 0 | 7 |
| White Cheddar | 1 oz | 120 | 90 | 10 | 6 | 30 | 180 | 0 | 0 | 6 |
| White Cheddar, Reduced Fat | 1 oz | 90 | 50 | 6 | 3.5 | 20 | 240 | 1 | 0 | 7 |
| **SWISS** | | | | | | | | | | |
| Baby Swiss | 1 oz | 110 | 80 | 9 | 6 | 25 | 110 | 0 | 0 | 7 |
| **Crisco** | | | | | | | | | | |
| **NO-STICK SPRAYS** | | | | | | | | | | |
| 100% Extra Virgin Olive Oil | 1/4 g | 0 | 0 | 0 | 0 | 0 | 0 | 0 | 0 | 0 |
| Butter Flavor | 1/4 g | 0 | 0 | 0 | 0 | 0 | 0 | 0 | 0 | 0 |
| Original | 1/4 g | 0 | 0 | 0 | 0 | 0 | 0 | 0 | 0 | 0 |
| **OILS** | | | | | | | | | | |
| 100% Extra Virgin Olive | 1 tbsp | 120 | 120 | 14 | 2 | 0 | 0 | 0 | 0 | 0 |
| Canola with Omega-3 DHA | 1 tbsp | 120 | 120 | 14 | 1 | 0 | 0 | 0 | 0 | 0 |
| Vegetable | 1 tbsp | 120 | 120 | 14 | 2 | 0 | 0 | 0 | 0 | 0 |
| **SHORTENING STICKS** | | | | | | | | | | |
| All-Vegetable | 1 tbsp | 110 | 110 | 12 | 3 | 0 | 0 | 0 | 0 | 0 |
| Butter Flavor, All-Vegetable | 1 tbsp | 110 | 110 | 12 | 3 | 0 | 0 | 0 | 0 | 0 |
| **Crystal Light** | | | | | | | | | | |
| **REFRESHMENT MIX** | | | | | | | | | | |
| Fruit Punch | 1 g | 5 | 0 | 0 | 0 | 0 | 10 | 0 | 0 | 0 |

| | SERVING SIZE | CAL | CAL FAT | TOT FAT (G) | SAT FAT (G) | CHOL (MG) | SOD (MG) | CARB (G) | FIBER (G) | PROT (G) |
|---|---|---|---|---|---|---|---|---|---|---|
| Lemonade | 2 g | 5 | 0 | 0 | 0 | 0 | 35 | 0 | 0 | 0 |
| Pink Lemonade | 2 g | 5 | 0 | 0 | 0 | 0 | 0 | 0 | 0 | 0 |
| Raspberry Ice | 1 g | 5 | 0 | 0 | 0 | 0 | 0 | 0 | 0 | 0 |
| Raspberry Lemonade | 1 g | 5 | 0 | 0 | 0 | 0 | 0 | 0 | 0 | 0 |
| **TEA MIX** | | | | | | | | | | |
| Green Peach Mango | 1 g | 5 | 0 | 0 | 0 | 0 | 5 | 0 | 0 | 0 |
| Iced | 1 g | 5 | 0 | 0 | 0 | 0 | 0 | 0 | 0 | 0 |
| Peach Iced | 1 g | 5 | 0 | 0 | 0 | 0 | 0 | 0 | 0 | 0 |
| Raspberry | 1 g | 5 | 0 | 0 | 0 | 0 | 0 | 0 | 0 | 0 |
| **Daisy Sour Cream** | | | | | | | | | | |
| Light | 2 tbsp | 40 | 25 | 2.5 | 2 | 10 | 25 | 2 | 0 | 2 |
| Regular | 2 tbsp | 60 | 45 | 5 | 3.5 | 20 | 15 | 1 | 0 | 1 |
| **Dannon** | | | | | | | | | | |
| **ALL NATURAL** | | | | | | | | | | |
| Coffee | 6 oz | 150 | 25 | 2.5 | 1.5 | 10 | 100 | 25 | 0 | 7 |
| Lemon | 6 oz | 150 | 25 | 2.5 | 1.5 | 10 | 100 | 25 | 0 | 7 |
| Plain, Nonfat | 6 oz | 80 | 0 | 0 | 0 | 5 | 120 | 12 | 0 | 9 |
| Plain, Regular | 6 oz | 160 | 70 | 8 | 5 | 20 | 120 | 12 | 0 | 9 |
| Vanilla | 6 oz | 150 | 25 | 2.5 | 1.5 | 10 | 100 | 25 | 0 | 7 |
| **FRUIT ON THE BOTTOM YOGURT** | | | | | | | | | | |
| Blueberry | 6 oz | 140 | 15 | 1.5 | 1 | 5 | 130 | 26 | <1 | 6 |
| Mixed Berry | 6 oz | 150 | 15 | 1.5 | 1.5 | 5 | 120 | 27 | <1 | 6 |
| Raspberry | 6 oz | 150 | 15 | 1.5 | 1 | 5 | 115 | 28 | <1 | 6 |
| Strawberry Banana | 6 oz | 150 | 15 | 1.5 | 1 | 5 | 95 | 26 | <1 | 6 |
| Strawberry | 6 oz | 150 | 15 | 1.5 | 1 | 5 | 110 | 28 | <1 | 6 |
| **LIGHT & FIT YOGURT** | | | | | | | | | | |
| Banana | 6 oz | 80 | 0 | 0 | 0 | <5 | 75 | 16 | n/a | 5 |
| Blackberry | 6 oz | 80 | 0 | 0 | 0 | <5 | 75 | 16 | n/a | 5 |
| Blueberry | 6 oz | 80 | 0 | 0 | 0 | <5 | 75 | 16 | n/a | 5 |
| Cherry Vanilla | 6 oz | 80 | 0 | 0 | 0 | <5 | 80 | 16 | n/a | 5 |
| Key Lime | 6 oz | 80 | 0 | 0 | 0 | <5 | 95 | 16 | n/a | 5 |
| Lemon Chiffon | 6 oz | 80 | 0 | 0 | 0 | <5 | 80 | 15 | n/a | 5 |
| Mixed Berry | 6 oz | 80 | 0 | 0 | 0 | <5 | 85 | 15 | n/a | 5 |
| Peach | 6 oz | 80 | 0 | 0 | 0 | <5 | 75 | 16 | n/a | 5 |
| Raspberry | 6 oz | 80 | 0 | 0 | 0 | <5 | 75 | 16 | n/a | 5 |
| Strawberry Banana | 6 oz | 80 | 0 | 0 | 0 | <5 | 75 | 16 | n/a | 5 |

| | SERVING SIZE | CAL | CAL FAT | TOT FAT (G) | SAT FAT (G) | CHOL (MG) | SOD (MG) | CARB (G) | FIBER (G) | PROT (G) |
|---|---|---|---|---|---|---|---|---|---|---|
| Strawberry Cheesecake | 6 oz | 80 | 0 | 0 | 0 | <5 | 75 | 15 | n/a | 5 |
| Strawberry | 6 oz | 80 | 0 | 0 | 0 | <5 | 80 | 16 | n/a | 5 |
| Vanilla | 6 oz | 80 | 0 | 0 | 0 | <5 | 75 | 16 | n/a | 5 |
| White Chocolate Raspberry | 6 oz | 80 | 0 | 0 | 0 | <5 | 75 | 16 | n/a | 5 |

## DiGiorno Pizza

| | SERVING SIZE | CAL | CAL FAT | TOT FAT (G) | SAT FAT (G) | CHOL (MG) | SOD (MG) | CARB (G) | FIBER (G) | PROT (G) |
|---|---|---|---|---|---|---|---|---|---|---|
| 12" Rising Crust—Four Cheese | 1/6 pizza | 310 | 100 | 11 | 5 | 25 | 850 | 40 | 2 | 15 |
| 12" Rising Crust—Three Meat | 1/6 pizza | 350 | 130 | 15 | 6 | 30 | 1010 | 41 | 2 | 16 |
| Cheese Stuffed Crust—Five Cheese | 5 oz | 390 | 160 | 17 | 9 | 45 | 1160 | 39 | 2 | 20 |
| Cheese Stuffed Crust—Pepperoni | 5 oz | 380 | 150 | 16 | 8 | 40 | 1040 | 40 | 3 | 19 |
| Classic Thin Crust—Four Cheese | 4-1/2 oz | 330 | 120 | 14 | 7 | 35 | 670 | 33 | 3 | 19 |
| Classic Thin Crust—Pepperoni | 4-1/2 oz | 340 | 140 | 16 | 7 | 35 | 800 | 33 | 3 | 17 |
| Crispy Flatbread Supreme | 4-1/2 oz | 380 | 200 | 22 | 9 | 45 | 980 | 28 | 4 | 16 |
| Deep Dish (Small Pizza)—Four Cheese | 4 oz | 290 | 150 | 16 | 8 | 20 | 440 | 26 | 2 | 12 |
| Deep Dish (Small Pizza)—Pepperoni | 4 oz | 300 | 150 | 17 | 8 | 25 | 470 | 26 | 2 | 12 |
| Thin Crispy Crust (Small Pizza)—Pepperoni | 8-1/2 oz | 590 | 220 | 24 | 11 | 50 | 1170 | 63 | 3 | 31 |
| Traditional Crust (Small Pizza)—Four Cheese | 26 oz | 720 | 270 | 30 | 12 | 35 | 1190 | 84 | 6 | 28 |
| Traditional Crust (Small Pizza)—Pepperoni | 10 oz | 770 | 320 | 35 | 14 | 45 | 1430 | 83 | 6 | 30 |
| Ultimate Toppings—Cheese | 4 oz | 320 | 120 | 13 | 7 | 35 | 820 | 34 | 2 | 16 |
| Ultimate Toppings—Pepperoni | 4 oz | 370 | 170 | 19 | 9 | 40 | 1080 | 34 | 2 | 17 |

## Doritos Tortilla Chips

| | SERVING SIZE | CAL | CAL FAT | TOT FAT (G) | SAT FAT (G) | CHOL (MG) | SOD (MG) | CARB (G) | FIBER (G) | PROT (G) |
|---|---|---|---|---|---|---|---|---|---|---|
| Baked Nacho Cheese | 1 oz | 120 | 30 | 3.5 | .5 | 0 | 230 | 21 | 2 | 2 |
| Cool Ranch | 1 oz | 150 | 70 | 8 | 1 | 0 | 180 | 18 | 2 | 2 |
| Nacho Cheese | 1 oz | 150 | 70 | 8 | 1.5 | 0 | 180 | 17 | 1 | 2 |

## Dove

### CHOCOLATES

| | SERVING SIZE | CAL | CAL FAT | TOT FAT (G) | SAT FAT (G) | CHOL (MG) | SOD (MG) | CARB (G) | FIBER (G) | PROT (G) |
|---|---|---|---|---|---|---|---|---|---|---|
| Promises Silky Smooth Milk Chocolate | 5 pieces | 220 | 110 | 13 | 8 | 5 | 25 | 24 | 1 | 2 |
| Promises Silky Smooth Dark Chocolate | 5 pieces | 210 | 120 | 14 | 7 | 5 | 10 | 21 | 2 | 3 |
| Silky Smooth Dark Chocolate Bar, Roasted Almond | 1 item | 180 | 100 | 12 | 6 | 5 | 10 | 18 | 2 | 3 |
| Silky Smooth Milk Chocolate Bar, Roasted Hazelnut | 1 item | 190 | 110 | 12 | 6 | 5 | 20 | 18 | 1 | 2 |

### ICE CREAM

| | SERVING SIZE | CAL | CAL FAT | TOT FAT (G) | SAT FAT (G) | CHOL (MG) | SOD (MG) | CARB (G) | FIBER (G) | PROT (G) |
|---|---|---|---|---|---|---|---|---|---|---|
| Ice Cream Bar, Milk Chocolate with Almonds | 1 item | 340 | 200 | 23 | 13 | 35 | 135 | 28 | 1 | 6 |
| Ice Cream, Beyond Vanilla | 1/2 cup | 240 | 140 | 15 | 10 | 50 | 60 | 23 | 2 | 4 |

## Dr. Pepper

| | SERVING SIZE | CAL | CAL FAT | TOT FAT (G) | SAT FAT (G) | CHOL (MG) | SOD (MG) | CARB (G) | FIBER (G) | PROT (G) |
|---|---|---|---|---|---|---|---|---|---|---|
| Original | 8 oz | 100 | 0 | 0 | 0 | 0 | 35 | 27 | 0 | 0 |

| | SERVING SIZE | CAL | CAL FAT | TOT FAT (G) | SAT FAT (G) | CHOL (MG) | SOD (MG) | CARB (G) | FIBER (G) | PROT (G) |
|---|---|---|---|---|---|---|---|---|---|---|
| **Drumstick** | | | | | | | | | | |
| Chocolate | 1 cone | 310 | 150 | 17 | 9 | 15 | 115 | 34 | 2 | 5 |
| Vanilla | 1 cone | 290 | 140 | 16 | 9 | 15 | 100 | 33 | 2 | 4 |
| Vanilla Caramel | 1 cone | 310 | 140 | 16 | 9 | 15 | 90 | 37 | 2 | 4 |
| Vanilla Fudge | 1 cone | 310 | 140 | 16 | 9 | 15 | 10 | 37 | 2 | 5 |
| **Duncan Hines** | | | | | | | | | | |
| **BROWNIE MIX (PREPARED)** | | | | | | | | | | |
| Dark Chocolate Premium Brownie | 1/18 package | 190 | 80 | 9 | 2 | 25 | 135 | 25 | 1 | <1 |
| Decadent Chocolate Marble Swirl Brownie | 1/18 package | 170 | 80 | 9 | 2 | 25 | 115 | 23 | 1 | <1 |
| Decadent Chocolate Peanut Butter Brownie | 1/16 package | 160 | 70 | 8 | 2.5 | 15 | 100 | 23 | 1 | <1 |
| Decadent Dark Fudge Chunk Brownie | 1/16 package | 160 | 60 | 7 | 1.5 | 15 | 120 | 24 | 1 | <1 |
| Decadent Triple Chocolate Brownie | 1/16 package | 180 | 70 | 8 | 2 | 15 | 115 | 25 | 1 | 2 |
| **CAKE MIX (PREPARED)** | | | | | | | | | | |
| Decadent Apple Caramel Cake | 1/12 package | 280 | 110 | 12 | 3 | 50 | 280 | 39 | 0 | 3 |
| Decadent Classic Carrot Cake | 1/12 package | 260 | 90 | 10 | 2.5 | 55 | 280 | 39 | 1 | 4 |
| Decadent Triple Chocolate Cake | 1/12 package | 270 | 110 | 12 | 3.5 | 55 | 300 | 39 | 2 | 4 |
| **FROSTING & GLAZES** | | | | | | | | | | |
| Whipped Chocolate Frosting | 3 tbsp | 140 | 60 | 7 | 2 | 0 | 70 | 20 | 0 | 0 |
| Whipped Cream Cheese Frosting | 3 tbsp | 160 | 70 | 8 | 2.5 | 0 | 70 | 22 | 0 | 0 |
| Whipped Fluffy White Frosting | 3 tbsp | 150 | 60 | 7 | 2 | 0 | 60 | 22 | 0 | 0 |
| Whipped Vanilla Frosting | 3 tbsp | 150 | 60 | 7 | 2 | 0 | 60 | 22 | 0 | 0 |
| **MUFFIN MIX (PREPARED)** | | | | | | | | | | |
| 100% Whole Grain Apple Cinnamon with Oatmeal Granola Topping | 1/12 package | 220 | 70 | 8 | 1.5 | 35 | 240 | 34 | 3 | 4 |
| 100% Whole Grain Blueberry Streusel | 1/12 package | 210 | 70 | 8 | 1.5 | 35 | 230 | 32 | 3 | 3 |
| **Edy's** | | | | | | | | | | |
| **FRUIT BARS** | | | | | | | | | | |
| Grape | 1 item | 80 | 0 | 0 | 0 | 0 | 0 | 20 | 0 | 0 |
| Lemonade | 1 item | 80 | 0 | 0 | 0 | 0 | 0 | 20 | 0 | 0 |
| Lime | 1 item | 80 | 0 | 0 | 0 | 0 | 0 | 20 | 0 | 0 |
| Variety Pack—Lime, Strawberry, Wildberry | 1 item | 60 | 0 | 0 | 0 | 0 | 0 | 13 | 0 | 0 |
| Variety Pack—Snack Size: Grape, Cherry, Tropical | 1 item | 50 | 0 | 0 | 0 | 0 | 0 | 13 | 0 | 0 |
| Variety Pack—Snack Size: Orange & Cream, Raspberry & Cream, Lime & Cream | 1 item | 45 | 5 | 0 | 0 | 0 | 15 | 9 | 0 | 0 |

| | SERVING SIZE | CAL | CAL FAT | TOT FAT (G) | SAT FAT (G) | CHOL (MG) | SOD (MG) | CARB (G) | FIBER (G) | PROT (G) |
|---|---|---|---|---|---|---|---|---|---|---|
| **ICE CREAM** | | | | | | | | | | |
| Dibs, Chocolate | 26 pieces | 360 | 230 | 25 | 16 | 15 | 85 | 30 | 2 | 3 |
| Dibs, Vanilla | 26 pieces | 340 | 220 | 24 | 15 | 15 | 70 | 30 | 1 | 2 |
| Fun Flavors—Chocolate Peanut Butter cup | 1/2 cup | 170 | 70 | 8 | 4 | 15 | 85 | 21 | 1 | 3 |
| Fun Flavors—Cookies 'N Cream | 1/2 cup | 130 | 40 | 4 | 2 | 10 | 80 | 20 | 0 | 1 |
| Fun Flavors—Nestle Butterfinger | 1/2 cup | 160 | 60 | 7 | 3 | 10 | 90 | 22 | 0 | 2 |
| Fun Flavors—Nestle Drumstick Sundae Cone | 1/2 cup | 160 | 60 | 7 | 4 | 10 | 60 | 21 | 0 | 2 |
| Fun Flavors—Nestle Toll House Cookie Dough | 1/2 cup | 150 | 50 | 6 | 4 | 15 | 65 | 23 | 0 | 2 |
| Fun Flavors—Nestle Vanilla Sandwich | 1/2 cup | 120 | 35 | 4 | 2 | 10 | 80 | 21 | 0 | 1 |
| Grand—Chocolate | 1/2 cup | 150 | 70 | 8 | 4.5 | 25 | 35 | 17 | 1 | 3 |
| Grand—Chocolate Chip | 1/2 cup | 160 | 80 | 9 | 6 | 25 | 45 | 18 | 0 | 2 |
| Grand—Coffee | 1/2 cup | 130 | 60 | 7 | 4 | 25 | 35 | 15 | 0 | 2 |
| Grand—French Vanilla | 1/2 cup | 150 | 80 | 9 | 5 | 50 | 35 | 16 | 0 | 2 |
| Grand—Mint Chocolate Chip | 1/2 cup | 160 | 80 | 9 | 6 | 25 | 45 | 18 | 0 | 2 |
| Grand—Neapolitan | 1/2 cup | 140 | 60 | 7 | 4 | 25 | 35 | 16 | 0 | 2 |
| Grand—Rocky Road | 1/2 cup | 190 | 100 | 11 | 5 | 30 | 35 | 19 | 1 | 3 |
| Grand—Vanilla | 1/2 cup | 140 | 70 | 8 | 4 | 25 | 35 | 15 | 0 | 2 |
| Grand—Vanilla Chocolate | 1/2 cup | 150 | 70 | 8 | 4.5 | 25 | 30 | 16 | 1 | 3 |
| Slow Churned—Chocolate | 1/2 cup | 100 | 30 | 4 | 2 | 20 | 30 | 15 | 0 | 3 |
| Slow Churned—Chocolate Chip | 1/2 cup | 120 | 40 | 4 | 3 | 20 | 50 | 17 | 0 | 3 |
| Slow Churned—Coffee | 1/2 cup | 105 | 30 | 3.5 | 2 | 20 | 45 | 15 | 0 | 3 |
| Slow Churned—Cookie Dough | 1/2 cup | 130 | 40 | 4.5 | 3 | 20 | 60 | 20 | 0 | 3 |
| Slow Churned —Cookies 'N Cream | 1/2 cup | 120 | 35 | 4 | 2 | 20 | 60 | 18 | 0 | 3 |
| Slow Churned—Neapolitan | 1/2 cup | 100 | 25 | 3 | 2 | 20 | 35 | 15 | 0 | 3 |
| Slow Churned—Rocky Road | 1/2 cup | 120 | 35 | 4 | 2 | 15 | 30 | 17 | 0 | 3 |
| Slow Churned—Strawberry | 1/2 cup | 110 | 25 | 3 | 1.5 | 15 | 40 | 18 | 0 | 2 |
| Slow Churned—Vanilla | 1/2 cup | 100 | 30 | 3.5 | 2 | 20 | 45 | 15 | 0 | 3 |
| **SHERBET** | | | | | | | | | | |
| Tropical Rainbow | 1/2 cup | 130 | 10 | 1 | .5 | 0 | 35 | 29 | 0 | 1 |
| **Egg Beaters** | | | | | | | | | | |
| Egg Whites | 3 tbsp | 25 | 0 | 0 | 0 | 0 | 75 | 1 | 0 | 5 |
| Original | 1/4 cup | 30 | 0 | 0 | 0 | 0 | 115 | 1 | 0 | 6 |
| **Entenmann's** | | | | | | | | | | |
| **BUNS** | | | | | | | | | | |
| Cheese Topped | 1 bun | 320 | 140 | 15 | 6 | 55 | 320 | 40 | 1 | 6 |
| Cinnamon Swirl | 1 bun | 320 | 130 | 14 | 5 | 45 | 280 | 44 | 2 | 5 |
| Crumb | 1 bun | 240 | 100 | 11 | 4 | 20 | 210 | 32 | 1 | 3 |

# store brands

| | SERVING SIZE | CAL | CAL FAT | TOT FAT (G) | SAT FAT (G) | CHOL (MG) | SOD (MG) | CARB (G) | FIBER (G) | PROT (G) |
|---|---|---|---|---|---|---|---|---|---|---|
| **CAKES** | | | | | | | | | | |
| All Butter Loaf Cake | 1/6 cake | 220 | 80 | 9 | 5 | 70 | 270 | 30 | 0 | 3 |
| Angel Food Cake | 1/6 cake | 160 | 0 | .5 | 0 | 0 | 240 | 35 | 0 | 3 |
| Cheese Filled Crumb Coffee Cake | 1/9 cake | 200 | 90 | 10 | 4 | 35 | 190 | 25 | <1 | 4 |
| Crumb Coffee Cake | 1/10 cake | 260 | 120 | 13 | 4 | 15 | 210 | 34 | 1 | 3 |
| Sour Cream Loaf Cake | 1/8 cake | 210 | 110 | 12 | 3.5 | 40 | 150 | 24 | 0 | 2 |
| Swiss Chocolate Chip Cake | 1/9 cake | 320 | 140 | 15 | 5 | 40 | 240 | 44 | 1 | 3 |
| **DANISHES** | | | | | | | | | | |
| Cheese Danish Twist | 1/8 Danish | 230 | 110 | 12 | 5 | 25 | 210 | 29 | <1 | 3 |
| Cherry Cheese Danish | 1/9 Danish | 200 | 80 | 9 | 3.5 | 25 | 170 | 25 | <1 | 3 |
| **DONUTS** | | | | | | | | | | |
| Frosted Mini Donuts | 1 donut | 160 | 100 | 11 | 7 | 5 | 90 | 15 | <1 | 1 |
| Glazed Donuts | 1 donut | 210 | 100 | 11 | 3 | 5 | 190 | 25 | <1 | 3 |
| Plain Donuts Softee Family Pack | 1 donut | 190 | 100 | 11 | 5 | 0 | 210 | 21 | <1 | 2 |
| Softees Frosted Donuts Bag | 3 donuts | 230 | 120 | 14 | 9 | 20 | 240 | 24 | <1 | 2 |
| Softees Powdered Donuts Bag | 4 donuts | 250 | 110 | 12 | 6 | 25 | 290 | 32 | <1 | 3 |
| **LITTLE BITES** | | | | | | | | | | |
| Banana Muffins | 1 pckg | 180 | 70 | 8 | 1.5 | 20 | 125 | 25 | 0 | 2 |
| Blueberry Muffins | 1 pckg | 180 | 70 | 8 | 1.5 | 25 | 190 | 25 | 0 | 2 |
| Chocolate Chip Muffins | 1 pckg | 190 | 80 | 9 | 2.5 | 20 | 135 | 26 | <1 | 2 |
| **OTHERS** | | | | | | | | | | |
| Éclairs | 1 éclair | 260 | 80 | 9 | 2.5 | 65 | 190 | 46 | 3 | 3 |
| Apple Puffs | 1 puff | 290 | 130 | 14 | 7 | 0 | 260 | 39 | 1 | 3 |
| Cheese Pastry Pockets | 1 pocket | 220 | 110 | 12 | 6 | 10 | n/a | n/a | <1 | n/a |
| Ultimate Cinnamon Pastry Twisters | 2 twisters | 70 | 20 | 2 | 1 | 0 | 55 | 11 | 0 | 1 |
| **PIES** | | | | | | | | | | |
| Apple Snack Pie | 1 pie | 430 | 220 | 24 | 13 | 0 | 320 | 50 | <1 | 0 |
| Cherry Snack Pie | 1 pie | 420 | 220 | 24 | 13 | 0 | 320 | 50 | <1 | 3 |
| **Equal** | | | | | | | | | | |
| Packet | 1 packet | 0 | 0 | 0 | 0 | 0 | 0 | <1 | 0 | 0 |
| Granular | 1 tsp | 0 | 0 | 0 | 0 | 0 | 0 | <1 | 0 | 0 |
| **Fleischmann's** | | | | | | | | | | |
| Margarine | 1 tbsp | 80 | 80 | 9 | 2 | 0 | 110 | 0 | 0 | 0 |
| Original Soft Spread | 1 tbsp | 60 | 60 | 7 | 1 | 0 | 35 | 0 | 0 | 0 |
| **Florida's Natural** | | | | | | | | | | |
| Original Orange | 8 fl oz | 110 | 0 | 0 | 0 | 0 | 0 | 26 | 0 | 2 |
| Ruby Red Grapefruit | 8 fl oz | 90 | 0 | 0 | 0 | 0 | 0 | 22 | 0 | 1 |

| | SERVING SIZE | CAL | CAL FAT | TOT FAT (G) | SAT FAT (G) | CHOL (MG) | SOD (MG) | CARB (G) | FIBER (G) | PROT (G) |
|---|---|---|---|---|---|---|---|---|---|---|
| **Fresh Gourmet** | | | | | | | | | | |
| **TRADITIONAL CROUTONS** | | | | | | | | | | |
| Classic Caesar | 6 pieces | 30 | 10 | 1 | 0 | 0 | 80 | 5 | 0 | 1 |
| Fat Free Garlic Caesar | 6 pieces | 30 | 5 | 0 | 0 | 0 | 55 | 5 | 0 | 1 |
| Fat Free Parmesan Ranch | 6 pieces | 30 | 5 | 0 | 0 | 0 | 80 | 5 | 0 | 1 |
| Italian Seasoned | 6 pieces | 30 | 10 | 1 | 0 | 0 | 80 | 5 | 0 | 1 |
| **Fritos** | | | | | | | | | | |
| **CORN CHIPS** | | | | | | | | | | |
| BBQ Flavored | 1 oz | 150 | 90 | 10 | 1.5 | 0 | 280 | 16 | 1 | 2 |
| Original | 1 oz | 160 | 90 | 10 | 1.5 | 0 | 170 | 15 | 1 | 2 |
| **DIPS** | | | | | | | | | | |
| Chili Cheese | 2 tbsp | 45 | 30 | 3 | 1 | 0 | 290 | 3 | <1 | 1 |
| Mild Cheddar Cheese | 2 tbsp | 50 | 30 | 3.5 | .5 | <5 | 340 | 4 | 0 | 1 |
| **Gardenburger** | | | | | | | | | | |
| **MEATLESS CHICKEN** | | | | | | | | | | |
| BBQ | 1 item | 250 | 72 | 8 | 1 | 0 | 890 | 30 | 5 | 14 |
| Buffalo Wings | 3 pieces | 180 | 108 | 12 | 1.5 | 0 | 1000 | 8 | 5 | 0 |
| Flame Grilled | 1 item | 100 | 22 | 2.5 | 0 | 0 | 360 | 5 | 3 | 13 |
| **VEGGIE BURGERS** | | | | | | | | | | |
| Original | 1 item | 100 | 30 | 3 | 1 | 10 | 400 | 18 | 5 | 5 |
| **Gold Peak Tea** | | | | | | | | | | |
| Sweetened | 8 fl oz | 80 | 0 | 0 | 0 | 0 | 25 | 21 | 0 | 0 |
| Unsweetened | 8 fl oz | 0 | 0 | 0 | 0 | 0 | 25 | 0 | 0 | 0 |
| **Good Humor** | | | | | | | | | | |
| **ICE CREAM BARS** | | | | | | | | | | |
| Dark & Milk Chocolate | 1 bar | 180 | 120 | 13 | 9 | 15 | 30 | 15 | 1 | 2 |
| Oreo | 1 bar | 250 | 140 | 15 | 8 | 15 | 150 | 28 | 1 | 3 |
| Reese's | 1 bar | 310 | 80 | 21 | 12 | 15 | 85 | 27 | 1 | 4 |
| **ICE CREAM SANDWICHES** | | | | | | | | | | |
| Chocolate Chip Cookie | 1 sandwich | 270 | 90 | 10 | 6 | 5 | 200 | 44 | 1 | 3 |
| Giant Neapolitan | 1 sandwich | 250 | 80 | 9 | 6 | 20 | 130 | 38 | 1 | 4 |
| Giant Vanilla | 1 sandwich | 250 | 80 | 9 | 6 | 20 | 125 | 38 | 1 | 0 |
| **Gorton's** | | | | | | | | | | |
| **FILLETS** | | | | | | | | | | |
| All Natural Cajun Blackened Gilled | 1 piece | 100 | 25 | 3 | .5 | 60 | 330 | 1 | 0 | 17 |

# store brands

| | SERVING SIZE | CAL | CAL FAT | TOT FAT (G) | SAT FAT (G) | CHOL (MG) | SOD (MG) | CARB (G) | FIBER (G) | PROT (G) |
|---|---|---|---|---|---|---|---|---|---|---|
| All Natural Italian Herb Grilled | 1 piece | 100 | 25 | 3 | .5 | 60 | 300 | 1 | 0 | 16 |
| All Natural Lemon Pepper Grilled | 1 piece | 100 | 25 | 3 | .5 | 70 | 290 | 1 | 0 | 17 |
| Beer Battered | 2 pieces | 250 | 160 | 18 | 4.5 | 25 | 550 | 16 | 1 | 7 |
| Grilled Tilapia, Roasted Garlic & Butter | 1 piece | 80 | 25 | 2.5 | .5 | 50 | 150 | <1 | 0 | 14 |
| Lemon Butter Grilled | 1 piece | 100 | 25 | 3 | .5 | 75 | 320 | 1 | 0 | 17 |
| Lemon Herb Breaded | 2 pieces | 240 | 120 | 13 | 2.5 | 25 | 720 | 21 | 0 | 9 |
| Lemon Pepper Battered | 2 pieces | 270 | 160 | 18 | 4.5 | 20 | 580 | 20 | 1 | 8 |
| Premium Tilapia Fish, Breaded | 1 piece | 250 | 110 | 12 | 3.5 | 25 | 480 | 23 | 1 | 12 |
| Salmon Classic Grilled | 1 piece | 100 | 25 | 3 | .5 | 35 | 270 | 2 | 0 | 15 |
| **TENDERS** | | | | | | | | | | |
| Beer Battered | 3 pieces | 230 | 130 | 14 | 3.5 | 20 | 650 | 18 | 2 | 7 |
| Extra Crunchy | 3 pieces | 190 | 70 | 10 | 2.5 | 30 | 610 | 22 | 0 | 8 |
| Original Batter | 3 pieces | 230 | 110 | 12 | 3 | 20 | 660 | 23 | 2 | 8 |
| **SHRIMP** | | | | | | | | | | |
| Beer Battered | 3-1/2 oz | 240 | 110 | 12 | 3.5 | 40 | 670 | 25 | 0 | 7 |
| Grilled, Classic | 1/2 cup, frzn | 110 | 15 | 1.5 | 0 | 50 | 920 | 5 | 0 | 18 |
| Scampi | 4 oz | 120 | 50 | 6 | 1 | 65 | 630 | 8 | <1 | 10 |
| **Goya** | | | | | | | | | | |
| **CANNED BEANS** | | | | | | | | | | |
| Black Beans | 1/2 cup | 90 | 5 | .5 | 0 | 0 | 460 | 19 | 6 | 7 |
| Blackeye Peas | 1/2 cup | 90 | 0 | 0 | 0 | 0 | 380 | 19 | 5 | 7 |
| Chickpeas | 1/2 cup | 100 | 20 | 2 | 0 | 0 | 360 | 20 | 7 | 6 |
| Kidney Beans in Sauce | 1/2 cup | 110 | 15 | 1.5 | n/a | n/a | 450 | 18 | 7 | 6 |
| Low Sodium Black Beans | 1/2 cup | 100 | 0 | 0 | 0 | 0 | 125 | 18 | 8 | 7 |
| Low Sodium Chickpeas | 1/2 cup | 100 | 5 | .5 | 0 | 0 | 120 | 20 | 7 | 6 |
| Low Sodium Pinto Beans | 1/2 cup | 100 | 0 | 0 | 0 | 0 | 115 | 18 | 7 | 6 |
| Low Sodium Red Kidney Beans | 1/2 cup | 110 | 0 | 0 | 0 | 0 | 110 | 19 | 8 | 8 |
| Navy Beans | 1/2 cup | 90 | 10 | 1 | 0 | 0 | 390 | 19 | 9 | 6 |
| Pinto Beans | 1/2 cup | 80 | 10 | 1 | 0 | 0 | 360 | 18 | 8 | 6 |
| Red Kidney Beans | 1/2 cup | 90 | 5 | 1 | 0 | 0 | 350 | 19 | 8 | 7 |
| Refried Pinto Beans, Traditional | 1/2 cup | 140 | 15 | 1.5 | 0 | 0 | 480 | 24 | 7 | 9 |
| Small White Beans | 1/2 cup | 90 | 0 | 0 | 0 | 0 | 360 | 19 | 6 | 6 |
| **RICE** | | | | | | | | | | |
| Chicken Flavored Rice Mix | 1/4 cup | 160 | 0 | 0 | 0 | 0 | 560 | 35 | 3 | 4 |
| Mexican Style Rice Mix, Chicken Flavor | 1/4 cup | 160 | 0 | 0 | 0 | 0 | 325 | 37 | 0 | 3 |
| Rice & Black Beans Rice Mix | 1/4 cup | 160 | 0 | 0 | 0 | 0 | 445 | 34 | 3 | 5 |
| Rice Primavera Rice Mix | 1/4 cup | 160 | 0 | 0 | 0 | 0 | 405 | 35 | 1 | 5 |

| | SERVING SIZE | CAL | CAL FAT | TOT FAT (G) | SAT FAT (G) | CHOL (MG) | SOD (MG) | CARB (G) | FIBER (G) | PROT (G) |
|---|---|---|---|---|---|---|---|---|---|---|
| Spanish Rice Mix | 1/4 cup | 160 | 5 | .5 | 0 | 0 | 830 | 34 | 1 | 4 |
| Yellow Rice Mix | 1/4 cup | 160 | 0 | 0 | 0 | 0 | 820 | 36 | 1 | 4 |

## Green Giant

### FROZEN BAGGED VEGETABLES IN SAUCE

| | SERVING SIZE | CAL | CAL FAT | TOT FAT (G) | SAT FAT (G) | CHOL (MG) | SOD (MG) | CARB (G) | FIBER (G) | PROT (G) |
|---|---|---|---|---|---|---|---|---|---|---|
| Alfredo Vegetables | 1 cup | 60 | 15 | 1.5 | .5 | 0 | 360 | 9 | 2 | 3 |
| Broccoli & Three Cheese Sauce | 1-1/4 cups | 45 | 15 | 1.5 | .5 | 0 | 420 | 7 | 2 | 3 |
| Broccoli and Carrots with Garlic Herbs | 1-1/4 cups | 40 | 5 | .5 | 0 | 0 | 200 | 7 | 2 | 2 |
| Broccoli Carrots Cauliflower & Cheese Sauce | 1 cup | 45 | 10 | 1 | 0 | 0 | 380 | 7 | 2 | 2 |
| Cauliflower & Three Cheese Sauce | 2-3/4 cups | 45 | 10 | 1.5 | 0 | 0 | 390 | 7 | 1 | 2 |
| Pasta, Broccoli & Alfredo Sauce | 2-1/4 cups | 220 | 35 | 4 | 1 | 5 | 710 | 38 | 3 | 9 |
| Pasta, Broccoli, Carrots, & Cheese Sauce | 2-3/4 cups | 220 | 30 | 3.5 | 1 | 0 | 880 | 36 | 3 | 8 |
| Pasta, Carrots, Broccoli, Sugar Snap Peas, & Garlic Sauce | 2 cups | 210 | 35 | 4 | 1.5 | 0 | 700 | 37 | 3 | 7 |
| Roasted Potatoes, Broccoli & Cheese Sauce | 1 cup | 110 | 15 | 2 | .5 | 0 | 640 | 20 | 2 | 4 |

### FROZEN VALLEY FRESH STEAMERS

| | SERVING SIZE | CAL | CAL FAT | TOT FAT (G) | SAT FAT (G) | CHOL (MG) | SOD (MG) | CARB (G) | FIBER (G) | PROT (G) |
|---|---|---|---|---|---|---|---|---|---|---|
| Asian Style Medley | 1 cup | 50 | 15 | 1.5 | .5 | 0 | 135 | 8 | 2 | 2 |
| Broccoli & Cheese Sauce | 1 cup | 45 | 10 | 1.5 | 0 | 0 | 380 | 7 | 2 | 2 |
| Broccoli Carrots Cauliflower & Cheese Sauce | 1 cup | 45 | 10 | 1 | 0 | 0 | 290 | 8 | 2 | 2 |
| Healthy Colors Market Blend | 1 cup | 40 | 10 | 1 | 0 | 0 | 210 | 7 | 2 | 1 |
| Healthy Colors Nature's Blend | 1 cup | 40 | 10 | 1 | 0 | 0 | 220 | 8 | 2 | 1 |
| Healthy Colors Valley Blend | 1-1/4 cups | 40 | 10 | 1 | .5 | 0 | 270 | 8 | 2 | 1 |
| Roasted Red Potatoes Green Beans & Rosemary Butter Sauce | 1-1/4 cups | 80 | 10 | 1 | .5 | 0 | 330 | 16 | 2 | 2 |

### FROZEN VEGETABLES

| | SERVING SIZE | CAL | CAL FAT | TOT FAT (G) | SAT FAT (G) | CHOL (MG) | SOD (MG) | CARB (G) | FIBER (G) | PROT (G) |
|---|---|---|---|---|---|---|---|---|---|---|
| Baby Brussels Sprouts & Butter Sauce | 2/3 cup | 60 | 10 | 1 | .5 | <5 | 320 | 9 | 3 | 3 |
| Baby Lima Beans & Butter Sauce | 2/3 cup | 100 | 15 | 1.5 | 1 | <5 | 420 | 18 | 5 | 5 |
| Baby Sweet Peas & Butter Sauce | 3/4 cup | 80 | 15 | 1.5 | 1 | <5 | 340 | 14 | 4 | 5 |
| Broccoli & Cheese Sauce | 2/3 cup | 60 | 25 | 2.5 | 1 | 0 | 460 | 7 | 2 | 2 |
| Broccoli Cauliflower Peas & Cheese Sauce | 2/3 cup | 60 | 25 | 2.5 | 1 | 0 | 440 | 8 | 2 | 2 |
| Broccoli Spears & Butter | 4 oz | 40 | 15 | 1.5 | 1 | 5 | 330 | 6 | 2 | 2 |
| Broccoli Spears, No Sauce | 3-1/2 oz | 25 | 0 | 0 | 0 | 0 | 120 | 4 | 2 | 2 |
| Cauliflower & Cheese Sauce | 1 pckg | 50 | 20 | 2.5 | 1 | 0 | 410 | 6 | 1 | 2 |
| Cheesy Rice & Broccoli | 1 pckg | 270 | 45 | 5 | 1.5 | 5 | 960 | 51 | 2 | 7 |

# store brands

| | SERVING SIZE | CAL | CAL FAT | TOT FAT (G) | SAT FAT (G) | CHOL (MG) | SOD (MG) | CARB (G) | FIBER (G) | PROT (G) |
|---|---|---|---|---|---|---|---|---|---|---|
| Chopped Spinach, No Sauce | 1/2 cup | 25 | 0 | 0 | 0 | 0 | 200 | 3 | 1 | 2 |
| Cream Style Corn | 1/2 cup | 110 | 10 | 1 | 0 | 0 | 320 | 24 | 2 | 2 |
| Creamed Spinach | 1/2 cup | 70 | 25 | 2.5 | 1.5 | 0 | 510 | 9 | 1 | 3 |
| Cut Broccoli, No Sauce | 2/3 cup | 20 | 0 | 0 | 0 | 0 | 105 | 4 | 2 | 1 |
| Cut Leaf Spinach & Butter | 1/2 cup | 30 | 10 | 1 | 0 | <5 | 330 | 4 | 2 | 2 |
| Green Bean Casserole | 2/3 cup | 110 | 70 | 8 | 3 | 0 | 450 | 9 | 1 | 2 |
| Honey Glazed Carrots | 1 cup | 90 | 30 | 3 | 1.5 | 0 | 180 | 15 | 3 | 1 |
| Niblets Corn & Butter Sauce | 1-1/4 cups | 80 | 15 | 1.5 | .5 | 0 | 270 | 15 | 2 | 2 |
| Roasted Potatoes w/Garlic & Herbs | 1 cup | 200 | 60 | 7 | 1.5 | 0 | 420 | 33 | 2 | 3 |
| Simply Steam Baby Vegetable Medley Seasoned | 1-1/2 cups | 50 | 5 | .5 | 0 | 0 | 280 | 11 | 1 | 2 |
| Simply Steam Broccoli & Carrots | 1-1/2 cups | 60 | 25 | 3 | 0 | 0 | 260 | 8 | 3 | 2 |
| Simply Steam Garden Vegetable Medley | 1 cup | 50 | 5 | .5 | 0 | 0 | 280 | 11 | 1 | 2 |
| Simply Steam No Sauce Asparagus Cuts | 2/3 cup | 20 | 0 | 0 | 0 | 0 | 90 | 3 | <1 | 2 |
| Simply Steam No Sauce Baby Lima Beans | 1/2 cup | 80 | 0 | 0 | 0 | 0 | 170 | 15 | 3 | 4 |
| Simply Steam No Sauce Baby Sweet Peas | 2/3 cup | 60 | 5 | .5 | 0 | 0 | 190 | 13 | 4 | 4 |
| Simply Steam No Sauce Green Beans & Almonds | 2/3 cup | 50 | 25 | 3 | 0 | 0 | 95 | 5 | 2 | 2 |
| Simply Steam No Sauce Niblets Corn | 2/3 cup | 70 | 5 | 1 | 0 | 0 | 55 | 13 | 2 | 2 |
| Simply Steam No Sauce Shoepeg White Corn | 1/2 cup | 70 | 10 | 1 | 0 | 0 | 45 | 15 | 2 | 2 |
| Simply Steam No Sauce Sugar Snap Peas | 2/3 cup | 45 | 0 | 0 | 0 | 0 | 95 | 10 | 2 | 2 |
| Simply Steam No Sauce Sweet Peas & Pearl Onions | 1-1/4 cup | 60 | 0 | 0 | 0 | 0 | 80 | 10 | 3 | 3 |
| Simply Steam Teriyaki Vegetables | 1-1/4 cups | 40 | 0 | 0 | 0 | 0 | 400 | 9 | 2 | 2 |
| **Grey Poupon** | | | | | | | | | | |
| Country Dijon Mustard | 1 tsp | 5 | 0 | 0 | 0 | 0 | 120 | 0 | 0 | 0 |
| Deli Mustard | 1 tsp | 5 | 0 | 0 | 0 | 0 | 50 | 0 | 0 | 0 |
| Hearty Spicy Brown Mustard | 1 tsp | 5 | 0 | 0 | 0 | 0 | 65 | 0 | 0 | 0 |
| **Gulden's Mustard** | | | | | | | | | | |
| Spicy Brown | 1 tsp | 5 | 0 | 0 | 0 | 0 | 50 | 0 | 0 | 0 |
| Yellow Squeeze | 1 tsp | 5 | 0 | 0 | 0 | 0 | 55 | 0 | 0 | 0 |
| Zesty Honey | 1 tsp | 10 | 0 | 0 | 0 | 0 | 35 | 2 | 0 | 0 |
| **Häagen-Dazs** | | | | | | | | | | |
| **BARS** | | | | | | | | | | |
| Chocolate & Dark Chocolate | 1 bar | 290 | 180 | 20 | 12 | 65 | 30 | 24 | 2 | 4 |
| Vanilla & Almonds | 1 bar | 310 | 200 | 22 | 13 | 65 | 40 | 22 | >1 | 5 |

| | SERVING SIZE | CAL | CAL FAT | TOT FAT (G) | SAT FAT (G) | CHOL (MG) | SOD (MG) | CARB (G) | FIBER (G) | PROT (G) |
|---|---|---|---|---|---|---|---|---|---|---|
| Vanilla & Dark Chocolate | 1 bar | 300 | 190 | 21 | 13 | 70 | 45 | 23 | 1 | 4 |
| Vanilla & Milk Chocolate | 1 bar | 290 | 190 | 21 | 14 | 75 | 55 | 22 | 0 | 4 |
| **FIVE ICE CREAM** | | | | | | | | | | |
| Caramel | 1/2 cup | 240 | 100 | 11 | 7 | 75 | 55 | 29 | 0 | 5 |
| Coffee | 1/2 cup | 220 | 100 | 12 | 7 | 70 | 50 | 23 | 0 | 5 |
| Milk Chocolate | 1/2 cup | 220 | 110 | 12 | 7 | 75 | 75 | 22 | <1 | 6 |
| Mint | 1/2 cup | 220 | 110 | 12 | 7 | 70 | 50 | 24 | 0 | 5 |
| Strawberry | 1/2 cup | 210 | 100 | 11 | 6 | 65 | 40 | 24 | 0 | 4 |
| Vanilla Bean | 1/2 cup | 220 | 100 | 11 | 7 | 70 | 50 | 24 | 0 | 5 |
| **FROZEN YOGURT** | | | | | | | | | | |
| Peach Low Fat | 1/2 cup | 170 | 20 | 2 | 1 | 40 | 40 | 31 | 0 | 8 |
| Raspberry Fat Free | 1/2 cup | 120 | 0 | 0 | 0 | 0 | 0 | 30 | 2 | 0 |
| Strawberry Fat Free | 1/2 cup | 120 | 0 | 0 | 0 | 0 | 0 | 31 | 1 | 0 |
| Vanilla Low Fat | 1/2 cup | 200 | 40 | 4.5 | 2.5 | 65 | 55 | 31 | 0 | 9 |
| **ICE CREAM** | | | | | | | | | | |
| Chocolate | 1/2 cup | 270 | 160 | 17 | 10 | 90 | 45 | 22 | 1 | 5 |
| Chocolate Chip Cookie Dough | 1/2 cup | 310 | 180 | 20 | 12 | 95 | 125 | 29 | 0 | 4 |
| Coffee | 1/2 cup | 270 | 160 | 18 | 11 | 120 | 70 | 21 | 0 | 5 |
| Cookies & Cream | 1/2 cup | 270 | 150 | 17 | 10 | 105 | 95 | 23 | 0 | 5 |
| Dulce de Leche | 1/2 cup | 290 | 150 | 17 | 10 | 100 | 95 | 28 | 0 | 5 |
| Mint Chip | 1/2 cup | 300 | 170 | 19 | 12 | 105 | 85 | 26 | <1 | 5 |
| Rocky Road | 1/2 cup | 300 | 160 | 18 | 9 | 90 | 75 | 29 | 1 | 5 |
| Strawberry | 1/2 cup | 250 | 140 | 16 | 10 | 95 | 65 | 23 | <1 | 4 |
| Vanilla | 1/2 cup | 270 | 160 | 18 | 11 | 120 | 70 | 21 | 0 | 5 |
| **SORBET** | | | | | | | | | | |
| Chocolate Lowfat | 1/2 cup | 130 | 5 | .5 | 0 | 0 | 70 | 28 | 2 | 2 |
| Coffee Lowfat | 1/2 cup | 200 | 40 | 4.5 | 2.5 | 65 | 50 | 31 | 0 | 8 |
| Dulche de Leche Lowfat | 1/2 cup | 190 | 25 | 2.5 | 2 | 5 | 75 | 35 | 0 | 6 |
| **Hamburger Helper** | | | | | | | | | | |
| **CHICKEN (NOT PREPARED)** | | | | | | | | | | |
| Creamy Chicken & Noodles | 1/4 pckg | 280 | 80 | .5 | 0 | 0 | 620 | 20 | <1 | 3 |
| Fettuccine Alfredo | 1/4 pckg | 280 | 70 | 3 | 1 | 0 | 700 | 25 | 1 | 4 |
| **COMPLETE MEALS (NOT PREPARED)** | | | | | | | | | | |
| Cheesy Chicken | 1/4 pckg | 210 | 50 | 5 | 1 | 10 | 850 | 31 | 1 | 9 |
| Chicken & Buttermilk Biscuits | 1/4 pckg | 270 | 80 | 9 | 3 | 10 | 220 | 36 | 2 | 7 |

| | SERVING SIZE | CAL | CAL FAT | TOT FAT (G) | SAT FAT (G) | CHOL (MG) | SOD (MG) | CARB (G) | FIBER (G) | PROT (G) |
|---|---|---|---|---|---|---|---|---|---|---|
| Chicken Fettuccine Alfredo | 1/4 pckg | 190 | 40 | 4.5 | 1 | 10 | 880 | 29 | 1 | 8 |
| Chicken with Cheesy Rice & Broccoli | 1/4 pckg | 210 | 45 | 5 | 1 | 10 | 820 | 34 | <1 | 7 |
| **OTHER ENTRÉES (NOT PREPARED)** | | | | | | | | | | |
| Cheesy Baked Potato | 1/4 pckg | 120 | 5 | .5 | 0 | 0 | 750 | 27 | 1 | 2 |
| Cheesy Hash Browns | 1/4 pckg | 170 | 10 | 1.5 | .5 | 1 | 870 | 36 | 2 | 3 |
| Cheesy Nacho | 1/4 pckg | 140 | 10 | 1 | 0 | 0 | 630 | 31 | 1 | 3 |
| Philly Cheese Steak | 1/4 pckg | 130 | 20 | 2 | 1 | 0 | 670 | 25 | 1 | 4 |
| **PASTA (NOT PREPARED)** | | | | | | | | | | |
| Beef | 1/4 pckg | 100 | 5 | .5 | 0 | 0 | 690 | 21 | 1 | 3 |
| Cheeseburger Macaroni | 1/4 pckg | 110 | 5 | .5 | 0 | 0 | 810 | 23 | <1 | 3 |
| Double Cheeseburger Macaroni | 1/4 pckg | 120 | 10 | 1 | 0 | 0 | 630 | 25 | 0 | 3 |
| Italian Lasagna | 1/4 pckg | 120 | 5 | .5 | 1 | 1 | 800 | 26 | <1 | 3 |
| Tomato Basil Penne | 1/4 pckg | 150 | 5 | 1 | 0 | 0 | 650 | 31 | 1 | 4 |
| **TUNA (NOT PREPARED)** | | | | | | | | | | |
| Cheesy Pasta | 1/4 pckg | 300 | 110 | 12 | 3 | 15 | 820 | 35 | 1 | 13 |
| Creamy Broccoli | 1/4 pckg | 290 | 110 | 12 | 3 | 20 | 870 | 34 | 2 | 14 |
| Creamy Parmesan | 1/4 pckg | 290 | 80 | 3 | 2.5 | 15 | 851 | 37 | 1 | 15 |
| Tuna Melt | 1/4 pckg | 300 | 90 | 10 | 3 | 15 | 1050 | 39 | <1 | 14 |
| **Healthy Choice** | | | | | | | | | | |
| **CAFÉ STEAMERS** | | | | | | | | | | |
| Chicken Margherita | 1 package | 330 | 80 | 8 | 1.5 | 30 | 500 | 42 | 4 | 21 |
| Chicken Pesto Classico | 1 package | 310 | 80 | 8 | 2 | 30 | 530 | 38 | 4 | 20 |
| Grilled Chicken Marinara | 1 package | 260 | 40 | 4 | 1.5 | 30 | 550 | 35 | 6 | 21 |
| Roasted Chicken Marsala | 1 package | 250 | 60 | 6 | 1.5 | 35 | 540 | 28 | 4 | 20 |
| Sweet Sesame Chicken | 1 package | 340 | 60 | 6 | 1 | 30 | 330 | 53 | 3 | 17 |
| **COMPLETE MEALS** | | | | | | | | | | |
| Beef Pot Roast | 1 package | 280 | 45 | 4.5 | 1.5 | 40 | 500 | 41 | 6 | 17 |
| Chicken Fettuccini Alfredo | 1 package | 300 | 70 | 7 | 2.5 | 45 | 580 | 39 | 7 | 20 |
| Chicken Parmigiana | 1 package | 350 | 90 | 10 | 2 | 25 | 580 | 49 | 7 | 16 |
| Classic Meatloaf | 1 package | 350 | 80 | 8 | 3 | 35 | 550 | 54 | 8 | 15 |
| Golden Roasted Turkey Breast | 1 package | 290 | 40 | 4.5 | 1 | 30 | 460 | 44 | 8 | 17 |
| Oven Roasted Chicken | 1 package | 250 | 45 | 5 | 1 | 35 | 540 | 35 | 5 | 14 |
| Sweet & Sour Chicken | 1 package | 420 | 90 | 9 | 2 | 20 | 480 | 71 | 6 | 14 |
| **FRENCH BREAD PIZZA** | | | | | | | | | | |
| Cheese | 1 pizza | 340 | 45 | 5 | 1.5 | 5 | 520 | 52 | 5 | 21 |
| Pepperoni | 1 pizza | 340 | 40 | 4.5 | 1.5 | 10 | 520 | 53 | 5 | 21 |

| | SERVING SIZE | CAL | CAL FAT | TOT FAT (G) | SAT FAT (G) | CHOL (MG) | SOD (MG) | CARB (G) | FIBER (G) | PROT (G) |
|---|---|---|---|---|---|---|---|---|---|---|
| **FROZEN TREATS** | | | | | | | | | | |
| Fudge Bar | 1 item | 80 | 15 | 1.5 | 1 | 5 | 65 | 13 | 4 | 3 |
| Vanilla Ice Cream Sandwich | 1 item | 150 | 15 | 1.5 | .5 | 5 | 120 | 30 | 0 | 4 |
| **PASTA** | | | | | | | | | | |
| Creamy Basil Pesto | 1 package | 240 | 70 | 7 | 2.5 | 10 | 510 | 35 | 5 | 9 |
| Mediterranean | 1 package | 340 | 40 | 4.5 | 2 | 10 | 410 | 62 | 12 | 12 |
| Tomato Basil Penne | 1 package | 280 | 60 | 6 | 2.5 | 10 | 600 | 44 | 7 | 13 |
| Tortellini Primavera Parmesan | 1 package | 230 | 45 | 5 | 2 | 20 | 490 | 37 | 6 | 9 |
| **SELECT ENTRÉES** | | | | | | | | | | |
| Chicken Alfredo Florentine | 1 package | 220 | 40 | 4.5 | 2 | 30 | 530 | 28 | 4 | 16 |
| Salisbury Steak | 1 package | 170 | 45 | 5 | 2 | 30 | 500 | 18 | 4 | 13 |
| Sesame Chicken | 1 package | 310 | 40 | 4.5 | 1 | 25 | 310 | 53 | 4 | 14 |
| **Hebrew National** | | | | | | | | | | |
| **BEEF FRANKS** | | | | | | | | | | |
| 97% Fat Free | 1 frank | 40 | 10 | 1 | 0 | 10 | 520 | 3 | 0 | 6 |
| Beef | 1 frank | 150 | 130 | 14 | 6 | 25 | 460 | 1 | 0 | 6 |
| Reduced Fat Beef | 1 frank | 110 | 80 | 9 | 3.5 | 20 | 490 | 2 | 0 | 5 |
| **KNOCKWURST & POLISH SAUSAGE** | | | | | | | | | | |
| Knockwurst | 1 item | 270 | 230 | 25 | 10 | 45 | 810 | 2 | 0 | 10 |
| Polish Sausage | 1 item | 250 | 210 | 23 | 9 | 40 | 870 | 1 | 0 | 10 |
| **SLICED LUNCH MEATS** | | | | | | | | | | |
| Beef Bologna | 1 slice | 80 | 70 | 8 | 3.5 | 15 | 240 | 0 | 0 | 3 |
| Beef Salami | 3 slices | 150 | 120 | 13 | 6 | 35 | 420 | 0 | 0 | 8 |
| Lean Beef Bologna | 4 slices | 90 | 45 | 5 | 2.5 | 20 | 440 | 1 | 0 | 8 |
| Lean Beef Salami | 4 slices | 90 | 50 | 5 | 3 | 25 | 480 | 1 | 0 | 9 |
| **Heinz** | | | | | | | | | | |
| **CONDIMENTS** | | | | | | | | | | |
| Sweet Relish | 1 tbsp | 20 | 0 | 0 | 0 | 0 | 95 | 5 | 0 | 0 |
| Tomato Ketchup | 1 tbsp | 15 | 0 | 0 | 0 | 0 | 190 | 4 | 0 | 0 |
| Yellow Mustard | 1 tbsp | 0 | 0 | 0 | 0 | 0 | 65 | 0 | 0 | 0 |
| **GRAVY** | | | | | | | | | | |
| Fat Free Roasted Turkey | 1/4 cup | 20 | 0 | 0 | 0 | 0 | 260 | 3 | 0 | 1 |
| Fat Free Savory Beef | 1/4 cup | 20 | 0 | 0 | 0 | 0 | 290 | 4 | 0 | 1 |
| Pork | 1/4 cup | 20 | 5 | .5 | 0 | 0 | 350 | 3 | 0 | 1 |
| Roasted Turkey | 1/4 cup | 25 | 10 | 1 | 0 | <5 | 290 | 3 | 0 | 1 |
| Savory Beef | 1/4 cup | 30 | 10 | 1 | .5 | <5 | 390 | 4 | 0 | 1 |

# store brands

| | SERVING SIZE | CAL | CAL FAT | TOT FAT (G) | SAT FAT (G) | CHOL (MG) | SOD (MG) | CARB (G) | FIBER (G) | PROT (G) |
|---|---|---|---|---|---|---|---|---|---|---|
| **Hellman's** | | | | | | | | | | |
| Real Mayonnaise | 1 tbsp | 90 | 90 | 10 | 1.5 | 5 | 90 | 0 | n/a | |
| **Heluva Good!** | | | | | | | | | | |
| **CHEESE SPREAD** | | | | | | | | | | |
| Cheddar & Horseradish | 2 tbsp | 90 | 60 | 7 | 3 | 20 | 210 | 3 | 0 | 5 |
| Port Wine | 2 tbsp | 90 | 60 | 7 | 3 | 20 | 210 | 3 | 0 | 5 |
| Sharp Cheddar | 2 tbsp | 90 | 60 | 7 | 3 | 20 | 210 | 3 | 0 | 5 |
| **DIPS** | | | | | | | | | | |
| Bacon Horseradish | 2 tbsp | 60 | 45 | 5 | 3 | 20 | 200 | 2 | 0 | 1 |
| Bodacious Onion | 2 tbsp | 60 | 45 | 5 | 3 | 20 | 210 | 3 | 0 | 1 |
| Buttermilk Ranch | 2 tbsp | 60 | 45 | 5 | 3 | 20 | 180 | 2 | 0 | 1 |
| Fat-Free French Onion | 2 tbsp | 25 | 0 | 0 | 0 | 0 | 210 | 3 | 0 | 1 |
| Fiesta Salsa | 2 tbsp | 60 | 45 | 5 | 3 | 20 | 230 | 3 | 0 | 1 |
| French Onion | 2 tbsp | 60 | 45 | 5 | 3 | 20 | 170 | 2 | 0 | 1 |
| Jalapeno Cheddar Dip | 2 tbsp | 60 | 45 | 5 | 3 | 20 | 210 | 2 | 0 | 1 |
| White Cheddar & Bacon | 2 tbsp | 60 | 45 | 5 | 3 | 20 | 160 | 2 | 0 | 1 |
| **Hershey's** | | | | | | | | | | |
| **CHOCOLATE BARS** | | | | | | | | | | |
| Milk Chocolate | 1 bar | 210 | 110 | 13 | 8 | 10 | 35 | 26 | 1 | 3 |
| Milk Chocolate with Almonds | 1 bar | 210 | 130 | 14 | 6 | 10 | 25 | 21 | 2 | 4 |
| Special Dark Chocolate | 1 bar | 180 | 110 | 12 | 8 | 5 | 15 | 25 | 3 | 2 |
| **KISSES** | | | | | | | | | | |
| Milk Chocolate | 9 pieces | 200 | 100 | 12 | 7 | 10 | 35 | 25 | 1 | 3 |
| **SYRUP** | | | | | | | | | | |
| Caramel | 2 tbsp | 110 | 0 | 0 | 0 | 0 | 125 | 27 | 0 | 1 |
| Genuine Chocolate | 2 tbsp | 100 | 0 | 0 | 0 | 0 | 15 | 24 | 1 | 1 |
| Strawberry | 2 tbsp | 100 | 0 | 0 | 0 | 0 | 10 | 26 | 0 | 0 |
| **Hi-C** | | | | | | | | | | |
| Blast Orange | 12 fl oz | 90 | 0 | 0 | 0 | 0 | 15 | 26 | 0 | 0 |
| Blast Strawberry | 12 fl oz | 100 | 0 | 0 | 0 | 0 | 15 | 27 | 0 | 0 |
| Flashin' Fruit Punch | 12 fl oz | 90 | 0 | 0 | 0 | 0 | 15 | 25 | 0 | 0 |
| Grabbin' Grape | 12 fl oz | 100 | 0 | 0 | 0 | 0 | 15 | 26 | 0 | 0 |
| Poppin' Lemonade | 12 fl oz | 100 | 0 | 0 | 0 | 0 | 15 | 27 | 0 | 0 |
| **Honest Tea** | | | | | | | | | | |
| Half & Half | 8 fl oz | 48 | 0 | 0 | 0 | 0 | 5 | 12 | 0 | 0 |
| Honey Green | 8 fl oz | 35 | 0 | 0 | 0 | 0 | 5 | 9 | 0 | 0 |
| Lemon Black | 8 fl oz | 40 | 0 | 0 | 0 | 0 | 5 | 10 | 0 | 0 |

| | SERVING SIZE | CAL | CAL FAT | TOT FAT (G) | SAT FAT (G) | CHOL (MG) | SOD (MG) | CARB (G) | FIBER (G) | PROT (G) |
|---|---|---|---|---|---|---|---|---|---|---|
| **Hood** | | | | | | | | | | |
| **COTTAGE CHEESE** | | | | | | | | | | |
| Country Style | 1/2 cup | 110 | 40 | 4.5 | 3 | 30 | 430 | 5 | 0 | 13 |
| Fat Free with Pineapple | 1/2 cup | 110 | 0 | 0 | 0 | 10 | 330 | 15 | 0 | 11 |
| Low Fat with Peaches | 1/2 cup | 110 | 10 | 1 | .5 | 10 | 310 | 18 | 0 | 10 |
| **FAT-FREE FROZEN YOGURT** | | | | | | | | | | |
| Chocolate | 1/2 cup | 90 | 0 | 0 | 0 | 0 | 65 | 19 | <1 | 4 |
| Strawberry | 1/2 cup | 80 | 0 | 0 | 0 | 0 | 45 | 18 | 0 | 3 |
| Vanilla | 1/2 cup | 90 | 0 | 0 | 0 | 0 | 60 | 19 | 0 | 3 |
| **FROZEN YOGURT** | | | | | | | | | | |
| Blueberry Tangy | 1/2 cup | 110 | 10 | 1 | .5 | <5 | 40 | 24 | 0 | 2 |
| Cherry Vanilla Tangy | 1/2 cup | 110 | 10 | 1 | .5 | <5 | 50 | 23 | 0 | 2 |
| Chocolate Chip Cookie Dough | 1/2 cup | 130 | 25 | 3 | 1.5 | <5 | 65 | 23 | <1 | 3 |
| Cookies & Cream | 1/2 cup | 110 | 10 | 1.5 | 0 | 0 | 85 | 22 | 0 | 3 |
| Strawberry Tangy | 1/2 cup | 110 | 10 | 1 | .5 | <5 | 40 | 24 | 0 | 2 |
| Vanilla Tangy | 1/2 cup | 110 | 10 | 1 | .5 | <5 | 45 | 23 | 0 | 2 |
| **ICE CREAM** | | | | | | | | | | |
| Chocolate | 1/2 cup | 140 | 60 | 6 | 4 | 25 | 50 | 18 | <1 | 3 |
| Chocolate Chip | 1/2 cup | 150 | 80 | 9 | 6 | 25 | 45 | 18 | 0 | 2 |
| Cookie Dough | 1/2 cup | 160 | 70 | 8 | 5 | 25 | 50 | 19 | 0 | 2 |
| Cookies 'n Cream | 1/2 cup | 150 | 70 | 8 | 4.5 | 25 | 70 | 19 | 0 | 2 |
| Golden Vanilla | 1/2 cup | 140 | 70 | 7 | 4.5 | 30 | 50 | 17 | 0 | 2 |
| Light Butter Pecan | 1/2 cup | 130 | 60 | 7 | 2 | 10 | 130 | 16 | <1 | 3 |
| Light Chocolate Chip | 1/2 cup | 120 | 40 | 4.5 | 3 | 10 | 50 | 18 | 0 | 3 |
| Light Coffee | 1/2 cup | 100 | 25 | 3 | 2 | 10 | 55 | 16 | 0 | 3 |
| Light Vanilla | 1/2 cup | 110 | 30 | 3 | 2 | 15 | 55 | 16 | 0 | 3 |
| Strawberry | 1/2 cup | 130 | 60 | 7 | 4.5 | 25 | 45 | 17 | 0 | 2 |
| **NOVELTIES** | | | | | | | | | | |
| Fudge Stix | 1 bar | 70 | 0 | 0 | 0 | 0 | 60 | 14 | 0 | 1 |
| Hoodsie Cup | 3 oz cup | 100 | 50 | 5 | 3.5 | 20 | 35 | 12 | 0 | 2 |
| Hoodsie Pop | 1 pop | 60 | 0 | 0 | 0 | 0 | 5 | 16 | 0 | 0 |
| Ice Cream Bar | 1 bar | 150 | 100 | 11 | 9 | 15 | 30 | 12 | <1 | 1 |
| Ice Cream Sandwiches | 1 sandwich | 170 | 50 | 6 | 3.5 | 20 | 140 | 28 | <1 | 2 |
| Orange Cream Bar | 1 bar | 90 | 15 | 1.5 | 1 | 5 | 40 | 19 | 0 | 1 |
| **SHERBET** | | | | | | | | | | |
| New England Creamery Orange | 1/2 cup | 110 | 0 | 0 | 0 | 0 | 35 | 27 | 0 | <1 |
| New England Creamery Rainbow | 1/2 cup | 110 | 0 | 0 | 0 | 0 | 35 | 27 | 0 | <1 |

| | SERVING SIZE | CAL | CAL FAT | TOT FAT (G) | SAT FAT (G) | CHOL (MG) | SOD (MG) | CARB (G) | FIBER (G) | PROT (G) |
|---|---|---|---|---|---|---|---|---|---|---|
| **Hormel** | | | | | | | | | | |
| **CHILI** | | | | | | | | | | |
| Chunky w/Beans | 8 oz | 260 | 60 | 7 | 3 | 30 | 900 | 33 | 7 | 16 |
| Less Sodium w/Beans | 8 oz | 260 | 60 | 7 | 3 | 30 | 880 | 33 | 7 | 16 |
| No Beans | 8 oz | 220 | 80 | 9 | 4 | 40 | 970 | 18 | 3 | 16 |
| Turkey Chili No Beans | 8 oz | 190 | 30 | 3 | 1 | 80 | 1230 | 16 | 3 | 23 |
| Vegetarian w/Beans | 8 oz | 190 | 10 | 1 | 0 | 0 | 780 | 35 | 10 | 11 |
| **CHILI MASTER** | | | | | | | | | | |
| Chili Roasted Tomato w/Beans | 8 oz | 210 | 55 | 6 | 2 | 25 | 990 | 25 | 7 | 14 |
| Chipotle Chicken Chili w/Beans | 8 oz | 240 | 65 | 7 | 2 | 50 | 970 | 28 | 7 | 17 |
| **PEPPERONI** | | | | | | | | | | |
| Original | 1 oz | 140 | 120 | 13 | 6 | 35 | 470 | 0 | 0 | 5 |
| Sticks | 1 oz | 140 | 120 | 13 | 5 | 30 | 500 | 0 | 0 | 5 |
| Turkey | 1 oz | 70 | 35 | 4 | 1.5 | 40 | 640 | 0 | 0 | 9 |
| **REFRIGERATED ENTRÉES** | | | | | | | | | | |
| Herb Rubbed Italian Style Beef Roast Au Jus | 5 oz | 220 | 100 | 11 | 5 | 85 | 350 | 2 | 0 | 28 |
| Sliced Meatballs & Gravy | 5 oz | 240 | 150 | 17 | 7 | 50 | 890 | 9 | 0 | 12 |
| Sliced Roast Beef & Gravy | 5 oz | 110 | 25 | 3 | 1.5 | 45 | 790 | 3 | 0 | 18 |
| Slow Simmered Pork Roast Au Jus | 5 oz | 180 | 60 | 7 | 2.5 | 85 | 600 | 1 | 0 | 28 |
| Turkey Meat Loaf | 5 oz | 190 | 45 | 5 | 2.5 | 50 | 1000 | 14 | 0 | 21 |
| **Hot Pockets** | | | | | | | | | | |
| Barbecue Recipe Beef | 1 item | 340 | 120 | 13 | 6 | 25 | 780 | 44 | 3 | 9 |
| Chicken Melt with Bacon | 1 item | 300 | 100 | 11 | 5 | 25 | 580 | 38 | 1 | 11 |
| Ham & Cheese | 1 item | 290 | 110 | 12 | 5 | 30 | 640 | 36 | 1 | 15 |
| Philly Steak & Cheese | 1 item | 310 | 120 | 13 | 7 | 30 | 590 | 37 | 1 | 10 |
| **BREAKFAST** | | | | | | | | | | |
| Ham, Egg, & Cheese | 1 item | 300 | 100 | 12 | 5 | 40 | 490 | 38 | 1 | 11 |
| Sausage, Egg, & Cheese | 1 item | 330 | 150 | 17 | 8 | 60 | 480 | 35 | 2 | 10 |
| **CHEESE STUFFED CRUST** | | | | | | | | | | |
| **PIZZERIA** | | | | | | | | | | |
| Pepperoni | 1/2 item | 260 | 120 | 13 | 5 | 20 | 620 | 26 | 1 | 9 |
| **MEXICAN STYLE** | | | | | | | | | | |
| Beef Taco | 1 item | 290 | 110 | 12 | 6 | 20 | 720 | 35 | 2 | 10 |
| Steak Fajita | 1 item | 290 | 110 | 12 | 6 | 25 | 700 | 34 | 2 | 9 |
| Three Cheese & Chicken Quesadilla | 1 item | 270 | 80 | 9 | 4.5 | 20 | 720 | 34 | 1 | 12 |
| **PANINI** | | | | | | | | | | |
| Bruschetta Chicken | 1/2 item | 190 | 60 | 6 | 2.5 | 30 | 620 | 25 | 3 | 9 |

| | SERVING SIZE | CAL | CAL FAT | TOT FAT (G) | SAT FAT (G) | CHOL (MG) | SOD (MG) | CARB (G) | FIBER (G) | PROT (G) |
|---|---|---|---|---|---|---|---|---|---|---|
| Deli Style Ham & Swiss | 1/2 item | 220 | 70 | 8 | 3.5 | 20 | 650 | 26 | 3 | 11 |
| Steak & Cheddar | 1/2 item | 258 | 100 | 11 | 6 | 25 | 660 | 26 | 2 | 11 |
| **PIZZERIA** | | | | | | | | | | |
| Four Cheese | 1 item | 330 | 120 | 13 | 6 | 25 | 750 | 39 | 1 | 13 |
| Four Meat & Four Cheese | 1 item | 340 | 140 | 16 | 7 | 30 | 610 | 38 | 2 | 10 |
| Pepperoni | 1 item | 340 | 150 | 17 | 8 | 25 | 730 | 37 | 2 | 10 |
| Sausage | 1 item | 340 | 140 | 16 | 7 | 20 | 570 | 39 | 2 | 9 |
| Supreme | 1 item | 330 | 140 | 15 | 6 | 25 | 590 | 38 | 3 | 10 |
| **SIDE SHOTS SOFT BAKED BUNS** | | | | | | | | | | |
| Buffalo Style Chicken | 2 items | 260 | 50 | 6 | 1.5 | 15 | 580 | 40 | 1 | 11 |
| Cheeseburger | 2 items | 300 | 90 | 10 | 3.5 | 15 | 640 | 40 | 1 | 12 |
| Sloppy Joe | 2 items | 270 | 70 | 7 | 2.5 | 15 | 710 | 39 | 2 | 10 |
| **SUBS** | | | | | | | | | | |
| Meatballs & Mozzarella | 1 item | 330 | 140 | 16 | 5 | 30 | 730 | 34 | 3 | 12 |
| Philly Steak & Cheese | 1 item | 330 | 120 | 13 | 5 | 30 | 730 | 34 | 1 | 11 |
| **Hunt's** | | | | | | | | | | |
| **BBQ SAUCE** | | | | | | | | | | |
| Honey Hickory | 2 tbsp | 50 | 0 | 0 | 0 | 0 | 420 | 13 | <1 | 0 |
| Original | 2 tbsp | 60 | 0 | 0 | 0 | 0 | 280 | 15 | <1 | 0 |
| **CANNED DICED TOMATOES** | | | | | | | | | | |
| Diced Plain | 1/2 cup | 30 | 0 | 0 | 0 | 0 | 280 | 6 | 2 | 1 |
| Diced with Basil, Garlic, & Oregano | 1/2 cup | 35 | 0 | 0 | 0 | 0 | 300 | 7 | 2 | 1 |
| **CRUSHED** | | | | | | | | | | |
| Plain | 1/2 cup | 45 | 0 | 0 | 0 | 0 | 230 | 9 | 3 | 2 |
| **TOMATO PASTE** | | | | | | | | | | |
| Plain | 2 tbsp | 30 | 0 | 0 | 0 | 0 | 105 | 7 | 2 | 1 |
| **TOMATO PUREE** | | | | | | | | | | |
| Plain | 1/4 cup | 40 | 0 | 0 | 0 | 0 | 125 | 8 | 3 | 2 |
| **TOMATO SAUCE** | | | | | | | | | | |
| No Salt Added | 1/4 cup | 20 | 0 | 0 | 0 | 0 | 20 | 5 | 2 | <1 |
| Plain | 1/4 cup | 20 | 0 | 0 | 0 | 0 | 410 | 4 | 1 | <1 |
| **SPAGHETTI SAUCE** | | | | | | | | | | |
| Four Cheese | 1/2 cup | 60 | 10 | 1 | 0 | 0 | 580 | 10 | 3 | 2 |
| Garlic & Herb | 1/2 cup | 40 | 10 | 1 | 0 | 0 | 610 | 8 | 3 | 1 |
| Meat Sauce | 1/2 cup | 60 | 10 | 1 | 0 | 0 | 610 | 10 | 3 | 2 |
| No Sugar Added | 1/2 cup | 35 | 0 | 0 | 0 | 0 | 580 | 7 | 3 | 1 |

| | SERVING SIZE | CAL | CAL FAT | TOT FAT (G) | SAT FAT (G) | CHOL (MG) | SOD (MG) | CARB (G) | FIBER (G) | PROT (G) |
|---|---|---|---|---|---|---|---|---|---|---|
| Traditional | 1/2 cup | 50 | 10 | 1 | 0 | 0 | 580 | 11 | 3 | 1 |
| **STEWED** | | | | | | | | | | |
| No Salt | 1/2 cup | 40 | 0 | 0 | 0 | 0 | 30 | 8 | 2 | 1 |
| Plain | 1/2 cup | 45 | 0 | 0 | 0 | 0 | 330 | 10 | 2 | 1 |
| **WHOLE CANNED TOMATOES** | | | | | | | | | | |
| No Salt Added | 1/2 cup | 30 | 0 | 0 | 0 | 0 | 20 | 6 | 2 | 1 |
| Plain | 1/2 cup | 25 | 0 | 0 | 0 | 0 | 180 | 5 | 2 | 1 |
| **International Delight** | | | | | | | | | | |
| Amaretto | 1 tbsp | 40 | 15 | 1.5 | 1 | 0 | 5 | 7 | 0 | 0 |
| Dulce de Leche | 1 tbsp | 45 | 20 | 2 | 1 | 0 | 5 | 7 | 0 | 0 |
| English Almond Toffee | 1 tbsp | 45 | 20 | 2 | 1 | 0 | 5 | 6 | 0 | 0 |
| French Vanilla | 1 tbsp | 45 | 20 | 2 | 1 | 0 | 5 | 6 | 0 | 0 |
| Hazelnut | 1 tbsp | 45 | 20 | 2 | 1 | 0 | 5 | 6 | 0 | 0 |
| Hershey's Chocolate Caramel | 1 tbsp | 45 | 20 | 2 | 1 | 0 | 5 | 7 | 0 | 0 |
| White Chocolate Macadamia | 1 tbsp | 45 | 20 | 2 | 1 | 0 | 5 | 6 | 0 | 0 |
| **COFFEEHOUSE INSPIRATIONS** | | | | | | | | | | |
| Caramel Macchiato | 1 tbsp | 40 | 15 | 1.5 | 1 | 0 | 5 | 7 | 0 | 0 |
| Skinny Caramel Macchiato | 1 tbsp | 30 | 0 | 0 | 0 | 0 | 5 | 7 | 0 | 0 |
| Skinny Vanilla Latte | 1 tbsp | 30 | 0 | 0 | 0 | 0 | 5 | 7 | 0 | 0 |
| Vanilla Latte | 1 tbsp | 40 | 15 | 1.5 | 1 | 0 | 5 | 7 | 0 | 0 |
| **Jack Link's** | | | | | | | | | | |
| **BEEF JERKY** | | | | | | | | | | |
| Beef Steak Original | 1 oz | 60 | 10 | 1 | .5 | 30 | 640 | 2 | 0 | 12 |
| Deli Cuts Sausage Bites Original | 7 pieces | 120 | 90 | 10 | 4 | 25 | 480 | 2 | 0 | 6 |
| Hickory Smoked | 1 oz | 80 | 10 | 1 | .5 | 25 | 650 | 5 | 0 | 14 |
| Jerky Chew Original | 1/3 oz | 30 | 0 | 0 | 0 | 0 | 450 | 0 | 0 | 9 |
| KC Masterpiece Barbecue | 1 oz | 80 | 10 | 1 | 0 | 25 | 430 | 8 | 0 | 11 |
| Original | 1 oz | 80 | 10 | 1 | 0 | 20 | 590 | 3 | 0 | 15 |
| Original Jack Pack | 2 oz | 230 | 150 | 16 | 8 | 45 | 800 | 10 | 0 | 11 |
| Tender Strips Original | 1 oz | 100 | 50 | 6 | 3 | 20 | 380 | 2 | 0 | 11 |
| Teriyaki | 1 oz | 80 | 10 | 1 | 0 | 20 | 600 | 5 | 0 | 14 |
| **JELL-O** | | | | | | | | | | |
| **COOK & SERVE PUDDING** | | | | | | | | | | |
| Chocolate | 1/6 packet | 90 | 0 | 0 | 0 | 0 | 110 | 22 | 1 | 1 |
| Lemon | 1/8 packet | 60 | 0 | 0 | 0 | 0 | 80 | 14 | 0 | 0 |
| Vanilla | 1/6 packet | 80 | 0 | 0 | 0 | 0 | 135 | 21 | 0 | 0 |

| | SERVING SIZE | CAL | CAL FAT | TOT FAT (G) | SAT FAT (G) | CHOL (MG) | SOD (MG) | CARB (G) | FIBER (G) | PROT (G) |
|---|---|---|---|---|---|---|---|---|---|---|
| **FAT-FREE/SUGAR-FREE INSTANT PUDDING** | | | | | | | | | | |
| Butterscotch, Sugar Free, Fat Free | 1/4 packet | 25 | 0 | 0 | 0 | 0 | 300 | 6 | 0 | 0 |
| Chocolate, Sugar Free | 1 snack cup | 60 | 10 | 1.5 | 1 | 0 | 180 | 13 | 1 | 2 |
| Chocolate, Sugar Free, Fat Free | 1/4 packet | 35 | 0 | 0 | 0 | 0 | 310 | 8 | 1 | 1 |
| Fat Free Chocolate | 1 snack cup | 100 | 0 | 0 | 0 | 0 | 180 | 23 | 1 | 2 |
| Fat Free Chocolate Vanilla Swirls | 1 snack cup | 100 | 0 | 10 | 0 | 0 | 190 | 23 | 1 | 2 |
| Fat Free Tapioca | 1 snack cup | 100 | 0 | 0 | 0 | 0 | 200 | 23 | 0 | 1 |
| Vanilla, Sugar Free, Fat Free | 1/4 packet | 25 | 0 | 0 | 0 | 0 | 300 | 6 | 0 | 0 |
| **INSTANT PUDDING** | | | | | | | | | | |
| Butterscotch | 1/4 packet | 90 | 0 | 0 | 0 | 0 | 400 | 23 | 0 | 0 |
| Chocolate | 1/4 packet | 100 | 0 | 0 | 0 | 0 | 420 | 25 | 1 | 0 |
| Vanilla | 1/4 packet | 90 | 0 | 0 | 0 | 0 | 350 | 23 | 0 | 0 |
| **GELATIN DESSERTS** | | | | | | | | | | |
| Cherry | 3/4 oz | 80 | 0 | 0 | 0 | 0 | 100 | 19 | 0 | 2 |
| Lemon | 3/4 oz | 80 | 0 | 0 | 0 | 0 | 120 | 19 | 0 | 2 |
| Lime | 3/4 oz | 80 | 0 | 0 | 0 | 0 | 100 | 19 | 0 | 2 |
| Orange | 3/4 oz | 80 | 0 | 0 | 0 | 0 | 80 | 19 | 0 | 2 |
| Strawberry | 3/4 oz | 80 | 0 | 0 | 0 | 0 | 90 | 19 | 0 | 2 |
| **GELATIN SNACK CUPS** | | | | | | | | | | |
| Strawberry | 1 snack cup | 70 | 0 | 0 | 0 | 0 | 40 | 17 | 0 | 0 |
| Strawberry & Orange | 1 snack cup | 70 | 0 | 0 | 0 | 0 | 40 | 17 | 0 | 1 |
| Strawberry & Raspberry | 1 snack cup | 70 | 0 | 0 | 0 | 0 | 40 | 17 | 0 | 1 |
| **NO-BAKE DESSERT MIXES** | | | | | | | | | | |
| Homestyle Cheesecake | 1/6 packet | 230 | 40 | 4.5 | 3 | 0 | 380 | 44 | 1 | 2 |
| Real Cheesecake | 1/8 packet | 290 | 130 | 15 | 7 | 0 | 330 | 39 | 2 | 4 |
| **PUDDING SNACK CUPS** | | | | | | | | | | |
| Chocolate Vanilla Swirls, Reduced Calorie, Sugar Free | 1 snack cup | 60 | 10 | 1.5 | 1 | 0 | 180 | 13 | 1 | 1 |
| Original Chocolate Vanilla Swirls | 1 snack cup | 110 | 15 | 1.5 | 1.5 | 0 | 190 | 24 | 1 | 2 |
| Original Tapioca | 1 snack cup | 110 | 10 | 1.5 | 1.5 | 0 | 200 | 25 | 0 | 1 |
| Original Vanilla | 1 snack cup | 110 | 10 | 1.5 | 1.5 | 0 | 190 | 23 | 0 | 1 |
| Pudding Snack Cups, Original Chocolate | 1 snack cup | 120 | 15 | 1.5 | 1.5 | 0 | 190 | 25 | 1 | 2 |
| Sugar Free Vanilla | 1 snack cup | 60 | 10 | 1 | 1 | 0 | 180 | 13 | 0 | 1 |
| **SUGAR-FREE/LOW-CALORIE SNACK CUPS** | | | | | | | | | | |
| Lime & Orange | 1 snack cup | 10 | 0 | 0 | 0 | 0 | 45 | 0 | 0 | 1 |

| | SERVING SIZE | CAL | CAL FAT | TOT FAT (G) | SAT FAT (G) | CHOL (MG) | SOD (MG) | CARB (G) | FIBER (G) | PROT (G) |
|---|---|---|---|---|---|---|---|---|---|---|
| Peach & Watermelon | 1 snack cup | 10 | 0 | 0 | 0 | 0 | 45 | 0 | 0 | 1 |
| Strawberry | 1 snack cup | 10 | 0 | 0 | 0 | 0 | 45 | 0 | 0 | 1 |
| **SUGAR-FREE/LOW-CALORIE GELATINS** | | | | | | | | | | |
| Cherry | 3/4 oz | 10 | 0 | 0 | 0 | 0 | 70 | 0 | 0 | 1 |
| Lemon | 3/4 oz | 10 | 0 | 0 | 0 | 0 | 55 | 0 | 0 | 1 |
| Lime | 3/4 oz | 10 | 0 | 0 | 0 | 0 | 60 | 0 | 0 | 1 |
| Orange | 3/4 oz | 10 | 0 | 0 | 0 | 0 | 65 | 0 | 0 | 1 |
| Strawberry | 3/4 oz | 10 | 0 | 0 | 0 | 0 | 45 | 0 | 0 | 1 |
| **Jet-Puffed** | | | | | | | | | | |
| **CRÈME** | | | | | | | | | | |
| Marshmallow | 1/2 oz | 40 | 0 | 0 | 0 | 0 | 0 | 11 | 0 | 0 |
| **MARSHMALLOWS** | | | | | | | | | | |
| Miniature | 1 oz | 100 | 0 | 0 | 0 | 25 | 25 | 23 | 0 | 1 |
| Original | 1 oz | 100 | 0 | 0 | 0 | 0 | 25 | 24 | 0 | 1 |
| **Jiffy Mix** | | | | | | | | | | |
| **BAKING MIXES** | | | | | | | | | | |
| All Purpose | 1/4 cup | 130 | 40 | 4.5 | 1 | 0 | 310 | 21 | <1 | 2 |
| Apple Cinnamon Muffin | 1/4 cup | 160 | 50 | 5 | 2 | <5 | 320 | 26 | 0 | 2 |
| Banana Muffin | 1/4 cup | 150 | 45 | 4.5 | 2 | <5 | 310 | 25 | <1 | 2 |
| Blueberry Muffin | 1/4 cup | 160 | 50 | 5 | 2 | <5 | 320 | 26 | 0 | 2 |
| Buttermilk Biscuit | 1/3 cup | 160 | 45 | 5 | 2 | <5 | 420 | 27 | <1 | 3 |
| Buttermilk Complete Pancake & Waffle | 1/3 cup | 170 | 40 | 4.5 | 2 | <5 | 380 | 30 | <1 | 3 |
| Corn Muffin | 1/4 cup | 150 | 40 | 4.5 | 2 | <5 | 340 | 27 | <1 | 2 |
| **DESSERT MIXES** | | | | | | | | | | |
| Chocolate Chip Cookie | 3 tbsp | 90 | 25 | 3 | 1.5 | 0 | 125 | 17 | 0 | 1 |
| Fudge Brownie | 1/8 item | 120 | 30 | 3.5 | 1 | 0 | 120 | 22 | <1 | 1 |
| Sugar Cookie | 3 tbsp | 90 | 10 | 1 | 0 | 0 | 80 | 19 | 0 | 2 |
| **Jiffy Pop** | | | | | | | | | | |
| Butter Popcorn | 4 cups | 140 | 70 | 7 | 1.5 | 0 | 220 | 19 | 3 | 3 |
| **Kashi** | | | | | | | | | | |
| **CEREAL** | | | | | | | | | | |
| 7 Whole Grain Flakes | 1 cup | 180 | 10 | 1 | 0 | 0 | 150 | 41 | 6 | 6 |
| Go Lean Crunch! | 1 cup | 190 | 25 | 3 | 0 | 0 | 100 | 37 | 8 | 9 |
| Go Lean Original | 1 cup | 140 | 10 | 1 | 0 | 0 | 85 | 30 | 10 | 13 |
| Good Friends Original | 1 cup | 160 | 15 | 1.5 | 0 | 0 | 110 | 42 | 12 | 5 |
| Granola Mountain Medley | 1/2 cup | 220 | 70 | 7 | 1.5 | 0 | 120 | 38 | 7 | 6 |

| | SERVING SIZE | CAL | CAL FAT | TOT FAT (G) | SAT FAT (G) | CHOL (MG) | SOD (MG) | CARB (G) | FIBER (G) | PROT (G) |
|---|---|---|---|---|---|---|---|---|---|---|
| Granola Summer Berry | 1/2 cup | 220 | 50 | 6 | 1 | 0 | 150 | 39 | 7 | 6 |
| Heart to Heart Golden Brown Maple Oatmeal | 1 packet | 160 | 20 | 2 | 0 | 0 | 100 | 33 | 5 | 4 |
| Heart to Heart Toasted Oat | 1 cup | 120 | 15 | 1.5 | 0 | 0 | 85 | 25 | 5 | 4 |
| Heart to Heart Warm Cinnamon Oat | 1 cup | 120 | 15 | 1.5 | 0 | 0 | 80 | 25 | 5 | 4 |
| Mighty Bites Honey Crunch | 1 cup | 120 | 15 | 1.5 | 0 | 0 | 160 | 23 | 3 | 5 |
| Strawberry Fields Original | 1 cup | 120 | 0 | 0 | 0 | 0 | 170 | 27 | 1 | 2 |

**FROZEN ENTRÉES & PIZZA**

| | SERVING SIZE | CAL | CAL FAT | TOT FAT (G) | SAT FAT (G) | CHOL (MG) | SOD (MG) | CARB (G) | FIBER (G) | PROT (G) |
|---|---|---|---|---|---|---|---|---|---|---|
| Chicken Florentine | 1 item | 290 | 80 | 9 | 4.5 | 45 | 550 | 31 | 5 | 22 |
| Pesto Pasta Primevera | 1 item | 290 | 100 | 11 | 2 | 5 | 750 | 37 | 7 | 11 |
| Sweet & Sour Chicken | 1 item | 320 | 35 | 3.5 | .5 | 35 | 380 | 55 | 6 | 18 |
| Original Crust Pizzas—Mediterranean | 1/3 item | 290 | 80 | 9 | 4 | 20 | 640 | 37 | 5 | 15 |
| Thin Crust Pizzas—Margherita | 1/3 item | 260 | 90 | 9 | 4 | 20 | 630 | 29 | 4 | 14 |

**GRANOLA BARS**

| | SERVING SIZE | CAL | CAL FAT | TOT FAT (G) | SAT FAT (G) | CHOL (MG) | SOD (MG) | CARB (G) | FIBER (G) | PROT (G) |
|---|---|---|---|---|---|---|---|---|---|---|
| Crunchy Honey Toasted 7-Grain | 1 item | 170 | 50 | 5 | .5 | 0 | 150 | 26 | 4 | 6 |
| Golean Chewy Oatmeal Raisin | 1 item | 280 | 45 | 5 | 3 | 0 | 140 | 49 | 6 | 13 |
| Golean Chewy Peanut Butter & Chocolate | 1 item | 290 | 60 | 6 | 4.5 | 0 | 280 | 48 | 6 | 13 |
| Golean Crunchy! Chocolate Almond | 1 item | 170 | 45 | 5 | 2.5 | 0 | 210 | 27 | 5 | 8 |
| Golean Crunchy! Chocolate Peanut | 1 item | 180 | 45 | 5 | 2 | 0 | 250 | 30 | 6 | 9 |
| Golean Roll! Chocolate Peanut | 1 item | 190 | 45 | 5 | 1.5 | 0 | 240 | 27 | 6 | 12 |
| Golean Roll! Chocolate Turtle | 1 item | 190 | 45 | 5 | 1.5 | 0 | 240 | 27 | 6 | 12 |
| TLC Chewy Cherry Dark Chocolate | 1 item | 120 | 15 | 2 | .5 | 0 | 65 | 24 | 4 | 5 |
| TLC Chewy Peanut Butter | 1 item | 140 | 45 | 5 | .5 | 0 | 85 | 19 | 4 | 7 |
| TLC Chewy Trail Mix | 1 item | 140 | 45 | 5 | .5 | 0 | 95 | 20 | 4 | 6 |

**TLC COOKIES**

| | SERVING SIZE | CAL | CAL FAT | TOT FAT (G) | SAT FAT (G) | CHOL (MG) | SOD (MG) | CARB (G) | FIBER (G) | PROT (G) |
|---|---|---|---|---|---|---|---|---|---|---|
| Happy Trail Mix | 1 item | 140 | 50 | 5 | 1 | 0 | 75 | 21 | 4 | 2 |
| Oatmeal Dark Chocolate | 1 item | 130 | 45 | 5 | 1.5 | 0 | 65 | 20 | 4 | 2 |

**TLC CRACKERS**

| | SERVING SIZE | CAL | CAL FAT | TOT FAT (G) | SAT FAT (G) | CHOL (MG) | SOD (MG) | CARB (G) | FIBER (G) | PROT (G) |
|---|---|---|---|---|---|---|---|---|---|---|
| Honey Sesame | 15 pieces | 120 | 30 | 3 | 0 | 0 | 140 | 22 | 2 | 3 |
| Original 7 Grain | 15 pieces | 120 | 30 | 3.5 | 0 | 0 | 160 | 21 | 2 | 3 |
| Whole Grains, Original | 7 pieces | 120 | 30 | 3.5 | 0 | 0 | 85 | 22 | 4 | 3 |

## Keebler

**BAKER'S TREASURES**

| | SERVING SIZE | CAL | CAL FAT | TOT FAT (G) | SAT FAT (G) | CHOL (MG) | SOD (MG) | CARB (G) | FIBER (G) | PROT (G) |
|---|---|---|---|---|---|---|---|---|---|---|
| Chocolate Chip Cookies | 2 cookies | 140 | 45 | 5 | 2 | <5 | 110 | 22 | <1 | 2 |
| Oatmeal Raisin Cookies | 2 cookies | 130 | 40 | 4.5 | 1.5 | <5 | 105 | 22 | 1 | 2 |

**CHIPS DELUXE COOKIES**

| | SERVING SIZE | CAL | CAL FAT | TOT FAT (G) | SAT FAT (G) | CHOL (MG) | SOD (MG) | CARB (G) | FIBER (G) | PROT (G) |
|---|---|---|---|---|---|---|---|---|---|---|
| Mini Rainbow Chocolate Chip | 1 cookie | 200 | 90 | 10 | 4 | 0 | 125 | 27 | <1 | 2 |

| | SERVING SIZE | CAL | CAL FAT | TOT FAT (G) | SAT FAT (G) | CHOL (MG) | SOD (MG) | CARB (G) | FIBER (G) | PROT (G) |
|---|---|---|---|---|---|---|---|---|---|---|
| Oatmeal Chocolate Chip | 2 cookies | 150 | 70 | 7 | 3 | 0 | 105 | 20 | 1 | 2 |
| **CLUB CRACKERS** | | | | | | | | | | |
| Cheddar Sandwich | 1 package | 190 | 80 | 9 | 2.5 | 0 | 290 | 24 | <1 | 3 |
| Original | 4 crackers | 70 | 25 | 3 | .5 | 0 | 125 | 9 | <1 | <1 |
| **FUDGE SHOPPE** | | | | | | | | | | |
| **COOKIES** | | | | | | | | | | |
| Fudge Sticks | 3 cookies | 150 | 70 | 8 | 5 | 0 | 40 | 20 | <1 | <1 |
| Fudge Stripes | 3 cookies | 150 | 70 | 7 | 4.5 | 0 | 110 | 21 | <1 | 1 |
| Grasshopper | 4 cookies | 150 | 60 | 7 | 4.5 | 0 | 75 | 20 | <1 | 1 |
| **SHORTBREAD COOKIES** | | | | | | | | | | |
| Sandies, Pecan | 2 cookies | 160 | 90 | 10 | 3 | <5 | 105 | 18 | <1 | 1 |
| **TOASTEDS CRACKERS** | | | | | | | | | | |
| Wheat | 5 crackers | 70 | 30 | 3 | .5 | 0 | 140 | 11 | <1 | 1 |
| Buttercrisp | 5 crackers | 80 | 35 | 4 | .5 | 0 | 150 | 10 | <1 | <1 |
| Toasted Onion | 5 crackers | 80 | 30 | 3.5 | .5 | 0 | 160 | 11 | <1 | 1 |
| Sesame | 5 crackers | 80 | 35 | 4 | .5 | 0 | 140 | 10 | <1 | 1 |
| Wheat | 5 crackers | 80 | 35 | 4 | .5 | 0 | 140 | 10 | 1 | 1 |
| **TOWN HOUSE CRACKERS** | | | | | | | | | | |
| Bistro Multigrain | 2 crackers | 80 | 25 | 3 | .5 | 0 | 130 | 11 | <1 | 1 |
| Flatbread Crisps—Italian Herb | 6 crisps | 70 | 20 | 2 | 0 | 0 | 130 | 12 | <1 | 1 |
| Flipsides Original | 5 crackers | 70 | 30 | 3.5 | .5 | 0 | 190 | 10 | <1 | 1 |
| Original | 5 crackers | 80 | 40 | 4.5 | 1 | 0 | 130 | 10 | <1 | <1 |
| Reduced Fat | 6 crackers | 60 | 15 | 1.5 | 0 | 0 | 160 | 11 | <1 | 1 |
| Toppers Original | 3 crackers | 70 | 30 | 3 | .5 | 0 | 135 | 9 | 0 | 1 |
| Wheat | 5 crackers | 80 | 35 | 4 | .5 | 0 | 170 | 10 | <1 | 1 |
| **VIENNA COOKIES** | | | | | | | | | | |
| Fingers | 2 cookies | 150 | 50 | 6 | 2 | 0 | 95 | 23 | <1 | 1 |
| **Kellogg's** | | | | | | | | | | |
| **ALL-BRAN CEREAL** | | | | | | | | | | |
| Complete Wheat Flakes | 3/4 cup | 90 | 5 | .5 | 0 | 0 | 210 | 23 | 5 | 3 |
| Original | 1/2 cup | 80 | 10 | 1 | 0 | 0 | 80 | 23 | 10 | 4 |
| **CORN FLAKES CEREAL** | | | | | | | | | | |
| Corn Flakes | 1 cup | 100 | 0 | 0 | 0 | 0 | 200 | 24 | 1 | 2 |
| Frosted Flakes | 3/4 cup | 110 | 0 | 0 | 0 | 0 | 140 | 27 | 1 | 1 |
| **LOW FAT GRANOLA** | | | | | | | | | | |
| With Raisins | 2/3 cup | 230 | 25 | 3 | 1 | 0 | 140 | 48 | 4 | 5 |
| Without Raisins | 1/2 cup | 190 | 25 | 2.5 | .5 | 0 | 110 | 40 | 3 | 4 |

| | SERVING SIZE | CAL | CAL FAT | TOT FAT (G) | SAT FAT (G) | CHOL (MG) | SOD (MG) | CARB (G) | FIBER (G) | PROT (G) |
|---|---|---|---|---|---|---|---|---|---|---|
| **MINI WHEATS CEREAL** | | | | | | | | | | |
| Original, Bite-Size | 24 pieces | 200 | 10 | 1 | 0 | 0 | 48 | 48 | 6 | 6 |
| Unfrosted, Bite-Size | 30 pieces | 200 | 15 | 1 | 0 | 0 | 200 | 45 | 6 | 5 |
| **RAISIN BRAN** | | | | | | | | | | |
| Raisin Bran Crunch | 1 cup | 190 | 10 | 1 | 0 | 0 | 210 | 45 | 4 | 3 |
| Raisin Bran Original | 1 cup | 190 | 1 | 0 | 0 | 0 | 250 | 46 | 7 | 5 |
| **RICE KRISPIES CEREAL** | | | | | | | | | | |
| Cocoa Krispies | 3/4 cup | 120 | 5 | 1 | .5 | 130 | 130 | 27 | <1 | 1 |
| Rice Krispies | 1-1/4 cups | 130 | 0 | 0 | 0 | 0 | 190 | 29 | <1 | 2 |
| **RICE KRISPIES TREAT BAR** | | | | | | | | | | |
| Original | 1 bar | 90 | 20 | 2.5 | 1 | 0 | 105 | 17 | 0 | 1 |
| Strawberry | 1 bar | 90 | 20 | 2 | .5 | 0 | 95 | 16 | 0 | 1 |
| **SMART START CEREAL** | | | | | | | | | | |
| Strong Heart Antioxidants | 1 cup | 190 | 5 | .5 | 0 | 0 | 280 | 43 | 3 | 3 |
| Strong Heart Toasted Oat | 1-1/4 cups | 220 | 20 | 2.5 | .5 | 0 | 140 | 48 | 5 | 6 |
| **SPECIAL K BARS** | | | | | | | | | | |
| Chocolatey Drizzle | 1 bar | 90 | 15 | 1.5 | 1 | 0 | 95 | 17 | 3 | 1 |
| Strawberry | 1 bar | 90 | 15 | 1.5 | 1 | 0 | 85 | 18 | 3 | 1 |
| Vanilla Crisp | 1 bar | 90 | 15 | 1.5 | 1 | 0 | 90 | 17 | 3 | 2 |
| **SPECIAL K CEREAL** | | | | | | | | | | |
| Chocolatey Delight | 3/4 cup | 120 | 20 | 2 | 2 | 0 | 180 | 25 | 3 | 2 |
| Low Fat Granola | 1/2 cup | 190 | 25 | 3 | .5 | 0 | 120 | 39 | 5 | 6 |
| Original | 1 cup | 120 | 5 | .5 | 0 | 0 | 220 | 23 | <1 | 6 |
| Red Berries | 1 cup | 110 | 0 | 0 | 0 | 0 | 190 | 27 | 3 | 2 |
| **SPECIAL K MEAL BAR** | | | | | | | | | | |
| Chocolate Peanut Butter | 1 bar | 180 | 50 | 6 | 3.5 | 0 | 250 | 25 | 5 | 10 |
| Chocolatey Chip | 1 bar | 170 | 40 | 4.5 | 3.5 | 0 | 180 | 26 | 5 | 10 |
| Strawberry | 1 bar | 170 | 45 | 5 | 4 | 0 | 160 | 25 | 5 | 10 |
| **SPECIAL K SNACK BAR** | | | | | | | | | | |
| Chocolate Delight | 1 bar | 110 | 25 | 3 | 2 | 0 | 85 | 16 | 1 | 4 |
| Chocolate Peanut | 1 bar | 110 | 30 | 3.5 | 2 | 0 | 70 | 15 | 1 | 4 |
| **Klondike** | | | | | | | | | | |
| **ICE CREAM BARS** | | | | | | | | | | |
| Double Chocolate | 1 bar | 240 | 130 | 14 | 11 | 10 | 75 | 27 | 1 | 3 |
| Krunch | 1 bar | 250 | 130 | 14 | 11 | 10 | 55 | 30 | 1 | 3 |
| Milk Chocolate Reese's Peanut Butter Cups | 1 bar | 260 | 150 | 16 | 11 | 10 | 90 | 26 | 1 | 3 |
| Oreo Cookies & Cream | 1 bar | 250 | 140 | 15 | 11 | 10 | 115 | 29 | 1 | 3 |

| | SERVING SIZE | CAL | CAL FAT | TOT FAT (G) | SAT FAT (G) | CHOL (MG) | SOD (MG) | CARB (G) | FIBER (G) | PROT (G) |
|---|---|---|---|---|---|---|---|---|---|---|
| Slim-a-Bear 100 Calorie French Vanilla Stick | 1 bar | 100 | 50 | 6 | 4.5 | 10 | 25 | 12 | 2 | 2 |
| Slim-a-Bear 100 Chocolate Fudge | 1 bar | 100 | 25 | 3 | 2 | 5 | 90 | 20 | 4 | 3 |
| **ICE CREAM SANDWICHES** | | | | | | | | | | |
| Classic Vanilla | 1 sandwich | 180 | 40 | 4.5 | 2.5 | 10 | 150 | 31 | <1 | 3 |
| Mrs. Field's Ice Cream Cookie Sandwich | 1 sandwich | 220 | 70 | 8 | 4 | <5 | 150 | 35 | <1 | 3 |
| Oreo Ice Cream Cookie Sandwich | 1 sandwich | 200 | 60 | 7 | 2 | 5 | 250 | 34 | <1 | 3 |
| Slim-a-Bear No Sugar Added Vanilla | 1 sandwich | 170 | 90 | 9 | 8 | 5 | 65 | 21 | 4 | 4 |
| **Knorr** | | | | | | | | | | |
| **ASIAN SIDES** | | | | | | | | | | |
| Chicken Fried Rice | 1/2 cup | 280 | 60 | 11 | 5 | 0 | 25 | 16 | 4 | 7 |
| Classic Chow Mein | 1/2 cup | 260 | 70 | 12 | 5 | 0 | 27 | 13 | 12 | 7 |
| **Cajun Sides** | | | | | | | | | | |
| Dirty Rice (prepared) | 1 cup | 250 | 15 | 2 | 0 | 2 | 35 | 17 | 8 | 8 |
| Garlic Butter Rice (prepared) | 1 cup | 260 | 35 | 15 | 6 | 3 | 30 | 16 | 4 | 7 |
| **FIESTA SIDES** | | | | | | | | | | |
| Mexican Rice (prepared) | 1/2 cup | 280 | 50 | 9 | 5 | 0 | 28 | 17 | 8 | 7 |
| Spanish Rice | 1/2 cup | 280 | 50 | 9 | 5 | 0 | 28 | 16 | 8 | 6 |
| **ITALIAN SIDES** | | | | | | | | | | |
| Creamy Garlic Shells | 2/3 cup | 320 | 90 | 20 | 15 | 5 | 26 | 15 | 8 | 10 |
| Scampi | 1/2 cup | 240 | 50 | 10 | 9 | 1 | 33 | 13 | 12 | 7 |
| **PREPARED RICE SIDES** | | | | | | | | | | |
| Beef | 1 cup | 240 | 20 | 3 | 3 | 0 | 39 | 16 | 4 | 6 |
| Cheddar Broccoli | 2/3 cup | 280 | 50 | 9 | 8 | 1 | 29 | 16 | 4 | 7 |
| Creamy Chicken | 1/2 cup | 280 | 50 | 9 | 8 | 0 | 25 | 16 | 4 | 6 |
| Rice Pilaf | 1 cup | 220 | 10 | 2 | 0 | 0 | 37 | 15 | 4 | 6 |
| **SIDES PLUS VEGGIES** | | | | | | | | | | |
| Roasted Chicken Rice with Harvest Vegetables | 3/4 cup | 320 | 70 | 12 | 8 | 2 | 31 | 19 | 16 | 8 |
| Vegetable Fried Rice | 1/2 cup | 300 | 70 | 12 | 5 | 0 | 29 | 17 | 12 | 6 |
| **Kraft** | | | | | | | | | | |
| **DELI DELUXE SLICES** | | | | | | | | | | |
| American | 1 slice | 70 | 50 | 6 | 3.5 | 20 | 310 | 0 | 0 | 4 |
| Cheddar | 1 slice | 110 | 80 | 9 | 5 | 30 | 440 | 1 | 0 | 6 |
| Swiss | 1 slice | 90 | 70 | 7 | 4.5 | 25 | 340 | 1 | 0 | 6 |
| **DIPS** | | | | | | | | | | |
| Bacon & Cheddar | 1 oz | 60 | 45 | 5 | 3.5 | 5 | 170 | 3 | 0 | 1 |
| Creamy Ranch | 1 oz | 60 | 40 | 4.5 | 3 | 0 | 190 | 3 | 0 | 1 |

| | SERVING SIZE | CAL | CAL FAT | TOT FAT (G) | SAT FAT (G) | CHOL (MG) | SOD (MG) | CARB (G) | FIBER (G) | PROT (G) |
|---|---|---|---|---|---|---|---|---|---|---|
| French Onion | 1 oz | 60 | 40 | 4.5 | 3 | 0 | 220 | 3 | 0 | 1 |
| Green Onion | 1 oz | 60 | 40 | 4.5 | 3 | 0 | 170 | 3 | 0 | 1 |
| Guacamole Flavor | 1 oz | 50 | 40 | 4.5 | 2.5 | 0 | 240 | 3 | 0 | 1 |
| **EASY MAC** | | | | | | | | | | |
| **MICROWAVABLE CUPS** | | | | | | | | | | |
| Big Packs Microwavable | 1 pouch | 350 | 60 | 6 | 3.5 | 10 | 830 | 63 | 2 | 10 |
| Original | 1 cup | 220 | 35 | 4 | 2 | 5 | 470 | 40 | 1 | 6 |
| Original Cheesy Made Easy | 1 cup | 220 | 35 | 4 | 2.5 | 5 | 670 | 40 | 1 | 6 |
| **GRATED CHEESE** | | | | | | | | | | |
| 100% Parmesan | 1 tsp | 20 | 15 | 1.5 | 1 | 5 | 85 | 0 | 0 | 2 |
| 100% Parmesan & Romano | 1 tsp | 20 | 15 | 1.5 | 1 | 5 | 85 | 0 | 0 | 2 |
| Reduced Fat Parmesan Style Topping | 1 tsp | 20 | 10 | 1 | .5 | 5 | 80 | 2 | 0 | 1 |
| **MACARONI & CHEESE** | | | | | | | | | | |
| **DELUXE DINNER** | | | | | | | | | | |
| Four Cheese | 1 item | 320 | 90 | 10 | 3 | 15 | 860 | 46 | 2 | 12 |
| Original Cheddar | 1 item | 320 | 90 | 6 | 3 | 35 | 870 | 45 | 1 | 12 |
| Sharp Cheddar | 1 item | 320 | 80 | 9 | 3 | 15 | 840 | 46 | 2 | 12 |
| **MAYONNAISE** | | | | | | | | | | |
| Fat Free | 1/2 oz | 10 | 0 | 0 | 0 | 0 | 120 | 2 | 0 | 0 |
| Light | 1/2 oz | 45 | 35 | 4 | .5 | 5 | 95 | 2 | 0 | 0 |
| Real | 1/2 oz | 90 | 90 | 10 | 1.5 | 5 | 70 | 0 | 0 | 0 |
| **SALAD DRESSING** | | | | | | | | | | |
| Balsamic Vinaigrette | 2 tbsp | 90 | 70 | 8 | 1 | 0 | 310 | 4 | 0 | 0 |
| Catalina | 2 tbsp | 130 | 100 | 11 | 1.5 | 0 | 380 | 7 | 0 | 0 |
| Classic Caesar | 2 tbsp | 130 | 110 | 12 | 2.5 | 15 | 380 | 2 | 0 | 2 |
| Classic Italian Vinaigrette | 2 tbsp | 60 | 35 | 4 | 0 | 0 | 430 | 5 | 0 | 0 |
| Creamy French | 2 tbsp | 150 | 120 | 14 | 2 | 0 | 260 | 5 | 0 | 1 |
| Free Classic Caesar | 2 tbsp | 50 | 0 | 0 | 0 | 0 | 350 | 11 | 0 | 1 |
| Free Italian | 2 tbsp | 20 | 0 | 0 | 0 | 0 | 380 | 4 | 0 | 0 |
| Honey Dijon | 2 tbsp | 100 | 80 | 9 | 1.5 | 0 | 250 | 6 | 0 | 0 |
| **SANDWICH SHOP MAYO** | | | | | | | | | | |
| Chipotle | 1/2 oz | 40 | 35 | 4 | .5 | 5 | 120 | 2 | 0 | 0 |
| Hot & Spicy | 1/2 oz | 100 | 100 | 11 | 1.5 | 5 | 85 | 0 | 0 | 0 |
| **SINGLES CHEESE** | | | | | | | | | | |
| American | 1 slice | 70 | 45 | 5 | 3 | 20 | 270 | 2 | 0 | 4 |
| American Fat Free | 1 slice | 25 | 0 | 0 | 0 | 5 | 250 | 2 | 0 | 4 |
| Pepperjack, 2% | 1 slice | 45 | 20 | 2.5 | 1.5 | 10 | 330 | 2 | 0 | 4 |

# store brands

| | SERVING SIZE | CAL | CAL FAT | TOT FAT (G) | SAT FAT (G) | CHOL (MG) | SOD (MG) | CARB (G) | FIBER (G) | PROT (G) |
|---|---|---|---|---|---|---|---|---|---|---|
| Sharp Cheddar, 2% | 1 slice | 45 | 25 | 3 | 1.5 | 10 | 250 | 1 | 0 | 4 |
| Sharp Cheddar, Fat Free | 1 slice | 25 | 0 | 0 | 0 | 5 | 250 | 2 | 0 | 4 |
| Swiss 2% | 1 slice | 45 | 20 | 2.5 | 1.5 | 10 | 270 | 2 | 0 | 4 |
| Swiss Fat Free | 1 slice | 25 | 0 | 0 | 0 | 5 | 250 | 2 | 0 | 4 |
| **Larabar** | | | | | | | | | | |
| Apple Pie | 1 bar | 190 | 90 | 10 | 1 | 0 | 10 | 24 | 5 | 4 |
| Banana Bread | 1 bar | 230 | 100 | 11 | 1 | 0 | 0 | 30 | 5 | 6 |
| Cherry Pie | 1 bar | 200 | 70 | 8 | .5 | 0 | 0 | 30 | 5 | 5 |
| Chocolate Coconut | 1 bar | 240 | 120 | 13 | 2.5 | 0 | 0 | 29 | 5 | 5 |
| Cinnamon Roll | 1 bar | 240 | 110 | 12 | 1 | 0 | 0 | 30 | 4 | 5 |
| Cocoa Mole | 1 bar | 220 | 80 | 9 | 1 | 0 | 0 | 33 | 6 | 4 |
| Coconut Cream Pie | 1 bar | 220 | 90 | 11 | 7 | 0 | 5 | 31 | 6 | 3 |
| Key Lime Pie | 1 bar | 220 | 90 | 10 | 3.5 | 0 | 0 | 31 | 4 | 4 |
| Lemon | 1 bar | 220 | 100 | 11 | 1.5 | 0 | 0 | 28 | 4 | 5 |
| Peanut Butter and Jelly | 1 bar | 210 | 90 | 10 | 2 | 0 | 60 | 27 | 4 | 6 |
| Peanut Butter Cookie | 1 bar | 220 | 110 | 12 | 2 | 0 | 45 | 23 | 4 | 7 |
| Pecan Pie | 1 bar | 220 | 130 | 14 | 1 | 0 | 0 | 24 | 4 | 3 |
| Tropical Fruit Tart | 1 bar | 210 | 110 | 12 | 7 | 0 | 0 | 25 | 5 | 3 |
| **The Laughing Cow** | | | | | | | | | | |
| **MINI BABYBEL** | | | | | | | | | | |
| Babybel Bonbel | 1 piece | 70 | 50 | 6 | 4 | 20 | 170 | 0 | 0 | 5 |
| Babybel Mild Cheddar | 1 piece | 70 | 45 | 5 | 3 | 20 | 140 | 0 | 0 | 5 |
| Babybel Original | 1 piece | 70 | 50 | 6 | 4 | 20 | 170 | 0 | 0 | 5 |
| Babybel Light | 1 piece | 50 | 25 | 3 | 1.5 | 15 | 160 | 0 | 0 | 6 |
| **LIGHT WEDGES** | | | | | | | | | | |
| Creamy Swiss Wedges | 1 piece | 35 | 10 | 1.5 | 1 | <5 | 210 | 1 | 0 | 2 |
| French Onion Wedges | 1 piece | 35 | 10 | 1.5 | 1 | <5 | 210 | 1 | 0 | 2 |
| Garlic & Herb Wedges | 1 piece | 35 | 10 | 1.5 | 1 | <5 | 210 | 1 | 0 | 2 |
| Mozzarella, Sun-Dried Tomato & Basil | 1 piece | 35 | 15 | 2 | 1 | 5 | 220 | 2 | 0 | 2 |
| Queso Fresco & Chipotle | 1 piece | 35 | 15 | 1.5 | 1 | 5 | 240 | 2 | 0 | 2 |
| **ORIGINAL WEDGES** | | | | | | | | | | |
| Original Creamy Swiss | 1 piece | 50 | 35 | 4 | 2.5 | 10 | 210 | 1 | 0 | 2 |
| **Lay's** | | | | | | | | | | |
| **POTATO CHIPS** | | | | | | | | | | |
| Barbecue Flavored | 1 oz | 150 | 90 | 10 | 1 | 0 | 200 | 15 | 1 | 2 |
| Cheddar & Sour Cream Flavored | 1 oz | 160 | 90 | 10 | 1 | <5 | 230 | 15 | <1 | 2 |
| Classic | 1 oz | 150 | 90 | 10 | 1 | 0 | 180 | 15 | 1 | 2 |

| | SERVING SIZE | CAL | CAL FAT | TOT FAT (G) | SAT FAT (G) | CHOL (MG) | SOD (MG) | CARB (G) | FIBER (G) | PROT (G) |
|---|---|---|---|---|---|---|---|---|---|---|
| Kettle Cooked Crinkle Cut Original | 1 oz | 150 | 70 | 8 | 1 | 0 | 110 | 18 | 1 | 2 |
| Kettle Cooked Original | 1 oz | 150 | 80 | 8 | 1 | 0 | 110 | 18 | 1 | 2 |
| Kettle Cooked Sea Salt & Vinegar Flavored | 1 oz | 150 | 70 | 8 | 1 | 0 | 250 | 16 | 2 | 2 |
| Light Original | 1 oz | 75 | 0 | 0 | 0 | 0 | 200 | 17 | 1 | 2 |
| Lightly Salted | 1 oz | 150 | 90 | 10 | 1 | 0 | 90 | 15 | 1 | 2 |
| Salt & Vinegar Flavored | 1 oz | 150 | 90 | 10 | 1 | 0 | 380 | 15 | 1 | 2 |
| Sour Cream & Onion Flavored | 1 oz | 160 | 90 | 10 | 1 | 0 | 210 | 15 | 1 | 2 |
| Wavy Original | 1 oz | 150 | 90 | 10 | 1 | 0 | 180 | 15 | 1 | 2 |
| **POTATO CRISPS** | | | | | | | | | | |
| Baked Original Crisps | 1 oz | 120 | 15 | 2 | 0 | 0 | 180 | 23 | 2 | 2 |
| Baked Sour Cream & Onion Flavored Crisps | 1 oz | 120 | 25 | 3 | .5 | 0 | 210 | 21 | 2 | 2 |
| Stax Original Flavored Crisps | 1 oz | 150 | 80 | 9 | 1 | 0 | 160 | 16 | 1 | 2 |
| Stax Sour Cream & Onion Flavored Crisps | 1 oz | 150 | 90 | 10 | 1 | 0 | 190 | 15 | 1 | 1 |

## Lean Cuisine—Entrées

### CAFÉ

| | SERVING SIZE | CAL | CAL FAT | TOT FAT (G) | SAT FAT (G) | CHOL (MG) | SOD (MG) | CARB (G) | FIBER (G) | PROT (G) |
|---|---|---|---|---|---|---|---|---|---|---|
| Chicken Carbonara | 1 entrée | 270 | 50 | 6 | 2 | 30 | 600 | 33 | 3 | 21 |
| Lemon Pepper Fish | 1 entrée | 290 | 70 | 8 | 2 | 25 | 520 | 40 | 2 | 15 |
| Orange Chicken | 1 entrée | 300 | 60 | 7 | 2 | 25 | 580 | 46 | 2 | 14 |
| Sweet & Sour Chicken | 1 entrée | 300 | 25 | 3 | 0 | 30 | 560 | 51 | 2 | 18 |
| Thai Style Chicken | 1 entrée | 260 | 35 | 4 | 1 | 35 | 540 | 35 | 0 | 21 |
| **CASUAL** | | | | | | | | | | |
| Chicken Club Panini | 1 entrée | 360 | 80 | 9 | 4 | 40 | 680 | 46 | 4 | 24 |
| Deluxe Pizza Traditional | 1 entrée | 340 | 70 | 8 | 2 | 20 | 510 | 49 | 4 | 17 |
| Pepperoni Pizza Traditional | 1 entrée | 350 | 70 | 8 | 3 | 20 | 630 | 50 | 3 | 20 |
| **COMFORT** | | | | | | | | | | |
| Beef Pot Roast | 1 entrée | 210 | 50 | 6 | 2 | 25 | 550 | 26 | 3 | 14 |
| Roasted Turkey & Vegetables | 1 entrée | 190 | 50 | 6 | 1 | 25 | 480 | 18 | 4 | 17 |
| **DINNERTIME SELECTS** | | | | | | | | | | |
| Chicken Fettuccini | 1 entrée | 330 | 50 | 6 | 3 | 40 | 770 | 42 | 4 | 26 |
| Grilled Chicken & Penne Pasta | 1 entrée | 330 | 45 | 5 | 2 | 30 | 500 | 53 | 6 | 18 |
| Roasted Turkey Breast | 1 entrée | 290 | 60 | 7 | 1 | 30 | 890 | 38 | 5 | 19 |
| Salisbury Steak | 1 entrée | 270 | 80 | 9 | 4 | 45 | 650 | 27 | 5 | 19 |
| **MARKET CREATIONS** | | | | | | | | | | |
| Chicken Alfredo | 1 entrée | 280 | 60 | 7 | 2 | 35 | 680 | 33 | 4 | 20 |
| Garlic Chicken | 1 entrée | 270 | 50 | 6 | 1 | 30 | 670 | 33 | 4 | 20 |
| Shrimp Scampi | 1 entrée | 250 | 60 | 7 | 4 | 58 | 690 | 32 | 4 | 15 |
| Sweet & Spicy Ginger Chicken | 1 entrée | 280 | 25 | 2 | 1 | 30 | 680 | 43 | 4 | 21 |

# store brands

| | SERVING SIZE | CAL | CAL FAT | TOT FAT (G) | SAT FAT (G) | CHOL (MG) | SOD (MG) | CARB (G) | FIBER (G) | PROT (G) |
|---|---|---|---|---|---|---|---|---|---|---|
| **SIMPLE FAVORITES** | | | | | | | | | | |
| Alfredo Pasta with Chicken & Broccoli | 1 entrée | 300 | 50 | 6 | 3 | 30 | 660 | 45 | 3 | 16 |
| Cheese Ravioli | 1 entrée | 220 | 45 | 5 | 3 | 35 | 620 | 33 | 3 | 11 |
| Chicken Chow Mein | 1 entrée | 240 | 35 | 4 | 1 | 25 | 550 | 39 | 3 | 13 |
| Chicken Fettuccini | 1 entrée | 270 | 50 | 6 | 3 | 40 | 690 | 32 | 0 | 22 |
| Classic Five Cheese Lasagna | 1 entrée | 360 | 70 | 8 | 3.5 | 20 | 600 | 51 | 4 | 21 |
| Lasagna with Meat Sauce | 1 entrée | 320 | 70 | 8 | 4 | 30 | 630 | 45 | 4 | 17 |
| Macaroni and Cheese | 1 entrée | 290 | 60 | 7 | 4 | 20 | 630 | 41 | 1 | 15 |
| Spaghetti with Meatballs | 1 entrée | 270 | 50 | 6 | 2 | 25 | 580 | 38 | 3 | 16 |
| **SPA CUISINE** | | | | | | | | | | |
| Butternut Squash Ravioli | 1 entrée | 270 | 60 | 7 | 2 | 19 | 590 | 42 | 5 | 10 |
| Ginger Garlic Stir Fry with Chicken | 1 entrée | 280 | 35 | 4 | 1 | 30 | 550 | 42 | 5 | 20 |
| Grilled Chicken Primavera | 1 entrée | 200 | 25 | 3 | 1 | 20 | 580 | 26 | 5 | 17 |
| **Lean Pockets** | | | | | | | | | | |
| Breakfast—Ham, Egg, & Cheese | 1 pocket | 270 | 70 | 7 | 3.5 | 60 | 460 | 40 | 1 | 11 |
| Breakfast—Sausage, Egg, & Cheese | 1 pocket | 280 | 70 | 8 | 3.5 | 55 | 430 | 40 | 2 | 11 |
| Cheeseburger | 1 pocket | 290 | 80 | 9 | 4 | 20 | 530 | 42 | 2 | 9 |
| Four Cheese Pizza | 1 pocket | 270 | 50 | 5 | 3 | 20 | 490 | 42 | 2 | 12 |
| Meatballs & Mozzarella | 1 pocket | 290 | 80 | 9 | 4 | 25 | 560 | 40 | 3 | 12 |
| Pepperoni Pizza | 1 pocket | 290 | 70 | 8 | 4 | 20 | 610 | 40 | 2 | 12 |
| Philly Steak & Cheese | 1 pocket | 270 | 70 | 8 | 4 | 25 | 630 | 39 | 2 | 10 |
| Soft Baked Subs—Italian Style Meatballs | 1 pocket | 250 | 60 | 7 | 2.5 | 20 | 590 | 35 | 3 | 12 |
| Stuffed Quesadilla—Grilled Chicken & Three Cheese | 1 pocket | 360 | 70 | 8 | 3.5 | 25 | 820 | 49 | 2 | 20 |
| Whole Grain—Chicken, Broccoli & Cheddar | 1 pocket | 250 | 60 | 7 | 3 | 20 | 420 | 40 | 4 | 10 |
| Whole Grain—Ham & Cheddar | 1 pocket | 270 | 70 | 8 | 4 | 25 | 540 | 39 | 3 | 11 |
| Whole Grain—Meatballs & Mozzarella | 1 pocket | 240 | 70 | 7 | 3.5 | 20 | 480 | 32 | 4 | 12 |
| Whole Grain—Three Cheese & Broccoli | 1 pocket | 240 | 50 | 6 | 3 | 15 | 430 | 41 | 4 | 12 |
| Whole Grain—Turkey & Ham with Cheese | 1 pocket | 260 | 70 | 8 | 3.5 | 20 | 500 | 38 | 3 | 10 |
| Whole Grain Pizzeria—Supreme Pizza | 1 pocket | 220 | 60 | 6 | 3 | 20 | 550 | 33 | 4 | 10 |
| **Lender's** | | | | | | | | | | |
| **FROZEN ORIGINAL BAGELS** | | | | | | | | | | |
| Blueberry | 1 bagel | 150 | 5 | .5 | 0 | 0 | 240 | 32 | 1 | 5 |
| Cinnamon Raisin | 1 bagel | 160 | 20 | 2 | 0 | 0 | 250 | 32 | 2 | 5 |
| Egg | 1 bagel | 150 | 10 | 1 | 0 | 15 | 300 | 30 | 1 | 6 |

| | SERVING SIZE | CAL | CAL FAT | TOT FAT (G) | SAT FAT (G) | CHOL (MG) | SOD (MG) | CARB (G) | FIBER (G) | PROT (G) |
|---|---|---|---|---|---|---|---|---|---|---|
| Soft | 1 bagel | 200 | 25 | 2.5 | .5 | 10 | 340 | 38 | 2 | 6 |
| Onion | 1 bagel | 140 | 5 | .5 | 0 | 0 | 290 | 30 | 1 | 5 |
| Plain | 1 bagel | 230 | 10 | 1 | 0 | 0 | 490 | 48 | 1 | 8 |
| **NEW YORK STYLE BAGELS** | | | | | | | | | | |
| 100% Whole Wheat | 1 bagel | 210 | 15 | 1.5 | 0 | 0 | 420 | 41 | 6 | 10 |
| Cinnamon Raisin | 1 bagel | 250 | 15 | 1.5 | .5 | 0 | 380 | 51 | 3 | 8 |
| Everything | 1 bagel | 250 | 15 | 1.5 | 0 | 20 | 490 | 49 | 2 | 9 |
| Plain | 1 bagel | 240 | 20 | 2 | 0 | 0 | 490 | 46 | 2 | 9 |
| **REFRIGERATED PREMIUM BAGELS** | | | | | | | | | | |
| 100% Whole Wheat | 1 bagel | 180 | 15 | 1.5 | 0 | 0 | 370 | 35 | 5 | 9 |
| Blueberry | 1 bagel | 210 | 15 | 1.5 | 0 | 0 | 320 | 41 | 1 | 7 |
| Cinnamon Raisin | 1 bagel | 200 | 15 | 1.5 | 0 | 0 | 290 | 40 | 2 | 6 |
| Egg | 1 bagel | 200 | 20 | 2 | .5 | 20 | 330 | 37 | 1 | 7 |
| Onion | 1 bagel | 200 | 15 | 1.5 | 0 | 0 | 330 | 38 | 2 | 7 |
| Premium Plain | 1 bagel | 210 | 15 | 1.5 | .5 | 0 | 440 | 43 | 2 | 7 |
| **Lightlife** | | | | | | | | | | |
| **BREAKFAST** | | | | | | | | | | |
| Gimme Lean Sausage | 2 oz | 60 | 0 | 0 | 0 | 0 | 310 | 7 | 3 | 7 |
| Smart Bacon | 1 slice | 20 | 10 | 1 | 0 | 0 | 140 | 0 | 0 | 2 |
| Smart Links Breakfast | 2 pieces | 100 | 25 | 3 | 0 | 0 | 500 | 8 | 3 | 10 |
| **CHICK'N & MORE** | | | | | | | | | | |
| Smart Cutlets Original | 1 piece | 110 | 5 | .5 | 0 | 0 | 360 | 8 | 3 | 17 |
| Smart Strips Chick'n | 3 pieces | 80 | 0 | 0 | 0 | 0 | 520 | 6 | 4 | 14 |
| Smart Strips Steak | 3 pieces | 80 | 0 | 0 | 0 | 0 | 570 | 6 | 5 | 14 |
| Smart Wings Buffalo | 4 pieces | 110 | 30 | 3 | 0 | 0 | 680 | 6 | 4 | 13 |
| **GROUNDS** | | | | | | | | | | |
| Gimme Lean Beef | 2 oz | 70 | 0 | 0 | 0 | 0 | 350 | 10 | 2 | 7 |
| Gimme Lean Sausage | 2 oz | 60 | 0 | 0 | 0 | 0 | 310 | 7 | 3 | 7 |
| Smart Ground Original | 1/3 package | 70 | 0 | 0 | 0 | 0 | 310 | 6 | 3 | 12 |
| **HOT DOGS & SAUSAGES** | | | | | | | | | | |
| Smart Dogs | 1 piece | 45 | 0 | 0 | 0 | 0 | 310 | 2 | 1 | 8 |
| Smart Sausages Italian Style | 1 piece | 140 | 70 | 7 | 1 | 0 | 500 | 7 | 1 | 13 |
| Tofu Pups | 1 piece | 60 | 25 | 2.5 | .5 | 0 | 300 | 2 | 1 | 8 |
| **LIGHT BURGERS** | | | | | | | | | | |
| Original | 1 piece | 120 | 15 | 1.5 | 0 | 0 | 500 | 12 | 3 | 16 |
| Veggie | 1 piece | 140 | 35 | 4 | .5 | 0 | 370 | 16 | 4 | 10 |

# store brands

| | SERVING SIZE | CAL | CAL FAT | TOT FAT (G) | SAT FAT (G) | CHOL (MG) | SOD (MG) | CARB (G) | FIBER (G) | PROT (G) |
|---|---|---|---|---|---|---|---|---|---|---|
| **SMART DELI** | | | | | | | | | | |
| Baked Ham Style | 4 slices | 70 | 10 | 1 | 0 | 0 | 390 | 3 | 0 | 12 |
| Bologna Style | 4 slices | 70 | 0 | 0 | 0 | 0 | 490 | 4 | 1 | 14 |
| Pepperoni Style | 13 slices | 50 | 10 | 1 | 0 | 0 | 240 | 2 | 1 | 9 |
| Roast Turkey Style | 4 slices | 100 | 30 | 3.5 | .5 | 0 | 300 | 5 | 2 | 13 |
| **Luna Bar** | | | | | | | | | | |
| Caramel Nut Brownie | 1 bar | 180 | 50 | 6 | 2.5 | 0 | 110 | 27 | 3 | 8 |
| Chocolate Raspberry | 1 bar | 170 | 45 | 5 | 2 | 0 | 135 | 27 | 5 | 8 |
| Cookies 'n Cream Delight | 1 bar | 180 | 45 | 5 | 2.5 | 0 | 140 | 28 | 4 | 8 |
| Dulce de Leche | 1 bar | 170 | 35 | 4 | 1.5 | 0 | 125 | 27 | 3 | 9 |
| Iced Oatmeal Raisin | 1 bar | 180 | 45 | 5 | 2 | 0 | 150 | 27 | 3 | 9 |
| Peanut Butter Cookie | 1 bar | 180 | 50 | 6 | 2 | 0 | 160 | 26 | 3 | 9 |
| Vanilla Almond | 1 bar | 190 | 60 | 6 | 2 | 0 | 210 | 25 | 3 | 10 |
| **Manwich** | | | | | | | | | | |
| Original | 1/4 cup | 40 | 0 | 0 | 0 | 0 | 410 | 9 | 2 | <1 |
| **Marie Callender's** | | | | | | | | | | |
| **CLASSIC ENTRÉES** | | | | | | | | | | |
| Beef & Broccoli | 1 entrée | 400 | 120 | 14 | 4.5 | 45 | 1200 | 52 | 3 | 22 |
| Beef Tips Dinner | 1 entrée | 310 | 60 | 7 | 2.5 | 45 | 890 | 41 | 7 | 21 |
| Fettuccine Chicken & Broccoli | 1 entrée | 650 | 360 | 40 | 16 | 70 | 1150 | 41 | 6 | 31 |
| Swedish Meatballs | 1 entrée | 540 | 250 | 28 | 11 | 60 | 1310 | 48 | 6 | 23 |
| **COMPLETE MEALS** | | | | | | | | | | |
| Chicken Parmesan Dinner | 1 entrée | 620 | 270 | 30 | 7 | 45 | 830 | 57 | 9 | 29 |
| Country Fried Chicken Dinner | 1 entrée | 570 | 240 | 27 | 9 | 70 | 1340 | 60 | 7 | 24 |
| Country Fried Pork Chop | 1 entrée | 470 | 180 | 20 | 7 | 60 | 1380 | 49 | 8 | 23 |
| Meat Loaf with Gravy | 1 entrée | 450 | 170 | 18 | 7 | 75 | 1090 | 41 | 6 | 29 |
| Old Fashioned Beef Pot Roast | 1 entrée | 260 | 60 | 6 | 2.5 | 45 | 1130 | 31 | 7 | 20 |
| Sweet & Sour Chicken | 1 entrée | 520 | 90 | 10 | 1.5 | 20 | 620 | 92 | 7 | 15 |
| Turkey with Stuffing | 1 entrée | 350 | 90 | 10 | 2.5 | 35 | 1200 | 43 | 9 | 23 |
| **HOME STYLE CREATIONS** | | | | | | | | | | |
| Classic Stroganoff | 1 entrée | 310 | 90 | 10 | 3.5 | 35 | 860 | 39 | 3 | 17 |
| Creamy Four Cheese Mac | 1 entrée | 470 | 220 | 24 | 10 | 40 | 980 | 44 | 5 | 19 |
| Meatball Lasagna | 1 entrée | 310 | 80 | 9 | 3 | 20 | 760 | 43 | 6 | 14 |
| Traditional Stuffing & Turkey | 1 entrée | 310 | 50 | 6 | 1.5 | 20 | 950 | 47 | 3 | 17 |
| **PASTA** | | | | | | | | | | |
| Chicken Carbonara | 1 entrée | 390 | 110 | 13 | 5 | 45 | 780 | 45 | 5 | 22 |
| Meat Lasagna | 1 entrée | 260 | 90 | 10 | 5 | 35 | 960 | 32 | 4 | 10 |

| | SERVING SIZE | CAL | CAL FAT | TOT FAT (G) | SAT FAT (G) | CHOL (MG) | SOD (MG) | CARB (G) | FIBER (G) | PROT (G) |
|---|---|---|---|---|---|---|---|---|---|---|
| Rigatoni Marinara Classic | 1 entrée | 460 | 210 | 24 | 9 | 45 | 990 | 41 | 7 | 19 |
| Spaghetti with Meat Sauce | 1 entrée | 490 | 130 | 14 | 4 | 20 | 1030 | 67 | 7 | 23 |
| Tortellini Romano | 1 entrée | 430 | 130 | 14 | 7 | 40 | 840 | 59 | 7 | 17 |
| **POT PIES** | | | | | | | | | | |
| Beef Pot Pie | 1 cup | 510 | 270 | 29 | 11 | 25 | 780 | 48 | 3 | 14 |
| Chicken Pot Pie | 1 cup | 520 | 280 | 31 | 11 | 30 | 800 | 45 | 3 | 14 |
| Turkey Pot Pie | 1 pie | 630 | 320 | 36 | 13 | 20 | 1180 | 58 | 4 | 19 |
| **Marzetti** | | | | | | | | | | |
| **CROUTONS** | | | | | | | | | | |
| Large Cut Fat Free Garlic & Onion | 2 tbsp | 30 | 0 | 0 | 0 | 0 | 85 | 5 | 0 | 1 |
| Large Cut Garlic & Butter | 2 tbsp | 35 | 15 | 1.5 | 0 | 0 | 55 | 4 | 0 | 1 |
| Large Cut Ranch | 2 tbsp | 35 | 15 | 1.5 | 0 | 0 | 95 | 4 | 0 | 1 |
| **DIPS** | | | | | | | | | | |
| Blue Cheese Veggie | 2 tbsp | 140 | 130 | 15 | 3 | 15 | 250 | 1 | 0 | 1 |
| Dill Veggie | 2 tbsp | 120 | 110 | 13 | 3.5 | 20 | 200 | 2 | 0 | 1 |
| Fat Free Caramel Apple | 2 tbsp | 100 | 0 | 0 | 0 | 0 | 105 | 25 | 0 | n/a |
| Fat Free Ranch Veggie | 2 tbsp | 30 | 0 | 0 | 0 | 0 | 330 | 6 | 0 | 1 |
| French Onion Veggie | 2 tbsp | 120 | 110 | 12 | 3 | 20 | 220 | 2 | 0 | 1 |
| Guacamole Veggie | 2 tbsp | 130 | 120 | 13 | 2.5 | 15 | 240 | 2 | 0 | 0 |
| Old Fashioned Caramel | 2 tbsp | 140 | 50 | 6 | 3 | 5 | 75 | 22 | 0 | 0 |
| Original Hummus | 2 tbsp | 70 | 50 | 6 | 1 | 0 | 110 | 4 | 1 | 2 |
| Ranch Veggie | 2 tbsp | 120 | 110 | 12 | 3.5 | 20 | 210 | 2 | 0 | 1 |
| Roasted Red Pepper Hummus | 2 tbsp | 70 | 50 | 5 | 1 | 0 | 150 | 4 | 1 | 2 |
| Strawberry Cream Cheese Fruit | 2 tbsp | 70 | 30 | 3.5 | 2 | 15 | 90 | 9 | 0 | 0 |
| **DRESSINGS** | | | | | | | | | | |
| Balsamic Vinaigrette | 2 tbsp | 100 | 80 | 9 | 1.5 | 0 | 340 | 4 | 0 | 0 |
| Chunky Blue Cheese | 2 tbsp | 150 | 140 | 15 | 3 | 15 | 320 | 1 | 0 | 1 |
| Classic Ranch | 2 tbsp | 160 | 150 | 17 | 2.5 | 10 | 200 | 1 | 0 | 1 |
| Country French | 2 tbsp | 160 | 130 | 14 | 2 | 5 | 180 | 7 | 0 | 0 |
| Creamy Caesar | 2 tbsp | 120 | 110 | 12 | 2 | 15 | 370 | 2 | 0 | 1 |
| Fat Free Honey Dijon | 2 tbsp | 50 | 0 | 0 | 0 | 0 | 290 | 12 | 0 | 0 |
| Fat Free Italian | 2 tbsp | 15 | 0 | 0 | 0 | 0 | 290 | 4 | 0 | 0 |
| Italian | 2 tbsp | 90 | 70 | 8 | 1 | 0 | 480 | 4 | 0 | 0 |
| Light Balsamic Vinaigrette | 2 tbsp | 45 | 30 | 3 | 0 | 0 | 350 | 5 | 0 | 0 |
| Light Chunky Blue Cheese | 2 tbsp | 80 | 70 | 7 | 1.5 | 15 | 340 | 4 | 1 | 1 |
| Light Classic Ranch | 2 tbsp | 80 | 70 | 8 | 1 | 10 | 250 | 2 | 0 | 1 |
| Ranch | 2 tbsp | 120 | 110 | 13 | 2 | 10 | 240 | 2 | 0 | 0 |

| | SERVING SIZE | CAL | CAL FAT | TOT FAT (G) | SAT FAT (G) | CHOL (MG) | SOD (MG) | CARB (G) | FIBER (G) | PROT (G) |
|---|---|---|---|---|---|---|---|---|---|---|
| Thousand Island | 2 tbsp | 150 | 130 | 15 | 2.5 | 15 | 250 | 5 | 0 | n/a |
| **Milky Way** | | | | | | | | | | |
| Fun Size | 2 bars | 150 | 50 | 6 | 4 | 5 | 55 | 24 | 0 | 1 |
| Original | 1 bar | 260 | 90 | 10 | 7 | 5 | 95 | 41 | 1 | 2 |
| **Minute Maid** | | | | | | | | | | |
| **FRUIT DRINKS** | | | | | | | | | | |
| Bright & Early | 8 fl oz | 110 | 0 | 0 | 0 | 0 | 20 | 30 | 0 | 0 |
| Cherry Limeade | 8 fl oz | 120 | 0 | 0 | 0 | 0 | 15 | 34 | 0 | 0 |
| Enhanced Pomegranate Berry Flavored Drink | 12 fl oz | 120 | 0 | 0 | 0 | 0 | 60 | 28 | 4 | 0 |
| Enhanced Pomegranate Flavored Tea | 8 fl oz | 40 | 0 | 0 | 0 | 0 | 20 | 9 | 0 | 0 |
| Enhanced Pomegranate Lemonade | 12 fl oz | 110 | 0 | 0 | 0 | 0 | 20 | 31 | 0 | 0 |
| Fruit Punch | 8 fl oz | 110 | 0 | 0 | 0 | 0 | 15 | 30 | 0 | 0 |
| Lemonade | 8 fl oz | 110 | 0 | 0 | 0 | 0 | 15 | 29 | 0 | 0 |
| Lemonade Iced Tea | 8 fl oz | 110 | 0 | 0 | 0 | 0 | 20 | 29 | 0 | 0 |
| Pineapple Orange | 8 fl oz | 120 | 0 | 0 | 0 | 0 | 15 | 29 | 0 | 1 |
| Pink Lemonade | 8 fl oz | 110 | 0 | 0 | 0 | 0 | 15 | 29 | 0 | 0 |
| Raspberry Lemonade | 8 fl oz | 120 | 0 | 0 | 0 | 0 | 15 | 32 | 0 | 0 |
| **JUICE** | | | | | | | | | | |
| Apple | 8 fl oz | 110 | 0 | 0 | 0 | 0 | 20 | 28 | 0 | 0 |
| Country Style Orange | 8 fl oz | 110 | 0 | 0 | 0 | 0 | 15 | 27 | 0 | 2 |
| Cranberry Apple Raspberry | 8 fl oz | 120 | 0 | 0 | 0 | 0 | 20 | 33 | 0 | 0 |
| Cranberry Grape | 8 fl oz | 150 | 0 | 0 | 0 | 0 | 20 | 38 | 0 | 0 |
| Grape | 10 fl oz | 150 | 0 | 0 | 0 | 0 | 25 | 39 | 0 | 0 |
| Grapefruit | 8 fl oz | 100 | 0 | 0 | 0 | 0 | 0 | 25 | 0 | 0 |
| Light Orange | 8 fl oz | 50 | 0 | 0 | 0 | 0 | 15 | 12 | 0 | 0 |
| Original Orange | 8 fl oz | 110 | 0 | 0 | 0 | 0 | 15 | 27 | 0 | 2 |
| Ruby Red Grapefruit | 8 fl oz | 130 | 0 | 0 | 0 | 0 | 20 | 34 | 0 | 0 |
| **Miracle Whip** | | | | | | | | | | |
| Fat Free | 1/2 oz | 15 | 0 | 0 | 0 | 0 | 125 | 3 | 0 | 0 |
| Light | 1/2 oz | 20 | 15 | 1.5 | 0 | 5 | 135 | 2 | 0 | 0 |
| Original | 1/2 oz | 40 | 35 | 3.5 | .5 | 5 | 105 | 2 | 0 | 0 |
| **Mission Tortillas** | | | | | | | | | | |
| 96% Fat Free Large Burrito Tortilla | 1 tortilla | 180 | 20 | 2.5 | .5 | 0 | 450 | 35 | 5 | 5 |
| 96% Fat Free Medium Soft Taco | 1 tortilla | 130 | 15 | 1.5 | 0 | 0 | 330 | 26 | 3 | 4 |
| 96% Fat Free Small Tortilla | 1 tortilla | 90 | 10 | 1 | 0 | 0 | 210 | 17 | 2 | 2 |
| Homestyle Tortilla | 1 tortilla | 180 | 35 | 4 | 1.5 | 0 | 490 | 31 | 3 | 5 |
| Large Burrito Tortilla | 1 tortilla | 210 | 45 | 5 | 2 | 0 | 630 | 36 | 1 | 6 |

| | SERVING SIZE | CAL | CAL FAT | TOT FAT (G) | SAT FAT (G) | CHOL (MG) | SOD (MG) | CARB (G) | FIBER (G) | PROT (G) |
|---|---|---|---|---|---|---|---|---|---|---|
| White Corn Tortilla | 2 tortillas | 90 | 10 | 1 | 0 | 0 | 10 | 18 | 3 | 2 |
| Yellow Corn Tortilla | 2 tortillas | 80 | 10 | 1 | 0 | 0 | 10 | 16 | 2 | 2 |
| **Monster** | | | | | | | | | | |
| **ENERGY DRINKS** | | | | | | | | | | |
| Absolutely Zero Energy | 8 fl oz | 0 | n/a | n/a | n/a | n/a | n/a | 1 | n/a | n/a |
| Lo-Carb Energy | 8 fl oz | 10 | n/a | n/a | n/a | n/a | n/a | 3 | n/a | n/a |
| M-80 Energy | 8 fl oz | 90 | n/a | n/a | n/a | n/a | n/a | 23 | n/a | n/a |
| Monster Energy | 8 fl oz | 100 | n/a | n/a | n/a | n/a | n/a | 27 | n/a | n/a |
| **JAVA MONSTER** | | | | | | | | | | |
| Loca Moca Energy | 8 fl oz | 100 | 15 | 1.5 | 1 | 10 | 340 | 17 | n/a | 5 |
| Mean Bean Energy | 8 fl oz | 100 | 15 | 1.5 | 1 | 10 | 340 | 17 | n/a | 5 |
| Originale Energy | 8 fl oz | 100 | 15 | 1.5 | 1 | 10 | 340 | 17 | n/a | 5 |
| **Morning Star Farms** | | | | | | | | | | |
| Chik Patties Original | 1 item | 140 | 45 | 5 | .5 | 0 | 590 | 16 | 2 | 8 |
| Chik'n Nuggets | 4 pieces | 190 | 80 | 9 | 1.5 | 0 | 600 | 19 | 4 | 12 |
| Garden Veggie Patties | 1 item | 110 | 30 | 3.5 | .5 | 0 | 350 | 9 | 3 | 10 |
| Grillers 1/4 Pounder | 1 item | 250 | 110 | 12 | 2 | 0 | 490 | 10 | 3 | 26 |
| Grillers California Turk'y Burger | 1 item | 90 | 45 | 5 | .5 | 0 | 390 | 7 | 5 | 9 |
| Grillers Chik'n Veggies Patties | 1 item | 80 | 30 | 3 | 0 | 0 | 350 | 7 | 5 | 9 |
| Grillers Original | 1 item | 130 | 50 | 6 | 1 | 0 | 260 | 5 | 2 | 15 |
| Grillers Prime Veggie Burgers | 1 item | 170 | 80 | 9 | 1 | 0 | 360 | 4 | 2 | 17 |
| Grillers Vegan Veggie Burgers | 1 item | 100 | 25 | 2.5 | 0 | 0 | 280 | 7 | 4 | 12 |
| Original Chick'n Tenders | 2 items | 190 | 60 | 7 | 1 | 0 | 580 | 20 | 3 | 12 |
| Veggie Bacon Strips | 2 items | 60 | 40 | 4.5 | .5 | 0 | 230 | 2 | 1 | 2 |
| Veggie Sausage Links | 2 items | 80 | 25 | 3 | .5 | 0 | 300 | 3 | 2 | 9 |
| Veggie Sausage Patties | 1 item | 80 | 25 | 3 | .5 | 0 | 260 | 3 | 1 | 10 |
| **Mott's** | | | | | | | | | | |
| **HEALTHY HARVEST SAUCE** | | | | | | | | | | |
| Granny Smith | 1 cup | 50 | 0 | 0 | 0 | 0 | 0 | 13 | 1 | 0 |
| Mixed Berry | 1 cup | 50 | 0 | 0 | 0 | 0 | 0 | 13 | 1 | 0 |
| Summer Strawberry | 1 cup | 50 | 0 | 0 | 0 | 0 | 0 | 13 | 1 | 0 |
| **MEDLEY JUICES** | | | | | | | | | | |
| Apple & Carrot Juice Blend | 8 oz | 110 | 0 | 0 | 0 | 0 | 80 | 25 | 0 | 0 |
| Grape Apple & Carrot Juice Blend | 8 oz | 140 | 0 | 0 | 0 | 0 | 80 | 33 | 0 | 0 |
| Tropical Fruit & Carrot Juice Blend | 8 oz | 140 | 0 | 0 | 0 | 0 | 90 | 32 | 0 | 0 |
| **ORIGINAL APPLE SAUCE** | | | | | | | | | | |
| Cinnamon Apple Sauce | 1 cup | 100 | 0 | 0 | 0 | 0 | 0 | 24 | 1 | 0 |

# store brands

| | SERVING SIZE | CAL | CAL FAT | TOT FAT (G) | SAT FAT (G) | CHOL (MG) | SOD (MG) | CARB (G) | FIBER (G) | PROT (G) |
|---|---|---|---|---|---|---|---|---|---|---|
| Natural Apple Sauce | 1 cup | 50 | 0 | 0 | 0 | 0 | 0 | 12 | 1 | 0 |
| Original Apple Sauce | 1 cup | 100 | 0 | 0 | 0 | 0 | 0 | 24 | 1 | 0 |
| **ORIGINAL JUICE** | | | | | | | | | | |
| 100% Apple Juice | 4 oz | 60 | 0 | 0 | 0 | 0 | 5 | 15 | 0 | 0 |
| 100% Juice, Fruit Punch | 4 oz | 60 | 0 | 0 | 0 | 0 | 5 | 16 | 0 | 0 |
| 100% Juice, Grape | 4 oz | 60 | 0 | 0 | 0 | 0 | 5 | 16 | 0 | 0 |
| **Mountain Dew** | | | | | | | | | | |
| Original | 8 fl oz | 110 | 0 | 0 | 0 | 0 | 35 | 29 | 0 | 0 |
| **Mrs. Smith's** | | | | | | | | | | |
| **COBBLERS** | | | | | | | | | | |
| Apple Crumb | 1/8 cobbler | 270 | 80 | 9 | 3.5 | 0 | 210 | 45 | 2 | 2 |
| Blackberry | 1/8 cobbler | 250 | 70 | 8 | 3.5 | 0 | 210 | 43 | 1 | 2 |
| Cherry Crumb | 1/8 cobbler | 270 | 80 | 9 | 4 | 0 | 200 | 46 | 1 | 2 |
| **CUSTARD PIES** | | | | | | | | | | |
| Classic Coconut Custard | 1/6 pie | 310 | 150 | 17 | 9 | 65 | 340 | 33 | 2 | 6 |
| Classic Pumpkin | 1/6 pie | 280 | 120 | 14 | 6 | 45 | 310 | 36 | 1 | 4 |
| **PREBAKED PIES** | | | | | | | | | | |
| Apple | 1/8 pie | 340 | 140 | 16 | 7 | 0 | 440 | 46 | 2 | 3 |
| Blueberry | 1/8 pie | 330 | 140 | 16 | 7 | 0 | 430 | 45 | 2 | 3 |
| Cherry | 1/8 pie | 350 | 140 | 16 | 7 | 0 | 360 | 48 | 1 | 3 |
| Peach | 1/8 pie | 330 | 140 | 16 | 7 | 0 | 420 | 43 | 1 | 3 |
| **Nabisco** | | | | | | | | | | |
| **CHEESE NIPS** | | | | | | | | | | |
| Cheddar | 1 oz | 150 | 60 | 6 | 1.5 | 0 | 340 | 19 | 1 | 3 |
| Cheddar, Reduced Fat | 1 oz | 130 | 30 | 3.5 | 1 | 0 | 350 | 21 | 1 | 3 |
| **CHIPS AHOY!** | | | | | | | | | | |
| Chocolate Chip | 1 oz | 160 | 70 | 8 | 2.5 | 0 | 105 | 21 | 1 | 2 |
| Chunky Chocolate | 1/2 oz | 80 | 40 | 4.5 | 1.5 | 0 | 55 | 11 | 1 | 1 |
| Chunky Peanut Butter | 1/2 oz | 90 | 45 | 5 | 2.5 | 0 | 75 | 10 | 0 | 1 |
| Chunky White Fudge | 1/2 oz | 90 | 40 | 4.5 | 1.5 | 0 | 60 | 11 | 0 | 1 |
| **NEWTONS COOKIES** | | | | | | | | | | |
| Fig | 1 oz | 110 | 20 | 2 | 0 | 0 | 125 | 22 | 1 | 1 |
| Fig, Fat Free | 1 oz | 90 | 0 | 0 | 0 | 0 | 125 | 22 | 1 | 1 |
| Raspberry | 1 oz | 100 | 15 | 1.5 | 0 | 0 | 110 | 21 | 0 | 1 |
| **NILLA WAFERS** | | | | | | | | | | |
| Reduced Fat | 1 oz | 120 | 15 | 2 | 0 | 0 | 110 | 24 | 0 | 1 |
| Wafers | 1 oz | 140 | 50 | 6 | 1.5 | 5 | 115 | 21 | 0 | 1 |

| | SERVING SIZE | CAL | CAL FAT | TOT FAT (G) | SAT FAT (G) | CHOL (MG) | SOD (MG) | CARB (G) | FIBER (G) | PROT (G) |
|---|---|---|---|---|---|---|---|---|---|---|
| **RITZ CRACKERS** | | | | | | | | | | |
| Hint of Salt | 1/2 oz | 80 | 35 | 4 | 1 | 0 | 35 | 10 | 0 | 1 |
| Original | 1/2 oz | 80 | 40 | 4.5 | 1 | 0 | 135 | 10 | 0 | 1 |
| Reduced Fat | 1/2 oz | 70 | 20 | 2 | 0 | 0 | 160 | 11 | 0 | 1 |
| **SIMPLY SOCIALS** | | | | | | | | | | |
| Original | 1/2 oz | 70 | 25 | 3 | .5 | 0 | 140 | 10 | 0 | 1 |
| Whole Wheat | 1/2 oz | 70 | 25 | 3 | .5 | 0 | 150 | 10 | 1 | 1 |
| **TOASTED CHIPS** | | | | | | | | | | |
| Main Street Original | 1 oz | 130 | 40 | 4.5 | .5 | 0 | 250 | 21 | 1 | 2 |
| Sweet Home Sour Cream & Onion | 1 oz | 130 | 50 | 6 | 1 | 0 | 270 | 19 | 0 | 2 |
| Wheat Thins Great Plains Multigrain | 1 oz | 120 | 35 | 4 | .5 | 0 | 240 | 20 | 1 | 2 |
| **TRISCUIT** | | | | | | | | | | |
| Cracked Pepper & Olive Oil | 1 oz | 120 | 35 | 4 | 1 | 0 | 140 | 20 | 3 | 3 |
| Fire Roasted Tomato | 1 oz | 120 | 35 | 4 | 1 | 0 | 150 | 20 | 3 | 3 |
| Garden Herb | 1 oz | 120 | 35 | 4 | 1 | 0 | 125 | 20 | 3 | 3 |
| Original | 1 oz | 120 | 40 | 4.5 | 1 | 0 | 180 | 19 | 3 | 3 |
| Reduced Fat | 1 oz | 120 | 25 | 3 | .5 | 0 | 160 | 21 | 3 | 3 |
| Roasted Garlic | 1 oz | 120 | 40 | 4.5 | 1 | 0 | 140 | 20 | 3 | 3 |
| Rosemary & Olive Oil | 1 oz | 120 | 35 | 4 | 1 | 0 | 135 | 20 | 3 | 3 |
| **WHEAT THINS** | | | | | | | | | | |
| Artisan Vermont White Cheddar | 12 crackers | 140 | 45 | 5 | 1 | <5 | 230 | 21 | 1 | 2 |
| Fiber Selects 5-Grain | 13 crackers | 120 | 40 | 4.5 | .5 | 0 | 220 | 22 | 5 | 2 |
| Fiber Selects Garden Vegetable | 15 crackers | 120 | 35 | 4 | .5 | 0 | 240 | 22 | 5 | 2 |
| Flatbread Garlic & Parsley | 2 crackers | 60 | 15 | 1.5 | 0 | 0 | 125 | 12 | <1 | 1 |
| Multigrain | 15 crackers | 140 | 40 | 4.5 | .5 | 0 | 200 | 22 | 2 | 2 |
| Original | 16 crackers | 140 | 45 | 5 | 1 | 0 | 230 | 22 | 2 | 2 |
| Ranch | 16 crackers | 140 | 50 | 5 | 1 | 0 | 190 | 21 | 2 | 2 |
| Reduced Fat | 16 crackers | 130 | 30 | 3.5 | .5 | 0 | 230 | 22 | 2 | 2 |
| Whole Grain | 16 crackers | 140 | 50 | 6 | 1 | 0 | 280 | 21 | 2 | 2 |
| **Nesquik** | | | | | | | | | | |
| **FLAVORED MILK** | | | | | | | | | | |
| Low Fat Chocolate | 1 cup | 170 | 25 | 2.5 | 1.5 | 10 | 160 | 29 | <1 | 8 |
| Low Fat Strawberry | 1 cup | 180 | 25 | 2.5 | 1.5 | 10 | 125 | 31 | 0 | 8 |
| Low Fat Vanilla | 1 cup | 170 | 20 | 2.5 | 1.5 | 10 | 130 | 30 | 0 | 8 |
| **SYRUP** | | | | | | | | | | |
| Chocolate | 1 tbsp | 50 | 0 | 0 | 0 | 0 | 30 | 13 | 0 | 0 |
| Strawberry | 1 tbsp | 50 | 0 | 0 | 0 | 0 | 0 | 13 | 0 | 0 |

# store brands

| | SERVING SIZE | CAL | CAL FAT | TOT FAT (G) | SAT FAT (G) | CHOL (MG) | SOD (MG) | CARB (G) | FIBER (G) | PROT (G) |
|---|---|---|---|---|---|---|---|---|---|---|
| **Nestea** | | | | | | | | | | |
| **ICED TEA** | | | | | | | | | | |
| Diet with Lemon Flavor | 8 fl oz | 0 | 0 | 0 | 0 | 0 | 30 | 0 | 0 | 0 |
| With Lemon Flavor | 8 fl oz | 80 | 0 | 0 | 0 | 0 | 30 | 23 | 0 | 0 |
| **ICED TEA MIXES** | | | | | | | | | | |
| Sweetened Iced Tea with Lemon | 1-1/3 tbsp | 60 | 0 | 0 | 0 | 0 | 0 | 15 | 0 | 0 |
| Unsweetened Regular | 2 tsp | 0 | 0 | 0 | 0 | 0 | 0 | <1 | 0 | 0 |
| **Nestlé Toll House** | | | | | | | | | | |
| Butterscotch Morsels | 1 tbsp | 70 | 35 | 4 | 3.5 | 0 | 15 | 9 | 0 | 0 |
| Chocolate Chunks Morsels | 1 tbsp | 60 | 30 | 3.5 | 2 | 0 | 0 | 8 | 0 | 0 |
| Milk Chocolate Morsels | 1 tbsp | 70 | 40 | 4 | 2.5 | 4 | 5 | 9 | 0 | 0 |
| Peanut Butter & Milk Chocolate Morsels | 1 tbsp | 70 | 40 | 4.5 | 3 | 0 | 25 | 9 | 0 | 1 |
| Premier White Morsels | 1 tbsp | 70 | 35 | 4 | 3.5 | 0 | 15 | 9 | 0 | 0 |
| **Newman's Own** | | | | | | | | | | |
| **BEVERAGES** | | | | | | | | | | |
| Virgin Lemonade | 8 fl oz | 110 | 0 | 0 | 0 | 0 | 40 | 27 | 0 | 0 |
| Virgin Lemon-Aided Iced Tea | 8 fl oz | 110 | 0 | 0 | 0 | 0 | 40 | 27 | 0 | 0 |
| Virgin Limeade | 8 fl oz | 140 | 0 | 0 | 0 | 0 | 35 | 34 | 0 | 0 |
| **DRESSING, REGULAR** | | | | | | | | | | |
| Balsamic Vinaigrette | 2 tbsp | 90 | 80 | 9 | 1 | 0 | 350 | 3 | 0 | 0 |
| Caesar | 2 tbsp | 150 | 140 | 16 | 2.5 | 0 | 420 | 1 | 0 | 1 |
| Family Recipe Italian | 2 tbsp | 130 | 120 | 13 | 2 | 0 | 400 | 1 | 0 | 1 |
| Olive Oil & Vinegar | 2 tbsp | 150 | 150 | 16 | 2.5 | 0 | 150 | 1 | 0 | 0 |
| Ranch | 2 tbsp | 150 | 140 | 16 | 2.5 | 10 | 310 | 2 | 0 | 0 |
| **LIGHTEN UP DRESSING** | | | | | | | | | | |
| Balsamic Vinaigrette | 2 tbsp | 45 | 40 | 4 | .5 | 0 | 390 | 2 | 0 | 0 |
| Caesar | 2 tbsp | 70 | 50 | 6 | 1 | 5 | 420 | 3 | 0 | 1 |
| Italian | 2 tbsp | 60 | 50 | 6 | 1 | 0 | 260 | 1 | 0 | 0 |
| Raspberry & Walnut | 2 tbsp | 70 | 45 | 5 | .5 | 0 | 120 | 7 | 0 | 0 |
| Red Wine Vinegar & Olive Oil | 2 tbsp | 50 | 40 | 4.5 | .5 | 0 | 390 | 2 | 0 | 0 |
| **MICROWAVE POPCORN** | | | | | | | | | | |
| Butter | 3-1/2 cups | 130 | 45 | 5 | 2 | 0 | 180 | 18 | 3 | 2 |
| Light Butter | 3-1/2 cups | 120 | 35 | 4 | 1.5 | 0 | 170 | 19 | 4 | 3 |
| Natural Flavor | 3-1/2 cups | 130 | 45 | 5 | 2 | 0 | 200 | 18 | 3 | 2 |
| **SALSA** | | | | | | | | | | |
| Bandito Chunky, Hot | 2 tbsp | 10 | 0 | 0 | 0 | 0 | 150 | 2 | <1 | 0 |
| Bandito Chunky, Medium | 2 tbsp | 10 | 0 | 0 | 0 | 0 | 105 | 2 | 1 | 0 |

| | SERVING SIZE | CAL | CAL FAT | TOT FAT (G) | SAT FAT (G) | CHOL (MG) | SOD (MG) | CARB (G) | FIBER (G) | PROT (G) |
|---|---|---|---|---|---|---|---|---|---|---|
| Bandito Chunky, Mild | 2 tbsp | 10 | 0 | 0 | 0 | 0 | 65 | 2 | 1 | 0 |
| Black Bean & Corn | 2 tbsp | 20 | 0 | 0 | 0 | 0 | 140 | 5 | 2 | 1 |
| Farmer's Garden | 3 tbsp | 15 | 0 | 0 | 0 | 0 | 220 | 4 | 0 | 1 |

## Northland
### JUICES
| | | | | | | | | | | |
|---|---|---|---|---|---|---|---|---|---|---|
| Blueberry Açaí | 8 fl oz | 130 | 0 | 0 | n/a | n/a | 15 | 32 | n/a | 0 |
| Blueberry Blackberry Açaí | 8 fl oz | 130 | 0 | 0 | n/a | n/a | 20 | 32 | n/a | 0 |
| Cranberry Grape | 8 fl oz | 140 | n/a | 0 | n/a | n/a | 35 | 36 | n/a | 0 |
| Organic Cranberry | 8 fl oz | 120 | n/a | 0 | n/a | n/a | 15 | 31 | n/a | 0 |
| Pure Pomegranate | 8 fl oz | 140 | 0 | 0 | n/a | n/a | 25 | 34 | n/a | 0 |

## Nutrigrain Bars
| | | | | | | | | | | |
|---|---|---|---|---|---|---|---|---|---|---|
| Apple Cinnamon | 1 bar | 120 | 30 | 3 | .5 | 0 | 110 | 24 | 3 | 2 |
| Blueberry | 1 bar | 120 | 30 | 3 | .5 | 0 | 110 | 24 | 3 | 2 |
| Cherry | 1 bar | 120 | 30 | 3 | .5 | 0 | 110 | 24 | 3 | 2 |
| Mixed Berry | 1 bar | 120 | 30 | 3 | .5 | 0 | 110 | 24 | 3 | 2 |
| Raspberry | 1 bar | 120 | 30 | 3 | .5 | 0 | 110 | 24 | 3 | 2 |
| Strawberry | 1 bar | 120 | 30 | 3 | .5 | 0 | 125 | 24 | 3 | 2 |

## Ocean Spray
### CRAISINS
| | | | | | | | | | | |
|---|---|---|---|---|---|---|---|---|---|---|
| Sweetened Dried Cranberries | 1/3 cup | 130 | 0 | 0 | 0 | 0 | n/a | 33 | 3 | 0 |

### CRANBERRY SAUCE
| | | | | | | | | | | |
|---|---|---|---|---|---|---|---|---|---|---|
| Jellied | 1/4 cup | 110 | 0 | 0 | 0 | 0 | n/a | 25 | 0 | 0 |

### JUICE & JUICE DRINKS
| | | | | | | | | | | |
|---|---|---|---|---|---|---|---|---|---|---|
| Cran-Apple Cranberry Apple Juice Drink | 8 fl oz | 130 | 0 | 0 | 0 | 0 | n/a | 32 | 0 | 0 |
| Cran-Cherry Cranberry Cherry Juice Drink | 8 fl oz | 120 | 0 | 0 | 0 | 0 | n/a | 30 | 0 | 0 |
| Cran-Grape Grape Cranberry Juice Drink | 8 fl oz | 120 | 0 | 0 | 0 | 0 | 35 | 31 | 0 | 0 |
| Cranberry Juice Cocktail | 8 fl oz | 120 | 0 | 0 | 0 | 0 | 35 | 30 | 0 | 0 |
| Diet Cranberry | 8 fl oz | 5 | 0 | 0 | 0 | 0 | 60 | 2 | 0 | 0 |
| Light Cranberry Juice Cocktail | 8 fl oz | 40 | 0 | 0 | 0 | 0 | 80 | 10 | 0 | 0 |
| Ruby Red Grapefruit Juice Cocktail | 8 fl oz | 110 | 0 | 0 | 0 | 0 | 65 | 28 | 0 | 0 |
| White Cranberry Juice Drink | 8 fl oz | 110 | 0 | 0 | 0 | 0 | 40 | 27 | 0 | 0 |

## Old El Paso
### REFRIED BEANS
| | | | | | | | | | | |
|---|---|---|---|---|---|---|---|---|---|---|
| Fat-free Refried Beans | 1/2 cup | 100 | 0 | 0 | 0 | 0 | 580 | 18 | 6 | 6 |
| Traditional Refried Beans | 1/2 cup | 90 | 5 | .5 | 0 | 0 | 580 | 16 | 5 | 5 |
| Vegetarian Refried Beans | 1/2 cup | 90 | 5 | .5 | 0 | 0 | 570 | 16 | 5 | 5 |

# store brands

| | SERVING SIZE | CAL | CAL FAT | TOT FAT (G) | SAT FAT (G) | CHOL (MG) | SOD (MG) | CARB (G) | FIBER (G) | PROT (G) |
|---|---|---|---|---|---|---|---|---|---|---|
| **SAUCES, SALSAS, & TOPPINGS** | | | | | | | | | | |
| Chopped Green Chiles | 2 tbsp | 10 | 0 | 0 | 0 | 0 | 120 | 2 | 0 | 0 |
| Hot Enchilada Sauce | 1/4 cup | 20 | 0 | 0 | 0 | 0 | 360 | 3 | 0 | 0 |
| Hot Taco Sauce | 1 tbsp | 5 | 0 | 0 | 0 | 0 | 90 | 1 | 0 | 0 |
| Medium Cheese 'n Salsa | 2 tbsp | 35 | 25 | 3 | .5 | 0 | 280 | 3 | 0 | 0 |
| Medium Enchilada Sauce | 1/4 cup | 20 | 0 | 0 | 0 | 0 | 360 | 3 | 0 | 0 |
| Medium Taco Sauce | 1 tbsp | 5 | 0 | 0 | 0 | 0 | 90 | 1 | 0 | 0 |
| Mild Cheese 'n Salsa | 2 tbsp | 35 | 25 | 3 | .5 | 0 | 280 | 3 | 0 | 0 |
| Mild Enchilada Sauce | 1/4 cup | 20 | 0 | 0 | 0 | 0 | 360 | 3 | 0 | 0 |
| Mild Green Chile Enchilada Sauce | 1/4 cup | 25 | 10 | 1.5 | 0 | 0 | 280 | 4 | 0 | 0 |
| Thick 'n Chunky Salsa, Hot | 2 tbsp | 10 | 0 | 0 | 0 | 0 | 230 | 2 | 0 | 0 |
| Thick 'n Chunky Salsa, Medium | 2 tbsp | 10 | 0 | 0 | 0 | 0 | 230 | 2 | 0 | 0 |
| Thick 'n Chunky Salsa, Mild | 2 tbsp | 10 | 0 | 0 | 0 | 0 | 230 | 2 | 0 | 0 |
| **SHELLS** | | | | | | | | | | |
| Soft Flour Tortillas | 2 items | 150 | 40 | 4.5 | 1 | 0 | 360 | 25 | 0 | 3 |
| Taco Shells | 3 items | 150 | 60 | 7 | 1.5 | 0 | 135 | 20 | 1 | 2 |
| Tostada Shells | 3 items | 150 | 60 | 7 | 3 | 0 | 135 | 19 | 1 | 2 |
| **Ore-Ida** | | | | | | | | | | |
| **CLASSIC FRIES** | | | | | | | | | | |
| Golden | 3 oz | 130 | 30 | 3.5 | 2 | 0 | 310 | 21 | 2 | 2 |
| Golden Crinkles | 3 oz | 120 | 35 | 3.5 | 2 | 0 | 310 | 20 | 2 | 2 |
| **EASY FRIES** | | | | | | | | | | |
| Golden | 3 oz | 180 | 70 | 8 | 1.5 | 0 | 450 | 25 | 2 | 2 |
| Golden Crinkles | 3 oz | 180 | 70 | 8 | 1.5 | 0 | 400 | 25 | 2 | 2 |
| **EXTRA CRISPY FRIES** | | | | | | | | | | |
| Fast Food | 3 oz | 160 | 60 | 6 | 1 | 0 | 440 | 23 | 2 | 2 |
| Tater Tots | 3 oz | 170 | 80 | 9 | 1.5 | 0 | 460 | 20 | 2 | 2 |
| **PREMIUM FRIES** | | | | | | | | | | |
| Country Style | 3 oz | 130 | 40 | 4.5 | 1 | 0 | 300 | 20 | 2 | 2 |
| Cripsy Crunchies! | 3 oz | 150 | 60 | 7 | 1 | 0 | 310 | 21 | 2 | 2 |
| Texas Crispers! | 3 oz | 150 | 50 | 6 | 1 | 0 | 230 | 21 | 2 | 2 |
| Waffle | 3 oz | 160 | 60 | 6 | 1.5 | 0 | 390 | 22 | 2 | 2 |
| **Oscar Mayer** | | | | | | | | | | |
| **BACON** | | | | | | | | | | |
| Bacon | 1/2 oz | 70 | 50 | 6 | 2 | 15 | 290 | 0 | 0 | 4 |
| Center Cut | 1/2 oz | 50 | 35 | 4 | 2 | 15 | 270 | 0 | 0 | 4 |

| | SERVING SIZE | CAL | CAL FAT | TOT FAT (G) | SAT FAT (G) | CHOL (MG) | SOD (MG) | CARB (G) | FIBER (G) | PROT (G) |
|---|---|---|---|---|---|---|---|---|---|---|
| Lower Sodium | 1/2 oz | 70 | 50 | 6 | 2.5 | 10 | 170 | 0 | 0 | 4 |
| Natural Hardwood Smoked | 1/2 oz | 70 | 50 | 6 | 2 | 15 | 290 | 0 | 0 | 4 |
| Natural Smoked Un-Cured | 1/2 oz | 70 | 50 | 5 | 2 | 15 | 250 | 0 | 0 | 6 |
| Ready-to-Serve Bacon | 1/2 oz | 70 | 50 | 6 | 2 | 15 | 320 | 0 | 0 | 5 |
| Ready-to-Serve Canadian Bacon, Fully Cooked | 1-4/5 oz | 60 | 15 | 2 | 1 | 30 | 480 | 1 | 0 | 9 |
| Real Bacon Bits & Pieces | 1/4 oz | 25 | 15 | 1.5 | .5 | 5 | 170 | 0 | 0 | 2 |
| **BOLOGNA** | | | | | | | | | | |
| 98% Fat Free | 1 oz | 25 | 0 | 0.5 | 0 | 10 | 240 | 3 | 0 | 3 |
| Beef | 1 oz | 90 | 70 | 8 | 3.5 | 20 | 310 | 1 | 0 | 3 |
| Chicken & Pork | 1 oz | 90 | 80 | 8 | 3 | 30 | 300 | 1 | 0 | 3 |
| Light Beef | 1 oz | 60 | 35 | 4 | 1.5 | 15 | 240 | 2 | 0 | 3 |
| **DELI CREATIONS** | | | | | | | | | | |
| **COMPLETE SANDWICHES** | | | | | | | | | | |
| Honey Ham & Swiss | 1 sandwich | 440 | 140 | 15 | 5 | 60 | 1410 | 50 | 3 | 28 |
| Oven Roasted Ham & Cheddar | 1 sandwich | 460 | 150 | 16 | 6 | 60 | 1410 | 51 | 3 | 29 |
| Steakhouse Cheddar | 1 sandwich | 430 | 140 | 16 | 6 | 60 | 1560 | 47 | 5 | 28 |
| Turkey & Cheddar Dijon | 1 sandwich | 430 | 140 | 15 | 5 | 50 | 1410 | 48 | 5 | 26 |
| Turkey Monterey | 1 sandwich | 450 | 150 | 17 | 6 | 55 | 1090 | 50 | 4 | 25 |
| **CHICKEN** | | | | | | | | | | |
| Breast Cuts Honey Roasted | 3 oz | 110 | 20 | 2 | .5 | 50 | 420 | 2 | 0 | 21 |
| Breast Cuts Oven Roasted | 3 oz | 110 | 20 | 2 | .5 | 60 | 410 | 0 | 0 | 22 |
| Breast Strips Grilled | 3 oz | 110 | 20 | 2 | .5 | 65 | 510 | 0 | 0 | 22 |
| Breast Strips Italian | 3 oz | 100 | 10 | 1 | 1 | 55 | 700 | 0 | 0 | 22 |
| White, Oven Roasted | 1 oz | 35 | 15 | 1.5 | .5 | 15 | 330 | 1 | 0 | 5 |
| **DELI FRESH MEATS** | | | | | | | | | | |
| Chicken Breast, Oven Roasted | 2 oz | 60 | 15 | 1.5 | .5 | 30 | 710 | 1 | 0 | 10 |
| Chicken Breast, Oven Roasted, Shaved | 2 oz | 70 | 10 | 1 | .5 | 35 | 540 | 2 | 0 | 12 |
| Chicken Breast, Shaved Rotisserie 98% Fat Free | 2 oz | 50 | 5 | 1 | 0 | 25 | 530 | 2 | 0 | 9 |
| Chicken Strips, Grilled | 3 oz | 100 | 15 | 1.5 | 1 | 55 | 690 | 0 | 0 | 22 |
| Chicken Strips, Southwestern Seasoned | 3 oz | 110 | 15 | 1.5 | 1 | 55 | 690 | 0 | 0 | 22 |
| Cured French-Dip Flavored Beef | 1-4/5 oz | 60 | 15 | 2 | .5 | 30 | 550 | 1 | 0 | 10 |
| Ham, Baked Cooked 96% Fat Free | 2 oz | 60 | 10 | 1 | 1 | 30 | 780 | 1 | 0 | 11 |
| Ham, Chopped | 1 oz | 60 | 35 | 4 | 1.5 | 15 | 300 | 2 | 0 | 4 |
| Ham, Honey Smoked Shaved | 2 oz | 70 | 15 | 1 | .5 | 35 | 820 | 2 | 0 | 11 |
| Ham, Natural Smoked | 2 oz | 60 | 10 | 1 | .5 | 35 | 490 | 1 | 0 | 12 |

# store brands

| | SERVING SIZE | CAL | CAL FAT | TOT FAT (G) | SAT FAT (G) | CHOL (MG) | SOD (MG) | CARB (G) | FIBER (G) | PROT (G) |
|---|---|---|---|---|---|---|---|---|---|---|
| Ham, Smoked 98% Fat Free | 1-7/10 oz | 45 | 10 | 1 | 0 | 25 | 340 | 0 | 0 | 9 |
| Honey Ham 96% Fat Free | 2 oz | 70 | 20 | 2 | 1 | 30 | 770 | 2 | 2 | 11 |
| Honey Smoked, Shaved 98% Fat Free | 1 oz | 50 | 5 | 1 | 0.5 | 20 | 470 | 2 | 0 | 9 |
| Roast Beef, Slow Roasted, Shaved | 1-4/5 oz | 60 | 15 | 2 | 1 | 30 | 530 | 0 | 0 | 10 |
| Turkey Breast, Honey Oven Roasted, Shaved | 2-1/5 oz | 70 | 10 | 1 | 0.5 | 30 | 600 | 3 | 0 | 11 |
| Turkey Breast, Mesquite 98% Fat Free | 2 oz | 50 | 10 | 1 | 0.5 | 20 | 440 | 2 | 0 | 8 |
| Turkey Breast, Oven Roasted | 1-4/5 oz | 45 | 10 | .5 | 0 | 20 | 460 | 1 | 0 | 8 |
| Turkey Breast, Oven Roasted, Shaved 98% Fat Free | 2 oz | 45 | 10 | .5 | 0 | 20 | 460 | 1 | 0 | 8 |
| Turkey, Oven Roasted White 95% Fat Free | 1 oz | 30 | 10 | 1 | 0 | 15 | 360 | 1 | 0 | 5 |
| **HOT DOGS & FRANKS** | | | | | | | | | | |
| Beef Frank | 1-1/2 oz | 130 | 110 | 12 | 5 | 30 | 470 | 1 | 0 | 5 |
| Beef, Classic Bun Length | 2 oz | 170 | 130 | 15 | 7 | 40 | 590 | 1 | 0 | 7 |
| Classic Cheese Dogs | 1-1/2 oz | 140 | 120 | 13 | 4 | 35 | 540 | 1 | 0 | 5 |
| Classic Cheese Turkey Frank | 1-1/2 oz | 90 | 60 | 7 | 2.5 | 40 | 490 | 2 | 1 | 6 |
| Classic Turkey Dog | 1-1/2 oz | 100 | 70 | 8 | 2.5 | 30 | 510 | 2 | 0 | 5 |
| **LUNCHABLE CRACKER STACKERS** | | | | | | | | | | |
| Bologna & American Cheese | 1 package | 390 | 200 | 22 | 9 | 60 | 900 | 33 | 2 | 14 |
| Ham & Cheddar | 1 package | 340 | 170 | 19 | 9 | 70 | 1110 | 23 | 1 | 20 |
| Ham & Swiss Cheese | 1 package | 340 | 160 | 18 | 9 | 70 | 1130 | 23 | 1 | 20 |
| Nachos Cheese Dip & Salsa | 1 package | 380 | 190 | 21 | 4.5 | 10 | 870 | 40 | 3 | 7 |
| Pizza, Pepperoni Flavored Sausage | 1 package | 310 | 120 | 13 | 6 | 30 | 760 | 31 | 3 | 16 |
| Turkey & American Cheese | 1 package | 380 | 170 | 19 | 8 | 45 | 850 | 38 | 2 | 14 |
| Turkey, Ham, Swiss, & Cheddar Deluxe | 1 package | 360 | 170 | 19 | 9 | 70 | 1750 | 26 | 1 | 20 |
| **SAUSAGE & SALAMI** | | | | | | | | | | |
| Beef Summer Sausage | 1 oz | 80 | 70 | 7 | 3.5 | 20 | 400 | 0 | 0 | 4 |
| Cotto Salami | 1 oz | 70 | 50 | 6 | 2 | 25 | 280 | 1 | 0 | 4 |
| Hard Salami | 1 oz | 100 | 70 | 8 | 3 | 25 | 510 | 1 | 0 | 7 |
| **TURKEY** | | | | | | | | | | |
| Bologna, Lower Fat | 1 oz | 50 | 35 | 4 | 1 | 20 | 270 | 1 | 0 | 3 |
| Breast, Hickory Smoked, 98% Fat Free | 1 oz | 30 | 5 | .5 | 0 | 10 | 260 | 1 | 0 | 5 |
| Cold Cuts, Turkey Breast, Smoked, Shaved | 1-4/5 oz | 45 | 10 | .5 | 0 | 20 | 460 | 1 | 0 | 8 |
| Oven Roasted White 95% Fat Free | 1 oz | 30 | 15 | 1.5 | 0 | 10 | 220 | 1 | 0 | 3 |
| Smoked Turkey | 2 slices | 60 | 20 | 2 | 1 | 25 | 470 | 1 | 0 | 9 |
| Smoked White 95 % Fat Free | 1 oz | 30 | 15 | 1.5 | 0 | 10 | 250 | 1 | 0 | 3 |
| Turkey Ham | 1 oz | 40 | 20 | 2.5 | 1 | 20 | 360 | 1 | 0 | 5 |

| | SERVING SIZE | CAL | CAL FAT | TOT FAT (G) | SAT FAT (G) | CHOL (MG) | SOD (MG) | CARB (G) | FIBER (G) | PROT (G) |
|---|---|---|---|---|---|---|---|---|---|---|
| **WIENERS** | | | | | | | | | | |
| 98% Fat Free | 2 oz | 40 | 0 | 0.5 | 0 | 15 | 470 | 3 | 0 | 5 |
| Bun Length | 2 oz | 170 | 140 | 16 | 5 | 45 | 680 | 1 | 0 | 6 |
| Light | 1-1/2 oz | 90 | 60 | 6 | 2 | 30 | 380 | 1 | 0 | 5 |
| Turkey, Chicken, & Pork | 1-1/2 oz | 130 | 110 | 12 | 4 | 35 | 540 | 1 | 0 | 5 |
| Wiener | 1-1/2 oz | 130 | 110 | 12 | 4 | 35 | 540 | 1 | 0 | 5 |
| **Ovaltine** | | | | | | | | | | |
| **POWDERED MIX** | | | | | | | | | | |
| Chocolate Malt | 4 tbsp | 80 | 0 | 0 | 0 | 0 | 115 | 18 | <1 | 1 |
| Malt | 4 tbsp | 80 | 0 | 0 | 0 | 0 | 55 | 18 | 0 | 2 |
| Rich Chocolate | 4 tbsp | 80 | 0 | 0 | 0 | 0 | 140 | 19 | 0 | <1 |
| **Pace** | | | | | | | | | | |
| Chunky Salsa | 2 tbsp | 10 | 0 | 0 | 0 | 0 | 230 | 3 | 1 | 0 |
| Picante Sauce | 2 tbsp | 10 | 0 | 0 | 0 | 0 | 250 | 3 | 1 | 0 |
| Salsa Verde | 2 tbsp | 15 | 0 | .5 | 0 | 0 | 230 | 2 | 0 | 0 |
| **PAM** | | | | | | | | | | |
| Canola Oil Cooking Spray | 1/4 g | 0 | 0 | 0 | 0 | 0 | 0 | 0 | 0 | 0 |
| Olive Oil Cooking Spray | 1/4 g | 0 | 0 | 0 | 0 | 0 | 0 | 0 | 0 | 0 |
| **Parkay** | | | | | | | | | | |
| **MARGARINE** | | | | | | | | | | |
| Light Spread | 1 tbsp | 45 | 45 | 5 | 1 | 0 | 75 | 0 | 0 | 0 |
| Original Spread | 1 tbsp | 70 | 70 | 7 | 1.5 | 0 | 80 | 0 | 0 | 0 |
| Spray | 1 g | 0 | 0 | 0 | 0 | 0 | 15 | 0 | 0 | 0 |
| **Pasta Roni** | | | | | | | | | | |
| Butter & Garlic Flavor, Prepared | 1 cup | 250 | 70 | 8 | 2 | 5 | 690 | 39 | 2 | 8 |
| Chicken & Broccoli Flavor, Prepared | 1 cup | 360 | 140 | 15 | 4 | 5 | 920 | 40 | 2 | 10 |
| Chicken Flavor, Prepared | 1 cup | 300 | 110 | 12 | 3 | 5 | 960 | 40 | 2 | 9 |
| Creamy Garlic, Prepared | 1 cup | 330 | 140 | 16 | 4.5 | 5 | 810 | 40 | 2 | 9 |
| Fettuccine Alfredo, Prepared | 1 cup | 450 | 220 | 24 | 7 | 5 | 1050 | 44 | 2 | 11 |
| Shells & White Cheddar, Prepared | 1 cup | 290 | 110 | 12 | 4 | 5 | 730 | 38 | 2 | 9 |
| White Cheddar & Broccoli, Prepared | 1 cup | 300 | 120 | 13 | 4 | 5 | 710 | 39 | 2 | 9 |
| **Pepperidge Farm** | | | | | | | | | | |
| **AMERICAN COLLECTION** | | | | | | | | | | |
| **COOKIES** | | | | | | | | | | |
| Nantucket Double Chocolate Chunk | 1 cookie | 140 | 63 | 7 | 3 | 10 | 65 | 19 | 0 | 1 |
| Soft Baked Captiva Dark Chocolate Brownie | 1 cookie | 140 | 45 | 6 | 3 | 10 | 75 | 22 | 0 | 1 |

| | SERVING SIZE | CAL | CAL FAT | TOT FAT (G) | SAT FAT (G) | CHOL (MG) | SOD (MG) | CARB (G) | FIBER (G) | PROT (G) |
|---|---|---|---|---|---|---|---|---|---|---|
| Soft Baked Caramel Milk Chocolate Chunk Caramel | 1 cookie | 140 | 54 | 6 | 3 | 5 | 75 | 21 | 1 | 1 |
| Soft Baked Milk Chocolate | 1 cookie | 150 | 63 | 7 | 3 | 5 | 70 | 21 | 1 | 1 |
| Soft Baked Nantucket Dark Chocolate Chunk | 1 cookie | 150 | 72 | 8 | 3.5 | 10 | 95 | 20 | 0 | 2 |
| Soft Baked Oatmeal | 1 cookie | 140 | 45 | 5 | 2 | 10 | 120 | 22 | 1 | 2 |
| Soft Baked Oatmeal Dark Chocolate Almond Cherry Chunk | 1 cookie | 140 | 45 | 5 | 2 | 5 | 70 | 22 | 1 | 2 |
| Soft Baked Oatmeal Dark Chocolate Chunk | 1 cookie | 140 | 54 | 6 | 2 | 1 | 70 | 21 | 1 | 2 |
| Soft Baked Santa Cruz Oatmeal Raisin | 1 cookie | 130 | 40 | 4.5 | 1.5 | 5 | 90 | 23 | 2 | 2 |
| Soft Baked Sausalito Milk Chocolate Chunk Macadamia Nut | 1 cookie | 160 | 72 | 8 | 3.5 | 10 | 85 | 19 | 0 | 2 |
| Soft Baked Snickerdoodle | 1 cookie | 140 | 45 | 5 | 2.5 | 10 | 95 | 22 | 1 | 2 |
| Soft Baked Sugar | 1 cookie | 140 | 45 | 5 | 2.5 | 10 | 90 | 22 | 0 | 2 |
| **CRACKERS** | | | | | | | | | | |
| Distinctive Cracker Entertaining Quartet | 4 crackers | 70 | 22 | 2.5 | .5 | 5 | 95 | 10 | 1 | 1 |
| Distinctive Entertaining Cracker Trio | 4 crackers | 70 | 27 | 3 | .5 | 5 | 110 | 11 | 1 | 1 |
| Golden Butter Distinctive | 4 crackers | 70 | 22 | 2.5 | 1 | 5 | 100 | 11 | 0 | 1 |
| Harvest Wheat Distinctive | 3 crackers | 80 | 32 | 3.5 | .5 | 0 | 125 | 11 | 1 | 1 |
| **DISTINCTIVE COOKIE COLLECTIONS** | | | | | | | | | | |
| Chocolate | 2 cookies | 130 | 63 | 7 | 3 | 5 | 70 | 16 | 1 | 1 |
| Distinctive Entertaining | 3 cookies | 140 | 63 | 7 | 3.5 | 10 | 75 | 18 | 1 | 2 |
| Ginger Family | 4 cookies | 160 | 45 | 5 | 3 | 5 | 135 | 26 | 1 | 2 |
| Golden Orchard | 3 cookies | 140 | 54 | 6 | 3.5 | 10 | 21 | 1 | 9 | 0 |
| **GOLDFISH CRACKERS** | | | | | | | | | | |
| Colors | 55 pieces | 140 | 45 | 5 | 1 | 5 | 260 | 20 | 1 | 4 |
| Made with Whole Grain, Cheddar | 55 pieces | 140 | 45 | 5 | 1 | 5 | 250 | 19 | 2 | 4 |
| Original | 55 pieces | 150 | 54 | 6 | .5 | 0 | 230 | 20 | 1 | 3 |
| Parmesan | 60 pieces | 130 | 36 | 4 | 1 | 0 | 280 | 20 | 1 | 4 |
| Pizza | 55 pieces | 140 | 45 | 5 | 1 | 0 | 230 | 20 | 1 | 3 |
| Racing Ranch Flavor Blasted | 54 pieces | 130 | 41 | 4.5 | 1 | 5 | 300 | 19 | 1 | 4 |
| **MILANO COOKIES** | | | | | | | | | | |
| Black & White | 3 cookies | 180 | 90 | 10 | 5 | 5 | 85 | 21 | 1 | 2 |
| Chocolate Mint | 2 cookies | 130 | 63 | 7 | 4 | 5 | 120 | 16 | 1 | 1 |
| Chocolate Raspberry | 2 cookies | 130 | 63 | 7 | 4 | 5 | 65 | 16 | 1 | 1 |
| Raspberry | 2 cookies | 130 | 63 | 7 | 4.5 | 5 | 40 | 16 | 1 | 1 |
| Strawberry | 2 cookies | 130 | 63 | 7 | 3.5 | 5 | 40 | 16 | 1 | 1 |

| | SERVING SIZE | CAL | CAL FAT | TOT FAT (G) | SAT FAT (G) | CHOL (MG) | SOD (MG) | CARB (G) | FIBER (G) | PROT (G) |
|---|---|---|---|---|---|---|---|---|---|---|
| **PIROUETTES** | | | | | | | | | | |
| Chocolate Fudge | 2 wafers | 120 | 36 | 4 | 2 | 0 | 30 | 17 | 1 | 2 |
| Chocolate Hazelnut | 2 wafers | 120 | 45 | 5 | 2 | 5 | 40 | 19 | 1 | 1 |
| French Vanilla | 2 wafers | 120 | 45 | 5 | 2.5 | 5 | 40 | 18 | 0 | 1 |
| Mint Chocolate | 2 wafers | 120 | 40 | 4.5 | 2.5 | 5 | 40 | 18 | 1 | 1 |
| **SWIRL BREADS** | | | | | | | | | | |
| Cinnamon Swirl Bread | 1 slice | 80 | 14 | 1.5 | 0 | 0 | 110 | 15 | 1 | 2 |
| Raisin Cinnamon Swirl Bread | 1 slice | 80 | 14 | 1.5 | 0 | 0 | 100 | 15 | 1 | 2 |
| **Peter Pan** | | | | | | | | | | |
| Creamy Original Peanut Butter | 2 tbsp | 210 | 150 | 17 | 3 | 0 | 140 | 6 | 2 | 8 |
| Creamy Reduced Fat Peanut Butter | 2 tbsp | 200 | 120 | 13 | 2 | 0 | 150 | 14 | 2 | 8 |
| Crunchy Original Peanut Butter | 2 tbsp | 200 | 140 | 16 | 3 | 0 | 110 | 6 | 3 | 8 |
| Crunchy Reduced Fat Peanut Butter | 2 tbsp | 200 | 120 | 13 | 2.5 | 0 | 150 | 14 | 2 | 8 |
| **Philadelphia Cream Cheese** | | | | | | | | | | |
| Chive & Onion | 2 tbsp | 90 | 80 | 9 | 5 | 35 | 150 | 2 | 0 | 2 |
| Fat Free | 2 tbsp | 30 | 0 | 0 | 0 | 5 | 200 | 2 | 0 | 4 |
| Garden Vegetable | 2 tbsp | 90 | 70 | 8 | 5 | 35 | 160 | 2 | 0 | 2 |
| Light | 2 tbsp | 70 | 45 | 5 | 3 | 20 | 140 | 2 | 0 | 2 |
| Neufchatel, 1/3 Less Fat | 2 tbsp | 70 | 60 | 6 | 4 | 20 | 120 | 1 | 0 | 2 |
| Original | 2 tbsp | 100 | 80 | 9 | 6 | 35 | 105 | 1 | 0 | 2 |
| Regular | 2 tbsp | 90 | 80 | 9 | 5 | 35 | 125 | 2 | 0 | 2 |
| Salmon | 2 tbsp | 90 | 70 | 8 | 5 | 30 | 210 | 2 | 0 | 2 |
| Strawberry | 2 tbsp | 90 | 70 | 7 | 4.5 | 30 | 110 | 5 | 0 | 1 |
| **Pillsbury** | | | | | | | | | | |
| **BISCUITS** | | | | | | | | | | |
| Grands! Buttermilk Biscuits, Frozen | 1 biscuit | 170 | 70 | 8 | 2.5 | 0 | 490 | 22 | <1 | 3 |
| Grands! Cheddar Garlic Biscuits, Frozen | 1 biscuit | 180 | 80 | 9 | 2.5 | <5 | 660 | 22 | <1 | 4 |
| Grands! Homestyle Buttermilk Biscuits | 1 biscuit | 180 | 70 | 7 | 1.5 | 0 | 580 | 25 | <1 | 3 |
| Grands! Homestyle Original Biscuits | 1 biscuit | 170 | 60 | 7 | 1.5 | 0 | 580 | 25 | <1 | 3 |
| Grands! Homestyle Reduced Fat Buttermilk Biscuits | 1 biscuit | 160 | 50 | 4 | 3.5 | 0 | 590 | 25 | <1 | 3 |
| **BREADS & ROLLS** | | | | | | | | | | |
| Dinner Rolls | 1 roll | 100 | 15 | 1.5 | 0 | 0 | 290 | 20 | <1 | 3 |
| Garlic Breadsticks | 2 breadsticks | 180 | 80 | 9 | 2.5 | 0 | 560 | 23 | <1 | 4 |
| Original Breadsticks | 2 breadsticks | 130 | 15 | 2 | 0 | 0 | 380 | 26 | <1 | 4 |
| Original Crescent Rolls | 1 roll | 110 | 60 | 6 | 2 | 0 | 220 | 11 | 0 | 2 |

| | SERVING SIZE | CAL | CAL FAT | TOT FAT (G) | SAT FAT (G) | CHOL (MG) | SOD (MG) | CARB (G) | FIBER (G) | PROT (G) |
|---|---|---|---|---|---|---|---|---|---|---|
| Original Crescent Rounds | 1 round | 110 | 60 | 6 | 2 | 0 | 220 | 11 | 0 | 2 |
| Reduced Fat Crescent Rolls | 1 roll | 90 | 35 | 4.5 | 1.5 | 0 | 220 | 12 | 0 | 2 |
| **CINNAMON ROLLS & TWISTS** | | | | | | | | | | |
| Caramel Rolls | 1 roll | 170 | 60 | 7 | 2 | 0 | 330 | 25 | <1 | 2 |
| Cinnamon Rolls with Icing | 1 roll | 140 | 45 | 5 | 1.5 | 0 | 340 | 23 | <1 | 2 |
| Flaky Twists with Icing | 1 twist | 180 | 80 | 9 | 2.5 | 0 | 310 | 22 | <1 | 2 |
| Grands! Cinnamon Rolls, Frozen | 1 roll | 290 | 100 | 11 | 3.5 | 0 | 460 | 45 | 1 | 4 |
| Reduced Fat Cinnamon Rolls with Icing | 1 roll | 130 | 30 | 3.5 | 2.5 | 0 | 340 | 24 | <1 | 2 |
| **DESSERTS** | | | | | | | | | | |
| Apple Toaster Strudel | 1 item | 190 | 80 | 8 | 3.5 | 5 | 180 | 26 | <1 | 3 |
| Blueberry Toaster Strudel | 1 item | 180 | 60 | 7 | 3 | 5 | 190 | 27 | <1 | 3 |
| Cherry Toaster Strudel | 1 item | 190 | 80 | 8 | 3.5 | 5 | 180 | 26 | <1 | 3 |
| Chocolate Chip Cookies | 1 oz | 130 | 60 | 6 | 2.5 | <5 | 95 | 18 | 0 | 1 |
| Peanut Butter Cookies | 1 oz | 120 | 50 | 6 | 1.5 | <5 | 135 | 16 | 0 | 2 |
| Raspberry Toaster Strudel | 1 item | 180 | 60 | 7 | 3 | 5 | 190 | 27 | <1 | 3 |
| Ready to Bake Chocolate Chip Cookies | 2 cookies | 170 | 70 | 8 | 2.5 | <5 | 125 | 23 | <1 | 2 |
| Ready to Bake Chocolate Chunk & Chip Cookies | 2 cookies | 170 | 70 | 8 | 2.5 | <5 | 125 | 23 | <1 | 2 |
| Ready to Bake Gingerbread Cookies | 1 oz | 130 | 60 | 6 | 1.5 | <5 | 105 | 18 | 0 | 2 |
| Ready to Bake Oatmeal Chocolate Chip Cookies | 2 cookies | 160 | 70 | 7 | 2.5 | <5 | 95 | 23 | 1 | 2 |
| Ready to Bake Pumpkin Shape Sugar Cookies | 2 cookies | 120 | 60 | 6 | 1.5 | <5 | 85 | 15 | 0 | 1 |
| Ready to Bake Sugar Cookies | 2 items | 170 | 70 | 8 | 3.5 | <5 | 100 | 22 | 0 | 2 |
| Simply Chocolate Chip Cookies | 1 item | 150 | 70 | 8 | 3.5 | 5 | 115 | 19 | 0 | 1 |
| Simply Peanut Butter Cookies | 1 item | 140 | 60 | 7 | 2 | 5 | 150 | 19 | <1 | 2 |
| Strawberry Toaster Strudel | 1 item | 180 | 60 | 7 | 3 | 5 | 190 | 27 | <1 | 3 |
| Sugar Cookies | 2 cookies | 120 | 50 | 5 | 1.5 | <5 | 95 | 18 | 0 | 1 |
| Wild Berry Toaster Strudel | 1 item | 180 | 60 | 7 | 3 | 5 | 190 | 27 | <1 | 3 |
| **Planters** | | | | | | | | | | |
| **CASHEWS** | | | | | | | | | | |
| Chocolate Lovers | 1-1/2 oz | 230 | 140 | 16 | 7 | 5 | 25 | 20 | 1 | 5 |
| Deluxe Jumbo | 1 oz | 170 | 110 | 13 | 2.5 | 0 | 115 | 8 | 1 | 5 |
| Deluxe Whole, Honey Roasted | 1 oz | 150 | 100 | 11 | 2 | 0 | 120 | 11 | 1 | 4 |
| Deluxe Whole, Lightly Salted | 1 oz | 160 | 110 | 13 | 2.5 | 0 | 60 | 9 | 1 | 5 |
| Deluxe Whole, Regular | 1 oz | 160 | 110 | 13 | 2.5 | 0 | 115 | 8 | 1 | 5 |

| | SERVING SIZE | CAL | CAL FAT | TOT FAT (G) | SAT FAT (G) | CHOL (MG) | SOD (MG) | CARB (G) | FIBER (G) | PROT (G) |
|---|---|---|---|---|---|---|---|---|---|---|
| **MIXED NUTS** | | | | | | | | | | |
| Cashew Lovers w/Macadamias & Pecans | 1 oz | 180 | 150 | 17 | 2.5 | 0 | 90 | 6 | 2 | 4 |
| Deluxe Lightly Salted | 1 oz | 170 | 140 | 15 | 2.5 | 0 | 50 | 6 | 2 | 5 |
| Deluxe Regular | 1 oz | 170 | 140 | 15 | 2.5 | 0 | 100 | 6 | 2 | 5 |
| Honey Roasted | 1 oz | 160 | 110 | 12 | 1.5 | 0 | 120 | 9 | 2 | 5 |
| Macadamia Lovers w/Almonds & Pecans | 1 oz | 190 | 170 | 19 | 2.5 | 0 | 80 | 4 | 3 | 3 |
| Pecan Lovers w/Cashews & Pistachios | 1 oz | 180 | 150 | 17 | 2 | 0 | 70 | 6 | 2 | 4 |
| Pistachio Lovers Mix w/Jumbo Cashews & Almonds | 1 oz | 160 | 120 | 13 | 1.5 | 0 | 80 | 7 | 3 | 6 |
| Regular | 1 oz | 170 | 130 | 15 | 2 | 0 | 110 | 5 | 2 | 6 |
| Select Cashew, Almond & Pecan | 1 oz | 170 | 130 | 15 | 2 | 0 | 95 | 7 | 2 | 5 |
| Select Macadamia, Cashew & Almond | 1 oz | 180 | 140 | 16 | 2.5 | 0 | 95 | 6 | 2 | 4 |
| Unsalted | 1 oz | 170 | 130 | 15 | 2 | 0 | 0 | 5 | 2 | 6 |
| **NUT-RITION** | | | | | | | | | | |
| Almonds, Lightly Salted | 1 oz | 170 | 130 | 15 | 1.5 | 0 | 40 | 6 | 3 | 6 |
| Almonds, Smoked, Lightly Salted | 1 oz | 170 | 130 | 15 | 1 | 0 | 120 | 6 | 3 | 6 |
| Antioxidant Mix | 1/4 cup | 160 | 100 | 11 | 5 | 0 | 0 | 15 | 2 | 4 |
| Digestive Health Mix | 1/4 cup | 140 | 70 | 8 | .5 | 0 | 60 | 15 | 5 | 3 |
| Energy Bar | 1 bar | 170 | 80 | 2 | 2 | 0 | 170 | 17 | 2 | 5 |
| Energy Mix | 1 oz | 190 | 130 | 15 | 2 | 0 | 120 | 12 | 3 | 5 |
| Heart Healthy Bar | 1 bar | 160 | 70 | 1 | 1.5 | 0 | 130 | 19 | 3 | 6 |
| Heart Healthy Mix | 1 oz | 170 | 140 | 16 | 1.5 | 0 | 45 | 5 | 3 | 6 |
| Omega-3 Mix | 1/4 cup | 160 | 90 | 10 | 1.5 | 0 | 0 | 15 | 2 | 3 |
| **PEANUTS** | | | | | | | | | | |
| Cocktail Peanuts, Honey Roasted | 1 oz | 160 | 110 | 12 | 1.5 | 0 | 115 | 8 | 2 | 6 |
| Cocktail Peanuts, Lightly Salted | 1 oz | 170 | 130 | 14 | 2 | 0 | 55 | 5 | 2 | 8 |
| Cocktail Peanuts, Regular | 1 oz | 170 | 130 | 14 | 2 | 0 | 115 | 5 | 2 | 7 |
| Cocktail Peanuts, Unsalted | 1 oz | 170 | 130 | 14 | 2 | 0 | 0 | 5 | 2 | 8 |
| Dry Roasted Peanuts, Regular | 1 oz | 160 | 120 | 14 | 2 | 0 | 190 | 5 | 2 | 8 |
| **TRAIL MIX** | | | | | | | | | | |
| Berry, Nut & Chocolate | 1 oz | 120 | 45 | 5 | 1 | 0 | 20 | 18 | 1 | 2 |
| Daybreak Blend Trail Mix Apple Cinnamon | 1 oz | 200 | 90 | 10 | 1 | 0 | 70 | 24 | 3 | 4 |
| Daybreak Blend Trail Mix Berry Almond | 1 oz | 180 | 70 | 7 | .5 | 0 | 55 | 27 | 3 | 3 |
| Energy Mix | 1-1/2 oz | 250 | 180 | 19 | 2.5 | 0 | 135 | 14 | 3 | 6 |
| Fruit & Nut | 1 oz | 140 | 80 | 9 | 3 | 0 | 15 | 14 | 2 | 3 |
| Mixed Nuts & Raisins | 1 oz | 160 | 100 | 12 | 2 | 0 | 20 | 11 | 2 | 6 |
| Nut & Chocolate | 1 oz | 170 | 90 | 11 | 2.5 | 0 | 15 | 16 | 2 | 4 |

| | SERVING SIZE | CAL | CAL FAT | TOT FAT (G) | SAT FAT (G) | CHOL (MG) | SOD (MG) | CARB (G) | FIBER (G) | PROT (G) |
|---|---|---|---|---|---|---|---|---|---|---|
| Nuts, Seeds, & Raisins | 1 oz | 160 | 100 | 12 | 1.5 | 0 | 15 | 11 | 2 | 6 |
| Spicy Nuts & Cajun Sticks | 1 oz | 150 | 100 | 11 | 1.5 | 0 | 270 | 10 | 2 | 5 |
| Sweet & Nutty | 1 oz | 160 | 90 | 10 | 2 | 0 | 35 | 15 | 2 | 5 |

### Polly-O Natural Cheese
**MOZZARELLA**

| | | | | | | | | | | |
|---|---|---|---|---|---|---|---|---|---|---|
| Fat Free | 1 oz | 40 | 0 | 0 | 0 | 5 | 240 | 1 | 0 | 7 |
| Part Skim | 1 oz | 70 | 45 | 5 | 3 | 15 | 200 | 1 | 0 | 6 |
| Whole Milk | 1 oz | 80 | 60 | 6 | 4 | 20 | 200 | 1 | 0 | 6 |

**RICOTTA**

| | | | | | | | | | | |
|---|---|---|---|---|---|---|---|---|---|---|
| Fat Free | 2 oz | 45 | 0 | 0 | 0 | 5 | 80 | 3 | 0 | 8 |
| Lite | 2 oz | 70 | 25 | 3 | 1.5 | 10 | 80 | 3 | 0 | 8 |
| Original | 2 oz | 110 | 70 | 8 | 5 | 25 | 65 | 2 | 0 | 7 |
| Part Skim | 2 oz | 90 | 50 | 6 | 4 | 20 | 65 | 2 | 0 | 8 |

**SNACK CHEESE**

| | | | | | | | | | | |
|---|---|---|---|---|---|---|---|---|---|---|
| Twist-Ums & String-Ums, Mozzarella | 1 item | 80 | 50 | 6 | 3.5 | 20 | 200 | 1 | 0 | 7 |
| Twist-Ums & String-Ums, Mozzarella and Cheddar | 1 item | 60 | 35 | 4 | 2.5 | 15 | 140 | 0 | 0 | 6 |

### Pom Wonderful

| | | | | | | | | | | |
|---|---|---|---|---|---|---|---|---|---|---|
| 100% Pomegranate Juice | 8 oz | 160 | 0 | 0 | 0 | 0 | 10 | 40 | 0 | 0 |

### Pop Secret

| | | | | | | | | | | |
|---|---|---|---|---|---|---|---|---|---|---|
| Butter | 1 cup | 40 | 25 | 2.5 | .5 | 0 | 66 | 4 | <1 | <1 |
| 94% Fat Free Butter | 1 cup | 20 | 0 | 0 | 0 | 0 | 45 | 4 | <1 | <1 |
| Extra Butter | 1 cup | 40 | 25 | 3 | .5 | 0 | 60 | 3 | <1 | <1 |
| Homestyle | 1 cup | 35 | 20 | 2 | 0 | 0 | 60 | 4 | <1 | <1 |
| Light Butter | 1 cup | 20 | 10 | 1 | 0 | 0 | 55 | 4 | <1 | <1 |
| Movie Theater Butter | 1 cup | 40 | 25 | 3 | .5 | 0 | 66 | 4 | <1 | <1 |

### Popsicle

| | | | | | | | | | | |
|---|---|---|---|---|---|---|---|---|---|---|
| Big Stick | 1 pop | 70 | n/a | 0 | n/a | n/a | 0 | 17 | n/a | 0 |
| Fire Cracker | 1 pop | 35 | n/a | 0 | n/a | n/a | 0 | 9 | n/a | 0 |
| Fudgsicle Triple Chocolate | 1 pop | 60 | 15 | 1.5 | 1 | 0 | 60 | 11 | 0 | 1 |
| Orange Cherry Grape | 1 pop | 45 | n/a | 0 | n/a | n/a | 0 | 11 | n/a | 0 |
| Rainbow | 1 pop | 45 | n/a | 0 | n/a | n/a | 0 | 11 | n/a | 0 |

### Post
**BRAN FLAKES**

| | | | | | | | | | | |
|---|---|---|---|---|---|---|---|---|---|---|
| Bran Flakes | 3/4 cup | 100 | 5 | .5 | 0 | 0 | 180 | 24 | 5 | 3 |

**GRAPE NUTS**

| | | | | | | | | | | |
|---|---|---|---|---|---|---|---|---|---|---|
| Original Cereal | 1/2 cup | 200 | 10 | 1 | 0 | 0 | 290 | 48 | 7 | 6 |

| | SERVING SIZE | CAL | CAL FAT | TOT FAT (G) | SAT FAT (G) | CHOL (MG) | SOD (MG) | CARB (G) | FIBER (G) | PROT (G) |
|---|---|---|---|---|---|---|---|---|---|---|
| Flakes | 3/4 cup | 110 | 10 | 1 | 0 | 0 | 125 | 24 | 3 | 3 |
| **HONEY BUNCHES OF OATS** | | | | | | | | | | |
| Honey Roasted Original | 3/4 cup | 120 | 15 | 1.5 | 0 | 0 | 150 | 25 | 2 | 2 |
| With Almonds | 3/4 cup | 130 | 20 | 2.5 | 0 | 0 | 140 | 26 | 2 | 2 |
| **RAISIN BRAN** | | | | | | | | | | |
| Original | 1 cup | 190 | 10 | 1 | 0 | 0 | 250 | 46 | 8 | 5 |
| **SELECTS CEREAL** | | | | | | | | | | |
| Banana Nut Crunch | 1 cup | 240 | 50 | 6 | .5 | 0 | 230 | 44 | 5 | 5 |
| Blueberry Morning | 1-1/4 cups | 220 | 25 | 3 | 0 | 0 | 210 | 45 | 2 | 3 |
| Great Grains, Raisins, Dates & Pecans | 3/4 cup | 200 | 35 | 4 | 0 | 0 | 150 | 40 | 5 | 4 |
| **SHREDDED WHEAT** | | | | | | | | | | |
| Lightly Frosted | 1 cup | 180 | 10 | 1 | 0 | 0 | 0 | 44 | 5 | 4 |
| Original | 2 pieces | 160 | 10 | 1 | 0 | 0 | 0 | 37 | 6 | 5 |
| Original Spoon Size | 1 cup | 170 | 10 | 1 | 0 | 0 | 0 | 40 | 6 | 6 |
| **TRAIL MIX CRUNCH** | | | | | | | | | | |
| Cranberry Vanilla | 1/2 cup | 190 | 35 | 4 | 0 | 0 | 135 | 36 | 4 | 4 |
| Raisin & Almond | 1/2 cup | 180 | 20 | 2.5 | 0 | 0 | 210 | 37 | 5 | 4 |
| **Powerade** | | | | | | | | | | |
| Fruit Punch | 8 fl oz | 50 | 0 | 0 | 0 | 0 | 100 | 14 | 0 | 0 |
| Grape | 8 fl oz | 50 | 0 | 0 | 0 | 0 | 100 | 14 | 0 | 0 |
| Lemon Lime | 8 fl oz | 50 | 0 | 0 | 0 | 0 | 100 | 14 | 0 | 0 |
| Orange | 8 fl oz | 50 | 0 | 0 | 0 | 0 | 100 | 14 | 0 | 0 |
| Zero Lemon Lime | 8 fl oz | 0 | 0 | 0 | 0 | 0 | 100 | 0 | 0 | 0 |
| Zero Orange | 8 fl oz | 0 | 0 | 0 | 0 | 0 | 100 | 0 | 0 | 0 |
| **Prego** | | | | | | | | | | |
| **TOMATO SAUCE** | | | | | | | | | | |
| Chunky Garden Tomato, Onion & Garlic Italian | 1/2 cup | 90 | 25 | 3 | 0 | 0 | 470 | 13 | 3 | 2 |
| Fresh Mushroom Italian | 1/2 cup | 70 | 15 | 1.5 | 0 | 0 | 480 | 13 | 3 | 2 |
| Italian Sausage & Garlic | 1/2 cup | 90 | 25 | 3 | 1 | 5 | 480 | 13 | 3 | 3 |
| Mushroom & Garlic Italian | 1/2 cup | 80 | 22 | 2.5 | 0 | 0 | 470 | 13 | 3 | 2 |
| Roasted Garlic & Herb Italian | 1/2 cup | 90 | 25 | 3 | 0 | 0 | 460 | 13 | 3 | 2 |
| Roasted Garlic Parmesan Italian | 1/2 cup | 70 | 10 | 1 | .5 | 5 | 480 | 13 | 3 | 3 |
| **Premium Saltine Crackers** | | | | | | | | | | |
| Fat Free | 1/2 oz | 60 | 0 | 0 | 0 | 0 | 200 | 13 | 0 | 2 |
| Low Sodium | 1/2 oz | 60 | 10 | 1.5 | 0 | 0 | 30 | 11 | 0 | 1 |

| | SERVING SIZE | CAL | CAL FAT | TOT FAT (G) | SAT FAT (G) | CHOL (MG) | SOD (MG) | CARB (G) | FIBER (G) | PROT (G) |
|---|---|---|---|---|---|---|---|---|---|---|
| Original | 1/2 oz | 60 | 10 | 1.5 | 0 | 0 | 190 | 11 | 0 | 1 |
| Soup and Oyster Crackers | 1/2 oz | 60 | 15 | 1.5 | 0 | 0 | 170 | 11 | 0 | 1 |
| **Progresso** | | | | | | | | | | |
| **SOUP** | | | | | | | | | | |
| Light Beef Pot Roast | 1 cup | 80 | 20 | 2 | .5 | 10 | 470 | 10 | 2 | 7 |
| Light Chicken & Dumpling | 1 cup | 80 | 15 | 1.5 | .5 | 20 | 690 | 12 | 2 | 6 |
| Light Chicken Noodle | 1 cup | 70 | 15 | 1.5 | .5 | 15 | 690 | 10 | 1 | 5 |
| Light Chicken Vegetable Rotini | 1 cup | 70 | 15 | 1.5 | 0 | 15 | 660 | 10 | 1 | 5 |
| Light Homestyle Vegetable and Rice | 1 cup | 60 | 0 | 0 | 0 | 0 | 470 | 14 | 4 | 2 |
| Light Vegetable | 1 cup | 60 | 0 | 0 | 0 | 0 | 470 | 14 | 4 | 2 |
| Light Vegetable and Noodle | 1 cup | 60 | 5 | .5 | 0 | 5 | 480 | 13 | 4 | 2 |
| Light Zesty Santa Fe Style Chicken | 1 cup | 80 | 10 | 1 | 0 | 10 | 460 | 12 | 2 | 5 |
| Light Zesty Southwestern Style Vegetable | 1 cup | 60 | 5 | 0 | 0 | 0 | 470 | 12 | 4 | 3 |
| Traditional 99% Fat Free Beef Barley | 1 cup | 120 | 15 | 1.5 | .5 | 10 | 720 | 20 | 4 | 7 |
| Traditional 99% Fat Free Chicken Noodle | 1 cup | 90 | 20 | 2 | .5 | 20 | 670 | 12 | 1 | 6 |
| Traditional 99% Fat Free New England Clam Chowder | 1 cup | 110 | 15 | 1.5 | 0 | 5 | 810 | 21 | 2 | 4 |
| Traditional Beef & Vegetable | 1 cup | 120 | 15 | 2 | 1 | 15 | 690 | 18 | 2 | 8 |
| Traditional Beef Barley | 1 cup | 120 | 25 | 2.5 | .5 | 15 | 690 | 17 | 2 | 8 |
| Traditional Chicken & Wild Rice | 1 cup | 100 | 15 | 1.5 | .5 | 15 | 870 | 15 | 1 | 6 |
| Traditional Chicken Barley | 1 cup | 80 | 10 | 1 | .5 | 15 | 690 | 11 | 2 | 7 |
| Traditional Chicken Cheese Enchilada Flavor | 1 cup | 170 | 100 | 11 | 3.5 | 25 | 890 | 9 | 1 | 8 |
| Traditional Chicken Noodle | 1 cup | 100 | 20 | 2.5 | .5 | 20 | 690 | 12 | 1 | 7 |
| Traditional Chicken Rice with Vegetables | 1 cup | 100 | 20 | 2 | .5 | 15 | 690 | 13 | 1 | 7 |
| Traditional Hearty Chicken & Rotini | 1 cup | 80 | 15 | 2 | .5 | 10 | 670 | 10 | <1 | 5 |
| Traditional Homestyle Chicken with Vegetables & Pearl Pasta | 1 cup | 100 | 20 | 2 | .5 | 10 | 690 | 14 | 1 | 7 |
| Traditional Italian Style Wedding | 1 cup | 120 | 35 | 4 | 1.5 | 15 | 690 | 11 | 2 | 7 |
| Traditional New England Clam Chowder | 1 cup | 180 | 80 | 9 | 2 | 15 | 890 | 20 | 1 | 6 |
| Traditional Potato Broccoli & Cheese Chowder | 1 cup | 210 | 110 | 12 | 3.5 | 15 | 860 | 20 | 2 | 5 |
| **Quaker** | | | | | | | | | | |
| **90 CALORIE BARS** | | | | | | | | | | |
| Chocolate Chip Chunk | 1 bar | 90 | 20 | 2 | .5 | 0 | 80 | 19 | 1 | 1 |
| Dark Chocolate Cherry Granola | 1 bar | 90 | 20 | 2 | .5 | 0 | 75 | 19 | 1 | 1 |
| Honey Nut Granola | 1 bar | 90 | 20 | 2 | 0 | 0 | 80 | 19 | 1 | 1 |
| Peanut Butter Granola | 1 bar | 90 | 20 | 2 | 0 | 0 | 120 | 18 | 1 | 2 |

| | SERVING SIZE | CAL | CAL FAT | TOT FAT (G) | SAT FAT (G) | CHOL (MG) | SOD (MG) | CARB (G) | FIBER (G) | PROT (G) |
|---|---|---|---|---|---|---|---|---|---|---|
| **CHEWY DIPPS BARS** | | | | | | | | | | |
| Caramel Nut Granola | 1 bar | 140 | 50 | 6 | 3.5 | 0 | 65 | 21 | 1 | 2 |
| Chocolate Chip Granola | 1 bar | 140 | 50 | 6 | 4 | 0 | 80 | 22 | 1 | 2 |
| Peanut Butter Granola | 1 bar | 150 | 60 | 7 | 3.5 | 0 | 105 | 19 | 1 | 3 |
| **INSTANT OATMEAL** | | | | | | | | | | |
| Apples & Cinnamon | 1 packet | 130 | 15 | 1.5 | 0 | 0 | 160 | 27 | 3 | 3 |
| Cinnamon & Spice | 1 packet | 160 | 25 | 2.5 | .5 | 0 | 210 | 32 | 3 | 4 |
| Maple & Brown Sugar | 1 packet | 160 | 25 | 2.5 | .5 | 0 | 260 | 32 | 3 | 4 |
| Original | 1 packet | 100 | 20 | 2 | 0 | 0 | 75 | 19 | 3 | 4 |
| Peaches & Cream | 1 packet | 130 | 20 | 2 | .5 | 0 | 180 | 27 | 2 | 3 |
| Raisin & Spice | 1 packet | 150 | 20 | 2 | 0 | 0 | 210 | 32 | 3 | 4 |
| Raisin Date & Walnut | 1 packet | 140 | 25 | 2.5 | 0 | 0 | 190 | 27 | 3 | 3 |
| Strawberries & Cream | 1 packet | 130 | 20 | 2 | .5 | 0 | 180 | 27 | 2 | 4 |
| **LIFE CEREAL** | | | | | | | | | | |
| Cinnamon | 3/4 cup | 120 | 15 | 1.5 | 0 | 0 | 150 | 25 | 2 | 3 |
| Original | 3/4 cup | 120 | 15 | 1.5 | 0 | 0 | 160 | 25 | 2 | 3 |
| **QUAKES** | | | | | | | | | | |
| Caramel Corn | 7 mini cakes | 60 | 0 | 0 | 0 | 0 | 150 | 13 | 0 | 1 |
| Cheddar Cheese | 9 mini cakes | 70 | 25 | 2.5 | 0 | 0 | 230 | 11 | 0 | 1 |
| Ranch | 10 mini cakes | 70 | 25 | 2.5 | 0 | 0 | 200 | 10 | 0 | 1 |
| Sour Cream & Onion | 10 mini cakes | 70 | 25 | 2.5 | 0 | 0 | 140 | 12 | 0 | 1 |
| **RICE CAKES** | | | | | | | | | | |
| Caramel Corn | 1 cake | 50 | 0 | 0 | 0 | 0 | 30 | 11 | 0 | 1 |
| Chocolate Crunch | 1 cake | 60 | 10 | 1 | 0 | 0 | 30 | 11 | 0 | 1 |
| Lightly Salted | 1 cake | 35 | 0 | 0 | 0 | 0 | 15 | 7 | 0 | 1 |
| Salt Free | 1 cake | 35 | 0 | 0 | 0 | 0 | 0 | 7 | 0 | 1 |
| **SIMPLE HARVEST** | | | | | | | | | | |
| Apples with Cinnamon Hot Cereal | 1 packet | 150 | 15 | 1.5 | 0 | 0 | 90 | 33 | 4 | 4 |
| Maple Brown Sugar with Pecans Hot Cereal | 1 packet | 160 | 30 | 3.5 | .5 | 0 | 75 | 30 | 4 | 4 |
| **Ragu** | | | | | | | | | | |
| **OLD WORLD STYLE SAUCE** | | | | | | | | | | |
| Marinara | 1/2 cup | 80 | 25 | 3 | 0 | 0 | 470 | 10 | 3 | 2 |
| Meat | 1/2 cup | 70 | 25 | 3 | .5 | 0 | 470 | 9 | 2 | 2 |
| Mushroom | 1/2 cup | 70 | 25 | 2.5 | 0 | 0 | 460 | 10 | 2 | 2 |
| Tomato & Mozzarella | 1/2 cup | 70 | 20 | 2 | .5 | 0 | 410 | 10 | 2 | 2 |

| | SERVING SIZE | CAL | CAL FAT | TOT FAT (G) | SAT FAT (G) | CHOL (MG) | SOD (MG) | CARB (G) | FIBER (G) | PROT (G) |
|---|---|---|---|---|---|---|---|---|---|---|
| Traditional | 1/2 cup | 80 | 25 | 2.5 | 0 | 0 | 480 | 11 | 3 | 2 |
| **WHITE SAUCE** | | | | | | | | | | |
| Classic Alfredo | 1/4 cup | 110 | 90 | 10 | 4 | 30 | 360 | 2 | 0 | 1 |
| Light Parmesan | 1/4 cup | 60 | 45 | 5 | 3 | 25 | 320 | 2 | 0 | 2 |
| **Reddi-Wip** | | | | | | | | | | |
| Fat Free Whipped Cream | 2 tbsp | 5 | 0 | 0 | 0 | 0 | 0 | 1 | 0 | 0 |
| Original Whipped Cream | 2 tbsp | 15 | 10 | 1 | .5 | <5 | 0 | <1 | 0 | 0 |
| **Reese's** | | | | | | | | | | |
| Peanut Butter Cups | 2 cups | 210 | 110 | 13 | 4.5 | 5 | 150 | 24 | 1 | 5 |
| **Rice-A-Roni** | | | | | | | | | | |
| **PREPARED RICE MIXES** | | | | | | | | | | |
| Broccoli Au Gratin Flavor | 1 cup | 350 | 140 | 16 | 5 | 5 | 910 | 46 | 2 | 8 |
| Chicken & Broccoli Flavor | 1 cup | 220 | 45 | 5 | 1 | 0 | 920 | 40 | 2 | 6 |
| Creamy Four Cheese Flavor | 1 cup | 270 | 110 | 12 | 3.5 | 5 | 740 | 37 | 1 | 6 |
| Fried Rice Flavor | 1 cup | 310 | 90 | 10 | 2 | 0 | 1350 | 50 | 2 | 7 |
| Long Grain & Wild Rice | 1 cup | 240 | 50 | 6 | 1 | 0 | 840 | 43 | 1 | 5 |
| Mexican Style | 1 cup | 250 | 70 | 8 | 1.5 | 0 | 720 | 40 | 2 | 6 |
| Nature's Way Long Grain & Wild Rice | 1 cup | 240 | 50 | 6 | 1 | 0 | 840 | 43 | 1 | 5 |
| Rice Pilaf | 1 cup | 310 | 80 | 9 | 1.5 | 0 | 1060 | 52 | 2 | 7 |
| Spanish Rice | 1 cup | 260 | 70 | 8 | 1.5 | 0 | 1250 | 44 | 3 | 6 |
| Whole Grain Blends Spanish | 1 cup | 250 | 60 | 8 | 1 | 0 | 760 | 42 | 3 | 5 |
| **Rold Gold** | | | | | | | | | | |
| **PRETZELS** | | | | | | | | | | |
| Classic Style | 1 oz | 110 | 0 | 0 | 0 | 0 | 450 | 23 | 1 | 2 |
| Classic Style Rods | 1 oz | 110 | 10 | 1 | 0 | 0 | 610 | 22 | 1 | 3 |
| Classic Style Thins | 1 oz | 110 | 10 | 1 | 0 | 0 | 560 | 23 | 1 | 2 |
| Hard Sourdough | 1 pretzel | 90 | 10 | 1 | 0 | 0 | 500 | 19 | 2 | 2 |
| **TWISTS** | | | | | | | | | | |
| Classic Style, Tiny | 1 oz | 110 | 10 | 1 | 0 | 0 | 450 | 23 | 1 | 2 |
| Honey Wheat, Braid | 1 oz | 110 | 10 | 1 | 0 | 0 | 230 | 23 | 1 | 2 |
| **Sabra** | | | | | | | | | | |
| Classic Babaganoush | 2 tbsp | 70 | 60 | 7 | 1 | 5 | 160 | 2 | 0 | 0 |
| Classic Hummus | 2 tbsp | 70 | 55 | 6 | 1 | 0 | 120 | 4 | 1 | 2 |
| Classic Tahini | 2 tbsp | 80 | 70 | 8 | 1 | 0 | 150 | 2 | <1 | 2 |
| Greek Olive Hummus | 2 tbsp | 70 | 60 | 6 | 1 | 0 | 130 | 4 | 1 | 2 |
| Hummus with Salsa | 2 tbsp | 60 | 50 | 5 | <1 | 0 | 135 | 3 | <1 | 1 |
| Luscious Lemon Hummus | 2 tbsp | 70 | 60 | 6 | 1 | 0 | 120 | 3 | 1 | 2 |

| | SERVING SIZE | CAL | CAL FAT | TOT FAT (G) | SAT FAT (G) | CHOL (MG) | SOD (MG) | CARB (G) | FIBER (G) | PROT (G) |
|---|---|---|---|---|---|---|---|---|---|---|
| Red Pepper Hummus | 2 tbsp | 70 | 50 | 6 | 1 | 0 | 120 | 4 | 1 | 2 |
| Roasted Garlic Hummus | 2 tbsp | 70 | 50 | 6 | 1 | 0 | 120 | 3 | 1 | 2 |
| Roasted Pine Nut Hummus | 2 tbsp | 80 | 60 | 9 | 1 | 0 | 125 | 4 | 1 | 2 |
| Spinach & Artichoke Hummus | 2 tbsp | 70 | 50 | 6 | 2 | 0 | 120 | 4 | 1 | 1 |
| Sun Dried Tomato Hummus | 2 tbsp | 70 | 50 | 6 | 1 | 0 | 120 | 4 | 1 | 2 |
| Tahini Hummus | 2 tbsp | 80 | 60 | 6 | 1 | 0 | 120 | 4 | 1 | 2 |
| **Shake 'n Bake** | | | | | | | | | | |
| BBQ Glaze for Chicken or Pork | 1/3 oz | 45 | 10 | 1 | 0 | 0 | 410 | 9 | 0 | 0 |
| Extra Crispy | 1/3 oz | 35 | 5 | .5 | 0 | 0 | 280 | 7 | 0 | 1 |
| Hot & Spicy | 1/3 oz | 40 | 10 | 1 | 0 | 0 | 180 | 7 | 0 | 1 |
| Italian | 1/3 oz | 35 | 5 | .5 | 0 | 0 | 280 | 7 | 0 | 1 |
| Original Chicken | 1/3 oz | 40 | 10 | 1 | 0 | 0 | 220 | 7 | 0 | 1 |
| Original Pork | 1/3 oz | 40 | 10 | 1 | 0 | 0 | 240 | 8 | 0 | 1 |
| **Silk** | | | | | | | | | | |
| **CREAMER** | | | | | | | | | | |
| Original | 1 tbsp | 15 | 10 | 1 | 0 | 0 | 10 | 1 | 0 | 0 |
| **LIGHT SOYMILK** | | | | | | | | | | |
| Chocolate | 1 cup | 90 | 15 | 1.5 | 0 | 0 | 80 | 15 | 2 | 3 |
| Original | 1 cup | 60 | 15 | 1.5 | 0 | 0 | 125 | 6 | 1 | 6 |
| Vanilla | 1 cup | 70 | 15 | 1.5 | 0 | 0 | 100 | 7 | 1 | 6 |
| **LIVE! SOY YOGURT** | | | | | | | | | | |
| Blueberry | 6 oz | 150 | 20 | 2 | 0 | 0 | 25 | 29 | 1 | 4 |
| Plain | 6 oz | 150 | 35 | 4 | .5 | 0 | 30 | 22 | 1 | 6 |
| Raspberry | 6 oz | 210 | 35 | 4 | .5 | 0 | 20 | 36 | 3 | 7 |
| Strawberry Banana | 6 oz | 150 | 20 | 2 | 0 | 0 | 25 | 29 | 1 | 4 |
| Vanilla | 6 oz | 150 | 25 | 3 | 0 | 0 | 20 | 25 | 1 | 5 |
| **PUREALMOND MILK** | | | | | | | | | | |
| Original | 1 cup | 60 | 25 | 2.5 | 0 | 0 | 150 | 8 | 1 | 1 |
| Vanilla | 1 cup | 90 | 25 | 2.5 | 0 | 0 | 150 | 16 | 1 | 1 |
| **SOYMILK** | | | | | | | | | | |
| Chocolate | 1 cup | 140 | 30 | 3.5 | .5 | 0 | 100 | 23 | 2 | 5 |
| Original | 1 cup | 100 | 35 | 4 | .5 | 0 | 120 | 8 | 1 | 7 |
| Vanilla | 1 cup | 100 | 30 | 3.5 | .5 | 0 | 95 | 11 | 1 | 6 |
| **Simply Orange** | | | | | | | | | | |
| **JUICES** | | | | | | | | | | |
| Original | 8 fl oz | 110 | 0 | 0 | 0 | 0 | 0 | 26 | 0 | 2 |
| Pulp Free | 8 fl oz | 110 | 0 | 0 | 0 | 0 | 0 | 26 | 0 | 2 |

# store brands

| | SERVING SIZE | CAL | CAL FAT | TOT FAT (G) | SAT FAT (G) | CHOL (MG) | SOD (MG) | CARB (G) | FIBER (G) | PROT (G) |
|---|---|---|---|---|---|---|---|---|---|---|
| Simply Apple | 8 fl oz | 120 | 0 | 0 | 0 | 0 | 5 | 30 | 0 | 2 |
| Simply Grapefruit | 8 fl oz | 90 | 0 | 0 | 0 | 0 | 10 | 21 | 0 | 1 |
| Simply Lemonade | 8 fl oz | 120 | 0 | 0 | 0 | 0 | 15 | 30 | 0 | 0 |
| With Calcium & Vitamin D | 8 fl oz | 110 | 0 | 0 | 0 | 0 | 0 | 27 | 0 | 2 |

## Simply Potatoes
### CUT POTATO PRODUCTS

| | | | | | | | | | | |
|---|---|---|---|---|---|---|---|---|---|---|
| Homestyle Slices | 2/3 cup | 90 | 0 | 0 | 0 | 0 | 75 | 21 | 2 | 2 |
| Red Wedges | 1/2 cup | 50 | 0 | 0 | 0 | 0 | 250 | 10 | 2 | 2 |
| Rosemary & Garlic Red Potato Wedges | 1/2 cup | 50 | 0 | 0 | 0 | 0 | 250 | 11 | 2 | 2 |
| Shredded Hash Browns | 1/2 cup | 70 | 0 | 0 | 0 | 0 | 55 | 16 | <2 | 1 |
| Southwest Style Hash Browns | 2/3 cup | 80 | 0 | 0 | 0 | 0 | 240 | 17 | 2 | 2 |

### MASHED POTATOES

| | | | | | | | | | | |
|---|---|---|---|---|---|---|---|---|---|---|
| Country Style | 1/2 cup | 100 | 20 | 2 | 1 | 5 | 95 | 18 | 2 | 2 |
| Garlic | 1/2 cup | 110 | 45 | 5 | 3 | 10 | 400 | 15 | 2 | 2 |
| Mashed Sweet Potatoes | 1/2 cup | 90 | 5 | 1 | 0 | 2 | 100 | 18 | 2 | 2 |
| Sour Cream and Chive | 1/2 cup | 110 | 40 | 4.5 | 2.5 | 10 | 330 | 16 | 2 | 3 |
| Traditional | 1/2 cup | 100 | 40 | 4 | 2.5 | 10 | 440 | 14 | 2 | 2 |

## Skinny Cow
### LOW FAT ICE CREAM
### SANDWICHES

| | | | | | | | | | | |
|---|---|---|---|---|---|---|---|---|---|---|
| No Sugar Added, Vanilla | 1 item | 140 | 20 | 2 | 1 | 15 | 115 | 30 | 5 | 4 |
| Vanilla, Chocolate | 1 item | 140 | 15 | 2 | 1 | 5 | 135 | 30 | 3 | 4 |

## Slim Jim

| | | | | | | | | | | |
|---|---|---|---|---|---|---|---|---|---|---|
| Beef & Cheese Jerky Twin Pack | 1 item | 150 | 100 | 11 | 6 | 45 | 630 | 3 | 0 | 9 |
| Hot Jerky | 1 oz | 150 | 120 | 13 | 5 | 20 | 430 | 2 | 1 | 6 |
| Mild Jerky | 1 oz | 160 | 130 | 14 | 6 | 20 | 490 | 2 | <1 | 7 |

## Smart Balance
### BUTTERY SPREADS

| | | | | | | | | | | |
|---|---|---|---|---|---|---|---|---|---|---|
| Heart Right Buttery Spread | 1 tbsp | 80 | 80 | 8 | 2.5 | 0 | 85 | 0 | 0 | 0 |
| Heart Right Light Buttery Spread | 1 tbsp | 45 | 45 | 5 | 1.5 | 0 | 80 | 0 | 0 | 0 |
| Omega-3 Light Buttery Spread | 1 tbsp | 50 | 50 | 5 | 1.5 | 0 | 80 | 0 | 0 | 0 |
| Organic Whipped Buttery Spread | 1 tbsp | 80 | 80 | 9 | 2.5 | 0 | 100 | 0 | 0 | 0 |
| Original | 1 tbsp | 80 | 80 | 9 | 2.5 | 0 | 90 | 0 | 0 | 0 |
| Whipped Buttery Spread | 1 tbsp | 60 | 60 | 7 | 2 | 0 | 30 | 0 | 0 | 0 |
| With Extra Virgin Olive Oil | 1 tbsp | 60 | 60 | 7 | 2 | 0 | 70 | 0 | 0 | 0 |

### PEANUT BUTTER

| | | | | | | | | | | |
|---|---|---|---|---|---|---|---|---|---|---|
| Rich Roast Chunky Peanut Butter | 2 tbsp | 190 | 145 | 16 | 3 | 0 | 145 | 8 | 2 | 7 |

| | SERVING SIZE | CAL | CAL FAT | TOT FAT (G) | SAT FAT (G) | CHOL (MG) | SOD (MG) | CARB (G) | FIBER (G) | PROT (G) |
|---|---|---|---|---|---|---|---|---|---|---|
| Rich Roast Creamy Peanut Butter | 2 tbsp | 190 | 145 | 16 | 3 | 0 | 145 | 8 | 2 | 7 |
| **POPCORN** | | | | | | | | | | |
| Light Butter | 2 tbsp | 120 | 40 | 4.5 | 1.5 | 0 | 290 | 18 | 4 | 3 |
| Smart 'n Healthy | 2 tbsp | 120 | 15 | 2 | 0 | 0 | 85 | 24 | 5 | 4 |
| Smart Movie Style Popcorn | 2 tbsp | 170 | 100 | 11 | 4 | 0 | 420 | 16 | 3 | 3 |
| **Smartfood** | | | | | | | | | | |
| White Cheddar Popcorn | 1 oz | 160 | 90 | 10 | 2 | <5 | 290 | 14 | 2 | 3 |
| **Snapple** | | | | | | | | | | |
| **JUICE & JUICE DRINKS** | | | | | | | | | | |
| 100% Juiced Fruit Punch | 11-1/2 fl oz | 170 | 0 | 0 | 0 | 0 | 15 | 42 | 0 | 0 |
| 100% Juiced Grape | 11-1/2 fl oz | 170 | 0 | 0 | 0 | 0 | 15 | 43 | 0 | 0 |
| 100% Juiced Green Apple | 11-1/2 fl oz | 160 | 0 | 0 | 0 | 0 | 20 | 41 | 0 | 0 |
| 100% Juiced Orange Mango | 11-1/2 fl oz | 170 | 0 | 0 | 0 | 0 | 15 | 41 | 0 | 0 |
| Açai Blackberry Fruit Juice | 8 fl oz | 110 | 0 | 0 | 0 | 0 | 5 | 27 | 0 | 0 |
| Lemonade Juice Drink | 8 fl oz | 90 | 0 | 0 | 0 | 0 | 45 | 24 | 0 | 0 |
| Kiwi-Strawberry Juice Drink | 8 fl oz | 110 | 0 | 0 | 0 | 0 | 10 | 27 | 0 | 0 |
| **TEAS** | | | | | | | | | | |
| Diet Lemon Tea | 8 fl oz | 10 | 0 | 0 | 0 | 0 | 5 | 0 | 0 | 0 |
| Green Tea | 8 fl oz | 60 | 0 | 0 | 0 | 0 | 5 | 15 | 0 | 0 |
| Lemon Tea | 8 fl oz | 80 | 0 | 0 | 0 | 0 | 5 | 21 | 0 | 0 |
| Peach Green Tea | 8 fl oz | 80 | 0 | 0 | 0 | 0 | 60 | 21 | 0 | 0 |
| **Snickers** | | | | | | | | | | |
| Original 2.7 oz Candy Bar | 1 bar | 280 | 130 | 14 | 5 | 5 | 140 | 35 | 1 | 4 |
| **Sprite** | | | | | | | | | | |
| Original | 8 fl oz | 100 | 0 | 0 | 0 | 0 | 45 | 26 | 0 | 0 |
| **Starbucks Ice Cream** | | | | | | | | | | |
| Coffee | 1/2 cup | 210 | 120 | 13 | 8 | 65 | 55 | 21 | 0 | 3 |
| Mocha Frappuccino | 1/2 cup | 220 | 120 | 13 | 8 | 55 | 65 | 23 | <1 | 3 |
| Signature Hot Chocolate | 1/2 cup | 203 | 120 | 13 | 8 | 50 | 60 | 25 | 1 | 3 |
| **Starkist** | | | | | | | | | | |
| **CANNED TUNA** | | | | | | | | | | |
| Chunk Light in Vegetable Oil | 2 oz | 80 | 35 | 4 | 1 | 20 | 170 | 0 | 0 | 10 |
| Chunk Light in Water | 2 oz | 50 | 10 | 1 | 0 | 25 | 180 | <1 | <1 | 10 |
| Chunk White Albacore Tuna | 2 oz | 70 | 20 | 2 | .5 | 25 | 190 | 0 | 0 | 12 |
| Low Sodium Chunk Light in Water | 2 oz | 60 | 5 | .5 | 0 | 25 | 100 | 0 | 0 | 15 |
| Very Low Sodium Chunk White Albacore in Water | 2 oz | 70 | 10 | 1 | 0 | 25 | 35 | 0 | 0 | 16 |

# store brands

| | SERVING SIZE | CAL | CAL FAT | TOT FAT (G) | SAT FAT (G) | CHOL (MG) | SOD (MG) | CARB (G) | FIBER (G) | PROT (G) |
|---|---|---|---|---|---|---|---|---|---|---|
| **TUNA CREATIONS** | | | | | | | | | | |
| Sweet & Spicy | 2 oz | 70 | 5 | 0 | 0 | 25 | 270 | 4 | n/a | 11 |
| Tomato Pesto | 2 oz | 70 | 15 | 2 | 0 | 15 | 190 | <1 | 0 | 13 |
| Zesty Lemon Pepper | 2 oz | 60 | 5 | .5 | 0 | 25 | 220 | 0 | n/a | 14 |
| **Stevia** | | | | | | | | | | |
| Packet | 1 packet | 0 | 0 | 0 | 0 | 0 | 0 | 0 | 0 | 0 |
| Packet with Fiber | 1 packet | 0 | 0 | 0 | 0 | 0 | 0 | 1 | 1 | 0 |
| **Stonyfield Organic** | | | | | | | | | | |
| Fat Free French Vanilla Yogurt | 6 oz | 130 | 0 | 0 | 0 | 0 | 110 | 25 | 0 | 7 |
| Low Fat Blueberry Yogurt | 6 oz | 120 | 10 | 1.5 | 1 | 5 | 90 | 21 | <1 | 6 |
| Low Fat Plain Yogurt | 6 oz | 90 | 15 | 1.5 | 1 | 0 | 110 | 11 | 0 | 7 |
| Low Fat Strawberry Yogurt | 6 oz | 120 | 10 | 1.5 | 1 | 5 | 90 | 21 | <1 | 6 |
| **Stove Top** | | | | | | | | | | |
| Chicken Stuffing Mix | 1 oz | 150 | 60 | 2.5 | 0 | 0 | 460 | 20 | 1 | 3 |
| Cornbread Stuffing Mix | 1 oz | 160 | 60 | 1 | 0 | 0 | 500 | 22 | 1 | 3 |
| Savory Herbs Stuffing Mix | 1 oz | 160 | 60 | 1 | 0 | 0 | 450 | 21 | 1 | 3 |
| Turkey Stuffing Mix | 1 oz | 160 | 60 | 1 | 0 | 0 | 440 | 21 | 1 | 3 |
| **Sunchips** | | | | | | | | | | |
| French Onion | 1 oz | 140 | 60 | 6 | 1 | 0 | 170 | 18 | 3 | 2 |
| Garden Salsa | 1 oz | 140 | 60 | 6 | 1 | 0 | 170 | 19 | 3 | 2 |
| Harvest Cheddar | 1 oz | 140 | 60 | 6 | 1 | 0 | 200 | 19 | 3 | 2 |
| Original | 1 oz | 140 | 50 | 6 | 1 | 0 | 120 | 19 | 3 | 2 |
| **Tastee Choice** | | | | | | | | | | |
| **ENTRÉES** | | | | | | | | | | |
| Shrimp and Asian Noodles | 1-1/2 cups | 410 | 110 | 12 | 3 | 80 | 1700 | 58 | 7 | 18 |
| Shrimp and Asian Style Vegetables | 1-1/2 cups | 130 | 20 | 2 | .5 | 125 | 1640 | 18 | 4 | 11 |
| Shrimp, Basmati Rice, and Regular Vegetables | 1-1/2 cups | 320 | 20 | 2 | .5 | 90 | 1470 | 58 | 4 | 16 |
| **MICRO CUISINE** | | | | | | | | | | |
| Lemon Herb Tilapia with Basmati Rice | 1 entrée | 446 | 162 | 18 | 13 | 24 | 809 | 52 | 26 | 19 |
| Shrimp Marinara with Linguine | 1 entrée | 332 | 33 | <4 | <1 | 79 | 763 | 51 | 4 | 23 |
| Shrimp Scampi with Linguine | 1 entrée | 368 | 87 | <10 | <8 | 65 | 577 | 48 | 8 | <22 |
| **Thomas'** | | | | | | | | | | |
| **BAGELS** | | | | | | | | | | |
| Cinnamon Raisin | 1 bagel | 250 | 15 | 1.5 | 0 | 0 | 410 | 50 | 4 | 8 |
| Egg | 1 bagel | 170 | 0 | 1.5 | .5 | 15 | 280 | 35 | 2 | 7 |

| | SERVING SIZE | CAL | CAL FAT | TOT FAT (G) | SAT FAT (G) | CHOL (MG) | SOD (MG) | CARB (G) | FIBER (G) | PROT (G) |
|---|---|---|---|---|---|---|---|---|---|---|
| Multi-Grain | 1 bagel | 250 | 25 | 3 | .5 | 0 | 480 | 51 | 8 | 10 |
| Onion | 1 bagel | 260 | 20 | 2 | .5 | 0 | 470 | 51 | 3 | 10 |
| Plain | 1 bagel | 260 | 20 | 2 | .5 | 0 | 500 | 51 | 2 | 9 |
| **ENGLISH MUFFINS** | | | | | | | | | | |
| Light Multi-Grain | 1 muffin | 100 | 10 | 1.5 | 0 | 0 | 170 | 24 | 8 | 6 |
| Plain | 1 muffin | 120 | 10 | 1 | 0 | 0 | 200 | 25 | 1 | 4 |
| Raisin | 1 muffin | 140 | 10 | 1 | 0 | 0 | 170 | 29 | 1 | 4 |
| **PITA BREAD** | | | | | | | | | | |
| Sahara 100% Whole Wheat | 1 pita | 130 | 0 | 1 | 0 | 0 | 310 | 28 | 5 | 7 |
| Sahara Original Style | 1 pita | 150 | 0 | 1 | 0 | 0 | 290 | 31 | 1 | 6 |
| **Tombstone** | | | | | | | | | | |
| **ORIGINAL PIZZA** | | | | | | | | | | |
| Deluxe | 1/5 pizza | 290 | 110 | 12 | 5 | 30 | 580 | 31 | 3 | 14 |
| Pepperoni | 1/2 pizza | 390 | 180 | 20 | 8 | 40 | 880 | 37 | 4 | 18 |
| Supreme | 1/5 pizza | 300 | 120 | 14 | 6 | 30 | 640 | 31 | 3 | 14 |
| **THIN CRUST PIZZA** | | | | | | | | | | |
| Cheese, Harvest Wheat | 1/3 pizza | 300 | 90 | 10 | 5 | 25 | 620 | 37 | 4 | 17 |
| Pepperoni | 1/4 pizza | 320 | 160 | 18 | 8 | 40 | 780 | 28 | 3 | 15 |
| Pepperoni, Harvest Wheat | 1/4 pizza | 260 | 90 | 10 | 4.5 | 25 | 610 | 29 | 3 | 15 |
| Sausage | 1/4 pizza | 330 | 150 | 17 | 7 | 40 | 760 | 29 | 3 | 17 |
| Supreme, Harvest Wheat | 1/4 pizza | 260 | 90 | 10 | 4.5 | 25 | 600 | 29 | 3 | 15 |
| Three Cheese | 1/4 pizza | 310 | 130 | 15 | 8 | 40 | 660 | 28 | 3 | 16 |
| **Total** | | | | | | | | | | |
| Whole Grain Cereal | 3/4 cup | 100 | 5 | .5 | 0 | 0 | 190 | 23 | 3 | 2 |
| **Tribe** | | | | | | | | | | |
| Classic Hummus | 2 tbsp | 60 | 35 | 3.5 | 0 | 0 | 130 | 4 | 1 | 2 |
| Cracked Chili Peppers Hummus | 2 tbsp | 60 | 30 | 3.5 | 0 | 0 | 135 | 4 | 1 | 2 |
| Roasted Eggplant Hummus | 2 tbsp | 45 | 25 | 3 | 0 | 0 | 150 | 3 | 1 | 2 |
| Roasted Garlic Hummus | 2 tbsp | 60 | 35 | 3.5 | 0 | 0 | 130 | 4 | 1 | 2 |
| Savory Dill Hummus | 2 tbsp | 60 | 35 | 3.5 | 0 | 0 | 120 | 4 | 1 | 2 |
| Scallion Hummus | 2 tbsp | 60 | 35 | 3.5 | 0 | 0 | 120 | 4 | 1 | 2 |
| Sundried Tomato & Basil Hummus | 2 tbsp | 60 | 35 | 3.5 | 0 | 0 | 130 | 4 | 1 | 2 |
| Sweet Roasted Red Peppers Hummus | 2 tbsp | 50 | 25 | 3 | 0 | 0 | 125 | 4 | 1 | 2 |
| Zesty Lemon Hummus | 2 tbsp | 60 | 35 | 3.5 | 0 | 0 | 125 | 4 | <1 | 2 |
| **Twizzlers** | | | | | | | | | | |
| Strawberry Twists | 4 pieces | 160 | 5 | .5 | 0 | 0 | 95 | 36 | 0 | 1 |

| | SERVING SIZE | CAL | CAL FAT | TOT FAT (G) | SAT FAT (G) | CHOL (MG) | SOD (MG) | CARB (G) | FIBER (G) | PROT (G) |
|---|---|---|---|---|---|---|---|---|---|---|
| **Tyson** | | | | | | | | | | |
| **ANY'TIZERS** | | | | | | | | | | |
| Buffalo Style Boneless Chicken Wings | 3 pieces | 150 | 70 | 7 | 1.5 | 30 | 680 | 8 | 0 | 12 |
| Buffalo Style Popcorn Chicken Bites | 8 pieces | 190 | 80 | 9 | 1.5 | 40 | 960 | 12 | 1 | 15 |
| Honey BBQ Boneless Wings | 3 pieces | 200 | 70 | 8 | 1.5 | 25 | 450 | 20 | 0 | 11 |
| Homestyle Chicken Fries | 7 pieces | 230 | 100 | 11 | 2.5 | 25 | 590 | 19 | 1 | 13 |
| Hot 'N Spicy Chicken Wings | 3 pieces | 220 | 130 | 15 | 3.5 | 110 | 560 | 1 | 0 | 20 |
| Variety Pack | 7 pieces | 230 | 100 | 11 | 2.5 | 25 | 590 | 19 | 1 | 13 |
| **BEEF MEALS & ENTRÉES** | | | | | | | | | | |
| Beef Steak Tips in Bourbon Sauce | 5 oz | 180 | 50 | 5 | 2 | 45 | 480 | 12 | 0 | 20 |
| Beef Tips in Gravy | 5 oz | 200 | 110 | 12 | 4.5 | 55 | 530 | 5 | 0 | 17 |
| Roast Beef in Brown Gravy | 5 oz | 130 | 35 | 4 | 2 | 50 | 600 | 5 | 0 | 17 |
| **CANNED CHICKEN** | | | | | | | | | | |
| Premium Chunk Chicken | 2 oz | 60 | 20 | 2.5 | .5 | 30 | 200 | 0 | 0 | 10 |
| Premium Chunk Chicken Breast (White) | 2 oz | 60 | 10 | 1 | 0 | 30 | 200 | 0 | 0 | 13 |
| **FULLY COOKED BEEF PRODUCTS** | | | | | | | | | | |
| Steak Fingers | 2 pieces | 250 | 160 | 18 | 5 | 20 | 540 | 14 | 1 | 8 |
| **FULLY COOKED CHICKEN PRODUCTS** | | | | | | | | | | |
| Breaded Chicken Breast Fillets | 1 piece | 240 | 80 | 9 | 1.5 | 45 | 680 | 20 | 0 | 19 |
| Chicken Breast Tenderloins | 1 piece | 150 | 60 | 7 | 1.5 | 20 | 370 | 12 | 1 | 10 |
| Chicken Nuggets | 5 pieces | 270 | 160 | 17 | 4 | 40 | 470 | 15 | 0 | 14 |
| Grilled & Ready Frozen Fully Cooked Chicken Breast Fillets | 1 piece | 110 | 10 | 1.5 | 0 | 60 | 230 | 1 | 0 | 24 |
| Honey BBQ Boneless Chicken Wyngs | 3 pieces | 210 | 110 | 12 | 2.5 | 25 | 400 | 13 | 0 | 11 |
| **GRILLED & READY** | | | | | | | | | | |
| Chicken Breast Strips | 3 oz | 100 | 15 | 2 | .5 | 50 | 470 | 1 | 0 | 21 |
| Fajita Chicken Strips | 3 oz | 110 | 35 | 4 | 1 | 55 | 540 | 1 | 0 | 17 |
| **HEAT 'N EAT ENTRÉES** | | | | | | | | | | |
| Chicken Breast Medallions in Italian Herb Sauce | 5 oz | 120 | 15 | 2 | .5 | 40 | 640 | 7 | 0 | 18 |
| **PORK MEALS & ENTRÉES** | | | | | | | | | | |
| Pork Loin in Sweet & Tangy Barbecue Sauce | 5 oz | 180 | 60 | 7 | 2.5 | 50 | 810 | 13 | 0 | 17 |
| Roast Pork in Gravy | 5 oz | 190 | 90 | 10 | 4 | 55 | 590 | 5 | 1 | 19 |

| | SERVING SIZE | CAL | CAL FAT | TOT FAT (G) | SAT FAT (G) | CHOL (MG) | SOD (MG) | CARB (G) | FIBER (G) | PROT (G) |
|---|---|---|---|---|---|---|---|---|---|---|
| **SKILLET CREATIONS** | | | | | | | | | | |
| Asian Style Chicken with Orange Sauce | 12 oz | 340 | 45 | 5 | 1.5 | 35 | 470 | 50 | 6 | 23 |
| Grilled Chicken Fajitas | 2 fajitas | 250 | 60 | 7 | 2 | 20 | 430 | 32 | 3 | 15 |
| Grilled Steak Fajitas | 2 fajitas | 300 | 70 | 8 | 3 | 25 | 430 | 38 | 4 | 19 |
| **Uncle Ben's** | | | | | | | | | | |
| **COUNTRY INN (PREPARED)** | | | | | | | | | | |
| Chicken Flavored | 1 cup | 200 | 10 | 1 | 0 | 0 | 940 | 41 | 1 | 6 |
| Country Inn Broccoli Au Gratin | 1 cup | 200 | 20 | 2 | 1 | 5 | 790 | 43 | 1 | 4 |
| Country Inn Chicken & Wild | 1 cup | 200 | 5 | 1 | .5 | 0 | 800 | 42 | 1 | 5 |
| Country Inn Pilaf | 1 cup | 200 | 5 | .5 | 0 | 0 | 640 | 43 | 1 | 5 |
| **LONG GRAIN & WILD RICE (PREPARED)** | | | | | | | | | | |
| Butter & Herb | 1 cup | 190 | 10 | 1 | 0 | 0 | 810 | 40 | 1 | 5 |
| Fast Cook Recipe | 1 cup | 190 | 5 | .5 | 0 | 0 | 680 | 41 | 1 | 5 |
| Herb Roasted Chicken | 1 cup | 190 | 10 | 1 | 0 | 0 | 640 | 39 | 3 | 5 |
| Original Recipe | 1 cup | 200 | 5 | 0 | 0 | 0 | 670 | 44 | 1 | 6 |
| **PREPARED RICE** | | | | | | | | | | |
| Chicken Whole Grain | 1 cup | 220 | 40 | 4 | .5 | 0 | 710 | 41 | 3 | 5 |
| Ready Chicken Whole Grain | 1 cup | 230 | 45 | 4.5 | .5 | 0 | 800 | 41 | 2 | 5 |
| Whole Grain & Wild Mushroom Recipe | 1 cup | 200 | 10 | 1.5 | 0 | 0 | 570 | 42 | 3 | 6 |
| **READY RICE (PREPARED)** | | | | | | | | | | |
| Garden Vegetable | 1 cup | 200 | 25 | 2.5 | 0 | 0 | 830 | 41 | 1 | 4 |
| Jasmine | 1 cup | 250 | 25 | 2.5 | 0 | 0 | 10 | 52 | 1 | 5 |
| Long Grain & Wild | 1 cup | 220 | 25 | 3 | 0 | 0 | 900 | 43 | 2 | 5 |
| Pilaf | 1 cup | 220 | 35 | 3.5 | .5 | 0 | 970 | 42 | 2 | 6 |
| Roasted Chicken | 1 cup | 220 | 30 | 3.5 | 0 | 0 | 960 | 41 | 2 | 5 |
| Spanish Style | 1 cup | 200 | 20 | 2.5 | 0 | 0 | 680 | 41 | 3 | 4 |
| Whole Grain Medley Brown & Wild | 1 cup | 220 | 30 | 3.5 | 0 | 0 | 730 | 42 | 3 | 6 |
| Whole Grain Medley Chicken Medley | 1 cup | 210 | 30 | 3.5 | 0 | 0 | 730 | 41 | 4 | 5 |
| Whole Grain Medley Roasted Garlic | 1 cup | 200 | 30 | 3 | 0 | 0 | 560 | 38 | 3 | 5 |
| **Utz** | | | | | | | | | | |
| **KETTLE CLASSIC POTATO CHIPS** | | | | | | | | | | |
| Jalapeno | 1 oz | 150 | 80 | 9 | 1.5 | 0 | 220 | 15 | 1 | 2 |
| Original | 1 oz | 150 | 80 | 9 | 1.5 | 0 | 120 | 15 | 1 | 2 |
| Reduced Fat | 1 oz | 130 | 50 | 6 | 1 | 0 | 120 | 18 | 1 | 2 |
| Salt & Malt Vinegar | 1 oz | 150 | 80 | 9 | 1.5 | 0 | 280 | 15 | 1 | 2 |

| | SERVING SIZE | CAL | CAL FAT | TOT FAT (G) | SAT FAT (G) | CHOL (MG) | SOD (MG) | CARB (G) | FIBER (G) | PROT (G) |
|---|---|---|---|---|---|---|---|---|---|---|
| **NATURAL POTATO CHIPS/ MEDLEY/PITA CHIPS** | | | | | | | | | | |
| Dark Russet | 1 oz | 150 | 80 | 7 | 1 | 0 | 120 | 15 | 1 | 2 |
| Lightly Salted | 1 oz | 140 | 70 | 8 | 1 | 0 | 75 | 15 | 1 | 2 |
| Reduced Fat | 1 oz | 130 | 50 | 6 | .5 | 0 | 95 | 18 | 1 | 2 |
| Sea Salt & Vinegar | 1 oz | 140 | 70 | 8 | 1 | 0 | 210 | 15 | 1 | 2 |
| **POPCORN/PUFF'N CORN** | | | | | | | | | | |
| Butter Popcorn | 2 cups | 170 | 110 | 12 | 3 | 0 | 250 | 13 | 2 | 2 |
| Cheese Popcorn | 2 cups | 160 | 100 | 11 | 1.5 | 5 | 300 | 14 | 3 | 2 |
| Hulless Cheese Puff'n Corn | 2 cups | 200 | 140 | 16 | 3 | 5 | 200 | 13 | 0 | 2 |
| Hulless Original Puff'n Corn | 2 cups | 200 | 150 | 17 | 3 | 0 | 150 | 11 | 0 | 0 |
| White Cheddar Popcorn | 2 cups | 150 | 80 | 9 | 1.5 | 5 | 240 | 15 | 3 | 3 |
| **PORK RINDS** | | | | | | | | | | |
| BBQ Pork Rinds | 1/2 oz | 80 | 45 | 5 | 1.5 | 20 | 210 | 0 | 0 | 8 |
| Pork Cracklins | 1/2 oz | 80 | 50 | 6 | 2 | 15 | 280 | 0 | 0 | 7 |
| Regular Pork Rinds | 1/2 oz | 80 | 50 | 5 | 1.5 | 20 | 230 | 0 | 0 | 8 |
| Salt & Vinegar Pork Rinds | 1/2 oz | 80 | 45 | 5 | 1.5 | 15 | 440 | 0 | 0 | 7 |
| **POTATO CHIPS** | | | | | | | | | | |
| BBQ | 1 oz | 150 | 90 | 10 | 2.5 | 0 | 240 | 15 | 1 | 2 |
| No Salt | 1 oz | 150 | 80 | 9 | 2 | 0 | 5 | 14 | 1 | 2 |
| Red Hot | 1 oz | 150 | 80 | 9 | 2 | 0 | 220 | 14 | 1 | 2 |
| Reduced Fat Sour Cream and Onion | 1 oz | 140 | 60 | <7 | 2 | 0 | 230 | 18 | 1 | 2 |
| Regular | 1 oz | 150 | 80 | 9 | 2 | 0 | 95 | 15 | 1 | 2 |
| Ripple | 1 oz | 150 | 90 | 10 | 2.5 | 0 | 95 | 14 | 1 | 2 |
| Salt & Pepper | 1 oz | 150 | 90 | 9 | 2 | 0 | 280 | 14 | 1 | 2 |
| Salt & Vinegar | 1 oz | 150 | 80 | 9 | 2 | 0 | 270 | 14 | 1 | 0 |
| Sour Cream & Onion | 1 oz | 160 | 90 | 10 | 3 | 0 | 170 | 14 | 1 | 2 |
| **V8** | | | | | | | | | | |
| **V-FUSION** | | | | | | | | | | |
| Açai Mixed Berry | 8 fl oz | 110 | 0 | 0 | 0 | 0 | 70 | 27 | 0 | 0 |
| Cranberry Blackberry | 8 fl oz | 110 | 0 | 0 | 0 | 0 | 90 | 26 | 0 | 0 |
| Light Peach Mango | 8 fl oz | 50 | 0 | 0 | 0 | 0 | 40 | 13 | 0 | 0 |
| Light Pomegranate Blueberry | 8 fl oz | 50 | 0 | 0 | 0 | 0 | 90 | 13 | 0 | 0 |
| Light Strawberry Banana | 8 fl oz | 50 | 0 | 0 | 0 | 0 | 40 | 12 | 0 | 0 |
| Passion Fruit Tangerine | 8 fl oz | 110 | 0 | 0 | 0 | 0 | 115 | 27 | 0 | 0 |
| Peach Mango | 8 fl oz | 120 | 0 | 0 | 0 | 0 | 70 | 28 | 0 | 0 |

| | SERVING SIZE | CAL | CAL FAT | TOT FAT (G) | SAT FAT (G) | CHOL (MG) | SOD (MG) | CARB (G) | FIBER (G) | PROT (G) |
|---|---|---|---|---|---|---|---|---|---|---|
| **100% VEGETABLE JUICE** | | | | | | | | | | |
| Original | 8 fl oz | 50 | 0 | 0 | 0 | 0 | 420 | 10 | 2 | 2 |
| **Van Camp's** | | | | | | | | | | |
| Baked Beanee Weenees | 1 item | 290 | 70 | 8 | 2.5 | 40 | 1160 | 42 | 6 | 13 |
| Chili with Beans | 1 cup | 350 | 160 | 18 | 8 | 35 | 900 | 31 | 7 | 17 |
| Chili, No Beans | 1 cup | 390 | 230 | 26 | 11 | 50 | 1080 | 20 | 6 | 20 |
| Homestyle Baked Beans | 1/2 cup | 160 | 10 | 1 | 0 | 0 | 470 | 30 | 5 | 7 |
| Original Beanee Weenees | 1 item | 240 | 70 | 8 | 3 | 40 | 990 | 29 | 8 | 14 |
| Pork and Beans, Maple & Brown Sugar | 1/2 cup | 160 | 10 | 1 | 0 | 0 | 440 | 30 | 8 | 7 |
| **The Vermont Bread Co.** | | | | | | | | | | |
| **BREAD** | | | | | | | | | | |
| Cinnamon Raisin | 1 slice | 70 | 0 | 0 | 0 | 0 | 125 | 17 | 2 | 3 |
| Oat Bran Oatmeal | 1 slice | 70 | 10 | 1 | 0 | 0 | 120 | 14 | 2 | 3 |
| Old Fashioned White | 1 slice | 70 | 5 | 1 | 0 | 0 | 120 | 15 | 0 | 2 |
| Old Style Pumpernickel | 1 slice | 90 | 0 | 0 | 0 | 0 | 190 | 19 | <1 | 3 |
| Old Style Rye | 1 slice | 90 | 0 | 0 | 0 | 0 | 190 | 19 | <1 | 4 |
| Sweet | 1 slice | 70 | 0 | 0 | 0 | 0 | 160 | 16 | 2 | 3 |
| Sunflower Sesame | 1 slice | 70 | 0 | .5 | 0 | 0 | 150 | 14 | 2 | 3 |
| Whole Wheat | 1 slice | 70 | 5 | .5 | 0 | 0 | 150 | 14 | 2 | 3 |
| Whole Wheat Sourdough | 1 slice | 70 | 0 | 0 | 0 | 0 | 125 | 15 | 2 | 3 |
| **BUNS** | | | | | | | | | | |
| Organic Burger | 1 slice | 170 | 20 | 2 | 0 | 0 | 390 | 34 | 1 | 5 |
| Organic Hot Dog | 1 slice | 150 | 15 | 2 | 0 | 0 | 350 | 31 | 1 | 4 |
| **ORGANIC BREAD** | | | | | | | | | | |
| Multigrain | 1 slice | 70 | 0 | 0 | 0 | 0 | 130 | 15 | 1 | 3 |
| Oat | 1 slice | 70 | 0 | 0 | 0 | 0 | 140 | 15 | 1 | 3 |
| Wheat | 1 slice | 70 | 0 | 0 | 0 | 0 | 150 | 15 | 1 | 3 |
| **Weight Watchers** | | | | | | | | | | |
| **SMART ONES BREAKFAST** | | | | | | | | | | |
| Breakfast Quesadilla | 1 entrée | 230 | 70 | 7 | 3.5 | 15 | 730 | 29 | 6 | 12 |
| Cheesy Scramble with Hashbrowns | 1 entrée | 210 | 80 | 9 | 4 | 70 | 510 | 18 | 3 | 15 |
| English Muffin Sandwich | 1 entrée | 210 | 50 | 5 | 2.5 | 15 | 610 | 27 | 2 | 13 |
| Ham and Cheese Scramble | 1 entrée | 220 | 80 | 9 | 4 | 65 | 610 | 13 | 2 | 21 |
| **SMART ONES DESSERTS** | | | | | | | | | | |
| Brownie à La Mode | 1 brownie | 200 | 35 | 4 | 2.5 | 25 | 160 | 36 | 3 | 5 |
| Chocolate Chip Cookie Dough Sundae | 1 sundae | 170 | 30 | 3 | 1.5 | 5 | 100 | 32 | 1 | 3 |

| | SERVING SIZE | CAL. | CAL. FAT | TOT FAT (G) | SAT FAT (G) | CHOL (MG) | SOD (MG) | CARB (G) | FIBER (G) | PROT (G) |
|---|---|---|---|---|---|---|---|---|---|---|
| Chocolate Éclair | 1 éclair | 140 | 35 | 4 | 1 | 30 | 180 | 24 | 1 | 3 |
| Peanut Butter Cup Sundae | 1 sundae | 170 | 50 | 5 | 2.5 | 5 | 90 | 28 | 3 | 4 |
| Strawberry Shortcake | 1 shortcake | 170 | 60 | 6 | 3 | 35 | 280 | 26 | <1 | 4 |
| **SMART ONES ENTRÉES** | | | | | | | | | | |
| Angel Hair Marinara | 1 entrée | 230 | 35 | 4 | 1 | 0 | 640 | 40 | 4 | 9 |
| Beef & Asian Style Vegetables | 1 entrée | 220 | 50 | 5 | 2 | 30 | 550 | 27 | 3 | 17 |
| Broccoli & Cheddar Roasted Potatoes | 1 entrée | 240 | 60 | 7 | 3.5 | 10 | 520 | 35 | 4 | 10 |
| Chicken Bruschetta Grilled Flatbread | 1 entrée | 310 | 70 | 8 | 1.5 | 20 | 570 | 42 | 4 | 17 |
| Chicken Enchiladas Monterey | 1 entrée | 310 | 90 | 10 | 3 | 25 | 730 | 41 | 5 | 12 |
| Chicken Fettuccini | 1 entrée | 290 | 50 | 6 | 2.5 | 60 | 720 | 40 | 3 | 20 |
| Chicken Marinara with Mozzarella Cheese & Grilled Flatbread | 1 entrée | 290 | 60 | 6 | 1.5 | 20 | 640 | 41 | 3 | 18 |
| Chicken Marsala with Broccoli | 1 entrée | 160 | 50 | 6 | 1.5 | 40 | 590 | 11 | 3 | 16 |
| Chicken Oriental | 1 entrée | 230 | 10 | 1.5 | .5 | 25 | 700 | 41 | 2 | 14 |
| Chicken Parmesan | 1 entrée | 290 | 50 | 5 | 1.5 | 40 | 630 | 35 | 4 | 26 |
| Cranberry Turkey Medallions | 1 entrée | 250 | 20 | 2 | 1 | 30 | 460 | 43 | 4 | 16 |
| Creamy Parmesan Chicken | 1 entrée | 210 | 40 | 4.5 | 1.5 | 30 | 730 | 24 | 4 | 18 |
| Four Cheese Pizza | 1 entrée | 370 | 70 | 7 | 3 | 10 | 690 | 57 | 4 | 18 |
| Home Style Beef Pot Roast | 1 entrée | 180 | 40 | 4.5 | 2 | 25 | 670 | 18 | 4 | 17 |
| Honey Mango Barbeque Chicken | 1 entrée | 240 | 35 | 4 | 1 | 35 | 520 | 32 | 3 | 18 |
| Lasagna Bake with Meat Sauce | 1 entrée | 270 | 40 | 4 | 1.5 | 15 | 540 | 43 | 3 | 14 |
| Macaroni & Cheese | 1 entrée | 270 | 20 | 2 | 1 | <5 | 790 | 52 | 2 | 11 |
| Meatloaf | 1 entrée | 240 | 70 | 8 | 2.5 | 45 | 820 | 22 | 3 | 21 |
| Orange Sesame Chicken | 1 entrée | 320 | 70 | 8 | 1.5 | 20 | 680 | 48 | 2 | 14 |
| Pasta Primavera | 1 entrée | 250 | 35 | 4 | 2 | 5 | 610 | 41 | 4 | 11 |
| Pepperoni Pizza | 1 entrée | 390 | 80 | 8 | 3 | 20 | 730 | 58 | 4 | 20 |
| Roast Beef in Gravy | 1 entrée | 230 | 100 | 11 | 3.5 | 40 | 530 | 18 | 2 | 16 |
| Roast Turkey Medallions w/Mushroom Gravy | 1 entrée | 220 | 10 | 2 | 0 | 55 | 550 | 38 | 3 | 13 |
| Roasted Chicken with Sour Cream & Chive Mashed Potatoes | 1 entrée | 180 | 35 | 4 | 1 | 40 | 820 | 20 | 2 | 17 |
| Salisbury Steak, 9 oz | 1 entrée | 200 | 70 | 7 | 2.5 | 55 | 740 | 12 | 4 | 20 |
| Santa Fe Style Rice & Beans | 1 entrée | 310 | 70 | 7 | 3 | 15 | 660 | 51 | 4 | 10 |
| Savory Steak & Ranch Grilled Flatbread | 1 entrée | 300 | 70 | 8 | 2 | 20 | 570 | 41 | 4 | 18 |
| Shrimp Marinara | 1 entrée | 190 | 15 | 2 | 0 | 20 | 650 | 34 | 4 | 10 |
| Slow Roasted Turkey Breast | 1 entrée | 200 | 60 | 7 | 2 | 40 | 710 | 18 | 2 | 17 |
| Spaghetti with Meat Sauce | 1 entrée | 290 | 45 | 5 | 2 | 15 | 720 | 44 | 5 | 16 |
| Stuffed Turkey Breast | 1 entrée | 260 | 50 | 5 | 1.5 | 20 | 700 | 39 | 4 | 14 |

| | SERVING SIZE | CAL | CAL FAT | TOT FAT (G) | SAT FAT (G) | CHOL (MG) | SOD (MG) | CARB (G) | FIBER (G) | PROT (G) |
|---|---|---|---|---|---|---|---|---|---|---|
| Sweet & Sour Chicken | 1 entrée | 210 | 20 | 2 | 0 | 20 | 510 | 31 | 2 | 16 |
| Teriyaki Chicken & Vegetables | 1 entrée | 230 | 20 | 2.5 | .5 | 25 | 620 | 39 | 3 | 14 |
| Thai Style Chicken & Rice Noodles | 1 entrée | 260 | 35 | 4 | .5 | 25 | 620 | 42 | 2 | 15 |
| Three Cheese Macaroni | 1 entrée | 300 | 50 | 6 | 2.5 | 10 | 570 | 48 | 3 | 14 |
| Traditional Lasagna with Meat Sauce | 1 entrée | 300 | 50 | 6 | 3 | 25 | 780 | 43 | 5 | 17 |

**SMART ONES SNACKS**

| | SERVING SIZE | CAL | CAL FAT | TOT FAT (G) | SAT FAT (G) | CHOL (MG) | SOD (MG) | CARB (G) | FIBER (G) | PROT (G) |
|---|---|---|---|---|---|---|---|---|---|---|
| Cheese Pizza Minis | 4 pieces | 270 | 60 | 7 | 3.5 | 10 | 480 | 38 | 5 | 13 |
| Fiesta Quesadilla | 1 quesadilla | 230 | 50 | 5 | 3 | 10 | 610 | 35 | 9 | 10 |
| Mini Cheeseburgers | 1 item | 200 | 80 | 9 | 4 | 25 | 360 | 20 | 3 | 10 |

## Wise
**CHEESE FLAVORED CORN SNACKS**

| | SERVING SIZE | CAL | CAL FAT | TOT FAT (G) | SAT FAT (G) | CHOL (MG) | SOD (MG) | CARB (G) | FIBER (G) | PROT (G) |
|---|---|---|---|---|---|---|---|---|---|---|
| Cheese Balls | 1 oz | 150 | 70 | 8 | 2 | 0 | 320 | 17 | 0 | 2 |
| Puffed Cheez Doodles | 1 oz | 150 | 70 | 8 | 2 | 0 | 320 | 17 | 0 | 2 |

**POTATO CHIPS**

| | SERVING SIZE | CAL | CAL FAT | TOT FAT (G) | SAT FAT (G) | CHOL (MG) | SOD (MG) | CARB (G) | FIBER (G) | PROT (G) |
|---|---|---|---|---|---|---|---|---|---|---|
| Barbeque Flavored | 1 oz | 150 | 90 | 10 | 3 | 0 | 210 | 14 | 1 | 2 |
| Cheddar & Sour Cream Flavored Ridgies | 1 oz | 150 | 80 | 9 | 2.5 | 0 | 190 | 15 | 1 | 2 |
| Honey Barbeque Flavored | 1 oz | 150 | 90 | 10 | 2.5 | 0 | 190 | 15 | 1 | 1 |
| Jalapeno Cheddar Flavored | 1 oz | 150 | 90 | 10 | 2.5 | 0 | 220 | 14 | <1 | 2 |
| Lightly Salted | 1 oz | 150 | 90 | 10 | 3 | 0 | 80 | 14 | 1 | 2 |
| New York Deli Kettle Cooked | 1 oz | 150 | 80 | 9 | 2.5 | 0 | 170 | 15 | 1 | 2 |
| New York Deli Salt & Vinegar Flavored Kettle Cooked | 1 oz | 140 | 70 | 8 | 2 | 0 | 240 | 16 | 1 | 2 |
| Rippled | 1 oz | 150 | 90 | 10 | 3 | 0 | 160 | 14 | 1 | 2 |
| Sour Cream & Onion Flavored Ridgies | 1 oz | 150 | 90 | 10 | 2.5 | 0 | 220 | 14 | 1 | 2 |

## Wish-Bone
**CREAMY**

| | SERVING SIZE | CAL | CAL FAT | TOT FAT (G) | SAT FAT (G) | CHOL (MG) | SOD (MG) | CARB (G) | FIBER (G) | PROT (G) |
|---|---|---|---|---|---|---|---|---|---|---|
| Chunky Blue Cheese | 2 tbsp | 150 | 140 | 15 | 2.5 | <5 | 270 | 1 | 0 | 0 |
| Creamy Caesar | 2 tbsp | 180 | 160 | 18 | 3 | 10 | 290 | 1 | 0 | <1 |
| Creamy Italian | 2 tbsp | 110 | 90 | 10 | 1.5 | 0 | 240 | 4 | 0 | <1 |
| Deluxe French | 2 tbsp | 130 | 100 | 11 | 1.5 | 0 | 170 | 5 | 0 | 0 |
| Ranch | 2 tbsp | 130 | 120 | 13 | 2 | 5 | 250 | 2 | 0 | 0 |
| Russian | 2 tbsp | 110 | 50 | 6 | 1 | 0 | 340 | 14 | 0 | 0 |
| Sweet & Spicy French | 2 tbsp | 140 | 110 | 12 | 2 | 0 | 340 | 6 | 0 | 0 |
| Thousand Island | 2 tbsp | 130 | 110 | 12 | 2 | 10 | 300 | 6 | 0 | 0 |

**FAT FREE**

| | SERVING SIZE | CAL | CAL FAT | TOT FAT (G) | SAT FAT (G) | CHOL (MG) | SOD (MG) | CARB (G) | FIBER (G) | PROT (G) |
|---|---|---|---|---|---|---|---|---|---|---|
| Chunky Blue Cheese | 2 tbsp | 30 | 0 | 0 | 0 | 0 | 280 | 7 | <1 | <1 |

| | SERVING SIZE | CAL | CAL FAT | TOT FAT (G) | SAT FAT (G) | CHOL (MG) | SOD (MG) | CARB (G) | FIBER (G) | PROT (G) |
|---|---|---|---|---|---|---|---|---|---|---|
| Italian | 2 tbsp | 15 | 0 | 0 | 0 | 0 | 350 | 3 | 0 | 0 |
| Ranch | 2 tbsp | 30 | 0 | 0 | 0 | 0 | 280 | 6 | <1 | 0 |
| Red Wine Vinaigrette | 2 tbsp | 35 | 0 | 0 | 0 | 0 | 230 | 7 | 0 | 0 |
| **LIGHT** | | | | | | | | | | |
| Asian with Sesame & Ginger Vinaigrette | 2 tbsp | 70 | 45 | 5 | 1 | 0 | 300 | 5 | 0 | 0 |
| Blue Cheese | 2 tbsp | 40 | 20 | 2 | 0 | 0 | 310 | 6 | 0 | <1 |
| Cream Caesar | 2 tbsp | 45 | 20 | 2 | .5 | 10 | 310 | 7 | 0 | <1 |
| Honey Dijon | 2 tbsp | 50 | 20 | 2 | 0 | 0 | 260 | 8 | <1 | 0 |
| Italian | 2 tbsp | 35 | 25 | 2.5 | 0 | 0 | 340 | 3 | 0 | 0 |
| Parmesan Peppercorn Ranch | 2 tbsp | 45 | 20 | 2 | 0 | <5 | 270 | 7 | <1 | 0 |
| Ranch | 2 tbsp | 40 | 20 | 2 | 0 | 0 | 290 | 5 | 0 | 0 |
| Thousand Island | 2 tbsp | 60 | 20 | 2 | 0 | 5 | 280 | 9 | 0 | 0 |
| **OIL & VINEGAR** | | | | | | | | | | |
| Balsamic Vinaigrette | 2 tbsp | 60 | 45 | 5 | .5 | 0 | 280 | 3 | 0 | 0 |
| Italian Dressing | 2 tbsp | 80 | 60 | 7 | 1 | 0 | 340 | 4 | 0 | 0 |
| Red Wine Vinaigrette | 2 tbsp | 70 | 45 | 5 | .5 | 0 | 230 | 6 | 0 | 0 |
| **SALAD SPRITZERS** | | | | | | | | | | |
| Balsamic Breeze Vinaigrette | 10 sprays | 10 | 10 | 1 | 0 | 0 | 130 | 1 | 0 | 0 |
| Italian Vinaigrette | 10 sprays | 10 | 10 | 1 | 0 | 0 | 100 | 1 | 0 | 0 |
| Ranch | 10 sprays | 15 | 10 | 1 | 0 | 0 | 70 | <1 | 0 | 0 |
| Raspberry Bliss Vinaigrette | 10 sprays | 10 | 0 | .5 | 0 | 0 | 95 | 2 | 0 | 0 |
| **WESTERN** | | | | | | | | | | |
| Fat Free | 2 tbsp | 50 | 0 | 0 | 0 | 0 | 280 | 12 | 0 | 0 |
| Light | 2 tbsp | 70 | 20 | 2 | 0 | 0 | 270 | 13 | 0 | 0 |
| Original | 2 tbsp | 160 | 110 | 12 | 1.5 | 0 | 230 | 11 | 0 | 0 |
| **Wonder** | | | | | | | | | | |
| **BREAD** | | | | | | | | | | |
| Classic White | 1 slice | 70 | 5 | 1 | 0 | 0 | 150 | 14 | 0 | 2 |
| Light Wheat | 2 slices | 80 | 10 | .5 | 0 | 0 | 240 | 18 | 5 | 5 |
| Light White | 2 slices | 80 | 10 | .5 | 0 | 0 | 260 | 18 | 5 | 4 |
| Stone Ground 100% Whole Wheat | 2 slices | 180 | 20 | 2.5 | .5 | 0 | 400 | 32 | 4 | 7 |
| Texas Toast | 1 slice | 100 | 10 | 1 | 0 | 0 | 200 | 19 | <1 | 3 |
| Whole Grain Wheat | 2 slices | 130 | 15 | 1.5 | 0 | 0 | 320 | 26 | 4 | 6 |
| Whole Grain White | 2 slices | 140 | 20 | 2 | .5 | 0 | 200 | 25 | 3 | 6 |
| **BUNS** | | | | | | | | | | |
| Classic White Hamburger Buns | 1 bun | 110 | 15 | 1.5 | 0 | 0 | 210 | 21 | <1 | 3 |
| Classic White Hot Dog Buns | 1 bun | 110 | 15 | 1.5 | 0 | 0 | 210 | 21 | <1 | 3 |

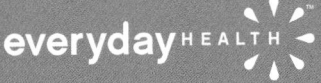

restaurants

# restaurants

| | SERVING SIZE | CAL | CAL FAT | TOT FAT (G) | SAT FAT (G) | CHOL (MG) | SOD (MG) | CARB (G) | FIBER (G) | PROT (G) |
|---|---|---|---|---|---|---|---|---|---|---|
| **A&W** | | | | | | | | | | |
| **BURGERS & CHICKEN** | | | | | | | | | | |
| Original Bacon Double Cheeseburger | 1 burger | 760 | 410 | 45 | 17 | 165 | 1570 | 45 | 4 | 44 |
| Original Double Cheeseburger | 1 burger | 680 | 340 | 38 | 14 | 150 | 1330 | 44 | 4 | 40 |
| Hamburger | 1 burger | 380 | 170 | 19 | 6 | 55 | 860 | 33 | 3 | 21 |
| Cheeseburger | 1 burger | 420 | 190 | 21 | 7 | 70 | 1040 | 37 | 4 | 23 |
| Chicken Strips | 3 pieces | 500 | 260 | 29 | 5 | 55 | 1050 | 32 | 2 | 28 |
| Grilled Chicken Sandwich | 1 sandwich | 400 | 140 | 15 | 3 | 90 | 820 | 31 | 4 | 35 |
| Crunchy Shrimp | 21 pieces | 340 | 170 | 19 | 5 | 110 | 820 | 34 | 2 | 13 |
| **HOT DOGS** | | | | | | | | | | |
| Coney Chili Cheese Dog | 1 hot dog | 380 | 210 | 23 | 9 | 10 | 1100 | 28 | 2 | 14 |
| Cheese Dog | 1 hot dog | 350 | 200 | 22 | 9 | 5 | 940 | 26 | 1 | 12 |
| Plain | 1 hot dog | 310 | 170 | 19 | 8 | 0 | 740 | 23 | 1 | 11 |
| **SIDES** | | | | | | | | | | |
| Breaded Onion Rings | 4 oz | 350 | 150 | 16 | 3.5 | 0 | 710 | 45 | 2 | 5 |
| Cheese Curds | 5 oz | 570 | 360 | 40 | 21 | 105 | 1220 | 27 | 2 | 27 |
| Chili | as served | 190 | 50 | 6 | 0 | 20 | 640 | 22 | 5 | 12 |
| Chili Fries | 6 oz | 370 | 130 | 15 | 4 | 10 | 790 | 49 | 5 | 8 |
| Cheese Fries | 6 oz | 390 | 160 | 18 | 4.5 | 5 | 870 | 50 | 4 | 4 |
| Corn Dog Nuggets, Small | 5 pieces | 180 | 70 | 8 | 2 | 25 | 520 | 20 | 1 | 5 |
| **SWEETS & TREATS** | | | | | | | | | | |
| Blue Raspberry Slushee, Medium | 20 fl oz | 570 | 0 | 0 | 0 | 0 | 65 | 142 | 0 | 0 |
| Chocolate Fudge Blendrrr, Medium | 20 fl oz | 560 | 290 | 32 | 27 | 10 | 125 | 92 | 2 | 4 |
| Chocolate Milkshake, Medium | 20 fl oz | 880 | 330 | 36 | 23 | 155 | 250 | 125 | 3 | 14 |
| Diet Root Beer Float, Medium | 20 fl oz | 170 | 45 | 5 | 3 | 40 | 105 | 30 | 0 | 2 |
| Diet Root Beer Freeze, Medium | 20 fl oz | 340 | 90 | 10 | 6 | 40 | 230 | 53 | 1 | 9 |
| Hot Fudge Sundae | 1 sundae | 350 | 100 | 11 | 6 | 30 | 140 | 54 | 1 | 8 |
| Limeade, Strawberry, Medium | 20 fl oz | 420 | 0 | 0 | 0 | 0 | 60 | 105 | 0 | 0 |
| Orange Freeze, Medium | 20 fl oz | 600 | 90 | 10 | 6 | 40 | 230 | 142 | n/a | 9 |
| Root Beer Float, Medium | 20 fl oz | 350 | 45 | 5 | 3 | 40 | 105 | 77 | 0 | 2 |
| Root Beer Freeze, Medium | 20 fl oz | 480 | 90 | 10 | 6 | 40 | 230 | 89 | 1 | 9 |
| Strawberry Banana Smoothie, Medium | 20 fl oz | 420 | 50 | 6 | 4.5 | 25 | 100 | 86 | 0 | 3 |
| Strawberry Smoothie, Medium | 20 fl oz | 370 | 50 | 6 | 4.5 | 25 | 90 | 74 | 0 | 3 |
| Vanilla Milkshake, Medium | 20 fl oz | 900 | 350 | 39 | 24 | 170 | 260 | 121 | 0 | 15 |
| **Applebee's** | | | | | | | | | | |
| **APPETIZERS** | | | | | | | | | | |
| Appetizer Sampler | as served | 2400 | 1413 | 157 | 45 | n/a | 5740 | 158 | 16 | 91 |

| | SERVING SIZE | CAL | CAL FAT | TOT FAT (G) | SAT FAT (G) | CHOL (MG) | SOD (MG) | CARB (G) | FIBER (G) | PROT (G) |
|---|---|---|---|---|---|---|---|---|---|---|
| Boneless Buffalo Wings, Classic | as served | 1170 | 621 | 69 | 16 | n/a | 3790 | 66 | 8 | 70 |
| Buffalo Chicken Wings, Classic | as served | 710 | 441 | 49 | 14 | n/a | 2030 | 7 | 2 | 60 |
| Chili Cheese Nachos | as served | 1680 | 963 | 107 | 39 | n/a | 3850 | 133 | 17 | 48 |
| Crunchy Onion Rings | as served | 1230 | 531 | 59 | 11 | n/a | 2160 | 161 | 12 | 14 |
| Mozzarella Sticks | as served | 940 | 414 | 46 | 20 | n/a | 2800 | 84 | 6 | 45 |
| Potato Skins | as served | 1380 | 873 | 97 | 49 | n/a | 1860 | 70 | 8 | 59 |
| Spinach & Artichoke Dip | as served | 1470 | 864 | 96 | 23 | n/a | 2440 | 122 | 16 | 33 |
| **ENTRÉES** | | | | | | | | | | |
| 9 oz House Sirloin | 1 entrée | 310 | 117 | 13 | 5 | n/a | 970 | 0 | 0 | 48 |
| 12 oz New York Strip | 1 entrée | 590 | 351 | 39 | 18 | n/a | 550 | 0 | 0 | 60 |
| Asiago Peppercorn Steak w/Sides | 1 entrée | 390 | 126 | 14 | 6 | n/a | 1520 | 26 | 5 | 43 |
| Chicken Fried Chicken w/Sides | 1 entrée | 1250 | 540 | 60 | 12 | n/a | 3450 | 114 | 12 | 62 |
| Chicken Parmesan w/Sides | 1 entrée | 1330 | 549 | 61 | 20 | n/a | 3400 | 114 | 12 | 81 |
| Chicken Tenders Basket w/Sides | 1 entrée | 1000 | 531 | 59 | 11 | n/a | 2140 | 81 | 7 | 36 |
| Garlic Herb Salmon | 1 entrée | 750 | 333 | 37 | 11 | n/a | 2640 | 59 | 6 | 46 |
| Hand-Battered Fish & Chips | 1 entrée | 1560 | 945 | 105 | 18 | n/a | 1960 | 106 | 10 | 47 |
| Shrimp 'N Parmesan Sirloin | 1 entrée | 540 | 252 | 28 | 14 | n/a | 2100 | 5 | 0 | 66 |
| Sizzling Asian Shrimp | 1 entrée | 710 | 315 | 15 | 3 | n/a | 3830 | 117 | 7 | 30 |
| Sizzling Bourbon Street Steak | 1 entrée | 700 | 369 | 41 | 10 | n/a | 2310 | 31 | 4 | 54 |
| Sizzling Chicken w/Spicy Queso Blanco | 1 entrée | 550 | 198 | 22 | 8 | n/a | 2500 | 37 | 6 | 53 |
| Sizzling Riblets Basket | 1 entrée | 1040 | 504 | 56 | 18 | n/a | 2640 | 56 | 5 | 62 |
| Sizzling Skillet Fajitas—Combo | 1 entrée | 1100 | 441 | 49 | 22 | n/a | 4790 | 104 | 10 | 59 |
| **PASTA & BOWLS** | | | | | | | | | | |
| Crispy Orange Chicken | 1 entrée | 2030 | 720 | 80 | 15 | n/a | 4480 | 264 | 15 | 84 |
| Shrimp Fettuccine Alfredo | 1 entrée | 1440 | 765 | 85 | 41 | n/a | 3320 | 110 | 9 | 63 |
| **SANDWICHES & BURGERS** | | | | | | | | | | |
| Bacon Cheddar Cheeseburger | 1 burger | 940 | 540 | 60 | 22 | n/a | 1610 | 48 | 1 | 55 |
| Bacon Cheese Chicken Grill | 1 sandwich | 720 | 297 | 33 | 11 | n/a | 1810 | 47 | 1 | 60 |
| BBQ Pulled Pork Sliders | as served | 1020 | 432 | 48 | 15 | n/a | 2040 | 89 | 3 | 55 |
| California Turkey Club | 1 sandwich | 1050 | 567 | 63 | 18 | n/a | 3600 | 62 | 4 | 56 |
| Cheeseburger Sliders | as served | 1240 | 720 | 80 | 25 | n/a | 2260 | 81 | 3 | 51 |
| Hamburger | 1 burger | 770 | 414 | 46 | 15 | n/a | 1170 | 47 | 1 | 44 |
| Oriental Chicken Rollup | 1 sandwich | 1060 | 486 | 54 | 11 | n/a | 2640 | 110 | 6 | 31 |
| Philly Burger | 1 burger | 1090 | 567 | 63 | 25 | n/a | 2520 | 70 | 5 | 60 |
| Veggie | 1 burger | 530 | 189 | 21 | 0 | n/a | 1390 | 61 | 8 | 26 |
| **SIDES** | | | | | | | | | | |
| Chili Cheese Fries | as served | 630 | 315 | 35 | 12 | n/a | 1670 | 59 | 7 | 18 |

| | SERVING SIZE | CAL | CAL FAT | TOT FAT (G) | SAT FAT (G) | CHOL (MG) | SOD (MG) | CARB (G) | FIBER (G) | PROT (G) |
|---|---|---|---|---|---|---|---|---|---|---|
| Crunchy Onion Rings | as served | 540 | 270 | 30 | 6 | n/a | 750 | 62 | 6 | 7 |
| French Fries | as served | 400 | 171 | 19 | 3.5 | n/a | 740 | 51 | 4 | 5 |
| Loaded Baked Potato | as served | 450 | 315 | 35 | 21 | n/a | 680 | 28 | 2 | 10 |
| **SOUPS & SALADS** | | | | | | | | | | |
| Chicken Noodle Soup | 1 bowl | 140 | 36 | 4 | 1 | n/a | 990 | 15 | 1 | 12 |
| Chili | 1 bowl | 480 | 261 | 29 | 13 | n/a | 1190 | 21 | 3 | 34 |
| Crispy Shrimp Caesar, w/o Dressing | 1 salad | 610 | 279 | 31 | 8 | n/a | 1520 | 54 | 7 | 31 |
| French Onion Soup | 1 bowl | 280 | 135 | 15 | 10 | n/a | 1230 | 18 | 3 | 16 |
| Grilled Chicken Caesar, w/o Dressing | 1 salad | 370 | 90 | 10 | 3.5 | n/a | 900 | 21 | 5 | 52 |
| Santa Fe Chicken, w/o Dressing | 1 salad | 910 | 486 | 54 | 18 | n/a | 2250 | 51 | 10 | 58 |

# Arby's
## CHICKEN & TURKEY

| | SERVING SIZE | CAL | CAL FAT | TOT FAT (G) | SAT FAT (G) | CHOL (MG) | SOD (MG) | CARB (G) | FIBER (G) | PROT (G) |
|---|---|---|---|---|---|---|---|---|---|---|
| Crispy Chicken Sandwich | 1 sandwich | 530 | 220 | 25 | 4 | 60 | 1310 | 52 | 4 | 25 |
| Popcorn Chicken, Regular | 1 sandwich | 360 | 150 | 16 | 2.5 | 40 | 980 | 27 | 2 | 26 |
| Prime-Cut Chicken, Large | as served | 610 | 250 | 28 | 4.0 | 85 | 1940 | 52 | 3 | 35 |
| Roast Chicken Bacon & Swiss Sandwich | 1 sandwich | 470 | 170 | 19 | 5 | 65 | 1310 | 43 | 2 | 32 |
| Roast Chicken Club | 1 sandwich | 500 | 210 | 23 | 7 | 70 | 1320 | 41 | 2 | 31 |
| Roast Chicken Sandwich | 1 sandwich | 400 | 150 | 16 | 3.0 | 50 | 870 | 40 | 3 | 24 |

## ROAST BEEF SANDWICHES & MELTS

| | SERVING SIZE | CAL | CAL FAT | TOT FAT (G) | SAT FAT (G) | CHOL (MG) | SOD (MG) | CARB (G) | FIBER (G) | PROT (G) |
|---|---|---|---|---|---|---|---|---|---|---|
| All-American Roastburger | 1 burger | 390 | 140 | 15 | 5 | 45 | 1730 | 44 | 2 | 20 |
| Arby's Melt | 1 sandwich | 370 | 120 | 13 | 4 | 50 | 1150 | 40 | 2 | 23 |
| Beef 'n Cheddar- Regular | 1 sandwich | 420 | 160 | 18 | 5 | 50 | 1260 | 43 | 2 | 23 |
| Classic Italian Toasted Sub | 1 sandwich | 590 | 270 | 30 | 8 | 55 | 1870 | 57 | 3 | 24 |
| French Dip & Swiss Toasted Sub w/Au Jus | 1 sandwich | 500 | 140 | 15 | 6 | 60 | 2220 | 61 | 2 | 29 |
| Philly Beef Toasted Sub | 1 sandwich | 560 | 220 | 25 | 7 | 65 | 1490 | 56 | 3 | 29 |
| Reuben Sandwich | 1 sandwich | 700 | 290 | 32 | 9 | 65 | 1870 | 64 | 4 | 39 |
| Roast Ham & Swiss Melt Sandwich | 1 sandwich | 710 | 270 | 30 | 8 | 75 | 2010 | 78 | 5 | 36 |
| Super Roast Beef Sandwich | 1 sandwich | 420 | 150 | 17 | 5 | 45 | 1080 | 45 | 3 | 23 |
| Turkey Bacon Club Toasted Sub | 1 sandwich | 560 | 200 | 23 | 6 | 60 | 1720 | 56 | 3 | 32 |
| Ultimate BLT Sandwich | 1 sandwich | 820 | 400 | 44 | 9 | 45 | 1690 | 78 | 5 | 32 |

## SALADS

| | SERVING SIZE | CAL | CAL FAT | TOT FAT (G) | SAT FAT (G) | CHOL (MG) | SOD (MG) | CARB (G) | FIBER (G) | PROT (G) |
|---|---|---|---|---|---|---|---|---|---|---|
| Chopped Farmhouse Crispy Chicken Salad | 1 salad | 430 | 210 | 24 | 8 | 65 | 1150 | 30 | 4 | 27 |
| Chopped Farmhouse Roasted Chicken Salad | 1 salad | 250 | 120 | 13 | 7 | 60 | 680 | 11 | 3 | 23 |
| Chopped Farmhouse Turkey & Ham | 1 salad | 250 | 120 | 14 | 7 | 60 | 910 | 9 | 4 | 23 |

| | SERVING SIZE | CAL | CAL FAT | TOT FAT (G) | SAT FAT (G) | CHOL (MG) | SOD (MG) | CARB (G) | FIBER (G) | PROT (G) |
|---|---|---|---|---|---|---|---|---|---|---|
| **SIDES** | | | | | | | | | | |
| Curly Fries, Medium | 6 oz | 600 | 280 | 31 | 4 | 25 | 1550 | 74 | 5 | 6 |
| Homestyle Fries, Medium | 6 oz | 480 | 190 | 21 | 3 | 0 | 1360 | 69 | 5 | 5 |
| Jalapeño Bites | 8 pieces | 470 | 250 | 27 | 10 | 40 | 1180 | 49 | 4 | 8 |
| Loaded Potato Bites | 5 Pieces | 340 | 180 | 20 | 6 | 5 | 760 | 29 | 2 | 10 |
| Mozzarella Sticks | 4 pieces | 440 | 200 | 23 | 9 | 5 | 1190 | 39 | 2 | 21 |
| Potato Cakes, Medium | 3 Pieces | 390 | 210 | 23 | 3.5 | 0 | 600 | 42 | 3 | 3 |
| Steakhouse Onion Rings | 4-3/5 oz | 460 | 210 | 24 | 3 | 0 | 1400 | 56 | 3 | 6 |

## Atlanta Bread Company

### BAKERY & BREADS

| | SERVING SIZE | CAL | CAL FAT | TOT FAT (G) | SAT FAT (G) | CHOL (MG) | SOD (MG) | CARB (G) | FIBER (G) | PROT (G) |
|---|---|---|---|---|---|---|---|---|---|---|
| Almond Croissant | 1 croissant | 620 | 310 | 35 | 12 | 55 | 330 | 67 | 4 | 13 |
| Apple Danish | 1 danish | 460 | 160 | 18 | 11 | 70 | 340 | 67 | 2 | 6 |
| Asiago Loaf | 1 slice | 80 | 10 | 1 | .5 | 5 | 180 | 14 | 1 | 3 |
| Blueberry Muffin | 1 muffin | 320 | 130 | 15 | 2.5 | 70 | 250 | 41 | 1 | 5 |
| Chocolate Chip Muffin | 1 muffin | 640 | 270 | 31 | 8 | 105 | 390 | 83 | 3 | 9 |
| Chocolate Chunk Cookie | 1 cookie | 430 | 190 | 21 | 10 | 30 | 180 | 58 | 2 | 5 |
| Ciabatta | 1 ciabatta | 270 | 20 | 2 | 1 | 5 | 500 | 55 | 2 | 10 |
| Double Chocolate Brownie | 1 brownie | 450 | 170 | 19 | 3.5 | 50 | 135 | 73 | 8 | 6 |
| French Roll | 1 roll | 160 | 5 | .5 | 0 | 0 | 370 | 34 | 1 | 6 |
| Low Fat Apple Muffin | 1 muffin | 230 | 20 | 2.5 | .5 | 55 | 290 | 48 | 1 | 5 |
| Nine Grain Bread | 1 slice | 120 | 15 | 2 | .5 | 0 | 240 | 22 | 2 | 5 |
| Sourdough Baguette | 1 slice | 90 | 0 | 0 | 0 | 0 | 190 | 18 | 1 | 3 |

### BREAKFAST

| | SERVING SIZE | CAL | CAL FAT | TOT FAT (G) | SAT FAT (G) | CHOL (MG) | SOD (MG) | CARB (G) | FIBER (G) | PROT (G) |
|---|---|---|---|---|---|---|---|---|---|---|
| Bacon, Egg & Cheese Sandwich | 1 sandwich | 490 | 190 | 21 | 7 | 280 | 950 | 52 | 2 | 23 |
| Chive Cream Cheese | 2 oz | 170 | 140 | 15 | 10 | 50 | 180 | 6 | 1 | 4 |
| Egg & Cheese Sandwich | 1 sandwich | 440 | 150 | 17 | 6 | 270 | 790 | 52 | 2 | 20 |
| Everything Bagel | 1 bagel | 350 | 35 | 3.5 | .5 | 0 | 1660 | 66 | 4 | 13 |
| French Toast w/Maple Syrup | 2 slices | 640 | 100 | 11 | 4 | 210 | 550 | 121 | 3 | 15 |
| Ham & Swiss Omelet | 1 omelet | 500 | 320 | 35 | 17 | 645 | 1280 | 3 | 0 | 50 |
| Honey Raisin Walnut Cream Cheese | 2 oz | 190 | 130 | 14 | 9 | 40 | 150 | 14 | 1 | 3 |
| Plain Bagel | 1 bagel | 300 | 10 | 1.5 | 0 | 0 | 500 | 60 | 3 | 11 |
| Sesame Seed Bagel | 1 bagel | 390 | 80 | 9 | 0 | 0 | 530 | 63 | 4 | 15 |
| Three Cheese Omelet | 1 omelet | 1100 | 760 | 85 | 44 | 770 | 1990 | 6 | 0 | 81 |
| Whole Grain Bagel | 1 bagel | 260 | 15 | 1.5 | 0 | 0 | 450 | 52 | 4 | 10 |

### PIZZA

| | SERVING SIZE | CAL | CAL FAT | TOT FAT (G) | SAT FAT (G) | CHOL (MG) | SOD (MG) | CARB (G) | FIBER (G) | PROT (G) |
|---|---|---|---|---|---|---|---|---|---|---|
| Chicken Pesto Calzone | 1 calzone | 840 | 300 | 33 | 7 | 60 | 1700 | 95 | 5 | 40 |

| | SERVING SIZE | CAL | CAL FAT | TOT FAT (G) | SAT FAT (G) | CHOL (MG) | SOD (MG) | CARB (G) | FIBER (G) | PROT (G) |
|---|---|---|---|---|---|---|---|---|---|---|
| Four Cheese Pizza | 1/2 pizza | 530 | 210 | 23 | 12 | 55 | 1240 | 46 | 3 | 35 |
| Pepperoni Pizza | 1/2 pizza | 340 | 90 | 10 | 5 | 25 | 790 | 44 | 3 | 18 |
| **SANDWICHES** | | | | | | | | | | |
| ABC Special | 1 sandwich | 750 | 340 | 38 | 10 | 105 | 1980 | 57 | 3 | 45 |
| Chicken Pesto Panini | 1 sandwich | 710 | 240 | 26 | 9 | 80 | 1000 | 80 | 4 | 40 |
| Turkey Bacon Rustica | 1 sandwich | 960 | 500 | 56 | 19 | 130 | 2480 | 62 | 3 | 53 |
| Veggie on Nine Grain | 1 sandwich | 500 | 220 | 25 | 8 | 35 | 820 | 52 | 5 | 18 |
| **SOUPS & SALADS** | | | | | | | | | | |
| Balsamic Bleu | 1 salad | 330 | 160 | 18 | 6 | 25 | 410 | 35 | 5 | 10 |
| Baja Chicken Enchilada | 1-1/4 cup | 330 | 170 | 19 | 9 | 70 | 1560 | 23 | 4 | 16 |
| Caesar | 1 salad | 150 | 80 | 9 | 6 | 5 | 390 | 7 | 2 | 14 |
| Chicken Peppercorn | 1-1/4 cup | 430 | 300 | 34 | 18 | 120 | 1530 | 13 | 0 | 15 |
| Classic Beef Chili | 1-1/4 cup | 290 | 90 | 10 | 4 | 45 | 1110 | 33 | 10 | 19 |
| Classic Chicken Noodle | 1-1/4 cup | 130 | 10 | 1.5 | 0 | 20 | 1050 | 15 | 1 | 11 |
| Garden Vegetable | 1-1/4 cup | 90 | 5 | .5 | 0 | 0 | 1090 | 16 | 4 | 3 |
| Greek | 1 salad | 240 | 150 | 16 | 8 | 30 | 1370 | 15 | 4 | 11 |

## Au Bon Pain
### BAKERY

| | SERVING SIZE | CAL | CAL FAT | TOT FAT (G) | SAT FAT (G) | CHOL (MG) | SOD (MG) | CARB (G) | FIBER (G) | PROT (G) |
|---|---|---|---|---|---|---|---|---|---|---|
| Blondie | 1 blondie | 530 | 288 | 32 | 10 | 35 | 630 | 57 | 3 | 6 |
| Blueberry Muffin | 1 muffin | 490 | 153 | 17 | 2 | 20 | 510 | 74 | 2 | 9 |
| Chocolate Chip Brownie | 1 brownie | 440 | 189 | 21 | 6 | 85 | 240 | 62 | 2 | 4 |
| Chocolate Chip Cookie | 1 cookie | 280 | 117 | 13 | 7 | 30 | 210 | 40 | 2 | 3 |
| Plain Bagel | 1 bagel | 280 | 9 | 1 | 0 | 0 | 430 | 56 | 2 | 11 |
| Plain Croissant | 1 croissant | 310 | 153 | 17 | 9 | 55 | 220 | 31 | 1 | 7 |
| **BREAD** | | | | | | | | | | |
| Artisan Sundried Tomato Bread | 2 slices | 270 | 9 | 1 | 0 | 0 | 750 | 57 | 2 | 10 |
| Asiago Breadstick | 1 breadstick | 190 | 36 | 4 | 3 | 10 | 350 | 28 | 1 | 9 |
| Ciabatta, Small | 1 roll | 180 | 9 | 1 | 0 | 0 | 480 | 38 | 2 | 6 |
| Farm House Rolls | 1 roll | 360 | 63 | 7 | 1 | 0 | 670 | 63 | 3 | 12 |
| Focaccia | 1 roll | 360 | 63 | 7 | 1 | 0 | 700 | 62 | 3 | 12 |
| Rosemary Garlic Bread Stick | 1 breadstick | 190 | 45 | 5 | 1 | 0 | 720 | 31 | 2 | 6 |
| Whole Wheat Multigrain Bread | 2 pieces | 260 | 27 | 3 | 0 | 0 | 630 | 53 | 9 | 11 |
| **HOT & COLD BAR** | | | | | | | | | | |
| Cajun Chicken Penne | 1 oz | 40 | 18 | 2 | 1 | 10 | 105 | 4 | 0 | 3 |
| Chicken Broccoli Alfredo Penne | 12 oz | 680 | 387 | 43 | 18 | 165 | 1100 | 38 | 2 | 28 |
| Italian Sausage, Peppers & Onions | 1 oz | 25 | 9 | 1 | 0 | 5 | 80 | 1 | 0 | 2 |
| Macaroni & Cheese | 1 oz | 40 | 27 | 3 | 2 | 10 | 115 | 3 | 0 | 2 |

| | SERVING SIZE | CAL | CAL. FAT | TOT FAT (G) | SAT FAT (G) | CHOL (MG) | SOD (MG) | CARB (G) | FIBER (G) | PROT (G) |
|---|---|---|---|---|---|---|---|---|---|---|
| Meat Lasagna | 10-7/10 oz | 470 | 216 | 24 | 11 | 100 | 1080 | 41 | 5 | 22 |
| **SALADS** | | | | | | | | | | |
| Chef's | 1 salad | 260 | 144 | 16 | 8 | 65 | 1070 | 7 | 3 | 25 |
| Chicken BLT | 1 salad | 300 | 144 | 16 | 7 | 285 | 860 | 7 | 3 | 34 |
| Grilled Chicken Caesar Asiago | 1 salad | 290 | 117 | 13 | 6 | 65 | 740 | 18 | 3 | 27 |
| Mandarin Sesame Chicken | 1 salad | 310 | 153 | 17 | 1 | 30 | 410 | 29 | 3 | 20 |
| Tuna Garden | 1 salad | 270 | 117 | 13 | 2 | 45 | 530 | 19 | 5 | 21 |
| Turkey Cobb | 1 salad | 340 | 171 | 19 | 8 | 260 | 940 | 16 | 4 | 27 |
| **SANDWICHES** | | | | | | | | | | |
| Bacon & Bagel Sandwich | 1 sandwich | 340 | 54 | 6 | 2 | 15 | 650 | 58 | 2 | 16 |
| Black Bean Burger | 1 sandwich | 560 | 162 | 18 | 5 | 5 | 970 | 76 | 13 | 30 |
| Caprese Sandwich | 1 sandwich | 680 | 288 | 32 | 15 | 75 | 1200 | 65 | 4 | 30 |
| Egg on a Bagel w/Bacon & Cheese | 1 sandwich | 570 | 207 | 23 | 10 | 415 | 920 | 59 | 2 | 32 |
| Ham & Swiss, Tomatoes & Romaine, Farmhouse Roll | 1/2 sandwich | 320 | 117 | 13 | 5 | 45 | 950 | 34 | 2 | 21 |
| Steakhouse on Ciabatta | 1 sandwich | 590 | 169 | 18 | 8 | 70 | 1850 | 72 | 3 | 36 |
| Turkey & Swiss on a Farmhouse Roll | 1/2 sandwich | 320 | 99 | 11 | 5 | 40 | 700 | 34 | 2 | 22 |
| **SOUPS & STEWS, MEDIUM** | | | | | | | | | | |
| Beef & Vegetable Stew | 12 fl oz | 310 | 144 | 16 | 3 | 55 | 1070 | 25 | 3 | 18 |
| Beef Chili | 12 fl oz | 300 | 117 | 13 | 4 | 40 | 1110 | 28 | 7 | 18 |
| Black Bean Soup | 12 fl oz | 280 | 18 | 2 | 0 | 0 | 1100 | 51 | 28 | 17 |
| Broccoli Cheddar Soup | 12 fl oz | 300 | 189 | 21 | 10 | 50 | 990 | 20 | 2 | 11 |
| Italian Wedding Soup | 12 fl oz | 190 | 90 | 10 | 4 | 15 | 1010 | 16 | 2 | 8 |
| Split Pea w/Ham Soup | 12 fl oz | 250 | 18 | 2 | 0 | 10 | 1220 | 41 | 15 | 18 |
| Vegetarian Lentil Soup | 12 fl oz | 170 | 18 | 2 | 0 | 0 | 1200 | 31 | 11 | 9 |

## Auntie Anne's
### DIPS

| | SERVING SIZE | CAL | CAL. FAT | TOT FAT (G) | SAT FAT (G) | CHOL (MG) | SOD (MG) | CARB (G) | FIBER (G) | PROT (G) |
|---|---|---|---|---|---|---|---|---|---|---|
| Caramel Dipping Sauce | 1-1/2 oz | 130 | 25 | 3 | 2 | 5 | 95 | 23 | 0 | 1 |
| Cream Cheese | 1-1/4 oz | 80 | 50 | 6 | 4.5 | 20 | 120 | 1 | 0 | 3 |
| Light Cream Cheese Dipping Sauce | 1-1/4 oz | 70 | 54 | 6 | 4 | 25 | 140 | 1 | 0 | 3 |
| Melted Cheese Dip | 2 oz | 150 | 100 | 12 | 3 | 20 | 850 | 6 | 0 | 5 |
| Sweet Mustard Dipping Sauce | as served | 60 | 20 | 2 | 1 | 35 | 0 | 10 | 0 | 2 |
| **DRINKS** | | | | | | | | | | |
| ICEE (average of all flavors) | 21 fl oz | 160 | 0 | 0 | 0 | 0 | 10 | 42 | 0 | 0 |
| Lemonade Mixer (average all flavors) | 20 fl oz | 315 | 0 | 0 | 0 | 0 | 23 | 79 | 0 | 0 |
| **PRETZELS** | | | | | | | | | | |
| Bacon, Egg & Cheese Pretzel Pocket | 1 item | 580 | 210 | 23 | 10 | 190 | 790 | 71 | 2 | 23 |

# restaurants

| | SERVING SIZE | CAL | CAL FAT | TOT FAT (G) | SAT FAT (G) | CHOL (MG) | SOD (MG) | CARB (G) | FIBER (G) | PROT (G) |
|---|---|---|---|---|---|---|---|---|---|---|
| Cinnamon Sugar Soft Pretzel | 1 pretzel | 470 | 108 | 12 | 7 | 25 | 400 | 84 | 2 | 8 |
| Jalapeno Pretzel | 1 pretzel | 330 | 45 | 5 | 3 | 10 | 1060 | 63 | 2 | 8 |
| Jumbo Pretzel Dog | 1 item | 610 | 260 | 29 | 13 | 65 | 1150 | 67 | 2 | 19 |
| Original Cinnamon Sugar Pretzel Stix | 6 stixs | 470 | 100 | 12 | 7 | 25 | 400 | 84 | 2 | 8 |
| Original Glazin' Raisin Soft Pretzel | 1 pretzel | 360 | 45 | 5 | 3 | 10 | 390 | 69 | 2 | 8 |
| Original Soft Pretzel | 1 pretzel | 340 | 45 | 5 | 3 | 10 | 1060 | 63 | 2 | 8 |
| Party Pretzel | 1 pretzel | 180 | 25 | 2.5 | 1.5 | 5 | 510 | 34 | 1 | 4 |
| Pepperoni Pretzel | 1 pretzel | 480 | 150 | 16 | 8 | 40 | 860 | 65 | 2 | 15 |
| Pepperoni Pretzel Pocket | 1 item | 650 | 240 | 27 | 12 | 65 | 1120 | 75 | 2 | 11 |
| Pretzel Stix | 6 stixs | 340 | 45 | 5 | 3 | 10 | 990 | 65 | 2 | 8 |
| Turkey & Cheddar Pretzel Pocket | 1 item | 470 | 90 | 10 | 5 | 50 | 1050 | 73 | 2 | 20 |

## Back Yard Burgers
### BURGERS

| | SERVING SIZE | CAL | CAL FAT | TOT FAT (G) | SAT FAT (G) | CHOL (MG) | SOD (MG) | CARB (G) | FIBER (G) | PROT (G) |
|---|---|---|---|---|---|---|---|---|---|---|
| American Cheeseburger 1/3 lb | 1 burger | 730 | 390 | 44 | 16 | 115 | 1300 | 47 | 3 | 39 |
| Bleu Cheeseburger 1/3 lb | 1 burger | 780 | 420 | 47 | 19 | 125 | 1430 | 47 | 3 | 42 |
| Burger 1/3 lb | 1 burger | 680 | 350 | 39 | 14 | 105 | 1040 | 47 | 3 | 36 |
| Pepper Jack Cheeseburger 1/3 lb | 1 burger | 740 | 400 | 45 | 17 | 120 | 1370 | 47 | 3 | 39 |
| Swiss Cheeseburger 1/3 lb | 1 burger | 790 | 430 | 48 | 19 | 135 | 1170 | 47 | 3 | 44 |

### CHICKEN SANDWICHES

| | SERVING SIZE | CAL | CAL FAT | TOT FAT (G) | SAT FAT (G) | CHOL (MG) | SOD (MG) | CARB (G) | FIBER (G) | PROT (G) |
|---|---|---|---|---|---|---|---|---|---|---|
| Blackened | 1 sandwich | 540 | 210 | 24 | 4 | 60 | 1810 | 53 | 4 | 32 |
| Crispy | 1 sandwich | 590 | 220 | 26 | 5 | 35 | 1360 | 65 | 4 | 25 |
| Grilled | 1 sandwich | 350 | 40 | 4.5 | .5 | 55 | 1280 | 47 | 3 | 31 |

### SIDES

| | SERVING SIZE | CAL | CAL FAT | TOT FAT (G) | SAT FAT (G) | CHOL (MG) | SOD (MG) | CARB (G) | FIBER (G) | PROT (G) |
|---|---|---|---|---|---|---|---|---|---|---|
| Chili | as served | 150 | 80 | 9 | 3 | 25 | 690 | 8 | 1 | 8 |
| Seasoned Fries, Regular | as served | 640 | 400 | 45 | 7 | 0 | 1160 | 58 | 6 | 6 |

## Baja Fresh
### BURRITOS

| | SERVING SIZE | CAL | CAL FAT | TOT FAT (G) | SAT FAT (G) | CHOL (MG) | SOD (MG) | CARB (G) | FIBER (G) | PROT (G) |
|---|---|---|---|---|---|---|---|---|---|---|
| Baja Burrito, Chicken | 1 burrito | 790 | 340 | 38 | 15 | 120 | 2140 | 65 | 8 | 52 |
| Baja Burrito, Shrimp | 1 burrito | 760 | 330 | 37 | 15 | 295 | 2230 | 66 | 7 | 47 |
| Bare Burrito Bowl Chicken | 1 burrito | 640 | 60 | 7 | 1 | 75 | 2330 | 97 | 20 | 45 |
| Bare Burrito Bowl Veggie & Cheese | 1 burrito | 580 | 90 | 10 | 4 | 15 | 1950 | 101 | 20 | 19 |
| Bean & Cheese Burrito, Chicken | 1 burrito | 970 | 310 | 35 | 18 | 135 | 2230 | 96 | 21 | 67 |
| Bean & Cheese Burrito, No Meat | 1 burrito | 840 | 290 | 33 | 17 | 65 | 1790 | 96 | 20 | 39 |
| Bean & Cheese Burrito, Shrimp | 1 burrito | 950 | 310 | 34 | 17 | 310 | 2320 | 96 | 20 | 61 |
| Burrito Mexicano, Chicken | 1 burrito | 790 | 120 | 13 | 3.5 | 75 | 2270 | 117 | 20 | 50 |
| Burrito Mexicano, Shrimp | 1 burrito | 770 | 110 | 13 | 3.5 | 245 | 2370 | 117 | 18 | 44 |
| Burrito Mexicano, Steak | 1 burrito | 860 | 190 | 21 | 7 | 75 | 2400 | 118 | 18 | 47 |

| | SERVING SIZE | CAL | CAL FAT | TOT FAT (G) | SAT FAT (G) | CHOL (MG) | SOD (MG) | CARB (G) | FIBER (G) | PROT (G) |
|---|---|---|---|---|---|---|---|---|---|---|
| Burrito Ultimo, Chicken | 1 burrito | 880 | 330 | 36 | 18 | 140 | 2190 | 84 | 9 | 54 |
| Diablo Shrimp Burrito | 1 burrito | 1000 | 300 | 34 | 12 | 275 | 2930 | 130 | 19 | 56 |
| Fajita Steak w/Flour Tortillas | 1 burrito | 1240 | 400 | 45 | 15 | 135 | 3440 | 149 | 25 | 65 |
| Grilled Veggie Burrito | 1 burrito | 800 | 300 | 33 | 17 | 65 | 1880 | 94 | 16 | 32 |
| **Fajitas (average of all)** | 1 entrée | 1119 | 312 | 35 | 11 | 162 | 2947 | 142 | 25 | 61 |
| **Nachos (average of all)** | as served | 2033 | 1013 | 113 | 42 | 211 | 2871 | 164 | 31 | 84 |
| **Quesadillas (average of all)** | 1 item | 1306 | 718 | 80 | 38 | 225 | 2461 | 86 | 9 | 64 |
| **SIDES** | | | | | | | | | | |
| Black Beans Side | as served | 360 | 20 | 2.5 | 1 | 5 | 1120 | 61 | 26 | 23 |
| Chips & Guacamole | as served | 1340 | 720 | 83 | 8 | 0 | 950 | 141 | 20 | 21 |
| Chips & Salsa Baja | as served | 810 | 330 | 37 | 4 | 0 | 1140 | 98 | 14 | 13 |
| **SOUPS & SALADS** | | | | | | | | | | |
| Baja Ensalada, Charbroiled Chicken | 1 salad | 310 | 60 | 7 | 2 | 110 | 1210 | 18 | 7 | 46 |
| Baja Ensalada, Charbroiled Shrimp | 1 salad | 230 | 50 | 6 | 2 | 250 | 1110 | 18 | 6 | 28 |
| Chicken Tortilla w/Charbroiled Chicken | as served | 320 | 130 | 14 | 4 | 40 | 2760 | 29 | 4 | 17 |
| Mango Chipotle Chicken Salad | 1 salad | 930 | 460 | 2.5 | 9 | 90 | 1960 | 67 | 10 | 42 |
| Tostada Salad, Charbroiled Chicken | 1 salad | 1140 | 490 | 55 | 14 | 115 | 2370 | 98 | 27 | 60 |
| Tostada Salad, Charbroiled Shrimp | 1 salad | 1120 | 490 | 55 | 14 | 285 | 2460 | 99 | 25 | 55 |
| Tostada Salad, No Meat | 1 salad | 1010 | 470 | 53 | 13 | 40 | 1930 | 98 | 25 | 32 |
| **Tacos (average of all)** | 1 taco | 230 | 81 | 9 | 3 | 44 | 420 | 25 | 2 | 13 |
| **Baskin Robbins** | | | | | | | | | | |
| **31° BELOW BLENDS** | | | | | | | | | | |
| Chocolate OREO | 16 oz | 1290 | 490 | 55 | 29 | 85 | 1080 | 187 | 3 | 22 |
| HEATH | 16 oz | 1160 | 490 | 54 | 31 | 115 | 860 | 151 | 1 | 21 |
| Reese's Peanut Butter Cup | 16 oz | 1220 | 600 | 67 | 28 | 90 | 870 | 134 | 5 | 33 |
| Strawberry Soft Serve Sundae | 10 oz | 450 | 160 | 18 | 11 | 65 | 310 | 59 | 1 | 12 |
| **BRIGHT CHOICES** | | | | | | | | | | |
| Butter Almond Crunch Ice Cream, Reduced Fat, No Sugar Added | 2-1/2 oz | 140 | 60 | 7 | 3 | 15 | 90 | 19 | 3 | 4 |
| Frozen Yogurt, Fat Free Vanilla | 2-1/2 oz | 90 | 0 | 0 | 0 | 0 | 65 | 20 | 0 | 4 |
| Lemon Cream Pie Ice Cream, Reduced Fat No Sugar Added | 2-1/2 oz | 130 | 45 | 5 | 2.5 | 20 | 70 | 23 | 2 | 3 |
| Light Mint OREO Ice Cream | 2-1/2 oz | 150 | 40 | 4.5 | 2.5 | 15 | 90 | 25 | 1 | 3 |
| Light Raspberry Chip Ice Cream | 2-1/2 oz | 140 | 35 | 4 | 2.5 | 15 | 60 | 24 | 1 | 3 |
| Sorbet, Pink Grapefruit | 2-1/2 oz | 80 | 0 | 0 | 0 | 0 | 10 | 21 | 0 | 0 |
| **CAPPUCCINO BLASTS** | | | | | | | | | | |
| Caramel | 16 oz | 510 | 140 | 16 | 10 | 60 | 310 | 87 | 0 | 7 |

# restaurants

| | SERVING SIZE | CAL | CAL FAT | TOT FAT (G) | SAT FAT (G) | CHOL (MG) | SOD (MG) | CARB (G) | FIBER (G) | PROT (G) |
|---|---|---|---|---|---|---|---|---|---|---|
| Mocha w/whipped Cream | 16 oz | 400 | 120 | 13 | 8 | 50 | 95 | 65 | 0 | 6 |
| Original | 16 oz | 310 | 110 | 12 | 7 | 45 | 100 | 47 | 0 | 6 |
| **FLOATS, FREEZES, & SHAKES** | | | | | | | | | | |
| Chocolate Shake | 16 oz | 660 | 290 | 32 | 20 | 115 | 230 | 78 | 1 | 14 |
| Freeze (with Orange Sherbet) | 16 oz | 370 | 35 | 4 | 2.5 | 15 | 120 | 82 | 0 | 3 |
| Vanilla Ice Cream & Root Beer Float | 16 fl oz | 470 | 180 | 20 | 13 | 80 | 130 | 69 | 0 | 6 |
| Vanilla Shake | 16 oz | 680 | 300 | 33 | 21 | 130 | 370 | 84 | 0 | 13 |
| Very Berry Strawberry Shake | 16 oz | 560 | 210 | 23 | 15 | 90 | 210 | 76 | 1 | 12 |
| **Fruit Creams (average of all)** | 16 oz | 633 | 163 | 18 | 11 | 67 | 333 | 107 | 1 | 14 |
| **HAND SCOOPED ICE CREAM** | | | | | | | | | | |
| Chocolate Chip Cookie Dough | 2-1/2 oz | 190 | 80 | 9 | 6 | 30 | 85 | 23 | 0 | 3 |
| Chocolate Fudge | 2-1/2 oz | 170 | 90 | 10 | 6 | 30 | 90 | 22 | 0 | 3 |
| Fudge Brownie | 2-1/2 oz | 190 | 100 | 11 | 7 | 30 | 90 | 22 | 1 | 3 |
| Mississippi Mud | 2-1/2 oz | 170 | 70 | 8 | 5 | 30 | 95 | 24 | 0 | 3 |
| New York Cheesecake | 2-1/2 oz | 170 | 90 | 10 | 6 | 30 | 75 | 19 | 0 | 3 |
| Old Fashioned Butter Pecan | 2-1/2 oz | 170 | 100 | 11 | 6 | 35 | 60 | 15 | 1 | 3 |
| Reese's Peanut Butter Cup | 2-1/2 oz | 190 | 100 | 11 | 6 | 30 | 80 | 19 | 0 | 4 |
| Rocky Road | 2-1/2 oz | 180 | 90 | 10 | 5 | 30 | 75 | 22 | 0 | 3 |
| Strawberry Shortcake | 2-1/2 oz | 170 | 80 | 9 | 6 | 30 | 100 | 22 | 0 | 3 |
| Vanilla | 2-1/2 oz | 170 | 90 | 10 | 6 | 40 | 45 | 17 | 0 | 3 |
| **Sherbet & Ice (average of all)** | 2-1/2 oz | 98 | 8 | 1 | .6 | 3 | 17 | 21.8 | 0 | 4 |
| **Soft Serve Ice Cream (average of all)** | 6 oz | 287 | 100 | 11 | 7 | 40 | 200 | 38 | 0 | 8 |
| **SUNDAES** | | | | | | | | | | |
| Classic Brownie | 1 sundae | 920 | 430 | 47 | 22 | 150 | 460 | 119 | 2 | 12 |
| Classic Banana Split | 1 sundae | 1010 | 310 | 34 | 20 | 115 | 240 | 173 | 8 | 12 |
| Premium Chocolate Chip Cookie Dough | 1 sundae | 990 | 380 | 43 | 28 | 105 | 540 | 138 | 2 | 13 |
| **Ben & Jerry's** | | | | | | | | | | |
| BerryBerry Extraordinary Sorbet | 1/2 cup | 100 | 0 | 0 | 0 | 0 | 5 | 27 | 1 | 0 |
| Cake Batter Ice Cream | 1/2 cup | 260 | 140 | 16 | 10 | 65 | 75 | 27 | <1 | 4 |
| Cherry Garcia Ice Cream | 1/2 cup | 240 | 120 | 13 | 9 | 60 | 35 | 28 | <1 | 4 |
| Chocolate Chip Cookie Dough Ice Cream | 1/2 cup | 270 | 130 | 14 | 8 | 65 | 60 | 33 | 0 | 4 |
| Chocolate Peanut Butter Swirl Ice Cream | 1/2 cup | 250 | 100 | 17 | 7 | 25 | 100 | 22 | 2 | 6 |
| Chunky Monkey Ice Cream | 1/2 cup | 290 | 160 | 18 | 10 | 65 | 35 | 29 | 1 | 4 |
| Coffee Coffee BuzzBuzzBuzz Ice Cream | 1/2 cup | 230 | 100 | 14 | 10 | 50 | 40 | 23 | 1 | 4 |
| Low Fat Frozen Yogurt Half Baked | 1/2 cup | 180 | 25 | 3 | 1.5 | 20 | 95 | 35 | 1 | 4 |
| Low Fat Frozen Yogurt Vanilla | 1/2 cup | 130 | 15 | 2 | 1 | 20 | 70 | 25 | 0 | 4 |

| | SERVING SIZE | CAL | CAL FAT | TOT FAT (G) | SAT FAT (G) | CHOL (MG) | SOD (MG) | CARB (G) | FIBER (G) | PROT (G) |
|---|---|---|---|---|---|---|---|---|---|---|
| Phish Food Ice Cream | 1/2 cup | 280 | 120 | 13 | 8 | 35 | 80 | 39 | 2 | 4 |
| Vanilla Heath Bar Crunch Ice Cream | 1/2 cup | 280 | 150 | 17 | 10 | 65 | 95 | 30 | 0 | 4 |

## Biggby Coffee
### DESSERTS

| | SERVING SIZE | CAL | CAL FAT | TOT FAT (G) | SAT FAT (G) | CHOL (MG) | SOD (MG) | CARB (G) | FIBER (G) | PROT (G) |
|---|---|---|---|---|---|---|---|---|---|---|
| Blueberry Muffin | 1 muffin | 530 | 250 | 28 | 5 | 110 | 500 | 63 | 0 | 6 |
| Blueberry Scone | 1 scone | 470 | 190 | 21 | 12 | 105 | 350 | 49 | 2 | 6 |
| Brownie | 1 brownie | 330 | 160 | 18 | 9 | 60 | 120 | 39 | 2 | 4 |
| Chocolate Chip Cookie | 1 cookie | 470 | 200 | 22 | 13 | 75 | 320 | 63 | 3 | 6 |
| Chocolate Chip Muffin | 1 muffin | 610 | 290 | 33 | 8 | 110 | 500 | 73 | 2 | 7 |

### REDUCED CALORIE
### DRINKS

| | SERVING SIZE | CAL | CAL FAT | TOT FAT (G) | SAT FAT (G) | CHOL (MG) | SOD (MG) | CARB (G) | FIBER (G) | PROT (G) |
|---|---|---|---|---|---|---|---|---|---|---|
| Banana Berry Freeze | 16 fl oz | 275 | 20 | 3 | 0 | 0 | 33 | 66 | 3 | 2 |
| Banana Freeze | 16 fl oz | 264 | 20 | 3 | 0 | 0 | 32 | 63 | 3 | 2 |
| Cocoa Carmella | 16 fl oz | 196 | 5 | 1 | 0 | 8 | 173 | 36 | 1 | 7 |
| Dark Hot Chocolate | 16 fl oz | 269 | 105 | 11 | 6 | 41 | 120 | 35 | 2 | 7 |
| Double Chocolate Freeze | 16 fl oz | 241 | 31 | 3 | 0 | 0 | 204 | 48 | 2 | 5 |
| Double Dark Hot Chocolate | 16 fl oz | 307 | 0 | 0 | 0 | 7 | 324 | 46 | 3 | 14 |
| Iced Chai Latte | 16 fl oz | 188 | 0 | 0 | 0 | 7 | 144 | 34 | 0 | 12 |
| Iced Hazelnut Mocha | 16 fl oz | 159 | 0 | 0 | 0 | 5 | 228 | 28 | 1 | 11 |
| Iced Latte | 16 fl oz | 100 | 0 | 0 | 0 | 6 | 138 | 14 | 0 | 11 |
| Iced Mocha Mocha | 16 fl oz | 175 | 0 | 0 | 0 | 5 | 249 | 30 | 2 | 11 |
| Iced Vanilla Bean | 16 fl oz | 93 | 0 | 0 | 0 | 6 | 127 | 16 | 0 | 10 |
| Latte | 16 fl oz | 112 | 0 | 0 | 0 | 7 | 103 | 10 | 0 | 13 |

### REGULAR DRINKS

| | SERVING SIZE | CAL | CAL FAT | TOT FAT (G) | SAT FAT (G) | CHOL (MG) | SOD (MG) | CARB (G) | FIBER (G) | PROT (G) |
|---|---|---|---|---|---|---|---|---|---|---|
| Caramel Marvel | 16 fl oz | 378 | 132 | 15 | 8 | 55 | 332 | 52 | 0 | 11 |
| Caramel Steamer | 16 fl oz | 283 | 109 | 12 | 6 | 44 | 225 | 36 | 0 | 7 |
| Chai Freeze | 16 fl oz | 430 | 57 | 6 | 1 | 9 | 95 | 86 | 0 | 5 |
| Chai Latte | 16 fl oz | 346 | 68 | 8 | 5 | 23 | 103 | 53 | 0 | 14 |
| Double Chocolate Freeze | 16 fl oz | 529 | 166 | 17 | 8 | 42 | 139 | 90 | 3 | 5 |
| Frozen Caramel Marvel | 16 fl oz | 453 | 150 | 16 | 7 | 36 | 188 | 76 | 0 | 2 |
| Frozen Hazelnut Mocha | 16 fl oz | 440 | 144 | 15 | 7 | 33 | 76 | 75 | 2 | 2 |
| Frozen Hot Chocolate | 16 fl oz | 529 | 166 | 17 | 8 | 42 | 139 | 90 | 3 | 5 |
| Frozen Latte | 16 fl oz | 330 | 60 | 6 | 0 | 0 | 81 | 69 | 0 | 3 |
| Frozen Mocha Mocha | 16 fl oz | 439 | 146 | 15 | 7 | 33 | 83 | 75 | 2 | 2 |
| Frozen White Lightning | 16 fl oz | 459 | 147 | 15 | 7 | 33 | 146 | 77 | 0 | 2 |
| Frozen Wild Zebra | 16 fl oz | 449 | 146 | 15 | 7 | 33 | 115 | 76 | 1 | 2 |
| Iced Chai Latte | 16 fl oz | 323 | 59 | 7 | 4 | 33 | 144 | 50 | 0 | 12 |

# restaurants

| | SERVING SIZE | CAL | CAL FAT | TOT FAT (G) | SAT FAT (G) | CHOL (MG) | SOD (MG) | CARB (G) | FIBER (G) | PROT (G) |
|---|---|---|---|---|---|---|---|---|---|---|
| Iced Hazelnut Mocha | 16 fl oz | 401 | 155 | 16 | 10 | 59 | 151 | 54 | 3 | 9 |
| Iced Vanilla Bean | 16 fl oz | 214 | 52 | 6 | 3 | 29 | 127 | 31 | 0 | 10 |
| Mint Mocha | 16 fl oz | 368 | 123 | 13 | 8 | 50 | 166 | 53 | 3 | 11 |
| Mocha Mocha | 16 fl oz | 357 | 126 | 13 | 8 | 50 | 175 | 50 | 3 | 11 |
| Nutty Buddy | 16 fl oz | 234 | 62 | 7 | 4 | 34 | 151 | 32 | 0 | 12 |
| Orange Freeze | 16 fl oz | 352 | 40 | 4 | 0 | 0 | 58 | 78 | 0 | 2 |
| Tea Latte | 16 fl oz | 265 | 71 | 8 | 5 | 40 | 174 | 36 | 0 | 14 |
| Teddy Bear | 16 fl oz | 382 | 129 | 14 | 8 | 52 | 301 | 52 | 0 | 11 |
| Vanilla Bean | 16 fl oz | 240 | 62 | 7 | 4 | 34 | 151 | 34 | 0 | 12 |
| Vanilla Freeze | 16 fl oz | 415 | 40 | 4 | 0 | 2 | 95 | 88 | 0 | 5 |
| White Hot Chocolate | 16 fl oz | 412 | 137 | 15 | 8 | 55 | 292 | 55 | 0 | 13 |
| White Lightning | 16 fl oz | 387 | 127 | 13 | 8 | 50 | 269 | 53 | 0 | 11 |
| Wild Zebra | 16 fl oz | 372 | 126 | 13 | 8 | 50 | 222 | 52 | 2 | 11 |

## Blimpie
### 6" SUB SANDWICHES

| | SERVING SIZE | CAL | CAL FAT | TOT FAT (G) | SAT FAT (G) | CHOL (MG) | SOD (MG) | CARB (G) | FIBER (G) | PROT (G) |
|---|---|---|---|---|---|---|---|---|---|---|
| Blimpie Best | 1 sandwich | 450 | 150 | 17 | 6 | 50 | 1330 | 49 | 3 | 24 |
| BLT | 1 sandwich | 430 | 200 | 22 | 5 | 25 | 960 | 43 | 2 | 15 |
| Club | 1 sandwich | 410 | 120 | 13 | 4 | 45 | 1050 | 49 | 3 | 23 |
| Hot Pastrami | 1 sandwich | 430 | 140 | 16 | 7 | 65 | 1350 | 42 | 1 | 30 |
| Meatball | 1 sandwich | 580 | 280 | 31 | 13 | 75 | 1960 | 50 | 4 | 27 |
| Reuben | 1 sandwich | 530 | 180 | 20 | 6 | 70 | 1740 | 52 | 3 | 34 |
| Roast Beef & Provolone | 1 sandwich | 430 | 130 | 14 | 5 | 55 | 980 | 46 | 3 | 28 |
| Tuna | 1 sandwich | 470 | 190 | 21 | 3 | 55 | 770 | 43 | 2 | 24 |
| Turkey & Provolone | 1 sandwich | 410 | 120 | 13 | 4 | 40 | 1310 | 49 | 3 | 24 |
| Veggie & Cheese | 1 sandwich | 460 | 190 | 21 | 9 | 40 | 1420 | 50 | 3 | 19 |

### SOUPS & SALADS

| | SERVING SIZE | CAL | CAL FAT | TOT FAT (G) | SAT FAT (G) | CHOL (MG) | SOD (MG) | CARB (G) | FIBER (G) | PROT (G) |
|---|---|---|---|---|---|---|---|---|---|---|
| Chicken Caesar | 1 salad | 190 | 70 | 8 | 4 | 65 | 460 | 6 | 3 | 25 |
| Chicken Noodle | 8-3/5 oz | 130 | 30 | 4 | 1 | 30 | 1040 | 18 | 2 | 7 |
| Garden Vegetable | 8-3/5 oz | 80 | 5 | 1 | 0 | 0 | 620 | 14 | 3 | 5 |
| Italian Style Wedding | 8-3/5 oz | 130 | 30 | 4 | 1.5 | 10 | 900 | 17 | 0 | 7 |
| Minestrone | 8-3/5 oz | 90 | 25 | 3 | 0 | 0 | 1150 | 14 | 4 | 4 |
| Tuna | 1 salad | 270 | 170 | 19 | 2.5 | 55 | 370 | 6 | 3 | 18 |

## Bob Evans
### BREAKFAST

| | SERVING SIZE | CAL | CAL FAT | TOT FAT (G) | SAT FAT (G) | CHOL (MG) | SOD (MG) | CARB (G) | FIBER (G) | PROT (G) |
|---|---|---|---|---|---|---|---|---|---|---|
| Border Scramble Omelet | 1 omelet | 635 | 414 | 46 | 18 | 769 | 1519 | 14 | 2 | 39 |
| Country Biscuit Breakfast | 1 omelet | 594 | 351 | 39 | 18 | 262 | 1524 | 41 | 1 | 21 |
| Farmer's Market Omelet | 1 omelet | 631 | 405 | 45 | 21 | 772 | 2129 | 14 | 1 | 37 |

| | SERVING SIZE | CAL | CAL FAT | TOT FAT (G) | SAT FAT (G) | CHOL (MG) | SOD (MG) | CARB (G) | FIBER (G) | PROT (G) |
|---|---|---|---|---|---|---|---|---|---|---|
| Garden Harvest Omelet | 1 omelet | 542 | 342 | 38 | 17 | 752 | 1762 | 14 | 2 | 30 |
| Ham & Cheddar Omelet | 1 omelet | 515 | 324 | 36 | 13 | 765 | 1808 | 4 | 0 | 40 |
| Meat Lovers BoBurrito | 1 burrito | 805 | 468 | 52 | 19 | 561 | 1883 | 40 | 3 | 44 |
| Plenty-o-Pancakes | 1 entrée | 712 | 162 | 18 | 11 | 0 | 1280 | 130 | 0 | 8 |
| Pot Roast Hash | 14 oz | 749 | 441 | 49 | 16 | 552 | 1307 | 32 | 3 | 43 |
| Sausage & Cheddar Omelet | 1 omelet | 552 | 387 | 43 | 16 | 752 | 1253 | 4 | 0 | 35 |
| Sausage Biscuit Bowl | 1 bowl | 998 | 549 | 61 | 28 | 501 | 3166 | 76 | 4 | 32 |
| Sunshine Skillet | 1 entrée | 565 | 315 | 35 | 13 | 501 | 1763 | 34 | 3 | 26 |
| Sweet Cream Waffle-No Topping | 1 entrée | 378 | 90 | 10 | 5 | 117 | 795 | 61 | 2 | 9 |
| Turkey Sausage Breakfast | 1 entrée | 362 | 63 | 7 | 2 | 31 | 1009 | 48 | 5 | 27 |
| Western Omelet | 1 omelet | 529 | 324 | 36 | 13 | 765 | 1809 | 8 | 1 | 41 |
| **BURGERS & SANDWICHES** | | | | | | | | | | |
| Biscuit Sandwich | 1 sandwich | 584 | 351 | 39 | 17 | 268 | 1475 | 33 | 1 | 22 |
| Big Farm Burger | 1 burger | 745 | 270 | 30 | 11 | 94 | 967 | 49 | 3 | 24 |
| Big Farm Cheeseburger | 1 burger | 850 | 342 | 38 | 17 | 124 | 1437 | 50 | 3 | 30 |
| Pot Roast Sandwich | 1 sandwich | 644 | 288 | 32 | 12 | 103 | 1342 | 52 | 2 | 35 |
| Turkey Bacon Melt | 1 sandwich | 569 | 243 | 27 | 11 | 86 | 1952 | 49 | 2 | 30 |
| Turkey Club Wrap | 1 wrap | 695 | 306 | 34 | 13 | 93 | 2246 | 58 | 5 | 37 |
| **ENTRÉES** | | | | | | | | | | |
| Chicken & Broccoli Alfredo | 1 entrée | 871 | 414 | 46 | 17 | 162 | 2183 | 62 | 6 | 53 |
| Chicken Parmesan w/Meat Sauce | 1 entrée | 1134 | 495 | 55 | 19 | 156 | 2739 | 94 | 6 | 64 |
| Chick-N-Noodles Deep Dish Dinner | 1 entrée | 699 | 261 | 29 | 15 | 113 | 2233 | 66 | 3 | 30 |
| Country Fried Steak | 1 entrée | 496 | 297 | 33 | 11 | 51 | 1217 | 31 | 0 | 18 |
| Fried Chicken Strips | 1 strip | 137 | 72 | 8 | 1 | 8 | 301 | 10 | 0 | 7 |
| Garlic Butter Grilled Chicken | 1 entrée | 180 | 54 | 6 | 2 | 89 | 738 | 1 | 0 | 31 |
| Grilled Chicken Breast | 1 entrée | 165 | 45 | 5 | 2 | 85 | 635 | 0 | 0 | 29 |
| Meatloaf | 1 entrée | 330 | 144 | 16 | 6 | 113 | 1144 | 15 | 1 | 13 |
| Pot Roast Stroganoff | 1 entrée | 813 | 387 | 43 | 15 | 178 | 1782 | 65 | 2 | 42 |
| Salmon | 1 entrée | 243 | 72 | 8 | 2 | 101 | 101 | 0 | 0 | 40 |
| Sirloin Steak | 1 entrée | 421 | 261 | 29 | 9 | 77 | 638 | 3 | 0 | 33 |
| Spaghetti w/Meat Sauce | 1 entrée | 778 | 324 | 36 | 12 | 12 | 2002 | 81 | 5 | 32 |
| Turkey & Dressing | 1 entrée | 688 | 297 | 33 | 10 | 115 | 3096 | 54 | 3 | 42 |
| Wildfire Grilled Chicken Breast | 1 entrée | 236 | 54 | 6 | 2 | 89 | 766 | 15 | 1 | 54 |
| **SALADS** | | | | | | | | | | |
| Cobb | 1 salad | 517 | 279 | 31 | 17 | 318 | 1673 | 10 | 3 | 51 |
| Country Spinach | 1 salad | 428 | 225 | 25 | 8 | 273 | 1297 | 12 | 5 | 44 |
| Cranberry Pecan Chicken | 1 salad | 639 | 324 | 36 | 13 | 129 | 1511 | 33 | 5 | 46 |

# restaurants

| | SERVING SIZE | CAL | CAL FAT | TOT FAT (G) | SAT FAT (G) | CHOL (MG) | SOD (MG) | CARB (G) | FIBER (G) | PROT (G) |
|---|---|---|---|---|---|---|---|---|---|---|
| Heritage Chef | 1 salad | 398 | 225 | 25 | 12 | 260 | 1324 | 11 | 3 | 34 |
| Specialty Garden | 1 salad | 124 | 63 | 7 | 3 | 16 | 334 | 10 | 1 | 6 |
| Wildfire Fried Chicken | 1 salad | 711 | 306 | 34 | 9 | 46 | 1332 | 70 | 7 | 32 |
| Wildfire Grilled Chicken | 1 salad | 389 | 117 | 13 | 5 | 85 | 963 | 37 | 6 | 32 |

## Bojangles
### CAJUN SPICED CHICKEN

| | SERVING SIZE | CAL | CAL FAT | TOT FAT (G) | SAT FAT (G) | CHOL (MG) | SOD (MG) | CARB (G) | FIBER (G) | PROT (G) |
|---|---|---|---|---|---|---|---|---|---|---|
| Breast | 1 breast | 278 | 153 | 17 | n/a | 75 | 565 | 12 | 1 | 33 |
| Leg | 1 leg | 122 | 144 | 16 | n/a | 96 | 530 | 11 | 1 | 10 |
| Thigh | 1 thigh | 310 | 207 | 23 | n/a | 67 | 465 | 11 | 1 | 16 |
| Wing | 1 wing | 160 | 225 | 25 | n/a | 94 | 630 | 11 | 1 | 9 |

### INDIVIDUAL FIXIN'S

| | SERVING SIZE | CAL | CAL FAT | TOT FAT (G) | SAT FAT (G) | CHOL (MG) | SOD (MG) | CARB (G) | FIBER (G) | PROT (G) |
|---|---|---|---|---|---|---|---|---|---|---|
| Macaroni & Cheese | as served | 198 | 126 | 14 | 5 | 26 | 418 | 12 | 1 | 7 |
| Potatoes w/o Gravy | as served | 80 | 9 | 1 | 0 | 0 | 380 | 16 | 1 | 2 |
| Seasoned Fries | as served | 344 | 171 | 19 | 5 | 13 | 480 | 39 | 4 | 5 |

### SANDWICHES

| | SERVING SIZE | CAL | CAL FAT | TOT FAT (G) | SAT FAT (G) | CHOL (MG) | SOD (MG) | CARB (G) | FIBER (G) | PROT (G) |
|---|---|---|---|---|---|---|---|---|---|---|
| Bacon, Egg, & Cheese Biscuit | 1 sandwich | 550 | 378 | 42 | 14 | 160 | 1250 | 27 | 1 | 17 |
| Cajun Filet Biscuit | 1 sandwich | 454 | 189 | 21 | 6 | 41 | 949 | 46 | 1 | 20 |
| Egg Biscuit | 1 sandwich | 400 | 270 | 30 | 6 | 120 | 630 | 26 | 1 | 8 |
| Plain Biscuit | 1 sandwich | 243 | 108 | 12 | 3 | 2 | 663 | 29 | 2 | 4 |
| Sausage Biscuit | 1 sandwich | 350 | 207 | 23 | 7 | 20 | 810 | 26 | 1 | 9 |
| Steak Biscuit | 1 sandwich | 649 | 441 | 49 | 13 | 34 | 1126 | 37 | 1 | 14 |

## Boston Market
### INDIVIDUAL PLATES

| | SERVING SIZE | CAL | CAL FAT | TOT FAT (G) | SAT FAT (G) | CHOL (MG) | SOD (MG) | CARB (G) | FIBER (G) | PROT (G) |
|---|---|---|---|---|---|---|---|---|---|---|
| 1 Thigh & 1 Drumstick | 5 oz | 290 | 150 | 17 | 5 | 210 | 950 | 0 | 0 | 37 |
| 1 Thigh & 2 Drumsticks | 6 oz | 290 | 100 | 11 | 3.5 | 240 | 1010 | 0 | 0 | 45 |
| 2 Thighs & 1 Drumstick | 9 oz | 490 | 260 | 29 | 8 | 335 | 1600 | 0 | 0 | 60 |
| BBQ Chicken Slider | 3-1/2 oz | 240 | 60 | 6 | 2 | 30 | 720 | 36 | 0 | 11 |
| Beef Brisket | 7 oz | 400 | 210 | 23 | 6 | 165 | 990 | 1 | 0 | 48 |
| Meatloaf, Regular | 7-1/2 oz | 480 | 270 | 30 | 13 | 145 | 1090 | 25 | 6 | 28 |
| Pastry Top Chicken Pot Pie | 15 oz | 810 | 430 | 48 | 24 | 140 | 1280 | 60 | 4 | 33 |
| Quarter White Rotisserie Chicken | 6-1/2 oz | 320 | 110 | 12 | 4 | 200 | 900 | 0 | 0 | 52 |
| Quarter White Rotisserie Chicken, no skin | 7 oz | 240 | 35 | 4 | 1 | 180 | 890 | 1 | 0 | 50 |
| Roasted Turkey Breast | 5 oz | 180 | 30 | 3 | 1 | 70 | 620 | 0 | 0 | 38 |
| Turkey Slider | 3 oz | 280 | 140 | 15 | 3.5 | 30 | 510 | 24 | 0 | 14 |
| USDA Choice All Beef Meatloaf | 7-1/2 oz | 480 | 270 | 30 | 13 | 145 | 1090 | 25 | 6 | 28 |

### SIDES

| | SERVING SIZE | CAL | CAL FAT | TOT FAT (G) | SAT FAT (G) | CHOL (MG) | SOD (MG) | CARB (G) | FIBER (G) | PROT (G) |
|---|---|---|---|---|---|---|---|---|---|---|
| Creamed Spinach | 7 oz | 280 | 210 | 23 | 15 | 70 | 580 | 12 | 4 | 9 |

| | SERVING SIZE | CAL | CAL FAT | TOT FAT (G) | SAT FAT (G) | CHOL (MG) | SOD (MG) | CARB (G) | FIBER (G) | PROT (G) |
|---|---|---|---|---|---|---|---|---|---|---|
| Green Beans | 3 oz | 60 | 35 | 3.5 | 1.5 | 0 | 180 | 7 | 3 | 2 |
| Macaroni & Cheese | 7-4/5 oz | 300 | 100 | 11 | 7 | 30 | 1100 | 35 | 2 | 11 |
| Mashed Potatoes | 7-4/5 oz | 270 | 100 | 11 | 5 | 25 | 820 | 36 | 4 | 6 |
| Sweet Corn | 6-1/5 oz | 170 | 35 | 4 | 1 | 0 | 95 | 37 | 2 | 6 |
| **SOUPS & SALADS** | | | | | | | | | | |
| Asian Salad | 1 salad | 570 | 270 | 31 | 5 | 100 | 1280 | 33 | 5 | 40 |
| Broccoli Cheddar Soup | 15 oz | 480 | 300 | 33 | 21 | 95 | 1490 | 25 | 4 | 22 |
| Caesar w/o Chicken Salad | 1 salad | 500 | 350 | 39 | 9 | 30 | 1190 | 25 | 3 | 14 |
| Chicken Tortilla Soup w/o Toppings | 12-4/5 oz | 160 | 70 | 8 | 1.5 | 45 | 1690 | 13 | 2 | 10 |
| Mediterranean Salad | 1 salad | 670 | 400 | 45 | 10 | 125 | 1380 | 27 | 11 | 40 |
| Southwest Santa Fe Salad | 1 salad | 690 | 380 | 42 | 9 | 125 | 1560 | 41 | 5 | 41 |

# Bruegger's
## BREADS

| | SERVING SIZE | CAL | CAL FAT | TOT FAT (G) | SAT FAT (G) | CHOL (MG) | SOD (MG) | CARB (G) | FIBER (G) | PROT (G) |
|---|---|---|---|---|---|---|---|---|---|---|
| Ciabatta Bread | 1 roll | 250 | 27 | 3 | 0 | 0 | 730 | 48 | 2 | 9 |
| Everything Bagel | 1 bagel | 310 | 20 | 3 | 0 | 0 | 710 | 62 | 4 | 12 |
| Fortified Multi-Grain Bagel | 1 bagel | 340 | 20 | 3 | 0 | 0 | 500 | 66 | 6 | 12 |
| Hearty White Bread | 2 slices | 260 | 9 | 1 | 0 | 0 | 620 | 54 | 2 | 10 |
| Plain Bagel | 1 bagel | 300 | 20 | 2 | 0 | 0 | 530 | 60 | 4 | 12 |
| White Wrap | 1 wrap | 180 | 18 | 2 | 1 | 0 | 420 | 32 | 3 | 6 |
| Whole Wheat Bagel | 1 bagel | 310 | 30 | 4 | 0 | 0 | 560 | 61 | 7 | 13 |
| **DELI SANDWICHES** | | | | | | | | | | |
| BLT on Hearty White | 1 sandwich | 720 | 378 | 42 | 10 | 70 | 1550 | 62 | 0 | 23 |
| Chicken Breast on Hearty White | 1 sandwich | 610 | 36 | 4 | 1.5 | 60 | 1520 | 94 | 0 | 35 |
| Garden Veggie on Wheat Bread | 1 sandwich | 360 | 27 | 3 | 0 | 0 | 540 | 67 | 4 | 13 |
| Turkey on Honey Wheat | 1 sandwich | 560 | 135 | 15 | 7 | 75 | 2060 | 60 | 2 | 41 |
| **SOUP & SALADS** | | | | | | | | | | |
| Beef Chili | 8 oz | 190 | 72 | 8 | 3 | 25 | 880 | 18 | 6 | 10 |
| Caesar, No Dressing | 1 salad | 160 | 72 | 8 | 2.5 | 15 | 220 | 14 | 2 | 7 |
| Caesar w/Chicken, Caesar Dressing | 1 salad | 380 | 180 | 20 | 6 | 85 | 1420 | 23 | 2 | 28 |
| Fire Roasted Tomato | 8 oz | 130 | 54 | 6 | 3 | <5 | 920 | 17 | 2 | 2 |
| Mandarin Medley, No Dressing | 1 salad | 220 | 72 | 8 | 4.5 | 20 | 300 | 29 | 4 | 8 |
| Sesame, No Dressing | 1 salad | 120 | 45 | 5 | 0 | 0 | 75 | 12 | 2 | 4 |

# Buffalo Wild Wings
## APPETIZERS & SIDES

| | SERVING SIZE | CAL | CAL FAT | TOT FAT (G) | SAT FAT (G) | CHOL (MG) | SOD (MG) | CARB (G) | FIBER (G) | PROT (G) |
|---|---|---|---|---|---|---|---|---|---|---|
| Buffalo Chips Regular | as served | 257 | 58 | 5 | 1 | 0 | 35 | 47 | 5 | 5 |
| Cheeseburger Slammers | as served | 1559 | 815 | 92 | 34 | 219 | 1451 | 98 | 7 | 66 |
| French Fries Basket | as served | 560 | 180 | 20 | 6 | 0 | 1320 | 84 | 8 | 8 |

# restaurants

| | SERVING SIZE | CAL | CAL FAT | TOT FAT (G) | SAT FAT (G) | CHOL (MG) | SOD (MG) | CARB (G) | FIBER (G) | PROT (G) |
|---|---|---|---|---|---|---|---|---|---|---|
| Macaroni & Cheese | as served | 380 | 117 | 13 | 5 | 25 | 1240 | 49 | 3 | 16 |
| Mini Corn Dogs | 5 pieces | 357 | 108 | 12 | 3 | 38 | 735 | 25 | 1 | 7 |
| Onion Rings Regular | as served | 460 | 220 | 26 | 5 | 0 | 960 | 52 | 4 | 4 |
| Potato Wedges Regular | as served | 280 | 117 | 14 | 4 | 0 | 1073 | 40 | 5 | 5 |
| The Sampler | as served | 1520 | 680 | 76 | 20 | 200 | 3120 | 128 | 8 | 76 |
| Ultimate Nachos | as served | 960 | 440 | 52 | 14 | 60 | 2680 | 108 | 8 | 24 |
| **ENTRÉES** | | | | | | | | | | |
| Boneless Wings | 1 wing | 88 | 55 | 6 | 2 | 21 | 178 | 3 | 0 | 5 |
| Breaded Tenders | 1 tender | 170 | 100 | 11 | 3 | 18 | 573 | 15 | 1 | 5 |
| Buffalo Chicken | as served | 908 | 476 | 49 | 17 | 149 | 2298 | 56 | 4 | 53 |
| Chicken Tenders | 3 pieces | 510 | 300 | 32 | 8 | 55 | 1720 | 44 | 4 | 14 |
| Popcorn Shrimp | 1/2 lb | 587 | 267 | 29 | 4 | 80 | 1933 | 59 | 3 | 23 |
| Ribs & More Ribs | as served | 2380 | 1420 | 158 | 58 | 410 | 5320 | 88 | 6 | 144 |
| Traditional Wings | 1 wing | 72 | 47 | 5 | 1 | 26 | 66 | 0 | 0 | 6 |
| **BURGERS, SANDWICHES, & WRAPS** | | | | | | | | | | |
| Bacon Cheddar Burger | 1 burger | 860 | 520 | 57 | 24 | 160 | 1170 | 44 | 3 | 46 |
| Buffalo Ranch Chicken Sandwich | 1 sandwich | 800 | 450 | 49 | 13 | 25 | 1460 | 60 | 3 | 32 |
| Chicken Tender Wrap | 1 wrap | 1040 | 420 | 46 | 17 | 80 | 2800 | 125 | 11 | 37 |
| Cheeseburger | 1 burger | 780 | 460 | 51 | 22 | 145 | 870 | 44 | 3 | 42 |
| Honey BBQ Bacon Chicken Sandwich | 1 sandwich | 530 | 170 | 18 | 9 | 125 | 890 | 42 | 3 | 50 |
| **SAUCES & DRESSINGS** | | | | | | | | | | |
| Blazin' | 1 oz | 60 | 50 | 5 | 0 | 10 | 1280 | 2 | 0 | 0 |
| Bleu Cheese | 1 oz | 280 | 270 | 30 | 6 | 30 | 480 | 2 | 0 | 2 |
| Honey BBQ | 1 oz | 70 | 0 | 0 | 0 | 0 | 400 | 18 | 0 | 0 |
| Honey Mustard | 1 oz | 80 | 50 | 6 | 0 | 10 | 320 | 6 | 0 | 0 |
| Hot / Medium Mild Sauce | 1 oz | 50 | 40 | 4 | 0 | 10 | 1200 | 2 | 0 | 0 |
| **Burger King** | | | | | | | | | | |
| **BK SALAD COLLECTION** | | | | | | | | | | |
| Garden Salad - No Chicken | 1 salad | 70 | 35 | 4 | 2.5 | 10 | 100 | 7 | 3 | 4 |
| Side Salad | 1 salad | 40 | 20 | 2 | 1 | 5 | 45 | 2 | 1 | 3 |
| Tendercrisp Chicken Salad | 1 salad | 410 | 200 | 23 | 6 | 65 | 1060 | 27 | 4 | 27 |
| Tendergrill Chicken Garden Salad | 1 salad | 230 | 70 | 8 | 3.5 | 85 | 930 | 9 | 3 | 34 |
| **BURGERS & SANDWICHES** | | | | | | | | | | |
| Bacon Cheeseburger | 1 sandwich | 330 | 150 | 16 | 7 | 55 | 810 | 28 | 1 | 18 |
| BK Big Fish | 1 sandwich | 640 | 280 | 31 | 5 | 45 | 1560 | 67 | 3 | 23 |
| BK Double Stacker | 1 sandwich | 560 | 320 | 36 | 15 | 110 | 1040 | 29 | 1 | 30 |

| | SERVING SIZE | CAL | CAL FAT | TOT FAT (G) | SAT FAT (G) | CHOL (MG) | SOD (MG) | CARB (G) | FIBER (G) | PROT (G) |
|---|---|---|---|---|---|---|---|---|---|---|
| BK Quad Stacker | 1 sandwich | 920 | 570 | 63 | 28 | 220 | 1730 | 31 | 1 | 58 |
| BK Triple Stacker | 1 sandwich | 740 | 450 | 50 | 22 | 165 | 1390 | 30 | 1 | 43 |
| BK Veggie Burger | 1 burger | 410 | 150 | 16 | 2.5 | 5 | 1030 | 44 | 7 | 22 |
| Buck Double | 1 sandwich | 410 | 200 | 22 | 10 | 85 | 740 | 28 | 1 | 24 |
| Cheeseburger | 1 burger | 300 | 130 | 14 | 6 | 45 | 710 | 28 | 1 | 16 |
| Double Bacon Cheeseburger | 1 burger | 510 | 270 | 30 | 14 | 105 | 1150 | 29 | 1 | 31 |
| Double Cheeseburger | 1 burger | 450 | 230 | 26 | 12 | 95 | 960 | 29 | 1 | 26 |
| Double Hamburger | 1 burger | 360 | 160 | 18 | 8 | 70 | 520 | 28 | 1 | 22 |
| Double Whopper | 1 burger | 900 | 510 | 57 | 19 | 140 | 1050 | 51 | 3 | 47 |
| Hamburger | 1 burger | 260 | 90 | 10 | 4 | 35 | 490 | 28 | 1 | 13 |
| Original Chicken | 1 sandwich | 630 | 350 | 39 | 7 | 65 | 1390 | 46 | 3 | 24 |
| Original Chicken Club | 1 sandwich | 690 | 390 | 43 | 9 | 75 | 1590 | 48 | 3 | 29 |
| Rodeo Cheeseburger | 1 sandwich | 350 | 160 | 17 | 7 | 45 | 600 | 37 | 2 | 16 |
| Spicy Chick'n Crisp | 1 sandwich | 460 | 270 | 30 | 5 | 30 | 810 | 34 | 2 | 13 |
| Tendercrisp Chicken | 1 sandwich | 800 | 410 | 46 | 8 | 70 | 1640 | 68 | 3 | 32 |
| Triple Whopper | 1 burger | 1140 | 670 | 75 | 27 | 205 | 1110 | 51 | 3 | 67 |
| Whopper | 1 burger | 670 | 360 | 40 | 11 | 75 | 980 | 51 | 3 | 29 |
| Whopper Jr. | 1 burger | 340 | 170 | 19 | 5 | 40 | 510 | 28 | 2 | 14 |
| Whopper w/Cheese | 1 burger | 760 | 430 | 47 | 16 | 100 | 1410 | 53 | 3 | 33 |
| **SIDE ORDERS** | | | | | | | | | | |
| BK Chicken Fries | 6 pieces | 250 | 130 | 15 | 3.5 | 30 | 820 | 16 | 1 | 14 |
| Chicken Tenders | 4 pieces | 180 | 100 | 11 | 2 | 30 | 310 | 13 | 0 | 9 |
| Mozzarella Sticks | 4 pieces | 280 | 140 | 15 | 5 | 35 | 650 | 24 | 2 | 11 |
| Onion Rings—Medium | as served | 400 | 190 | 21 | 3.5 | 0 | 630 | 47 | 4 | 6 |
| Salted French Fries—Medium | as served | 440 | 200 | 22 | 4.5 | 0 | 670 | 56 | 5 | 5 |

## California Pizza Kitchen
### APPETIZERS

| | | | | | | | | | | |
|---|---|---|---|---|---|---|---|---|---|---|
| Avocado Club Egg Rolls | as served | 1172 | n/a | n/a | 19 | n/a | 1519 | 58 | 4 | 45 |
| Buffalo Chicken | as served | 483 | n/a | n/a | 11 | n/a | 2242 | 18 | 2 | 17 |
| Crispy Artichoke Hearts | as served | 302 | n/a | n/a | 4 | n/a | 509 | 14 | 3 | 7 |
| Garlic Cheese Focaccia w/Checca | as served | 951 | n/a | n/a | 11 | n/a | 2195 | 119 | 6 | 30 |
| Lettuce Wraps w/Chicken | as served | 711 | n/a | n/a | 2 | n/a | 1574 | 92 | 8 | 36 |
| Mediterranean Plate | as served | 398 | n/a | n/a | 4 | n/a | 827 | 36 | 3 | 8 |
| Singapore Shrimp Rolls | as served | 633 | n/a | n/a | 2 | n/a | 2434 | 105 | 5 | 15 |
| Spinach Artichoke Dip | as served | 873 | n/a | n/a | 15 | n/a | 1242 | 103 | 9 | 20 |

### ENTRÉES

| | | | | | | | | | | |
|---|---|---|---|---|---|---|---|---|---|---|
| Baja Fish Tacos | 1 entrée | 976 | n/a | n/a | 10 | n/a | 1796 | 95 | 8 | 36 |

# restaurants

| | SERVING SIZE | CAL | CAL FAT | TOT FAT (G) | SAT FAT (G) | CHOL (MG) | SOD (MG) | CARB (G) | FIBER (G) | PROT (G) |
|---|---|---|---|---|---|---|---|---|---|---|
| Chicken Marsala | 1 entrée | 1412 | n/a | n/a | 15 | n/a | 1960 | 113 | 6 | 89 |
| Chicken Piccata | 1 entrée | 1325 | n/a | n/a | 30 | n/a | 1178 | 99 | 5 | 82 |
| Wild Caught Mahi Mahi w/Spaghettini | 1 entrée | 1212 | n/a | n/a | 12 | n/a | 1259 | 77 | 8 | 67 |
| **PASTA ENTRÉES** | | | | | | | | | | |
| Asparagus & Spinach Spaghettini | 1 entrée | 1115 | n/a | n/a | 10 | n/a | 2078 | 119 | 10 | 32 |
| Baby Clam Linguini w/Tomato Basil Sauce | 1 entrée | 792 | n/a | n/a | 16 | n/a | 1452 | 93 | 5 | 28 |
| Broccoli Sun-Dried Tomato Fusilli | 1 entrée | 1287 | n/a | n/a | 14 | n/a | 1022 | 121 | 10 | 37 |
| Chicken Tequila Fettuccine | 1 entrée | 1225 | n/a | n/a | 42 | n/a | 1247 | 95 | 6 | 34 |
| Four Cheese Ravioli | 1 entrée | 947 | n/a | n/a | 41 | n/a | 987 | 49 | 2 | 28 |
| Garlic Cream Fettuccine | 1 entrée | 1300 | n/a | n/a | 51 | n/a | 586 | 89 | 4 | 28 |
| Jambalaya | 1 entrée | 1188 | n/a | n/a | 15 | n/a | 2206 | 106 | 8 | 62 |
| Kung Pao Spaghetti | 1 entrée | 1165 | n/a | n/a | 7 | n/a | 1230 | 135 | 11 | 33 |
| Pesto Cream Penne w/Shrimp | 1 entrée | 1328 | n/a | n/a | 50 | n/a | 1013 | 89 | 5 | 38 |
| Portobello Mushroom Ravioli w/Tomato Basil Sauce | 1 entrée | 718 | n/a | n/a | 10 | n/a | 1550 | 81 | 5 | 21 |
| Spaghetti Bolognese | 1 entrée | 890 | n/a | n/a | 8 | n/a | 745 | 117 | 5 | 33 |
| Thai Linguini | 1 entrée | 1521 | n/a | n/a | 20 | n/a | 2780 | 158 | 10 | 32 |
| Tomato Basil Spaghetti | 1 entrée | 886 | n/a | n/a | 5 | n/a | 805 | 118 | 5 | 21 |
| **PIZZA** | | | | | | | | | | |
| BBQ Chicken w Applewood Smoked Bacon | 1 pizza | 1316 | n/a | n/a | 25 | n/a | 3288 | 136 | 6 | 72 |
| Buffalo Chicken | 1 pizza | 1247 | n/a | n/a | 23 | n/a | 3377 | 124 | 8 | 61 |
| California Club | 1 pizza | 1560 | n/a | n/a | 26 | n/a | 3542 | 129 | 13 | 71 |
| Margherita Thin Crust | 1 pizza | 1105 | n/a | n/a | 20 | n/a | 2008 | 106 | 7 | 54 |
| Meat Cravers | 1 pizza | 1530 | n/a | n/a | 33 | n/a | 4134 | 127 | 7 | 77 |
| Original BBQ Chicken | 1 pizza | 1136 | n/a | n/a | 19 | n/a | 2568 | 136 | 6 | 60 |
| Pepperoni | 1 pizza | 1140 | n/a | n/a | 22 | n/a | 2637 | 122 | 7 | 47 |
| The Works | 1 pizza | 1430 | n/a | n/a | 29 | n/a | 3335 | 131 | 9 | 63 |
| Thin Crust | 1 pizza | 439 | n/a | n/a | 0 | n/a | 958 | 91 | 3 | 15 |
| Traditional Cheese | 1 pizza | 998 | n/a | n/a | 16 | n/a | 2161 | 122 | 7 | 42 |
| White | 1 pizza | 1103 | n/a | n/a | 21 | n/a | 2455 | 118 | 6 | 49 |
| **SALADS** | | | | | | | | | | |
| Classic Caesar | 1 salad | 553 | n/a | n/a | 14 | n/a | 1030 | 29 | 8 | 16 |
| CPK Cobb w Blue Cheese Dressing | 1 salad | 1076 | n/a | n/a | 22 | n/a | 1877 | 23 | 9 | 53 |
| Field Greens | 1 salad | 998 | n/a | n/a | 12 | n/a | 805 | 68 | 15 | 18 |
| Waldorf Chicken w Blue Cheese Dressing | 1 salad | 1570 | n/a | n/a | 30 | n/a | 2082 | 83 | 16 | 55 |

| | SERVING SIZE | CAL | CAL FAT | TOT FAT (G) | SAT FAT (G) | CHOL (MG) | SOD (MG) | CARB (G) | FIBER (G) | PROT (G) |
|---|---|---|---|---|---|---|---|---|---|---|
| **SANDWICHES ON HERB ONION FOCACCIA** | | | | | | | | | | |
| California Chicken Club | 1 sandwich | 1027 | n/a | n/a | 13 | n/a | 1479 | 91 | 7 | 45 |
| Grilled Chicken Caesar | 1 sandwich | 1027 | n/a | n/a | 13 | n/a | 2026 | 91 | 7 | 45 |
| Grilled Vegetable | 1 sandwich | 830 | n/a | n/a | 9 | n/a | 2531 | 96 | 7 | 22 |
| Italian Deli | 1 sandwich | 1218 | n/a | n/a | 23 | n/a | 2936 | 90 | 5 | 47 |
| Turkey Stack | 1 sandwich | 839 | n/a | n/a | 8 | n/a | 2772 | 93 | 5 | 45 |
| **Caribou Coffee** | | | | | | | | | | |
| **BAKERY** | | | | | | | | | | |
| Blackberry White Chocolate Scone | 1 scone | 470 | 190 | 21 | 11 | 30 | 540 | 63 | 2 | 6 |
| Blueberry Muffin | 1 muffin | 410 | 170 | 18 | 3.5 | 35 | 370 | 55 | 1 | 7 |
| Caramel High Rise Bar | 1 bar | 550 | 280 | 31 | 18 | 80 | 190 | 58 | 2 | 6 |
| Chocolate Chip Cookie | 1 cookie | 420 | 190 | 22 | 11 | 40 | 190 | 54 | 2 | 4 |
| Cinnamon Coffee Cake | 1 slice | 540 | 220 | 24 | 6 | 85 | 370 | 74 | 0 | 5 |
| Cinnamon Sugar Donut | 1 doughnut | 400 | 160 | 18 | 9 | 20 | 420 | 55 | 2 | 5 |
| French Toast Muffin | 1 muffin | 490 | 170 | 19 | 4.5 | 20 | 280 | 74 | 0 | 6 |
| Multi Grain Bagel | 1 bagel | 360 | 60 | 7 | 1 | 0 | 640 | 63 | 6 | 13 |
| Reduced Fat Banana Bread | 1 slice | 380 | 80 | 11 | 6 | 0 | 460 | 72 | 2 | 5 |
| Reduced Fat Blueberry Coffee Cake | 1 slice | 340 | 120 | 14 | 4 | 55 | 340 | 50 | 1 | 5 |
| Reduced Fat Cranberry Orange Scone | 1 scone | 430 | 100 | 11 | 6 | 35 | 460 | 79 | 3 | 4 |
| **COOLERS (No Whip Cream)** | | | | | | | | | | |
| Caramel | 16 fl oz | 400 | 50 | 5 | 5 | 0 | 95 | 86 | 0 | 3 |
| Espresso | 16 fl oz | 270 | 45 | 5 | 5 | 0 | 95 | 55 | 0 | 3 |
| Mocha, Milk Chocolate | 16 fl oz | 550 | 120 | 13 | 8 | 25 | 180 | 98 | 0 | 10 |
| Northern Lite Caramel | 16 fl oz | 110 | 20 | 2 | 2 | 0 | 135 | 38 | 8 | 3 |
| Northern Lite Mocha, Milk Choc | 16 fl oz | 200 | 40 | 4.5 | 3.5 | 0 | 150 | 60 | 11 | 6 |
| Northern Lite Vanilla | 16 fl oz | 110 | 20 | 2 | 2 | 0 | 135 | 38 | 8 | 3 |
| Vanilla | 16 fl oz | 380 | 50 | 5 | 5 | 0 | 95 | 83 | 0 | 3 |
| **LATTES** | | | | | | | | | | |
| Iced, 2% Milk, No Whip Cream | 16 fl oz | 150 | 60 | 6 | 4 | 25 | 140 | 14 | 0 | 12 |
| Made w/2% Milk | 16 fl oz | 200 | 70 | 8 | 5 | 30 | 170 | 19 | 0 | 14 |
| **MOCHAS (No Whip Cream)** | | | | | | | | | | |
| Campfire, 2% Milk, Milk Choc. | 16 fl oz | 520 | 210 | 24 | 13 | 15 | 130 | 68 | 0 | 11 |
| Iced, 2% Milk, Milk Choc. | 16 fl oz | 350 | 100 | 11 | 5 | 35 | 160 | 51 | 0 | 12 |
| **SMOOTHIES (No Whip Cream)** | | | | | | | | | | |
| Passion Fruit Green Tea | 16 fl oz | 290 | 0 | 0 | 0 | 0 | 40 | 70 | 0 | 2 |
| Strawberry Banana | 16 fl oz | 350 | 0 | 0 | 0 | 0 | 30 | 84 | 2 | 3 |

| | SERVING SIZE | CAL | CAL. FAT | TOT FAT (G) | SAT FAT (G) | CHOL (MG) | SOD (MG) | CARB (G) | FIBER (G) | PROT (G) |
|---|---|---|---|---|---|---|---|---|---|---|
| **SNOWDRIFTS (No Whip Cream)** | | | | | | | | | | |
| Cookies & Cream, 2% Milk, Milk Choc. | 16 fl oz | 630 | 160 | 18 | 8 | 40 | 320 | 103 | 1 | 15 |
| Mint, 2% Milk, Milk Choc. | 16 fl oz | 510 | 110 | 13 | 6 | 40 | 180 | 84 | 0 | 14 |
| **SPECIALTY BEVERAGES** | | | | | | | | | | |
| Breve | 16 fl oz | 510 | 400 | 45 | 28 | 145 | 180 | 18 | 0 | 13 |
| Caramel High Rise, 2% Milk, No Whip | 16 fl oz | 260 | 60 | 7 | 4.5 | 25 | 150 | 39 | 0 | 12 |
| Hot Apple Blast w/o Whip | 16 fl oz | 300 | 0 | 0 | 0 | 0 | 45 | 74 | 0 | 0 |
| Macchiato w 2% Milk | 16 fl oz | 20 | 5 | 1 | 0 | 0 | 30 | 1 | 0 | 3 |
| Mint Condition, 2% Milk Choc., No Whip | 16 fl oz | 520 | 210 | 23 | 13 | 125 | 70 | 0 | 0 | 6 |
| Reindeer Drink w 2% Milk | 16 fl oz | 310 | 80 | 9 | 6 | 35 | 190 | 43 | 0 | 15 |
| **TEA LATTES (No Whip Cream)** | | | | | | | | | | |
| Black Thai, 2% Milk | 16 fl oz | 260 | 60 | 7 | 4.5 | 30 | 150 | 37 | 0 | 12 |
| Blended Chai, 2% Milk | 16 fl oz | 242 | 35 | 4 | 3 | 17 | 95 | 40 | 0 | 7 |
| Iced Caramel Earl Grey, 2% Milk | 16 fl oz | 260 | 50 | 6 | 3.5 | 20 | 370 | 46 | 0 | 6 |
| Iced Chai, 2% Milk | 16 fl oz | 226 | 38 | 4 | 3 | 19 | 88 | 39 | 0 | 8 |

## Carinos

| | SERVING SIZE | CAL | CAL. FAT | TOT FAT (G) | SAT FAT (G) | CHOL (MG) | SOD (MG) | CARB (G) | FIBER (G) | PROT (G) |
|---|---|---|---|---|---|---|---|---|---|---|
| **APPETIZERS** | | | | | | | | | | |
| Baked Stuffed Mushrooms | as served | 463 | 332 | 37 | 23 | 173 | 1095 | 20 | 2 | 13 |
| Hand-Breaded Calamari | as served | 1233 | 231 | 26 | 6 | 653 | 5264 | 176 | 7 | 68 |
| Mozzarella w/Marinara | as served | 743 | 384 | 43 | 19 | 101 | 2234 | 57 | 2 | 33 |
| **ENTRÉES** | | | | | | | | | | |
| Angel Hair w/Artichokes | as served | 673 | 127 | 14 | 1 | 5 | 1780 | 113 | 11 | 22 |
| Baked Cheese Tortelloni | as served | 1004 | 405 | 45 | 27 | 189 | 2979 | 87 | 7 | 57 |
| Carino's Favorites Combo | as served | 1408 | 529 | 59 | 25 | 334 | 3408 | 128 | 10 | 89 |
| Chicken Fettuccine | as served | 958 | 337 | 37 | 20 | 136 | 2199 | 107 | 5 | 43 |
| Chicken Marsala | as served | 1427 | 907 | 101 | 30 | 189 | 2244 | 64 | 3 | 51 |
| Chicken Milano | as served | 1418 | 824 | 92 | 34 | 248 | 3447 | 65 | 3 | 79 |
| Chicken Penne Gorgonzola | as served | 1420 | 798 | 89 | 37 | 205 | 2114 | 107 | 6 | 47 |
| Chicken Scaloppini | as served | 1806 | 1337 | 149 | 60 | 396 | 2144 | 55 | 3 | 57 |
| Grilled Chicken Diavolo | as served | 600 | 170 | 19 | 4 | 111 | 1764 | 57 | 5 | 51 |
| Homemade 16-Layer Lasagna | as served | 902 | 417 | 46 | 23 | 243 | 2252 | 62 | 6 | 57 |
| Homemade Parmigiana—Chicken | as served | 1124 | 430 | 48 | 15 | 237 | 2863 | 102 | 6 | 72 |
| Lobster Ravioli | as served | 933 | 560 | 62 | 29 | 198 | 1905 | 64 | 5 | 26 |
| Shrimp Scampi | as served | 2051 | 1344 | 149 | 83 | 514 | 1157 | 115 | 7 | 46 |
| Skilletini- Chicken | as served | 1215 | 650 | 72 | 12 | 91 | 2195 | 94 | 6 | 47 |
| Spaghetti & Handmade Meatballs | as served | 1108 | 337 | 37 | 12 | 192 | 2551 | 136 | 11 | 55 |
| Spicy Shrimp & Chicken | as served | 1294 | 653 | 73 | 26 | 244 | 1805 | 106 | 5 | 53 |

| | SERVING SIZE | CAL | CAL FAT | TOT FAT (G) | SAT FAT (G) | CHOL (MG) | SOD (MG) | CARB (G) | FIBER (G) | PROT (G) |
|---|---|---|---|---|---|---|---|---|---|---|
| Stuffed Vegetable Rigatoni | as served | 907 | 377 | 42 | 14 | 116 | 2708 | 96 | 12 | 32 |
| **SALADS** | | | | | | | | | | |
| Chicken Gorgonzola & Sun Dried Tomato | as served | 655 | 368 | 41 | 10 | 70 | 1584 | 47 | 6 | 30 |
| Classic Grilled Chicken Caesar | as served | 726 | 483 | 54 | 8 | 89 | 1928 | 35 | 6 | 32 |
| Honey Pecan Crusted Salmon | as served | 794 | 403 | 45 | 7 | 117 | 1661 | 52 | 7 | 45 |
| Pecan Crusted Chicken | as served | 972 | 447 | 50 | 16 | 159 | 3417 | 86 | 6 | 41 |

## Carl's Jr

**SALADS**

| | SERVING SIZE | CAL | CAL FAT | TOT FAT (G) | SAT FAT (G) | CHOL (MG) | SOD (MG) | CARB (G) | FIBER (G) | PROT (G) |
|---|---|---|---|---|---|---|---|---|---|---|
| Cranberry, Apple, Walnut, Grilled Chicken | 11 oz | 300 | 100 | 11 | 4 | 70 | 840 | 25 | 4 | 26 |
| Garden Side | 5 oz | 50 | 20 | 3 | 2 | 5 | 75 | 5 | 2 | 3 |
| Hawaiian Grilled Chicken | 15 oz | 260 | 70 | 8 | 0 | 55 | 560 | 34 | 4 | 22 |
| Original Grilled Chicken | 13 oz | 200 | 60 | 6 | 3 | 70 | 610 | 13 | 3 | 24 |
| **SANDWICHES & BURGERS** | | | | | | | | | | |
| Bacon Swiss Crispy Chicken | 1 sandwich | 750 | 360 | 40 | 9 | 70 | 1990 | 62 | 4 | 36 |
| Big Carl | 1 burger | 920 | 530 | 59 | 23 | 145 | 1370 | 51 | 2 | 46 |
| Big Hamburger | 1 burger | 460 | 160 | 17 | 8 | 50 | 1090 | 54 | 3 | 24 |
| Carl's Catch Fish Sandwich | 1 sandwich | 710 | 330 | 37 | 6 | 40 | 1280 | 74 | 4 | 20 |
| Carl's Super star w/Cheese | 1 burger | 920 | 510 | 58 | 23 | 145 | 1640 | 54 | 3 | 47 |
| Charbroiled BBQ Chicken | 1 sandwich | 380 | 60 | 7 | 2 | 60 | 1010 | 49 | 2 | 34 |
| Charbroiled Chicken Club | 1 sandwich | 560 | 240 | 27 | 7 | 90 | 1280 | 44 | 2 | 39 |
| Chicken Strips | 3 pieces | 270 | 130 | 14 | 3 | 45 | 800 | 17 | 1 | 19 |
| Double Western Bacon Cheeseburger | 1 burger | 960 | 470 | 52 | 23 | 140 | 1750 | 70 | 3 | 52 |
| Green Burrito Crisp Burritos | 3 pieces | 540 | 230 | 25 | 9 | 35 | 1030 | 57 | 5 | 22 |
| Guacamole Bacon Six Dollar Burger | 1 burger | 1040 | 630 | 70 | 25 | 145 | 2240 | 53 | 4 | 49 |
| Hand Breaded Chicken Tenders | 3 pieces | 340 | 170 | 19 | 4 | 70 | 1160 | 14 | 1 | 28 |
| Jalapeño Burger | 1 burger | 720 | 410 | 46 | 15 | 85 | 1340 | 50 | 3 | 27 |
| Low Carb Six Dollar Burger | 1 burger | 570 | 380 | 43 | 18 | 120 | 1480 | 7 | 1 | 38 |
| Original Six Dollar Burger | 1 burger | 890 | 480 | 54 | 20 | 130 | 2040 | 58 | 3 | 45 |
| Single Teriyaki Burger | 1 burger | 610 | 260 | 29 | 11 | 65 | 1020 | 60 | 3 | 28 |
| Spicy Chicken Sandwich | 1 sandwich | 420 | 230 | 27 | 5 | 25 | 930 | 33 | 2 | 12 |
| **SIDES** | | | | | | | | | | |
| Chili Cheese Fries | 11 oz | 980 | 500 | 56 | 19 | 70 | 2350 | 88 | 8 | 28 |
| CrissCut Fries | 5 oz | 450 | 260 | 29 | 5 | 0 | 900 | 42 | 4 | 5 |
| Fried Zucchini | 5 oz | 330 | 160 | 18 | 3 | 0 | 610 | 36 | 2 | 6 |
| Natural-Cut French Fries—Medium | 4 oz | 460 | 200 | 22 | 5 | 0 | 1180 | 60 | 5 | 5 |
| Onion Rings | 5 oz | 530 | 250 | 28 | 5 | 0 | 590 | 61 | 3 | 8 |

| | SERVING SIZE | CAL | CAL FAT | TOT FAT (G) | SAT FAT (G) | CHOL (MG) | SOD (MG) | CARB (G) | FIBER (G) | PROT (G) |
|---|---|---|---|---|---|---|---|---|---|---|

## Carrabba's Italian Grill

### ANTIPASTI

| | | | | | | | | | | |
|---|---|---|---|---|---|---|---|---|---|---|
| Anitipasti Platter | as served | 1750 | n/a | n/a | n/a | n/a | n/a | n/a | n/a | n/a |
| Calamari, Regular | as served | 1380 | n/a | n/a | n/a | n/a | n/a | n/a | n/a | n/a |
| Cozze in Bianco, Regular | as served | 1780 | n/a | n/a | n/a | n/a | n/a | n/a | n/a | n/a |
| Crab Cakes | as served | 550 | n/a | n/a | n/a | n/a | n/a | n/a | n/a | n/a |
| Grilled Bruschette | as served | 1350 | n/a | n/a | n/a | n/a | n/a | n/a | n/a | n/a |
| Mozzarella Marinara, Regular | as served | 1150 | n/a | n/a | n/a | n/a | n/a | n/a | n/a | n/a |
| Shrimp Scampi | as served | 1360 | n/a | n/a | n/a | n/a | n/a | n/a | n/a | n/a |
| Zucchini Fritte, Regular | as served | 590 | n/a | n/a | n/a | n/a | n/a | n/a | n/a | n/a |

### BRICK OVEN PIZZA

| | | | | | | | | | | |
|---|---|---|---|---|---|---|---|---|---|---|
| Margherita | 1/2 pizza | 850 | n/a | n/a | n/a | n/a | n/a | n/a | n/a | n/a |
| Pepperoni | 1/2 pizza | 880 | n/a | n/a | n/a | n/a | n/a | n/a | n/a | n/a |

### FAMILY CLASSICS & COMBINATIONS

| | | | | | | | | | | |
|---|---|---|---|---|---|---|---|---|---|---|
| Chicken Gratella, Regular | 1 entrée | 280 | n/a | n/a | n/a | n/a | n/a | n/a | n/a | n/a |
| Chicken Parmesan, Regular | 1 entrée | 820 | n/a | n/a | n/a | n/a | n/a | n/a | n/a | n/a |
| Chicken Trio | 1 entrée | 1140 | n/a | n/a | n/a | n/a | n/a | n/a | n/a | n/a |
| Filet Fiorentini | 7 oz | 550 | n/a | n/a | n/a | n/a | n/a | n/a | n/a | n/a |
| Filet Marsala | 7 oz | 880 | n/a | n/a | n/a | n/a | n/a | n/a | n/a | n/a |
| Filet Scampi | 7 oz | 910 | n/a | n/a | n/a | n/a | n/a | n/a | n/a | n/a |
| Filet Spiedino | 7 oz | 850 | n/a | n/a | n/a | n/a | n/a | n/a | n/a | n/a |
| Grilled Salmon, Small | 1 entrée | 860 | n/a | n/a | n/a | n/a | n/a | n/a | n/a | n/a |
| Italian Classics | 1 entrée | 850 | n/a | n/a | n/a | n/a | n/a | n/a | n/a | n/a |
| Marsala, Chicken | 1 entrée | 610 | n/a | n/a | n/a | n/a | n/a | n/a | n/a | n/a |
| Marsala, Veal | 1 entrée | 580 | n/a | n/a | n/a | n/a | n/a | n/a | n/a | n/a |
| Spiendini De Mare | 1 entrée | 610 | n/a | n/a | n/a | n/a | n/a | n/a | n/a | n/a |
| "The Carrabba" Marsala | 1 entrée | 700 | n/a | n/a | n/a | n/a | n/a | n/a | n/a | n/a |

### SIDE ITEMS

| | | | | | | | | | | |
|---|---|---|---|---|---|---|---|---|---|---|
| Carrabba's Boule Bread | as served | 420 | n/a | n/a | n/a | n/a | n/a | n/a | n/a | n/a |
| Cavatappi Amatriciana | as served | 400 | n/a | n/a | n/a | n/a | n/a | n/a | n/a | n/a |
| Garlic Mashed Potatoes | as served | 532 | n/a | n/a | n/a | n/a | n/a | n/a | n/a | n/a |

### SIGNATURE PASTA

| | | | | | | | | | | |
|---|---|---|---|---|---|---|---|---|---|---|
| Chicken & Spinach Cannelloni | 1 entrée | 550 | n/a | n/a | n/a | n/a | n/a | n/a | n/a | n/a |
| Lasagne | 1 entrée | 880 | n/a | n/a | n/a | n/a | n/a | n/a | n/a | n/a |
| Linguine Pescatore | 1 entrée | 840 | n/a | n/a | n/a | n/a | n/a | n/a | n/a | n/a |
| Linguine w/Clams | 1 entrée | 1340 | n/a | n/a | n/a | n/a | n/a | n/a | n/a | n/a |

| | SERVING SIZE | CAL | CAL FAT | TOT FAT (G) | SAT FAT (G) | CHOL (MG) | SOD (MG) | CARB (G) | FIBER (G) | PROT (G) |
|---|---|---|---|---|---|---|---|---|---|---|
| Lobster Ravioli | 1 entrée | 730 | n/a | n/a | n/a | n/a | n/a | n/a | n/a | n/a |
| Manicotti Pasta | 1 entrée | 530 | n/a | n/a | n/a | n/a | n/a | n/a | n/a | n/a |
| Pasta Carrabba | 1 entrée | 1530 | n/a | n/a | n/a | n/a | n/a | n/a | n/a | n/a |
| Rigatoni Martino | 1 entrée | 1490 | n/a | n/a | n/a | n/a | n/a | n/a | n/a | n/a |
| Spaghetti w/Italian Sausage | 1 entrée | 1270 | n/a | n/a | n/a | n/a | n/a | n/a | n/a | n/a |
| Spaghetti w/Meatballs | 1 entrée | 1150 | n/a | n/a | n/a | n/a | n/a | n/a | n/a | n/a |
| **ZUPPE & INSALATE** | | | | | | | | | | |
| House Salad | 1 salad | 360 | n/a | n/a | n/a | n/a | n/a | n/a | n/a | n/a |
| Mediterranean Salad | 1 salad | 240 | n/a | n/a | n/a | n/a | n/a | n/a | n/a | n/a |
| Insalata Carrabba | 1 salad | 840 | n/a | n/a | n/a | n/a | n/a | n/a | n/a | n/a |
| Mama Mandola's Sicilian Chicken Soup, Bowl | 1 bowl | 620 | n/a | n/a | n/a | n/a | n/a | n/a | n/a | n/a |
| Minestrone, Bowl | 1 bowl | 280 | n/a | n/a | n/a | n/a | n/a | n/a | n/a | n/a |

## Carvel
### BLENDED DRINKS, SMALL

| | SERVING SIZE | CAL | CAL FAT | TOT FAT (G) | SAT FAT (G) | CHOL (MG) | SOD (MG) | CARB (G) | FIBER (G) | PROT (G) |
|---|---|---|---|---|---|---|---|---|---|---|
| Arctic Blender—Cookie Dough | 16 oz | 920 | 360 | 40 | 22 | 115 | 460 | 126 | 1 | 15 |
| Arctic Blender—Fried Ice Cream | 16 oz | 670 | 279 | 31 | 18 | 100 | 330 | 85 | 2 | 13 |
| Arctic Blender—Peanut Butter | 16 oz | 870 | 297 | 33 | 17 | 90 | 510 | 88 | 3 | 18 |
| Carvelanche—Butterfinger | 16 oz | 730 | 342 | 38 | 24 | 135 | 340 | 92 | 1 | 10 |
| Carvelanche—Cake Mix | 16 oz | 770 | 279 | 31 | 20 | 135 | 500 | 110 | 0 | 10 |
| Carvelanche—M&M'S | 16 oz | 760 | 351 | 39 | 18 | 135 | 230 | 88 | 0 | 11 |
| Carvelatte—Coffee | 16 oz | 670 | 288 | 32 | 20 | 115 | 340 | 84 | 0 | 14 |
| Carvelatte—Mocha | 16 oz | 610 | 225 | 25 | 15 | 90 | 280 | 88 | 1 | 10 |
| Float—Chocolate Ice Cream & Coke | 16 oz | 360 | 42 | 14 | 8 | 35 | 150 | 54 | 1 | 6 |
| Float—Chocolate Ice Cream & Soda Water | 16 oz | 420 | 135 | 15 | 8 | 35 | 220 | 69 | 1 | 6 |
| Float—Vanilla Ice Cream & Coke | 16 oz | 380 | 153 | 17 | 11 | 85 | 150 | 53 | 0 | 4 |
| Float—Vanilla Ice Cream & Soda Water | 16 oz | 440 | 162 | 18 | 11 | 85 | 220 | 68 | 0 | 4 |
| Iceberg—Barq's Root Beer | 16 oz | 550 | 243 | 27 | 18 | 120 | 290 | 67 | 0 | 10 |
| Thick Chocolate Shake | 1 shake | 650 | 243 | 27 | 16 | 70 | 320 | 93 | 2 | 14 |
| Thick Strawberry Shake | 1 shake | 600 | 351 | 39 | 26 | 190 | 350 | 70 | 0 | 13 |
| Thick Vanilla Shake | 1 shake | 660 | 279 | 31 | 20 | 150 | 280 | 86 | 0 | 11 |
| **DASHERS, SMALL** | | | | | | | | | | |
| Banana's Foster | 12 oz | 660 | 207 | 23 | 15 | 90 | 420 | 105 | 2 | 6 |
| Fudge Brownie | 12 oz | 850 | 405 | 45 | 21 | 135 | 420 | 102 | 4 | 10 |
| Mint Chocolate Chip | 12 oz | 770 | 378 | 42 | 24 | 100 | 290 | 95 | 4 | 9 |
| Peanut Butter Cup | 12 oz | 1060 | 540 | 60 | 20 | 55 | 670 | 95 | 7 | 22 |
| Strawberry Shortcake | 12 oz | 580 | 261 | 29 | 19 | 145 | 240 | 74 | 2 | 7 |

| | SERVING SIZE | CAL | CAL FAT | TOT FAT (G) | SAT FAT (G) | CHOL (MG) | SOD (MG) | CARB (G) | FIBER (G) | PROT (G) |
|---|---|---|---|---|---|---|---|---|---|---|
| **ICE CREAM CONES, SMALL** | | | | | | | | | | |
| Cake Cone w/Chocolate | 1 cone | 440 | 189 | 21 | 13 | 55 | 220 | 51 | 2 | 10 |
| Sugar Cone w/Chocolate | 1 cone | 460 | 189 | 21 | 13 | 55 | 250 | 59 | 2 | 11 |
| Waffle Cone w/Chocolate | 1 cone | 490 | 207 | 23 | 13 | 60 | 220 | 63 | 2 | 10 |
| **ICE CREAM CUPS, SMALL** | | | | | | | | | | |
| Chocolate | 1 cup | 410 | 189 | 21 | 13 | 55 | 220 | 48 | 2 | 10 |
| Classic Hot Fudge Sundae | 1 sundae | 540 | 270 | 30 | 22 | 115 | 220 | 60 | 2 | 7 |
| No Sugar Added Vanilla | 1 cup | 260 | 63 | 7 | 4.5 | 30 | 190 | 51 | 0 | 11 |
| Sherbet | 1 cup | 290 | 27 | 3 | 1.5 | 5 | 115 | 67 | 0 | 2 |
| Vanilla | 1 cup | 450 | 234 | 26 | 17 | 130 | 210 | 47 | 0 | 6 |

## Charley's Grilled Subs
### BREAKFAST

| | SERVING SIZE | CAL | CAL FAT | TOT FAT (G) | SAT FAT (G) | CHOL (MG) | SOD (MG) | CARB (G) | FIBER (G) | PROT (G) |
|---|---|---|---|---|---|---|---|---|---|---|
| Bacon, Egg, & Cheese Sandwich | 1 entrée | 540 | 234 | 26 | 9 | 492 | 1188 | 54 | 2 | 33 |
| Egg & Cheese Sandwich | 1 entrée | 470 | 145 | 17 | 6 | 482 | 948 | 54 | 2 | 29 |
| Ham Omelet | 1 entrée | 410 | 226 | 25.5 | 10 | 690 | 1289 | 10 | 0 | 42 |
| Ham, Egg, & Cheese Sandwich | 1 entrée | 540 | 165 | 19.5 | 7 | 512 | 1438 | 55 | 2 | 39 |
| Sausage Omelet | 1 entrée | 474 | 310 | 35 | 14 | 708 | 1219 | 8 | 0 | 42 |
| Veggie Omelet | 1 entrée | 359 | 208 | 24 | 8 | 656 | 801 | 13 | 1 | 33.5 |
| Western Omelet | 1 entrée | 521 | 218 | 25 | 8.5 | 669 | 1021 | 13 | 1 | 38 |
| **FRIES** | | | | | | | | | | |
| Cheddar | as served | 523 | 255 | 30 | 7 | 23 | 1022 | 55 | 2 | 14 |
| Ranch Bacon | as served | 530 | 228 | 25 | 5.5 | 33 | 1082 | 51 | 2 | 15 |
| Regular | as served | 453 | 210 | 25 | 4.5 | 0 | 322 | 41 | 2 | 5 |
| **SALADS** | | | | | | | | | | |
| Buffalo Chicken | 1 salad | 208 | 64 | 7.5 | 2 | 65 | 1333 | 14 | 2 | 25 |
| Fresh Garden | 1 salad | 58 | 14 | 2 | 0 | 0 | 383 | 9 | 2 | 0.5 |
| Grilled Chicken | 1 salad | 198 | 59 | 7 | 2 | 65 | 533 | 10 | 2 | 25 |
| Grilled Steak | 1 salad | 208 | 84 | 10 | 3 | 45 | 693 | 10 | 2 | 20 |
| **SUBS** | | | | | | | | | | |
| Bacon 3 Cheese | 1 sub | 635 | 250 | 32 | 14 | 92.5 | 1687 | 54 | 2 | 43 |
| BBQ Cheddar | 1 sub | 581 | 170 | 19.5 | 9.5 | 75 | 1718 | 68 | 3 | 36 |
| Chicken Bacon Club | 1 sub | 570 | 185 | 24.5 | 10 | 100 | 1347 | 53 | 2 | 45 |
| Chicken Buffalo | 1 sub | 526 | 140 | 16 | 6.5 | 85 | 1703 | 59 | 4 | 41.5 |
| Chicken Cordon Blue | 1 sub | 570 | 155 | 18 | 8.5 | 120 | 1210 | 54 | 2 | 53 |
| Chicken Teriyaki | 1 sub | 522 | 135 | 15.5 | 7.5 | 90 | 1281 | 58 | 3 | 43 |
| Italian Deli | 1 sub | 585 | 220 | 25 | 6 | 63 | 1890 | 53 | 2 | 37 |
| Philly Cheesesteak | 1 sub | 521 | 160 | 18.5 | 7.5 | 65 | 1448 | 56 | 3 | 36 |

| | SERVING SIZE | CAL | CAL FAT | TOT FAT (G) | SAT FAT (G) | CHOL (MG) | SOD (MG) | CARB (G) | FIBER (G) | PROT (G) |
|---|---|---|---|---|---|---|---|---|---|---|
| Philly Veggie | 1 sub | 449 | 130 | 15 | 8 | 38 | 1142 | 62 | 4 | 23 |
| Sicilian Steak | 1 sub | 640 | 270 | 30.5 | 11.5 | 95 | 1877 | 54 | 2 | 41 |
| Turkey Cheddar Melt | 1 sub | 470 | 100 | 11.5 | 5.5 | 80 | 1570 | 53 | 2 | 36 |

## Cheesecake Factory
### APPETIZERS

| | SERVING SIZE | CAL | CAL FAT | TOT FAT (G) | SAT FAT (G) | CHOL (MG) | SOD (MG) | CARB (G) | FIBER (G) | PROT (G) |
|---|---|---|---|---|---|---|---|---|---|---|
| Ahi Carpaccio | as served | 260 | n/a | n/a | n/a | n/a | n/a | n/a | n/a | n/a |
| Avocado Eggrolls | as served | 960 | n/a | n/a | n/a | n/a | n/a | n/a | n/a | n/a |
| Buffalo Blasts | as served | 900 | n/a | n/a | n/a | n/a | n/a | n/a | n/a | n/a |
| Buffalo Chicken Strips | as served | 1120 | n/a | n/a | n/a | n/a | n/a | n/a | n/a | n/a |
| Buffalo Wings | as served | 1180 | n/a | n/a | n/a | n/a | n/a | n/a | n/a | n/a |
| Chicken Pot Stickers | as served | 470 | n/a | n/a | n/a | n/a | n/a | n/a | n/a | n/a |
| Crabcakes | as served | 850 | n/a | n/a | n/a | n/a | n/a | n/a | n/a | n/a |
| Crispy Crab Wontons | as served | 650 | n/a | n/a | n/a | n/a | n/a | n/a | n/a | n/a |
| Crispy Taquitos | as served | 1080 | n/a | n/a | n/a | n/a | n/a | n/a | n/a | n/a |
| Factory Nachos | as served | 1660 | n/a | n/a | n/a | n/a | n/a | n/a | n/a | n/a |
| Fire Roasted Fresh Artichoke | as served | 1130 | n/a | n/a | n/a | n/a | n/a | n/a | n/a | n/a |
| Firecracker Salmon | as served | 660 | n/a | n/a | n/a | n/a | n/a | n/a | n/a | n/a |
| Fried Calamari | as served | 800 | n/a | n/a | n/a | n/a | n/a | n/a | n/a | n/a |
| Fried Macaroni & Cheese | as served | 1660 | n/a | n/a | n/a | n/a | n/a | n/a | n/a | n/a |
| Hot Spinach & Cheese Dip | as served | 1050 | n/a | n/a | n/a | n/a | n/a | n/a | n/a | n/a |
| Popcorn Shrimp | as served | 580 | n/a | n/a | n/a | n/a | n/a | n/a | n/a | n/a |
| Quesadilla | as served | 1170 | n/a | n/a | n/a | n/a | n/a | n/a | n/a | n/a |
| Roadside Sliders | as served | 730 | n/a | n/a | n/a | n/a | n/a | n/a | n/a | n/a |
| Southern Fried Chicken Sliders | as served | 1230 | n/a | n/a | n/a | n/a | n/a | n/a | n/a | n/a |
| Spicy Ahi Tempura Roll | as served | 620 | n/a | n/a | n/a | n/a | n/a | n/a | n/a | n/a |
| Sweet Corn Tamale Cakes | as served | 1760 | n/a | n/a | n/a | n/a | n/a | n/a | n/a | n/a |
| Tex Mex Eggrolls | as served | 760 | n/a | n/a | n/a | n/a | n/a | n/a | n/a | n/a |
| Thai Lettuce Wraps | as served | 970 | n/a | n/a | n/a | n/a | n/a | n/a | n/a | n/a |
| Vietnamese Shrimp Summer Rolls | as served | 790 | n/a | n/a | n/a | n/a | n/a | n/a | n/a | n/a |

### APPETIZER SALADS

| | SERVING SIZE | CAL | CAL FAT | TOT FAT (G) | SAT FAT (G) | CHOL (MG) | SOD (MG) | CARB (G) | FIBER (G) | PROT (G) |
|---|---|---|---|---|---|---|---|---|---|---|
| B.L.T. Salad | as served | 1490 | n/a | n/a | n/a | n/a | n/a | n/a | n/a | n/a |
| Boston House | as served | 1020 | n/a | n/a | n/a | n/a | n/a | n/a | n/a | n/a |
| Caesar Appetizer | as served | 910 | n/a | n/a | n/a | n/a | n/a | n/a | n/a | n/a |
| Caesar Appetizer Salad w/Chicken | as served | 1030 | n/a | n/a | n/a | n/a | n/a | n/a | n/a | n/a |
| Factory Chopped | as served | 870 | n/a | n/a | n/a | n/a | n/a | n/a | n/a | n/a |
| French Country | as served | 490 | n/a | n/a | n/a | n/a | n/a | n/a | n/a | n/a |
| Fresh Vegetable | as served | 900 | n/a | n/a | n/a | n/a | n/a | n/a | n/a | n/a |

# restaurants

| | SERVING SIZE | CAL | CAL FAT | TOT FAT (G) | SAT FAT (G) | CHOL (MG) | SOD (MG) | CARB (G) | FIBER (G) | PROT (G) |
|---|---|---|---|---|---|---|---|---|---|---|
| Fresh Vegetable Salad w/Chicken | as served | 1020 | n/a | n/a | n/a | n/a | n/a | n/a | n/a | n/a |
| Thai Noodle | as served | 970 | n/a | n/a | n/a | n/a | n/a | n/a | n/a | n/a |
| Tossed Green | as served | 670 | n/a | n/a | n/a | n/a | n/a | n/a | n/a | n/a |
| **CHEESECAKES** | | | | | | | | | | |
| Brownie Sundae | 1 slice | 1260 | n/a | n/a | n/a | n/a | n/a | n/a | n/a | n/a |
| Cherry | 1 slice | 850 | n/a | n/a | n/a | n/a | n/a | n/a | n/a | n/a |
| Chocolate Mousse | 1 slice | 930 | n/a | n/a | n/a | n/a | n/a | n/a | n/a | n/a |
| Chocolate Chip Cookie-Dough | 1 slice | 1130 | n/a | n/a | n/a | n/a | n/a | n/a | n/a | n/a |
| Chocolate Raspberry Truffle | 1 slice | 1060 | n/a | n/a | n/a | n/a | n/a | n/a | n/a | n/a |
| Craig's Crazy Carrot Cake | 1 slice | 1030 | n/a | n/a | n/a | n/a | n/a | n/a | n/a | n/a |
| Dulce De Leche Caramel | 1 slice | 1090 | n/a | n/a | n/a | n/a | n/a | n/a | n/a | n/a |
| Dutch Apple Caramel Streusel | 1 slice | 860 | n/a | n/a | n/a | n/a | n/a | n/a | n/a | n/a |
| Fresh Banana Cream | 1 slice | 930 | n/a | n/a | n/a | n/a | n/a | n/a | n/a | n/a |
| Fresh Strawberry | 1 slice | 710 | n/a | n/a | n/a | n/a | n/a | n/a | n/a | n/a |
| Godiva Chocolate | 1 slice | 1080 | n/a | n/a | n/a | n/a | n/a | n/a | n/a | n/a |
| Kahlua Cocoa Coffee | 1 slice | 860 | n/a | n/a | n/a | n/a | n/a | n/a | n/a | n/a |
| Key Lime | 1 slice | 850 | n/a | n/a | n/a | n/a | n/a | n/a | n/a | n/a |
| Lemon Raspberry Cream | 1 slice | 780 | n/a | n/a | n/a | n/a | n/a | n/a | n/a | n/a |
| Low Carb | 1 slice | 530 | n/a | n/a | n/a | n/a | n/a | n/a | n/a | n/a |
| Oreo | 1 slice | 860 | n/a | n/a | n/a | n/a | n/a | n/a | n/a | n/a |
| Original | 1 slice | 700 | n/a | n/a | n/a | n/a | n/a | n/a | n/a | n/a |
| Pineapple Upside-Down | 1 slice | 920 | n/a | n/a | n/a | n/a | n/a | n/a | n/a | n/a |
| Pumpkin | 1 slice | 1080 | n/a | n/a | n/a | n/a | n/a | n/a | n/a | n/a |
| Snickers Bar Chunks | 1 slice | 1020 | n/a | n/a | n/a | n/a | n/a | n/a | n/a | n/a |
| Stefanie's Ultimate Red Velvet Cake | 1 slice | 1550 | n/a | n/a | n/a | n/a | n/a | n/a | n/a | n/a |
| Tiramisu | 1 slice | 780 | n/a | n/a | n/a | n/a | n/a | n/a | n/a | n/a |
| Vanilla Bean | 1 slice | 890 | n/a | n/a | n/a | n/a | n/a | n/a | n/a | n/a |
| **EGGS & OMELETS** | | | | | | | | | | |
| Bourbon Street Omelet | 1 entrée | 1770 | n/a | n/a | n/a | n/a | n/a | n/a | n/a | n/a |
| Brioche Breakfast Sandwich | 1 entrée | 1600 | n/a | n/a | n/a | n/a | n/a | n/a | n/a | n/a |
| California Omelet | 1 entrée | 1960 | n/a | n/a | n/a | n/a | n/a | n/a | n/a | n/a |
| Energy Breakfast | 1 entrée | 690 | n/a | n/a | n/a | n/a | n/a | n/a | n/a | n/a |
| Factory Create An Omelet | 1 entrée | 2500 | n/a | n/a | n/a | n/a | n/a | n/a | n/a | n/a |
| Factory Huevos Rancheros | 1 entrée | 1160 | n/a | n/a | n/a | n/a | n/a | n/a | n/a | n/a |
| Mini Egg Breakfast | 1 entrée | 1410 | n/a | n/a | n/a | n/a | n/a | n/a | n/a | n/a |
| Morning Quesadilla | 1 entrée | 2140 | n/a | n/a | n/a | n/a | n/a | n/a | n/a | n/a |
| Shiitake, Spinach, & Goat Cheese Scramble | 1 entrée | 1710 | n/a | n/a | n/a | n/a | n/a | n/a | n/a | n/a |

| | SERVING SIZE | CAL | CAL FAT | TOT FAT (G) | SAT FAT (G) | CHOL (MG) | SOD (MG) | CARB (G) | FIBER (G) | PROT (G) |
|---|---|---|---|---|---|---|---|---|---|---|
| Spinach, Mushroom, Cheese & Bacon Omelet | 1 entrée | 1890 | n/a | n/a | n/a | n/a | n/a | n/a | n/a | n/a |
| Sunrise Fiesta Burrito | 1 entrée | 1780 | n/a | n/a | n/a | n/a | n/a | n/a | n/a | n/a |
| **FACTORY COMBINATIONS** | | | | | | | | | | |
| Chicken Madeira & Steak Diane | 1 entrée | 2070 | n/a | n/a | n/a | n/a | n/a | n/a | n/a | n/a |
| Herb Crusted Salmon & Shrimp Scampi | 1 entrée | 2000 | n/a | n/a | n/a | n/a | n/a | n/a | n/a | n/a |
| Shrimp Scampi & Steak Diane | 1 entrée | 2070 | n/a | n/a | n/a | n/a | n/a | n/a | n/a | n/a |
| Shrimp Scampi & Chicken Madeira | 1 entrée | 2040 | n/a | n/a | n/a | n/a | n/a | n/a | n/a | n/a |
| Steak Diane & Herb Crusted Salmon | 1 entrée | 2030 | n/a | n/a | n/a | n/a | n/a | n/a | n/a | n/a |
| **FISH & SEAFOOD** | | | | | | | | | | |
| Fresh Grilled Mahi Mahi | 1 entrée | 1370 | n/a | n/a | n/a | n/a | n/a | n/a | n/a | n/a |
| Fresh Grilled Salmon | 1 entrée | 1610 | n/a | n/a | n/a | n/a | n/a | n/a | n/a | n/a |
| Herb Crusted Filet Of Salmon | 1 entrée | 1400 | n/a | n/a | n/a | n/a | n/a | n/a | n/a | n/a |
| Jamaican Black Pepper Shrimp | 1 entrée | 1360 | n/a | n/a | n/a | n/a | n/a | n/a | n/a | n/a |
| Mahi Mahi Mediterranean | 1 entrée | 1210 | n/a | n/a | n/a | n/a | n/a | n/a | n/a | n/a |
| Miso Salmon | 1 entrée | 1740 | n/a | n/a | n/a | n/a | n/a | n/a | n/a | n/a |
| Shrimp & Chicken Gumbo | 1 entrée | 1570 | n/a | n/a | n/a | n/a | n/a | n/a | n/a | n/a |
| Shrimp Scampi | 1 entrée | 1630 | n/a | n/a | n/a | n/a | n/a | n/a | n/a | n/a |
| Wasabi Crusted Ahi Tuna | 1 entrée | 1640 | n/a | n/a | n/a | n/a | n/a | n/a | n/a | n/a |
| **GLAMBURGERS & SANDWICHES** | | | | | | | | | | |
| B.B.Q. Pulled Pork Sandwich | 1 sandwich | 1730 | n/a | n/a | n/a | n/a | n/a | n/a | n/a | n/a |
| Blackened Chicken Sandwich | 1 sandwich | 1880 | n/a | n/a | n/a | n/a | n/a | n/a | n/a | n/a |
| Blue Cheese B.L.T. Burger | 1 burger | 1550 | n/a | n/a | n/a | n/a | n/a | n/a | n/a | n/a |
| California Cheesesteak | 1 sandwich | 1720 | n/a | n/a | n/a | n/a | n/a | n/a | n/a | n/a |
| Chicken Parmesan Sandwich | 1 sandwich | 2240 | n/a | n/a | n/a | n/a | n/a | n/a | n/a | n/a |
| Chicken Salad Sandwich | 1 sandwich | 2010 | n/a | n/a | n/a | n/a | n/a | n/a | n/a | n/a |
| Classic Burger | 1 burger | 1900 | n/a | n/a | n/a | n/a | n/a | n/a | n/a | n/a |
| Club Sandwich | 1 sandwich | 1880 | n/a | n/a | n/a | n/a | n/a | n/a | n/a | n/a |
| Crab Cake Sandwich | 1 sandwich | 1600 | n/a | n/a | n/a | n/a | n/a | n/a | n/a | n/a |
| Cuban Sandwich | 1 sandwich | 1570 | n/a | n/a | n/a | n/a | n/a | n/a | n/a | n/a |
| Factory Burger | 1 burger | 1190 | n/a | n/a | n/a | n/a | n/a | n/a | n/a | n/a |
| Green Chile Cheeseburger | 1 burger | 1650 | n/a | n/a | n/a | n/a | n/a | n/a | n/a | n/a |
| Grilled Cheese Sandwich | 1 sandwich | 1510 | n/a | n/a | n/a | n/a | n/a | n/a | n/a | n/a |
| Grilled Chicken & Avocado Club | 1 sandwich | 2200 | n/a | n/a | n/a | n/a | n/a | n/a | n/a | n/a |
| Grilled Portabella On A Bun | 1 burger | 1830 | n/a | n/a | n/a | n/a | n/a | n/a | n/a | n/a |
| Grilled Shrimp & Bacon Club | 1 sandwich | 2350 | n/a | n/a | n/a | n/a | n/a | n/a | n/a | n/a |

# restaurants

| | SERVING SIZE | CAL | CAL FAT | TOT FAT (G) | SAT FAT (G) | CHOL (MG) | SOD (MG) | CARB (G) | FIBER (G) | PROT (G) |
|---|---|---|---|---|---|---|---|---|---|---|
| Grilled Turkey Burger | 1 burger | 1650 | n/a | n/a | n/a | n/a | n/a | n/a | n/a | n/a |
| Incredible Grilled Eggplant Sandwich | 1 sandwich | 1940 | n/a | n/a | n/a | n/a | n/a | n/a | n/a | n/a |
| Kobe Burger | 1 burger | 1580 | n/a | n/a | n/a | n/a | n/a | n/a | n/a | n/a |
| Memphis Burger | 1 burger | 1760 | n/a | n/a | n/a | n/a | n/a | n/a | n/a | n/a |
| Monterey Cheeseburger | 1 burger | 1830 | n/a | n/a | n/a | n/a | n/a | n/a | n/a | n/a |
| Navajo Sandwich | 1 sandwich | 1790 | n/a | n/a | n/a | n/a | n/a | n/a | n/a | n/a |
| Old Fashioned Burger | 1 burger | 1410 | n/a | n/a | n/a | n/a | n/a | n/a | n/a | n/a |
| Rene's Special Sandwich | 1 sandwich | 1810 | n/a | n/a | n/a | n/a | n/a | n/a | n/a | n/a |
| Smokehouse B.B.Q. Burger | 1 burger | 1840 | n/a | n/a | n/a | n/a | n/a | n/a | n/a | n/a |
| Sonoma Burger | 1 burger | 1870 | n/a | n/a | n/a | n/a | n/a | n/a | n/a | n/a |
| Spicy Chicken Sandwich | 1 sandwich | 1740 | n/a | n/a | n/a | n/a | n/a | n/a | n/a | n/a |
| **LUNCH SPECIALS** | | | | | | | | | | |
| Chicken Specials | 1 entrée | 1750 | n/a | n/a | n/a | n/a | n/a | n/a | n/a | n/a |
| Pasta | 1 entrée | 1710 | n/a | n/a | n/a | n/a | n/a | n/a | n/a | n/a |
| Renee's Special | 1 entrée | 1810 | n/a | n/a | n/a | n/a | n/a | n/a | n/a | n/a |
| Salad | 1 entrée | 1340 | n/a | n/a | n/a | n/a | n/a | n/a | n/a | n/a |
| Salmon | 1 entrée | 1390 | n/a | n/a | n/a | n/a | n/a | n/a | n/a | n/a |
| **PASTAS** | | | | | | | | | | |
| Bistro Shrimp | 1 entrée | 2730 | n/a | n/a | n/a | n/a | n/a | n/a | n/a | n/a |
| Cajun Jambalaya | 1 entrée | 1300 | n/a | n/a | n/a | n/a | n/a | n/a | n/a | n/a |
| Evelyn's Favorite | 1 entrée | 1680 | n/a | n/a | n/a | n/a | n/a | n/a | n/a | n/a |
| Farfalle w/Chicken & Roasted Garlic | 1 entrée | 2600 | n/a | n/a | n/a | n/a | n/a | n/a | n/a | n/a |
| Fettuccini Alfredo | 1 entrée | 2020 | n/a | n/a | n/a | n/a | n/a | n/a | n/a | n/a |
| Fettuccini Alfredo w/Chicken | 1 entrée | 2300 | n/a | n/a | n/a | n/a | n/a | n/a | n/a | n/a |
| Four Cheese | 1 entrée | 1300 | n/a | n/a | n/a | n/a | n/a | n/a | n/a | n/a |
| Garlic Noodles | 1 entrée | 1540 | n/a | n/a | n/a | n/a | n/a | n/a | n/a | n/a |
| Pasta Carbonara | 1 entrée | 2220 | n/a | n/a | n/a | n/a | n/a | n/a | n/a | n/a |
| Pasta Da Vinci | 1 entrée | 2000 | n/a | n/a | n/a | n/a | n/a | n/a | n/a | n/a |
| Pasta Marinara | 1 entrée | 1100 | n/a | n/a | n/a | n/a | n/a | n/a | n/a | n/a |
| Pasta w/Meat Sauce | 1 entrée | 1140 | n/a | n/a | n/a | n/a | n/a | n/a | n/a | n/a |
| Shrimp w/Angel Hair | 1 entrée | 1150 | n/a | n/a | n/a | n/a | n/a | n/a | n/a | n/a |
| Spicy Chicken Chipotle | 1 entrée | 1930 | n/a | n/a | n/a | n/a | n/a | n/a | n/a | n/a |
| Thai Chicken | 1 entrée | 1780 | n/a | n/a | n/a | n/a | n/a | n/a | n/a | n/a |
| **PIZZAS** | | | | | | | | | | |
| B.B.Q. Chicken | 1 pizza | 1580 | n/a | n/a | n/a | n/a | n/a | n/a | n/a | n/a |
| Cheese | 1 pizza | 1320 | n/a | n/a | n/a | n/a | n/a | n/a | n/a | n/a |
| Chicken & Mushroom | 1 pizza | 1670 | n/a | n/a | n/a | n/a | n/a | n/a | n/a | n/a |

| | SERVING SIZE | CAL | CAL FAT | TOT FAT (G) | SAT FAT (G) | CHOL (MG) | SOD (MG) | CARB (G) | FIBER (G) | PROT (G) |
|---|---|---|---|---|---|---|---|---|---|---|
| Four Seasons | 1 pizza | 1640 | n/a | n/a | n/a | n/a | n/a | n/a | n/a | n/a |
| Hawaiian | 1 pizza | 1380 | n/a | n/a | n/a | n/a | n/a | n/a | n/a | n/a |
| Pepperoni | 1 pizza | 1470 | n/a | n/a | n/a | n/a | n/a | n/a | n/a | n/a |
| Roasted Vegetables & Goat Cheese | 1 pizza | 1430 | n/a | n/a | n/a | n/a | n/a | n/a | n/a | n/a |
| Spicy Meat | 1 pizza | 1720 | n/a | n/a | n/a | n/a | n/a | n/a | n/a | n/a |
| The Everything | 1 pizza | 1590 | n/a | n/a | n/a | n/a | n/a | n/a | n/a | n/a |
| Tomato, Basil & Cheese | 1 pizza | 1330 | n/a | n/a | n/a | n/a | n/a | n/a | n/a | n/a |
| White Cheese | 1 pizza | 1530 | n/a | n/a | n/a | n/a | n/a | n/a | n/a | n/a |
| **SALADS** | | | | | | | | | | |
| Barbecue Ranch Chicken | 1 salad | 1740 | n/a | n/a | n/a | n/a | n/a | n/a | n/a | n/a |
| Caesar | 1 salad | 1360 | n/a | n/a | n/a | n/a | n/a | n/a | n/a | n/a |
| Chinese Chicken | 1 salad | 1730 | n/a | n/a | n/a | n/a | n/a | n/a | n/a | n/a |
| Cobb | 1 salad | 1610 | n/a | n/a | n/a | n/a | n/a | n/a | n/a | n/a |
| Grilled Chicken Tostada | 1 salad | 1540 | n/a | n/a | n/a | n/a | n/a | n/a | n/a | n/a |
| Herb Crusted Salmon | 1 salad | 780 | n/a | n/a | n/a | n/a | n/a | n/a | n/a | n/a |
| Luau | 1 salad | 1120 | n/a | n/a | n/a | n/a | n/a | n/a | n/a | n/a |
| Santa Fe | 1 salad | 1820 | n/a | n/a | n/a | n/a | n/a | n/a | n/a | n/a |
| Seared Tuna Tatkai | 1 salad | 550 | n/a | n/a | n/a | n/a | n/a | n/a | n/a | n/a |
| **SIDE DISHES** | | | | | | | | | | |
| Corn Succotash | as served | 300 | n/a | n/a | n/a | n/a | n/a | n/a | n/a | n/a |
| French Fries | as served | 560 | n/a | n/a | n/a | n/a | n/a | n/a | n/a | n/a |
| Macaroni & Cheese | as served | 1230 | n/a | n/a | n/a | n/a | n/a | n/a | n/a | n/a |
| Mashed Potatoes | as served | 560 | n/a | n/a | n/a | n/a | n/a | n/a | n/a | n/a |
| **SMALL PLATES & SNACKS** | | | | | | | | | | |
| Ahi Tartare | as served | 380 | n/a | n/a | n/a | n/a | n/a | n/a | n/a | n/a |
| Arugula Salad | 1 salad | 710 | n/a | n/a | n/a | n/a | n/a | n/a | n/a | n/a |
| Beets w/Goat Cheese | as served | 270 | n/a | n/a | n/a | n/a | n/a | n/a | n/a | n/a |
| Crispy Artichoke Hearts | as served | 680 | n/a | n/a | n/a | n/a | n/a | n/a | n/a | n/a |
| Crispy Crab Bites | as served | 380 | n/a | n/a | n/a | n/a | n/a | n/a | n/a | n/a |
| Crispy Fried Cheese | as served | 510 | n/a | n/a | n/a | n/a | n/a | n/a | n/a | n/a |
| Endive Salad | as served | 430 | n/a | n/a | n/a | n/a | n/a | n/a | n/a | n/a |
| Greek Salad | as served | 710 | n/a | n/a | n/a | n/a | n/a | n/a | n/a | n/a |
| Hand Battered Onion Rings | as served | 520 | n/a | n/a | n/a | n/a | n/a | n/a | n/a | n/a |
| Margherita Pizzette | as served | 650 | n/a | n/a | n/a | n/a | n/a | n/a | n/a | n/a |
| Mini Corn Dogs | as served | 550 | n/a | n/a | n/a | n/a | n/a | n/a | n/a | n/a |
| Roasted Pear & Blue Cheese Pizzette | as served | 680 | n/a | n/a | n/a | n/a | n/a | n/a | n/a | n/a |
| Sausage & Ricotta Pizzette | as served | 700 | n/a | n/a | n/a | n/a | n/a | n/a | n/a | n/a |

| | SERVING SIZE | CAL | CAL FAT | TOT FAT (G) | SAT FAT (G) | CHOL (MG) | SOD (MG) | CARB (G) | FIBER (G) | PROT (G) |
|---|---|---|---|---|---|---|---|---|---|---|
| Shitake Asparagus & Bacon Pizzette | as served | 640 | n/a | n/a | n/a | n/a | n/a | n/a | n/a | n/a |
| Shrimp Scampi Crostini | as served | 410 | n/a | n/a | n/a | n/a | n/a | n/a | n/a | n/a |
| Stuffed Mushrooms | as served | 520 | n/a | n/a | n/a | n/a | n/a | n/a | n/a | n/a |
| Sweet Corn Fritters | as served | 570 | n/a | n/a | n/a | n/a | n/a | n/a | n/a | n/a |
| White Bean Hummus | as served | 850 | n/a | n/a | n/a | n/a | n/a | n/a | n/a | n/a |
| Wild Mushroom Pizzette | as served | 600 | n/a | n/a | n/a | n/a | n/a | n/a | n/a | n/a |
| **SPECIAL MENU** | | | | | | | | | | |
| Bar-B-Que Salmon | 1 entrée | 1210 | n/a | n/a | n/a | n/a | n/a | n/a | n/a | n/a |
| Caramel Chicken | 1 entrée | 1790 | n/a | n/a | n/a | n/a | n/a | n/a | n/a | n/a |
| Cashew Chicken Salad | 1 entrée | 1360 | n/a | n/a | n/a | n/a | n/a | n/a | n/a | n/a |
| Chargrilled Coulotte Steak | 1 entrée | 1420 | n/a | n/a | n/a | n/a | n/a | n/a | n/a | n/a |
| Chicken Bellagio | 1 entrée | 2130 | n/a | n/a | n/a | n/a | n/a | n/a | n/a | n/a |
| Chicken Enchiladas | 1 entrée | 1540 | n/a | n/a | n/a | n/a | n/a | n/a | n/a | n/a |
| Fried Shrimp Platter | 1 entrée | 1830 | n/a | n/a | n/a | n/a | n/a | n/a | n/a | n/a |
| New Orleans Shrimp | 1 entrée | 1200 | n/a | n/a | n/a | n/a | n/a | n/a | n/a | n/a |
| Salisbury Chipped Steak | 1 entrée | 1300 | n/a | n/a | n/a | n/a | n/a | n/a | n/a | n/a |
| Shrimp Franchese | 1 entrée | 1390 | n/a | n/a | n/a | n/a | n/a | n/a | n/a | n/a |
| Tomato Basil Pasta | 1 entrée | 1740 | n/a | n/a | n/a | n/a | n/a | n/a | n/a | n/a |
| **SPECIALTIES** | | | | | | | | | | |
| Bang-Bang Chicken & Shrimp | 1 entrée | 1660 | n/a | n/a | n/a | n/a | n/a | n/a | n/a | n/a |
| Beer Battered Fish & Chips | 1 entrée | 1440 | n/a | n/a | n/a | n/a | n/a | n/a | n/a | n/a |
| Cajun Chicken "Littles" | 1 entrée | 1840 | n/a | n/a | n/a | n/a | n/a | n/a | n/a | n/a |
| Chicken & Biscuits | 1 entrée | 2580 | n/a | n/a | n/a | n/a | n/a | n/a | n/a | n/a |
| Chicken Madeira | 1 entrée | 1650 | n/a | n/a | n/a | n/a | n/a | n/a | n/a | n/a |
| Chicken Marsala & Mushrooms | 1 entrée | 2040 | n/a | n/a | n/a | n/a | n/a | n/a | n/a | n/a |
| Chicken Piccata | 1 entrée | 1860 | n/a | n/a | n/a | n/a | n/a | n/a | n/a | n/a |
| Crispy Chicken Costoletta | 1 entrée | 2540 | n/a | n/a | n/a | n/a | n/a | n/a | n/a | n/a |
| Crispy Spicy Beef | 1 entrée | 1760 | n/a | n/a | n/a | n/a | n/a | n/a | n/a | n/a |
| Factory Burrito Grande | 1 entrée | 1920 | n/a | n/a | n/a | n/a | n/a | n/a | n/a | n/a |
| Famous Factory Meatloaf | 1 entrée | 1630 | n/a | n/a | n/a | n/a | n/a | n/a | n/a | n/a |
| Fresh Fish Tacos | 1 entrée | 1620 | n/a | n/a | n/a | n/a | n/a | n/a | n/a | n/a |
| Grilled Chicken Medallions | 1 entrée | 1470 | n/a | n/a | n/a | n/a | n/a | n/a | n/a | n/a |
| Lemon-Herb Roasted Chicken | 1 entrée | 1710 | n/a | n/a | n/a | n/a | n/a | n/a | n/a | n/a |
| Orange Chicken | 1 entrée | 1800 | n/a | n/a | n/a | n/a | n/a | n/a | n/a | n/a |
| Shepherd's Pie | 1 entrée | 1770 | n/a | n/a | n/a | n/a | n/a | n/a | n/a | n/a |
| Spicy Cashew Chicken | 1 entrée | 2250 | n/a | n/a | n/a | n/a | n/a | n/a | n/a | n/a |
| Stuffed Chicken Tortillas | 1 entrée | 1950 | n/a | n/a | n/a | n/a | n/a | n/a | n/a | n/a |

| | SERVING SIZE | CAL | CAL FAT | TOT FAT (G) | SAT FAT (G) | CHOL (MG) | SOD (MG) | CARB (G) | FIBER (G) | PROT (G) |
|---|---|---|---|---|---|---|---|---|---|---|
| Teriyaki Chicken | 1 entrée | 1330 | n/a | n/a | n/a | n/a | n/a | n/a | n/a | n/a |
| Weight Management Grilled Chicken | 1 entrée | 590 | n/a | n/a | n/a | n/a | n/a | n/a | n/a | n/a |
| White Chicken Chili | 1 entrée | 850 | n/a | n/a | n/a | n/a | n/a | n/a | n/a | n/a |
| **SPECIALTY DESSERTS** | | | | | | | | | | |
| Black-Out Cake | 1 slice | 1270 | n/a | n/a | n/a | n/a | n/a | n/a | n/a | n/a |
| Carrot Cake | 1 slice | 1550 | n/a | n/a | n/a | n/a | n/a | n/a | n/a | n/a |
| Chocolate Tower Truffle Cake | 1 slice | 1670 | n/a | n/a | n/a | n/a | n/a | n/a | n/a | n/a |
| Factory Mud Pie | 1 slice | 2120 | n/a | n/a | n/a | n/a | n/a | n/a | n/a | n/a |
| Fresh Strawberry Shortcake | 1 slice | 1040 | n/a | n/a | n/a | n/a | n/a | n/a | n/a | n/a |
| Godiva Chocolate Brownie Sundae | 1 slice | 1100 | n/a | n/a | n/a | n/a | n/a | n/a | n/a | n/a |
| Lemoncello Cream Torte | 1 slice | 1060 | n/a | n/a | n/a | n/a | n/a | n/a | n/a | n/a |
| Tiramisu | 1 slice | 950 | n/a | n/a | n/a | n/a | n/a | n/a | n/a | n/a |
| Warm Apple Crisp | 1 slice | 1420 | n/a | n/a | n/a | n/a | n/a | n/a | n/a | n/a |
| **STEAKS & CHOPS** | | | | | | | | | | |
| Beef Ribs | 1 entrée | 2360 | n/a | n/a | n/a | n/a | n/a | n/a | n/a | n/a |
| Carne Asada Skirt Steak | 1 entrée | 1500 | n/a | n/a | n/a | n/a | n/a | n/a | n/a | n/a |
| Charbroiled Flat Iron Steak | 1 entrée | 1430 | n/a | n/a | n/a | n/a | n/a | n/a | n/a | n/a |
| Grilled Pork Chops | 1 entrée | 1910 | n/a | n/a | n/a | n/a | n/a | n/a | n/a | n/a |
| Grilled Rib-Eye Steak | 1 entrée | 1640 | n/a | n/a | n/a | n/a | n/a | n/a | n/a | n/a |
| Grilled Rib-Eye Steak, Cajun Style | 1 entrée | 1850 | n/a | n/a | n/a | n/a | n/a | n/a | n/a | n/a |
| Hibachi Steak | 1 entrée | 1700 | n/a | n/a | n/a | n/a | n/a | n/a | n/a | n/a |
| Steak Diane | 1 entrée | 1630 | n/a | n/a | n/a | n/a | n/a | n/a | n/a | n/a |
| **SUNDAY BRUNCH** | | | | | | | | | | |
| Brunch Combo | 1 entrée | 1530 | n/a | n/a | n/a | n/a | n/a | n/a | n/a | n/a |
| Buttermilk Pancakes | 1 entrée | 1210 | n/a | n/a | n/a | n/a | n/a | n/a | n/a | n/a |
| Eggs Benedict | 1 entrée | 1710 | n/a | n/a | n/a | n/a | n/a | n/a | n/a | n/a |
| French Toast | 1 entrée | 2080 | n/a | n/a | n/a | n/a | n/a | n/a | n/a | n/a |
| Giant Belgian Waffles | 1 entrée | 830 | n/a | n/a | n/a | n/a | n/a | n/a | n/a | n/a |
| Lemon-Ricotta Pancakes | 1 entrée | 1320 | n/a | n/a | n/a | n/a | n/a | n/a | n/a | n/a |
| Monte Cristo Sandwich | 1 entrée | 2640 | n/a | n/a | n/a | n/a | n/a | n/a | n/a | n/a |
| Smoked Salmon Platter | 1 entrée | 730 | n/a | n/a | n/a | n/a | n/a | n/a | n/a | n/a |
| Steak & Eggs | 1 entrée | 1920 | n/a | n/a | n/a | n/a | n/a | n/a | n/a | n/a |
| **WEIGHT MANAGEMENT SALADS** | | | | | | | | | | |
| Asian Chicken | 1 salad | 540 | n/a | n/a | n/a | n/a | n/a | n/a | n/a | n/a |
| Pear & Endive | 1 salad | 460 | n/a | n/a | n/a | n/a | n/a | n/a | n/a | n/a |
| Spicy Chicken | 1 salad | 440 | n/a | n/a | n/a | n/a | n/a | n/a | n/a | n/a |

# restaurants

| | SERVING SIZE | CAL | CAL FAT | TOT FAT (G) | SAT FAT (G) | CHOL (MG) | SOD (MG) | CARB (G) | FIBER (G) | PROT (G) |
|---|---|---|---|---|---|---|---|---|---|---|
| **Chick-fil-A** | | | | | | | | | | |
| **BREAKFAST** | | | | | | | | | | |
| Bacon, Egg & Cheese Biscuit | 6 oz | 500 | 240 | 27 | 12 | 230 | 1370 | 43 | 2 | 21 |
| Biscuit | 3 oz | 310 | 120 | 13 | 6 | 0 | 700 | 41 | 2 | 5 |
| Chicken Biscuit | 5 oz | 440 | 180 | 20 | 8 | 25 | 1240 | 47 | 3 | 17 |
| Chicken Breakfast Burrito | 7 oz | 450 | 180 | 20 | 8 | 260 | 990 | 43 | 2 | 24 |
| Cinnamon Cluster | 4 oz | 430 | 150 | 17 | 7 | 30 | 240 | 63 | 2 | 7 |
| Egg & Cheese Bagel (& Chicken) | 7 oz | 480 | 180 | 20 | 6 | 240 | 1230 | 49 | 3 | 29 |
| Hash Brown | 3 oz | 280 | 170 | 19 | 4 | 0 | 410 | 25 | 2 | 3 |
| Sausage Biscuit | 5 oz | 590 | 370 | 41 | 16 | 50 | 1250 | 42 | 2 | 16 |
| Sausage Breakfast Burrito | 7 oz | 510 | 260 | 29 | 12 | 270 | 970 | 40 | 2 | 23 |
| Yogurt Parfait | 8 oz | 230 | 25 | 3 | 2 | 10 | 60 | 44 | 0 | 6 |
| **CHICKEN** | | | | | | | | | | |
| Chargrilled Chicken Club Sandwich | 9 oz | 410 | 110 | 12 | 5 | 80 | 1460 | 39 | 3 | 37 |
| Chicken Salad Sandwich | 8 oz | 500 | 180 | 20 | 3.5 | 80 | 1240 | 52 | 4 | 29 |
| Chicken Sandwich | 6 oz | 430 | 150 | 17 | 3.5 | 65 | 1370 | 39 | 3 | 31 |
| Nuggets-12 Count | 6 oz | 400 | 160 | 17 | 3.5 | 105 | 1480 | 18 | 1 | 42 |
| Spicy Chicken Sandwich | 7 oz | 490 | 180 | 20 | 4 | 60 | 1730 | 46 | 4 | 31 |
| **SALADS** | | | | | | | | | | |
| Carrot & Raisin, Large | 9 oz | 390 | 160 | 18 | 2.5 | 10 | 240 | 60 | 5 | 2 |
| Chargrilled & Fruit | 12 oz | 230 | 60 | 6 | 3.5 | 55 | 650 | 23 | 4 | 22 |
| Chargrilled Chicken Garden | 10-1/2 oz | 180 | 60 | 6 | 3.5 | 55 | 650 | 11 | 4 | 22 |
| Chick-N-Strips | 14 oz | 470 | 200 | 23 | 6 | 85 | 1340 | 27 | 4 | 41 |
| Side | 4 oz | 70 | 40 | 4.5 | 3 | 15 | 110 | 5 | 2 | 5 |
| Southwest Chargrilled | 11-1/2 oz | 240 | 80 | 9 | 4 | 60 | 820 | 18 | 5 | 26 |
| **SIDES** | | | | | | | | | | |
| Hearty Breast of Chicken Soup | 15-1/2 oz | 220 | 50 | 6 | 2 | 40 | 1760 | 30 | 3 | 12 |
| Waffle Potato Fries | 4-1/2 oz | 430 | 210 | 23 | 4.5 | 0 | 210 | 50 | 5 | 5 |
| **Chili's** | | | | | | | | | | |
| **APPETIZERS** | | | | | | | | | | |
| Boneless Buffalo Wings w/Bleu Cheese | as served | 1060 | n/a | 81 | 14 | n/a | 3330 | 44 | 2 | 38 |
| Bottomless Tostado Chips w/Salsa | as served | 1020 | n/a | 51 | 10 | n/a | 1210 | 125 | 11 | 12 |
| Crispy Onion String & Jalapeno Stack w/Jalapeno Ranch | as served | 1020 | n/a | 86 | 13 | n/a | 1780 | 49 | 6 | 8 |
| Fried Cheese | as served | 730 | n/a | 39 | 17 | n/a | 2270 | 60 | 2 | 33 |
| Hot Spinach & Artichoke Dip w/Chips | as served | 1640 | n/a | 102 | 43 | n/a | 1630 | 41 | 11 | 31 |
| Loaded Nachos w/Beef | as served | 1150 | n/a | 82 | 38 | n/a | 3340 | 42 | 5 | 61 |

| | SERVING SIZE | CAL | CAL FAT | TOT FAT (G) | SAT FAT (G) | CHOL (MG) | SOD (MG) | CARB (G) | FIBER (G) | PROT (G) |
|---|---|---|---|---|---|---|---|---|---|---|
| Loaded Nachos w/Chicken | as served | 1060 | n/a | 66 | 32 | n/a | 2680 | 44 | 5 | 82 |
| Skillet Queso w/Chips | as served | 1500 | n/a | 73 | 30 | n/a | 3340 | 46 | 9 | 40 |
| Southwestern Eggrolls w/Avocado Ranch | as served | 910 | n/a | 57 | 14 | n/a | 1980 | 72 | 7 | 27 |
| Texas Cheese Fries w/Jalapeno Ranch | as served | 1930 | n/a | 135 | 62 | n/a | 5530 | 97 | 11 | 86 |
| Triple Dipper Big Mouth Bites w/Jalapeno Ranch | as served | 740 | n/a | 48 | 13 | n/a | 1760 | 46 | 1 | 30 |
| Triple Dipper Chicken Crispers No Dressing | as served | 320 | n/a | 14 | 5 | n/a | 1040 | 19 | 1 | 27 |
| Triple Dipper Hot Spinach & Artichoke Dip w/Chips | as served | 570 | n/a | 45 | 20 | n/a | 1230 | 20 | 2 | 16 |
| **BURGERS W/FRIES** | | | | | | | | | | |
| Classic Bacon Burger | 1 burger | 1520 | n/a | 88 | 26 | n/a | 3630 | 115 | 9 | 63 |
| Jalapeno Smokehouse w/Jalapeno Ranch | 1 burger | 2130 | n/a | 139 | 43 | n/a | 6460 | 127 | 10 | 92 |
| **ENTRÉES** | | | | | | | | | | |
| Cajun Pasta w/Grilled Shrimp, w/Sides | 1 entrée | 1310 | n/a | 75 | 40 | n/a | 3350 | 105 | 6 | 50 |
| Cheese Quesadilla, w/o Sides | 1 entrée | 460 | n/a | 24 | 12 | n/a | 1000 | 42 | 2 | 20 |
| Chicken Crispers w/Honey Mustard, w/Sides | 1 entrée | 1750 | n/a | 109 | 16 | n/a | 4690 | 136 | 10 | 54 |
| Classic Sirloin, w/o Sides | 1 entrée | 310 | n/a | 19 | 9 | n/a | 1440 | 4 | 1 | 31 |
| Country Fried Steak, w/Sides | 1 entrée | 1440 | n/a | 83 | 15 | n/a | 3220 | 123 | 10 | 52 |
| Fried Shrimp w/Tequila Lime Sauce, w/o Sides | 1 entrée | 400 | n/a | 28 | 5 | n/a | 1130 | 18 | 8 | 19 |
| Grilled Salmon w/Garlic & Herbs, w/o Sides | 1 entrée | 370 | n/a | 23 | 8 | n/a | 560 | 1 | 0 | 41 |
| Half Rack of Baby Back Ribs, w/o Sides | 1 entrée | 560 | n/a | 41 | 13 | n/a | 2050 | 17 | 1 | 28 |
| Macaroni & Cheese, w/o Sides | 1 entrée | 400 | n/a | 10 | 6 | n/a | 1160 | 68 | 3 | 14 |
| Monterey Chicken, w/o Sides | 1 entrée | 470 | n/a | 25 | 13 | n/a | 1140 | 13 | 2 | 50 |
| Original Ribs, w/o Sides | 1 entrée | 1110 | n/a | 81 | 27 | n/a | 4100 | 33 | 2 | 57 |
| **FAJITAS** | | | | | | | | | | |
| Beef w/o Tortillas & Condiments, w/Sides | 1 entrée | 470 | n/a | 25 | 5 | n/a | 2810 | 26 | 5 | 47 |
| Buffalo Chicken w/o Tortillas & Condiments, w/Sides | 1 entrée | 1040 | n/a | 76 | 17 | n/a | 4800 | 43 | 5 | 45 |
| TRIO w/o Tortillas & Condiments, w/Sides | 1 entrée | 530 | n/a | 26 | 7 | n/a | 2760 | 28 | 6 | 53 |
| Flame-Grilled Ribeye, w/o Sides | 1 entrée | 900 | n/a | 68 | 32 | n/a | 1980 | 18 | 2 | 50 |
| **SALADS** | | | | | | | | | | |
| Asian Salad w/Grilled Chicken | 1 salad | 540 | n/a | 33 | 5 | n/a | 2110 | 40 | 8 | 29 |
| Asian Salad w/Salmon | 1 salad | 650 | n/a | 42 | 9 | n/a | 2310 | 40 | 8 | 32 |
| Boneless Buffalo Chicken Salad | 1 salad | 1150 | n/a | 84 | 17 | n/a | 4410 | 52 | 7 | 45 |
| Caribbean Salad w/Grilled Chicken | 1 salad | 560 | n/a | 24 | 4 | n/a | 470 | 64 | 7 | 24 |
| Chicken Caesar Salad | 1 salad | 710 | n/a | 42 | 8 | n/a | 1010 | 25 | 6 | 58 |

# restaurants

| | SERVING SIZE | CAL | CAL. FAT | TOT FAT (G) | SAT FAT (G) | CHOL (MG) | SOD (MG) | CARB (G) | FIBER (G) | PROT (G) |
|---|---|---|---|---|---|---|---|---|---|---|
| Grilled BBQ Chicken Salad | 1 salad | 1060 | n/a | 63 | 19 | n/a | 2190 | 50 | 12 | 76 |
| House Salad No Dressing | 1 salad | 100 | n/a | 3 | 0 | n/a | 135 | 17 | 3 | 4 |
| Quesadilla Explosion Salad | 1 salad | 1400 | n/a | 88 | 26 | n/a | 2360 | 90 | 12 | 66 |
| **SANDWICHES** | | | | | | | | | | |
| BBQ Pulled Pork Sandwich w/Fries | 1 sandwich | 1250 | n/a | 53 | 14 | n/a | 3300 | 147 | 10 | 41 |
| Buffalo Chicken Ranch Sandwich w/Fries | 1 sandwich | 1560 | n/a | 86 | 14 | n/a | 4010 | 141 | 9 | 49 |
| Grilled Chicken Sandwich w/Fries | 1 sandwich | 1240 | n/a | 62 | 14 | n/a | 2510 | 114 | 9 | 56 |
| Smoked Turkey on Chile-Pepper Roll w/Fries | 1 sandwich | 1230 | n/a | 58 | 12 | n/a | 3230 | 118 | 7 | 39 |
| Steakhouse Sandwich w/Fries | 1 sandwich | 1080 | n/a | 51 | 20 | n/a | 3780 | 115 | 11 | 38 |
| **SOUPS & CHILIS** | | | | | | | | | | |
| Black Bean Soup | 1 cup | 150 | n/a | 4 | 2 | n/a | 740 | 20 | 5 | 8 |
| Broccoli Cheese Soup | 1 cup | 120 | n/a | 8 | 4 | n/a | 640 | 8 | 1 | 5 |
| Chicken Enchilada Soup | 1 cup | 220 | n/a | 13 | 5 | n/a | 670 | 11 | 1 | 14 |
| Loaded Baked Potato Soup | 1 cup | 140 | n/a | 7 | 5 | n/a | 580 | 14 | 1 | 6 |
| Southwestern Vegetable Soup | 1 cup | 110 | n/a | 5 | 3 | n/a | 600 | 11 | 2 | 4 |
| **TACOS** | | | | | | | | | | |
| Crispy Chicken Tacos w/Corn Tortillas | 1 taco | 1120 | n/a | 48 | 13 | n/a | 2820 | 115 | 13 | 59 |
| Crispy Shrimp Tacos w/Corn Tortillas | 1 taco | 830 | n/a | 28 | 5 | n/a | 2620 | 111 | 21 | 34 |
| Crispy Shrimp Tacos w/Flour Tortillas | 1 taco | 950 | n/a | 33 | 7 | n/a | 3260 | 126 | 21 | 37 |
| Pulled Pork Tacos w/Corn Tortillas | 1 taco | 800 | n/a | 22 | 8 | n/a | 2870 | 99 | 12 | 52 |
| Pulled Pork Tacos w/Flour Tortillas | 1 taco | 920 | n/a | 27 | 9 | n/a | 3500 | 114 | 12 | 55 |
| Smoked Chicken Tacos w/Corn Tortillas | 1 taco | 700 | n/a | 15 | 6 | n/a | 3060 | 98 | 12 | 45 |
| Smoked Chicken Tacos w/Flour Tortillas | 1 taco | 820 | n/a | 20 | 8 | n/a | 3700 | 113 | 12 | 49 |
| **Chipotle Mexican Grill** | | | | | | | | | | |
| **INGREDIENTS** | | | | | | | | | | |
| Flour Tortilla (burrito) | 1 tortilla | 290 | 80 | 9 | 3 | 0 | 670 | 44 | 2 | 7 |
| Barbacoa | 4 oz | 170 | 60 | 7 | 2.5 | 60 | 510 | 2 | 0 | 24 |
| Black Beans | 4 oz | 120 | 10 | 1 | 0 | 0 | 250 | 23 | 11 | 7 |
| Carnitas | 4 oz | 190 | 70 | 8 | 2.5 | 70 | 540 | 1 | 0 | 27 |
| Chicken | 4 oz | 190 | 60 | 6.5 | 2 | 115 | 370 | 1 | 0 | 32 |
| Cilantro Lime Rice | 3 oz | 130 | 30 | 3 | .5 | 0 | 150 | 23 | 0 | 2 |
| Corn Salsa | 3-1/2 oz | 80 | 15 | 1.5 | 0 | 0 | 410 | 15 | 3 | 3 |
| Fajita Vegetables | 2-1/2 oz | 20 | 5 | .5 | 0 | 0 | 170 | 4 | 1 | 1 |
| Flour Tortilla (taco) | 1 tortilla | 90 | 25 | 2.5 | 1 | 0 | 200 | 13 | <1 | 2 |
| Pinto Beans | 4 oz | 120 | 10 | 1 | 0 | 5 | 330 | 22 | 10 | 7 |
| Steak | 4 oz | 190 | 60 | 6.5 | 2 | 65 | 320 | 2 | 0 | 30 |

# Chuck E Cheese

## PIZZA, MEDIUM

| | SERVING SIZE | CAL | CAL FAT | TOT FAT (G) | SAT FAT (G) | CHOL (MG) | SOD (MG) | CARB (G) | FIBER (G) | PROT (G) |
|---|---|---|---|---|---|---|---|---|---|---|
| All Meats Combo | 1 slice | 215 | 97 | 11 | 4 | 22 | 608 | 21 | 1 | 9 |
| BBQ Chicken | 1 slice | 185 | 51 | 6 | 2 | 13 | 460 | 24 | 1 | 8 |
| Cheese | 1 slice | 155 | 47 | 5 | 2 | 8 | 360 | 21 | 1 | 6 |
| Veggie Combo | 1 slice | 160 | 53 | 6 | 2 | 7 | 366 | 22 | 2 | 6 |

## PLATTERS

| | | | | | | | | | | |
|---|---|---|---|---|---|---|---|---|---|---|
| Sampler | 1/7 platter | 329 | 172 | 19 | 5 | 58 | 840 | 25 | 2 | 13 |
| Sandwich | 1 piece | 183 | 70 | 8 | 2 | 20 | 543 | 20 | 1 | 9 |
| Veggie | 1/8 platter | 129 | 96 | 11 | 2 | 12 | 264 | 7 | 2 | 2 |
| Wing | 1/6 platter | 300 | 168 | 20 | 4 | 104 | 1308 | 16 | 4 | 16 |

## OVEN BAKED SANDWICHES

| | | | | | | | | | | |
|---|---|---|---|---|---|---|---|---|---|---|
| Chicken Ciabatta | 1 sandwich | 715 | 252 | 28 | 7 | 86 | 1940 | 80 | 3 | 44 |
| Ham & Cheese | 1 sandwich | 685 | 241 | 27 | 8 | 68 | 2206 | 79 | 3 | 33 |
| Italian Sub | 1 sandwich | 790 | 349 | 39 | 12 | 83 | 2374 | 78 | 3 | 34 |

## SIDES & COMPLEMENTS

| | | | | | | | | | | |
|---|---|---|---|---|---|---|---|---|---|---|
| Breadsticks | 1 breadstick | 175 | 77 | 9 | 2 | 7 | 412 | 18 | 1 | 6 |
| Buffalo Wings | 1 wing | 75 | 42 | 5 | 1 | 26 | 327 | 4 | 1 | 4 |
| French Fries | 4 oz | 420 | 178 | 20 | 2 | 4 | 929 | 55 | 6 | 6 |
| Hot Dog | 1 hot dog | 310 | 168 | 19 | 7 | 32 | 1084 | 35 | 2 | 11 |
| Mozzarella Sticks | 1 piece | 93 | 55 | 6 | 2 | 7 | 211 | 6 | 0 | 4 |
| Side Pasta Salad | 6 oz | 150 | 35 | 4 | .5 | 0 | 280 | 24 | 1 | 4 |

# Church's Chicken

## CHICKEN

| | | | | | | | | | | |
|---|---|---|---|---|---|---|---|---|---|---|
| Breast | 1 piece | 200 | 99 | 11 | 3 | 80 | 450 | 3 | 1 | 21 |
| Nuggets | 5 pieces | 162 | 63 | 7 | 2 | 21 | 759 | 13 | 1 | 9 |
| Original Chicken Sandwich | 1 sandwich | 458 | 198 | 22 | 4 | 37 | 1241 | 48 | 3 | 16 |
| Original Leg | 1 piece | 110 | 54 | 6 | 2 | 55 | 280 | 3 | 0 | 10 |
| Original Thigh | 1 piece | 330 | 207 | 23 | 6 | 110 | 680 | 8 | 1 | 21 |
| Original Wing | 1 piece | 300 | 171 | 19 | 5 | 120 | 540 | 7 | 3 | 27 |
| Spicy Chicken Sandwich | 1 sandwich | 456 | 189 | 21 | 4 | 37 | 1292 | 47 | 3 | 15 |
| Spicy Tender Strips | 1 piece | 135 | 63 | 7 | 2 | 25 | 480 | 7 | 4 | 11 |
| Tender Strips | 1 piece | 120 | 54 | 6 | 2 | 35 | 440 | 6 | 0 | 12 |

## SIDES

| | | | | | | | | | | |
|---|---|---|---|---|---|---|---|---|---|---|
| Cole Slaw | 6 oz | 150 | 90 | 10 | 2 | 5 | 170 | 15 | 2 | 1 |
| French Fries | 3-1/2 oz | 290 | 126 | 14 | 3 | 0 | 320 | 38 | 4 | 3 |
| Jalapeño Cheese Bombs | 4 pieces | 240 | 90 | 10 | 6 | 30 | 970 | 29 | 3 | 8 |

# restaurants

| | SERVING SIZE | CAL | CAL FAT | TOT FAT (G) | SAT FAT (G) | CHOL (MG) | SOD (MG) | CARB (G) | FIBER (G) | PROT (G) |
|---|---|---|---|---|---|---|---|---|---|---|
| Macaroni & Cheese | 6 oz | 221 | 90 | 10 | 5 | 9 | 799 | 24 | 2 | 7 |
| Regular Mashed Potatoes & Gravy | 6 oz | 70 | 18 | 2 | 0 | 1 | 480 | 12 | 1 | 2 |

## CiCi's
### PIZZA, 12″

| | | | | | | | | | | |
|---|---|---|---|---|---|---|---|---|---|---|
| Buffalo Chicken | 1 slice | 140 | 40.5 | 4.5 | 1.5 | 10 | 460 | 19 | 1 | 6 |
| Cheese | 1 slice | 150 | 36 | 4 | 2 | 10 | 330 | 19 | 1 | 6 |
| Deep Dish | 1 slice | 170 | 54 | 6 | 3 | 15 | 330 | 19 | 1 | 7 |
| Macaroni & Cheese | 1 slice | 170 | 27 | 3 | 1 | 5 | 260 | 29 | 1 | 6 |
| Pepperoni | 1 slice | 160 | 40.5 | 4.5 | 2 | 10 | 370 | 20 | 1 | 6 |
| Sausage | 1 slice | 140 | 45 | 5 | 2 | 10 | 420 | 20 | 1 | 6 |
| Thin Crust Italiano | 2 slices | 190 | 99 | 11 | 4 | 20 | 470 | 17 | 1 | 7 |
| Zesty Veggie | 1 slice | 130 | 36 | 4 | 1 | 5 | 320 | 20 | 1 | 4 |

### SIDES

| | | | | | | | | | | |
|---|---|---|---|---|---|---|---|---|---|---|
| Garlic Bread | 1 slice | 100 | 45 | 5 | 1.5 | 5 | 120 | 10 | 0 | 4 |

## Cinnabon

| | | | | | | | | | | |
|---|---|---|---|---|---|---|---|---|---|---|
| Bites, 4 ct. | 1 bun | 350 | 130 | 15 | 7 | 5 | 330 | 51 | 1 | 5 |
| Classic | 1 bun | 880 | 320 | 36 | 17 | 20 | 830 | 127 | 2 | 13 |
| Classic Pack, 4 pk | 4 buns | 3760 | 1430 | 160 | 76 | 85 | 3470 | 538 | 9 | 52 |
| Combo Pack, 4 pk | 4 buns | 4050 | 1620 | 181 | 78 | 95 | 3650 | 563 | 11 | 54 |
| Frosting Cup | 1 item | 180 | 100 | 11 | 6 | 10 | 105 | 20 | 0 | 1 |
| Minibon | 1 bun | 350 | 130 | 14 | 7 | 5 | 330 | 51 | 1 | 5 |
| Pecanbon Bites, 4 ct. | 1 bun | 480 | 220 | 25 | 9 | 10 | 410 | 60 | 2 | 6 |
| Pecanbon Pack, 4 pk | 4 buns | 4330 | 1810 | 202 | 81 | 110 | 3840 | 587 | 14 | 57 |
| Stix | 5 stixs | 390 | 190 | 21 | 9 | 20 | 440 | 46 | 1 | 6 |

## Cold Stone Creamery
### CAKES & COOKIES

| | | | | | | | | | | |
|---|---|---|---|---|---|---|---|---|---|---|
| Cookie Sandwich Kiss 'N' Tell | 1 sandwich | 550 | 230 | 25 | 13 | 55 | 490 | 74 | 1 | 5 |
| Cupcake Double Chocolate Devotion | 1 sandwich | 360 | 170 | 19 | 13 | 15 | 160 | 45 | 2 | 4 |
| Cupcake Sweet Cream | 1 cupcake | 390 | 190 | 21 | 15 | 30 | 135 | 48 | 2 | 8 |
| Ice Cream Cake Cookie Dough Delirium, 6″ | 1 slice | 520 | 240 | 26 | 15 | 55 | 220 | 62 | 1 | 6 |
| Ice Cream Cake Cookies & Creamery, 6″ | 1 slice | 400 | 180 | 20 | 12 | 45 | 300 | 48 | 1 | 6 |

### ICE CREAM, FROZEN
### YOGURT, & SORBET

| | | | | | | | | | | |
|---|---|---|---|---|---|---|---|---|---|---|
| Black Cherry | 8 oz | 530 | 270 | 30 | 19 | 120 | 120 | 58 | 0 | 8 |
| Blueberry | 8 oz | 510 | 280 | 31 | 21 | 120 | 90 | 53 | 0 | 9 |
| Chocolate | 8 oz | 520 | 290 | 32 | 20 | 125 | 160 | 53 | 2 | 9 |
| Chocolate Cake Batter | 8 oz | 550 | 270 | 30 | 18 | 110 | 340 | 68 | 2 | 9 |

| | SERVING SIZE | CAL | CAL FAT | TOT FAT (G) | SAT FAT (G) | CHOL (MG) | SOD (MG) | CARB (G) | FIBER (G) | PROT (G) |
|---|---|---|---|---|---|---|---|---|---|---|
| Chocolate Peanut Butter | 8 oz | 660 | 400 | 45 | 21 | 35 | 320 | 58 | 4 | 16 |
| Coffee | 8 oz | 530 | 280 | 31 | 20 | 125 | 125 | 54 | 0 | 8 |
| Cookie Batter | 8 oz | 580 | 280 | 33 | 19 | 65 | 430 | 68 | 1 | 7 |
| Fudge Brownie Batter | 8 oz | 550 | 270 | 30 | 19 | 45 | 200 | 69 | 2 | 8 |
| Mint | 8 oz | 530 | 270 | 30 | 19 | 120 | 120 | 57 | 0 | 8 |
| Peach | 8 oz | 500 | 210 | 23 | 16 | 90 | 70 | 71 | 0 | 7 |
| Pecan Praline | 8 oz | 530 | 270 | 30 | 19 | 115 | 150 | 58 | 0 | 8 |
| Raspberry Sorbet | 8 oz | 260 | 0 | 0 | 0 | 0 | 30 | 67 | 0 | 0 |
| Strawberry Mango Banana Sorbet | 8 oz | 350 | 0 | 0 | 0 | 0 | 25 | 87 | 1 | 0 |
| Tart & Tangy Frozen Yogurt | 8 oz | 230 | 0 | 0 | 0 | 0 | 115 | 53 | 0 | 5 |
| Tart & Tangy Berry Frozen Yogurt | 8 oz | 240 | 0 | 0 | 0 | 0 | 105 | 58 | 0 | 5 |
| Vanilla Bean | 8 oz | 530 | 280 | 31 | 19 | 120 | 120 | 52 | 0 | 8 |
| **MIX-INS** | | | | | | | | | | |
| Apple Pie Filling | 3/4 oz | 90 | 0 | 0 | 0 | 0 | 25 | 16 | 1 | 0 |
| Chocolate Chips | 1 oz | 130 | 60 | 7 | 4.5 | 0 | 0 | 16 | 1 | 1 |
| Chocolate Shavings | 1/2 oz | 90 | 45 | 5 | 3 | 0 | 0 | 9 | 2 | 1 |
| Cookie Dough | 1 oz | 180 | 70 | 8 | 2.5 | 5 | 150 | 26 | 0 | 1 |
| Graham Cracker Pie Crust | 1 oz | 130 | 50 | 6 | 2.5 | 0 | 135 | 17 | 1 | 1 |
| Peanut Butter | 3/4 oz | 150 | 120 | 13 | 2.5 | 0 | 125 | 5 | 1 | 6 |
| **SHAKES & SMOOTHIES** | | | | | | | | | | |
| Shake, Cherry CheeseShake, Love it Size | 20 fl oz | 1290 | 590 | 66 | 42 | 260 | 310 | 157 | 1 | 19 |
| Shake, Lotta Caramel Latte Love it Size | 20 fl oz | 1530 | 650 | 72 | 45 | 280 | 530 | 200 | 0 | 20 |
| Shake, Sinless Milk & Cookies | 20 fl oz | 710 | 80 | 9 | 2 | 0 | 580 | 147 | 1 | 28 |
| Shake, Sinless Very Vanilla | 20 fl oz | 590 | 10 | 1 | .5 | 5 | 390 | 135 | 0 | 27 |
| Sinless Smoothie, Strawberry Bananza | 20 fl oz | 220 | 15 | 1.5 | 0 | 0 | 45 | 57 | 6 | 3 |
| Smoothie, Banana Strawberry | 20 fl oz | 450 | 50 | 6 | 3.5 | 0 | 250 | 102 | 6 | 4 |
| Smoothie, Raspberry Banana | 20 fl oz | 460 | 45 | 5 | 3.5 | 0 | 250 | 105 | 8 | 4 |
| **Cosi** | | | | | | | | | | |
| **FLATBREAD PIZZAS** | | | | | | | | | | |
| Cheese—Original Crust | 1 pizza | 709 | 219 | 24 | 9 | 49 | 397 | 90 | 4 | 35 |
| Cheese—Thin Crust | 1 pizza | 495 | 213 | 24 | 9 | 49 | 315 | 47 | 3 | 27 |
| Margherita—Original Crust | 1 pizza | 741 | 240 | 27 | 10 | 57 | 410 | 91 | 5 | 38 |
| Margherita—Thin Crust | 1 pizza | 527 | 234 | 26 | 10 | 57 | 328 | 47 | 3 | 30 |
| Pepperoni—Thin Crust | 1 pizza | 637 | 323 | 36 | 14 | 79 | 852 | 47 | 3 | 33 |
| Pepperoni—Original Crust | 1 pizza | 851 | 329 | 37 | 14 | 79 | 934 | 90 | 4 | 41 |
| **SALADS** | | | | | | | | | | |
| Bombay Chicken w/Dressing | 1 salad | 481 | 292 | 32 | 5 | 61 | 1094 | 17 | 4 | 25 |

# restaurants

| | SERVING SIZE | CAL | CAL FAT | TOT FAT (G) | SAT FAT (G) | CHOL (MG) | SOD (MG) | CARB (G) | FIBER (G) | PROT (G) |
|---|---|---|---|---|---|---|---|---|---|---|
| Cobb Salad w/Dressing | 1 salad | 708 | 482 | 55 | 12 | 120 | 1347 | 17 | 2 | 39 |
| Chicken Caesar w/Dressing | 1 salad | 621 | 396 | 44 | 10 | 103 | 1670 | 20 | 2 | 39 |
| Greek w/Dressing | 1 salad | 517 | 419 | 47 | 10 | 22 | 1480 | 19 | 4 | 11 |
| Mediterranean Shrimp | 1 salad | 357 | 281 | 31 | 7 | 101 | 1508 | 17 | 5 | 19 |
| Signature Salad w/Dressing | 1 salad | 611 | 401 | 45 | 5 | 32 | 664 | 44 | 5 | 12 |
| Steakhouse w/Bleu Cheese Dressing | 1 salad | 614 | 442 | 49 | 18 | 99 | 836 | 14 | 5 | 28 |
| Tuscan Steak w/Dressing | 1 salad | 532 | 309 | 34 | 17 | 86 | 1542 | 26 | 6 | 30 |
| Wild Alaskan Salmon w/Dressing | 1 salad | 457 | 245 | 27 | 6 | 266 | 1372 | 24 | 7 | 35 |
| **SANDWICHES** | | | | | | | | | | |
| Buffalo Bleu | 1 sandwich | 565 | 226 | 25 | 4 | 90 | 923 | 47 | 3 | 36 |
| Fire-Roasted Veggie | 1 sandwich | 324 | 68 | 8 | 4 | 16 | 259 | 44 | 4 | 11 |
| Grilled Chicken TBM | 1 sandwich | 691 | 328 | 36 | 8 | 104 | 367 | 47 | 3 | 46 |
| Grilled Chicken TBM Light | 1 sandwich | 531 | 152 | 17 | 7 | 104 | 483 | 50 | 3 | 46 |
| Hummus & Veggie | 1 sandwich | 397 | 59 | 7 | 0 | 0 | 532 | 72 | 7 | 13 |
| Italiano | 1 sandwich | 747 | 377 | 42 | 16 | 103 | 2210 | 49 | 3 | 49 |
| Market w/Turkey | 1 sandwich | 687 | 290 | 32 | 13 | 95 | 885 | 62 | 2 | 38 |
| Sesame Ginger Chicken | 1 sandwich | 480 | 63 | 7 | 1 | 71 | 1272 | 69 | 4 | 35 |
| Shrimp Remoulade | 1 sandwich | 456 | 180 | 20 | 6 | 150 | 825 | 48 | 3 | 21 |
| Tandoori Chicken | 1 sandwich | 541 | 204 | 23 | 2 | 58 | 819 | 48 | 2 | 36 |
| Tandoori Chicken Light | 1 sandwich | 376 | 27 | 3 | 1 | 58 | 889 | 50 | 2 | 35 |
| Tuna | 1 sandwich | 539 | 57 | 6 | 2 | 77 | 948 | 52 | 4 | 53 |
| Turkey Light | 1 sandwich | 390 | 48 | 5 | 1 | 35 | 526 | 62 | 2 | 26 |
| Tuscan Pesto Chicken | 1 sandwich | 510 | 159 | 6 | 6 | 98 | 452 | 49 | 4 | 39 |

# Country/Old Country/ Hometown/Granny's Buffet

### BREADS & MUFFINS

| | SERVING SIZE | CAL | CAL FAT | TOT FAT (G) | SAT FAT (G) | CHOL (MG) | SOD (MG) | CARB (G) | FIBER (G) | PROT (G) |
|---|---|---|---|---|---|---|---|---|---|---|
| Banana Walnut Muffin | 1 muffin | 270 | 120 | 13 | 2 | 0 | 290 | 35 | 1 | 5 |
| Biscuits | 1 biscuit | 180 | 99 | 11 | 4.5 | <5 | 340 | 16 | 1 | 3 |
| Blueberry Muffin | 1 muffin | 230 | 80 | 9 | 1.5 | 0 | 290 | 34 | 1 | 4 |
| Cinnamon Bread | 1 slice | 160 | 20 | 2.5 | .5 | 0 | 140 | 32 | 1 | 3 |
| Cinnamon Rolls | 1 roll | 140 | 45 | 5 | 1 | 0 | 115 | 23 | 1 | 2 |
| Corn Muffin | 1 muffin | 320 | 110 | 12 | 2 | 35 | 630 | 49 | 1 | 6 |
| Cornbread | 1 piece | 160 | 54 | 6 | 1 | 15 | 320 | 25 | 1 | 3 |
| French Bread Loaf | 1 slice | 70 | 5 | .5 | 0 | 0 | 160 | 14 | 2 | 3 |
| Garlic Bread | 1 slice | 70 | 30 | 3 | .5 | 0 | 110 | 9 | 0 | 2 |
| Garlic Cheese Biscuit | 1 biscuit | 220 | 126 | 14 | 6 | 10 | 630 | 20 | 1 | 5 |

| | SERVING SIZE | CAL | CAL FAT | TOT FAT (G) | SAT FAT (G) | CHOL (MG) | SOD (MG) | CARB (G) | FIBER (G) | PROT (G) |
|---|---|---|---|---|---|---|---|---|---|---|
| Hot Dog Bun | 1 bun | 120 | 20 | 2 | 1 | 0 | 210 | 22 | 3 | 4 |
| Wheat Bread Loaf | 1 slice | 70 | 10 | 1 | 0 | 0 | 130 | 12 | 1 | 3 |
| **BREAKFAST** | | | | | | | | | | |
| Buttermilk Pancakes | 1 pancake | 120 | 20 | 2 | .5 | 5 | 380 | 19 | 0 | 3 |
| French Toast | 1 slice | 220 | 80 | 9 | 2 | 105 | 270 | 29 | 1 | 8 |
| Hashbrown Patties | 1 piece | 110 | 60 | 7 | 1.5 | 0 | 220 | 13 | 2 | 1 |
| Plain Omelet | 1 omelet | 140 | 100 | 11 | 3 | 360 | 150 | 2 | 0 | 10 |
| Potatoes O'Brien | as served | 150 | 50 | 6 | 1 | 0 | 270 | 25 | 2 | 2 |
| Waffles | 1 waffle | 120 | 50 | 6 | 3 | 50 | 180 | 15 | 1 | 2 |
| **DESSERTS** | | | | | | | | | | |
| Cappuccino Cake | 1 slice | 180 | 90 | 10 | 4.5 | 30 | 210 | 18 | 0 | 3 |
| Chocolate Haystacks | 1 piece | 160 | 70 | 8 | 4 | 0 | 90 | 19 | 2 | 3 |
| Chocolate Marble Cake | 1 slice | 180 | 63 | 7 | 2 | 20 | 190 | 26 | 1 | 2 |
| Dessert Pizza | 1 slice | 100 | 40 | 4 | 2 | 10 | 45 | 17 | 1 | 1 |
| Reduced Sugar Apple Pie | 1 slice | 180 | 63 | 7 | 3.5 | 0 | 160 | 28 | 2 | 3 |
| Reduced Sugar Banana Cream Pie | 1 slice | 180 | 100 | 11 | 9 | 0 | 150 | 20 | 1 | 2 |
| Reduced Sugar Chocolate Cream Pie | 1 slice | 180 | 110 | 11 | 9 | 0 | 260 | 19 | 1 | 2 |
| Rocky Road Pudding | 3 oz | 150 | 20 | 2.5 | .5 | 0 | 135 | 27 | 1 | 2 |
| **MAIN DISHES** | | | | | | | | | | |
| BBQ Baked Chicken Pizza | 1 slice | 250 | 60 | 7 | 3.5 | 30 | 800 | 32 | 1 | 15 |
| BBQ Beef Ribs | 1 tong | 300 | 210 | 23 | 9 | 60 | 350 | 7 | 0 | 17 |
| BBQ Pork Ribs | 1 rib | 140 | 80 | 9 | 3.5 | 35 | 320 | 5 | 0 | 9 |
| Beef Stroganoff | 1 spoon | 190 | 70 | 8 | 2.5 | 55 | 200 | 19 | 1 | 13 |
| Carved Grilled Pork Loin | 3 oz | 140 | 90 | 10 | 3.5 | 45 | 370 | 0 | 0 | 13 |
| Carved Ham | 3 oz | 100 | 45 | 5 | 3 | 40 | 990 | 0 | 0 | 14 |
| Carved Roast Beef | 3 oz | 230 | 135 | 15 | 7 | 70 | 55 | 0 | 0 | 23 |
| Carved Salmon Filet | 3 oz | 190 | 100 | 11 | 2 | 55 | 390 | 0 | 0 | 19 |
| Carved Sirloin Steak | 3 oz | 180 | 80 | 9 | 3.5 | 70 | 170 | 0 | 0 | 25 |
| Cheese Pizza | 1 slice | 150 | 40 | 4 | 2 | 10 | 350 | 22 | 1 | 8 |
| Chicken Alfredo | 1 spoon | 230 | 130 | 14 | 4 | 35 | 530 | 16 | 1 | 10 |
| Chicken Strips | as served | 170 | 90 | 10 | 2.5 | 25 | 430 | 10 | 0 | 10 |
| Clam Strips | 1 tong | 320 | 180 | 20 | 3.5 | 15 | 630 | 28 | 2 | 9 |
| Country BBQ Chicken Breast | 1 breast | 310 | 140 | 16 | 5 | 165 | 780 | 6 | 2 | 40 |
| Country BBQ Chicken Drumstick | 1 drumstick | 100 | 50 | 6 | 1.5 | 55 | 280 | 2 | 0 | 10 |
| Country BBQ Chicken Wing | 1 wing | 80 | 40 | 4.5 | 1 | 40 | 280 | 3 | 1 | 10 |
| Country Fried Steak w/o Gravy | 1 steak | 210 | 120 | 13 | 4 | 25 | 630 | 15 | 1 | 9 |
| County Pasta Gratin | 1 spoon | 160 | 40 | 4 | 1 | 20 | 720 | 24 | 1 | 8 |

# restaurants

| | SERVING SIZE | CAL | CAL FAT | TOT FAT (G) | SAT FAT (G) | CHOL (MG) | SOD (MG) | CARB (G) | FIBER (G) | PROT (G) |
|---|---|---|---|---|---|---|---|---|---|---|
| Creamy Penne Carbonara | 1 spoon | 260 | 150 | 17 | 5 | 35 | 870 | 17 | 2 | 11 |
| Enchiladas | 1 enchilada | 250 | 160 | 18 | 9 | 45 | 560 | 12 | 1 | 13 |
| Fire Grilled Chicken Alfredo | 1 spoon | 220 | 130 | 14 | 4 | 40 | 480 | 14 | 2 | 10 |
| Fried Fish | 1 piece | 80 | 40 | 4 | .5 | 10 | 200 | 9 | 1 | 3 |
| Grilled BBQ Pork Steak | 1 piece | 150 | 80 | 9 | 3 | 50 | 540 | 3 | 0 | 14 |
| Grilled BBQ Smoked Sausage | 1 spoon | 170 | 120 | 13 | 6 | 20 | 520 | 8 | 1 | 6 |
| Grilled Pork Steak | 1 item | 140 | 80 | 9 | 3 | 50 | 440 | 0 | 0 | 14 |
| Hand Breaded Fried Chicken Breast | 1 piece | 360 | 200 | 22 | 6 | 170 | 470 | 0 | 2 | 41 |
| Hand Breaded Fried Chicken Drumstick | 1 piece | 100 | 60 | 7 | 2 | 60 | 120 | 0 | 0 | 10 |
| Hand Breaded Fried Chicken Wing | 1 piece | 90 | 50 | 6 | 1.5 | 45 | 115 | 0 | 0 | 10 |
| Honey BBQ Pork Riblets | 1 piece | 120 | 80 | 9 | 3 | 35 | 170 | 3 | 0 | 8 |
| Honey Glazed Baked Ham | 1 slice | 120 | 50 | 5 | 2.5 | 40 | 990 | 1 | 0 | 16 |
| Macaroni & Cheese | 1 spoon | 110 | 20 | 2.5 | 1 | 5 | 500 | 18 | 1 | 4 |
| Meatloaf | 3 oz | 180 | 100 | 11 | 4.5 | 60 | 44 | 7 | 0 | 12 |
| Orange Chicken | 1 spoon | 340 | 200 | 22 | 4.5 | 55 | 520 | 26 | 1 | 12 |
| Oven Roasted Rotisserie Style Turkey | 3 oz | 100 | 40 | 4 | 1 | 40 | 450 | 1 | 0 | 14 |
| Pepperoni & Sausage Calzone | 1 slice | 150 | 36 | 6 | 3 | 45 | 390 | 15 | 0 | 7 |
| Perfect Pot Roast | 1 spoon | 160 | 60 | 7 | 2.5 | 40 | 780 | 9 | 1 | 15 |
| Pot Roast Stroganoff | as served | 130 | 50 | 6 | 2 | 25 | 540 | 15 | 1 | 6 |
| Roasted Jerk Chicken Breast | 1 piece | 320 | 160 | 18 | 5 | 165 | 820 | 0 | 0 | 40 |
| Rotisserie Chicken Breast | 1 piece | 310 | 150 | 17 | 5 | 165 | 680 | 1 | 2 | 40 |
| Steak Fajita | 1 spoon | 120 | 50 | 6 | 2 | 40 | 300 | 2 | 1 | 14 |
| Tostada | 1 tostada | 110 | 36 | 6 | .5 | 0 | 85 | 14 | 1 | 1 |
| **SIDES** | | | | | | | | | | |
| Au Gratin Potatoes | 1 spoon | 110 | 45 | 5 | 3.5 | 15 | 330 | 10 | 1 | 5 |
| Candied Yams | 1 spoon | 140 | 10 | 1.5 | 0 | 0 | 450 | 33 | 2 | 1 |
| Cauliflower Au Gratin | 1 spoon | 50 | 20 | 2 | .5 | 0 | 410 | 8 | 2 | 2 |
| Cheesy Hashbrowns | 1 spoon | 140 | 70 | 8 | 5 | 25 | 310 | 10 | 1 | 6 |
| French Fries | 1 spoon | 170 | 80 | 9 | 1.5 | 0 | 400 | 23 | 2 | 2 |
| Green Bean Casserole | 1 spoon | 100 | 60 | 7 | 2.5 | 0 | 440 | 10 | 2 | 2 |
| Grilled Cowboy Potatoes | 1 spoon | 180 | 80 | 9 | 1.5 | 0 | 640 | 23 | 4 | 3 |
| **SOUPS & SALADS** | | | | | | | | | | |
| BLT Salads | 1 spoon | 120 | 110 | 12 | 2 | 15 | 180 | 2 | 1 | 2 |
| Caesar Salads | 1 cup | 70 | 36 | 6 | 1 | 5 | 110 | 4 | 1 | 1 |
| California Coleslaw Salads | 1 spoon | 100 | 0 | 0 | 0 | 0 | 85 | 24 | 1 | 1 |
| Carrot & Raisin Salads | 1 spoon | 140 | 80 | 9 | 1.5 | 10 | 115 | 17 | 2 | 1 |
| Chicken Caesar Salad | 1 cup | 90 | 60 | 7 | 1.5 | 20 | 120 | 3 | 1 | 6 |

| | SERVING SIZE | CAL | CAL FAT | TOT FAT (G) | SAT FAT (G) | CHOL (MG) | SOD (MG) | CARB (G) | FIBER (G) | PROT (G) |
|---|---|---|---|---|---|---|---|---|---|---|
| Chicken Noodle Soup | 4 oz | 80 | 20 | 2 | .5 | 20 | 300 | 8 | 1 | 6 |
| Chicken Pasta Salad | 1 spoon | 240 | 171 | 19 | 3.5 | 30 | 320 | 13 | 1 | 6 |
| Italian Pasta Salad | 1 salad | 190 | 120 | 13 | 4 | 20 | 520 | 14 | 1 | 6 |
| Italian Sausage & Bean Soup | 4 oz | 50 | 20 | 2.5 | 1 | 5 | 480 | 6 | 1 | 2 |
| Macaroni Vegetable Salad | 1 spoon | 240 | 140 | 16 | 3 | 45 | 330 | 21 | 1 | 5 |
| Marinated Green Bean Salad | 1 spoon | 120 | 100 | 11 | 1.5 | 2 | 380 | 19 | 1 | 4 |
| Marinated Vegetables Salad | 1 spoon | 50 | 30 | 3.5 | .5 | 0 | 150 | 5 | 2 | 2 |
| Minestrone | 4 oz | 60 | 10 | 1 | 0 | 0 | 370 | 11 | 1 | 3 |
| New England Clam Chowder | 4 oz | 150 | 100 | 11 | 8 | 5 | 440 | 12 | 1 | 2 |
| Oriental Chicken w/o Dressing Salad | 1 spoon | 50 | 10 | 1.5 | 0 | 15 | 45 | 6 | 1 | 5 |
| Orzo Pasta w/Feta Cheese Salad | 1 spoon | 150 | 70 | 8 | 2 | 6 | 440 | 17 | 2 | 4 |
| Potato Salad | 1 spoon | 120 | 60 | 7 | 1 | 25 | 300 | 15 | 1 | 2 |
| Seafood Salad | 1 spoon | 310 | 230 | 26 | 3.5 | 40 | 500 | 15 | 1 | 4 |
| Seven Layer Salad | 1 spoon | 190 | 150 | 17 | 4.5 | 30 | 250 | 4 | 1 | 5 |
| Sicilian Pasta Salad | 1 spoon | 140 | 60 | 7 | 1.5 | 2 | 430 | 16 | 1 | 4 |
| Strawberry Walnut Salad | 1 spoon | 90 | 60 | 7 | .5 | 0 | 5 | 6 | 2 | 2 |
| Tarragon Potato Salad | 1 spoon | 120 | 60 | 7 | 1.5 | 10 | 160 | 13 | 1 | 1 |
| Three Bean Salad | 1 spoon | 90 | 40 | 4.5 | .5 | 0 | 480 | 12 | 3 | 2 |
| Waldorf Salad | 1 spoon | 110 | 60 | 7 | 1 | 5 | 40 | 12 | 1 | 2 |
| Vegetable Beef Soup | 1 spoon | 50 | 20 | 2 | .5 | 10 | 240 | 7 | 1 | 3 |

## Culver's
### BURGERS

| | SERVING SIZE | CAL | CAL FAT | TOT FAT (G) | SAT FAT (G) | CHOL (MG) | SOD (MG) | CARB (G) | FIBER (G) | PROT (G) |
|---|---|---|---|---|---|---|---|---|---|---|
| Butter Burger "The Original", Single | 1 burger | 346 | 104 | 12 | 5 | 65 | 700 | 35 | 1 | 19 |
| Butter Burger, Low Carb | 1 burger | 477 | 315 | 35 | 14 | 165 | 972 | 2 | 0 | 37 |
| Deluxe, Single | 1 burger | 494 | 243 | 27 | 14 | 93 | 857 | 34 | 1 | 22 |
| Mushroom & Swiss, Single | 1 burger | 431 | 176 | 20 | 9 | 85 | 551 | 32 | 1 | 25 |
| Sourdough Melt, Single | 1 burger | 414 | 176 | 20 | 10 | 85 | 600 | 33 | 0 | 25 |
| Veggie Burger | 1 burger | 464 | 171 | 15 | 10 | 35 | 1202 | 56 | 4 | 13 |
| Wisconsin Swiss Melt, Single | 1 burger | 404 | 176 | 20 | 9 | 85 | 575 | 33 | 2 | 26 |

### ENTRÉES

| | SERVING SIZE | CAL | CAL FAT | TOT FAT (G) | SAT FAT (G) | CHOL (MG) | SOD (MG) | CARB (G) | FIBER (G) | PROT (G) |
|---|---|---|---|---|---|---|---|---|---|---|
| BBQ Chicken | 1 entrée | 337 | 63 | 7 | 2 | 63 | 1186 | 43 | 2 | 19 |
| BBQ Pork | 1 entrée | 392 | 90 | 10 | 4 | 51 | 1099 | 47 | 2 | 22 |
| Beef Pot Roast Dinner | 1 entrée | 745 | 323 | 36 | 25 | 134 | 1710 | 73 | 8 | 33 |
| Chicken Salad on Grilled Sourdough | 1 entrée | 525 | 249 | 28 | 8 | 101 | 1087 | 34 | 1 | 34 |
| Chili Cheese Hot Dog | 1 entrée | 505 | 292 | 33 | 13 | 84 | 1350 | 36 | 0 | 22 |
| Chopped Steak Dinner | 1 entrée | 849 | 445 | 49 | 24 | 189 | 1277 | 63 | 8 | 41 |
| Crispy Chicken Filet Sandwich | 1 sandwich | 579 | 311 | 35 | 12 | 55 | 1056 | 50 | 3 | 21 |

# restaurants

| | SERVING SIZE | CAL | CAL FAT | TOT FAT (G) | SAT FAT (G) | CHOL (MG) | SOD (MG) | CARB (G) | FIBER (G) | PROT (G) |
|---|---|---|---|---|---|---|---|---|---|---|
| Fish 'n Chips, 6 piece | 1 entrée | 1381 | 746 | 84 | 17 | 105 | 1050 | 104 | 4 | 45 |
| Flame Roasted Chicken Sandwich | 1 sandwich | 309 | 77 | 9 | 3 | 65 | 980 | 36 | 1 | 27 |
| Pork Tenderloin, Grilled | 1 entrée | 458 | 153 | 17 | 8 | 100 | 972 | 33 | 2 | 35 |
| Shaved Prime Rib Sandwich | 1 sandwich | 507 | 256 | 28 | 15 | 76 | 1215 | 35 | 0 | 34 |
| Tuna Salad on Grilled Sourdough | 1 sandwich | 501 | 241 | 27 | 7 | 63 | 1063 | 35 | 1 | 31 |
| Turkey Sourdough BLT | 1 sandwich | 562 | 280 | 32 | 16 | 106 | 1923 | 36 | 0 | 34 |
| Ultimate Grilled Cheese | 1 sandwich | 290 | 121 | 14 | 10 | 60 | 1360 | 38 | 0 | 16 |
| **SIDES** | | | | | | | | | | |
| Chili Cheddar Fries | as served | 607 | 264 | 29 | 8 | 32 | 482 | 72 | 5 | 15 |
| Crinkle Cut Fries, Small | as served | 275 | 108 | 12 | 2 | 0 | 40 | 38 | 3 | 4 |
| Mashed Potatoes | as served | 120 | 8 | 1 | 0 | 6 | 204 | 24 | 2 | 2 |
| Onion Rings, Breaded | 1 serving | 630 | 324 | 36 | 4 | 0 | 1070 | 70 | 3 | 7 |
| **SOUPS & SALADS** | | | | | | | | | | |
| Boston Clam Chowder | 11 oz | 252 | 99 | 11 | 3 | 24 | 1344 | 25 | 1 | 12 |
| Chicken & Dumpling | 11 oz | 300 | 194 | 22 | 9 | 54 | 1248 | 19 | 1 | 9 |
| Chicken Noodle | 11 oz | 112 | 18 | 2 | 1 | 69 | 1550 | 14 | 1 | 9 |
| Classic Caesar w/Flame Roasted Chicken | 1 salad | 340 | 142 | 16 | 7 | 91 | 1445 | 14 | 3 | 34 |
| Corn Chowder | 11 oz | 276 | 117 | 13 | 3 | 18 | 996 | 35 | 4 | 7 |
| Cream of Broccoli | 11 oz | 185 | 90 | 10 | 5 | 30 | 1548 | 16 | 1 | 8 |
| French Onion | 11 oz | 129 | 59 | 7 | 2 | 6 | 2010 | 11 | 0 | 7 |
| Garden Fresco Salad | 1 salad | 229 | 88 | 10 | 4 | 32 | 375 | 19 | 5 | 16 |
| Italian Wedding Style | 11 oz | 275 | 54 | 6 | 3 | 12 | 1475 | 44 | 2 | 11 |
| Minestrone | 11 oz | 100 | 9 | 1 | 0 | 0 | 1175 | 19 | 4 | 4 |
| Vegetable Beef & Barley Soup | 11 oz | 112 | 36 | 4 | 1 | 13 | 1300 | 14 | 3 | 7 |

# Currito
## BREAKFAST

| | | | | | | | | | | |
|---|---|---|---|---|---|---|---|---|---|---|
| Bacon/Egg | 1 entrée | 473 | 206 | 22.9 | 8.9 | 254.6 | 1163 | 46 | 2 | 23.1 |
| Egg/Cheese | 1 entrée | 433 | 175 | 19.4 | 7.7 | 248.6 | 1049.9 | 46 | 2 | 21 |
| Huevos Rancheros | 1 entrée | 505 | 181 | 20.1 | 7.7 | 248.6 | 1311.6 | 57 | 6.6 | 25.5 |
| Truck Stop | 1 entrée | 524 | 218 | 24.3 | 9 | 254.6 | 1239.5 | 56 | 2.7 | 23.8 |

## BURRITOS, REGULAR

| | | | | | | | | | | |
|---|---|---|---|---|---|---|---|---|---|---|
| Classic | 1 burrito | 784 | 250 | 27.7 | 11.9 | 50 | 2878.6 | 105 | 7.4 | 26.3 |
| Bangkok | 1 burrito | 655 | 180 | 20 | 4.1 | 0 | 2013.1 | 106 | 4.6 | 16.2 |
| Buffalo | 1 burrito | 811 | 396 | 44 | 15.5 | 55.6 | 2025.3 | 92 | 3.3 | 13.6 |
| Cajun | 1 burrito | 805 | 226 | 25.1 | 10.8 | 30.4 | 5425.4 | 126 | 11.1 | 22.8 |
| Mediterranean | 1 burrito | 828 | 304 | 33.7 | 10.6 | 37.5 | 3027.3 | 107 | 8.6 | 23.2 |
| Summer | 1 burrito | 837 | 252 | 28.1 | 11.8 | 50 | 2596.3 | 115 | 9.6 | 27.9 |

| | SERVING SIZE | CAL | CAL FAT | TOT FAT (G) | SAT FAT (G) | CHOL (MG) | SOD (MG) | CARB (G) | FIBER (G) | PROT (G) |
|---|---|---|---|---|---|---|---|---|---|---|
| Teriyaki | 1 burrito | 650 | 141 | 15.6 | 3 | 0 | 2205.9 | 111 | 7.6 | 15.1 |
| **SALAD** | | | | | | | | | | |
| Caesar | 1 salad | 336 | 150 | 16.7 | 6.6 | 114.6 | 763.7 | 7 | 0.8 | 37.8 |
| Chinese Chicken | 1 salad | 488 | 239 | 26.5 | 4.2 | 59.5 | 648.8 | 31 | 5.4 | 31.2 |
| House | 1 salad | 35 | 4 | 0.4 | 0.1 | 0 | 20.6 | 7 | 2.9 | 1.9 |
| **SMOOTHIES, SMALL** | | | | | | | | | | |
| Berry Blitz | 1 smoothie | 191 | 5.1 | 0.6 | 0.1 | 0 | 20 | 47.5 | 3.5 | 0.7 |
| Cape Codder | 1 smoothie | 237 | 3.5 | 0.4 | 0 | 0 | 33.5 | 57.4 | 2.6 | 2.1 |
| Jimmy Carter | 1 smoothie | 464 | 95.7 | 10.6 | 2.3 | 3.4 | 289.7 | 76.1 | 2.2 | 1.8 |
| Mango Passion | 1 smoothie | 251 | 4.1 | 0.5 | 0.1 | 0 | 42.1 | 60.1 | 2.2 | 2.7 |
| Milkshake | 1 smoothie | 431 | 2.8 | 0.3 | 0.2 | 3.4 | 250.6 | 89.3 | 0 | 15.9 |
| Soy Smoothie | 1 smoothie | 182 | 41.5 | 4.6 | 0.6 | 0 | 29.6 | 32.2 | 5.5 | 7 |
| Strawbana | 1 smoothie | 241 | 12.3 | 1.4 | 0.7 | 2.7 | 40.9 | 58.5 | 3.5 | 1.7 |
| Triathlete | 1 smoothie | 167 | 2.5 | 0.3 | 0.1 | 0 | 25.4 | 40.9 | 2.5 | 0.7 |
| **SNACK BURRITOS** | | | | | | | | | | |
| Cheese | 1 burrito | 403 | 189 | 21 | 10.7 | 50 | 625 | 35 | 1 | 16 |
| Chix & Cheese | 1 burrito | 476 | 190 | 21.2 | 7.3 | 85.4 | 713.2 | 36 | 1.5 | 33.3 |
| Steak & Cheese | 1 burrito | 521 | 255 | 28.4 | 10.5 | 78.6 | 679.5 | 36 | 1.5 | 28.5 |
| PB&J | 1 burrito | 696 | 303 | 33.7 | 6.7 | 0 | 359 | 81 | 4.3 | 17.7 |
| Nutella | 1 burrito | 608 | 253 | 28.2 | 5.5 | 0 | 345 | 79 | 4.8 | 9.8 |

# D'Angelo
## SOUPS & SMALL SALADS

| | SERVING SIZE | CAL | CAL FAT | TOT FAT (G) | SAT FAT (G) | CHOL (MG) | SOD (MG) | CARB (G) | FIBER (G) | PROT (G) |
|---|---|---|---|---|---|---|---|---|---|---|
| Beef Stew | as served | 220 | 72 | 8 | 3.5 | 30 | 820 | 23 | 2 | 12 |
| Broccoli & Cheddar | as served | 250 | 171 | 19 | 11 | 60 | 840 | 12 | 2 | 9 |
| Chicken Caesar Salad | 1 salad | 670 | 477 | 53 | 11 | 115 | 2070 | 21 | 5 | 36 |
| Chicken Noodle | as served | 110 | 27 | 3 | 1 | 25 | 830 | 14 | 1 | 6 |
| Cobb Salad | 1 salad | 330 | 162 | 18 | 8 | 75 | 800 | 14 | 6 | 30 |
| Greek Salad | 1 salad | 780 | 630 | 70 | 14 | 40 | 1550 | 23 | 6 | 14 |
| Hearty Vegetable | as served | 40 | 0 | 0 | 0 | 0 | 270 | 7 | 2 | 2 |
| Italian Wedding | as served | 120 | 54 | 6 | 2 | 15 | 920 | 11 | 2 | 6 |
| NE Clam Chowder | as served | 320 | 162 | 18 | 10 | 60 | 700 | 31 | 1 | 9 |

## SUB SANDWICHES, SMALL

| | SERVING SIZE | CAL | CAL FAT | TOT FAT (G) | SAT FAT (G) | CHOL (MG) | SOD (MG) | CARB (G) | FIBER (G) | PROT (G) |
|---|---|---|---|---|---|---|---|---|---|---|
| BLT & Cheese | 1 sandwich | 500 | 207 | 23 | 11 | 45 | 1510 | 51 | 6 | 23 |
| Cheeseburger | 1 sandwich | 530 | 225 | 25 | 10 | 80 | 1430 | 49 | 5 | 28 |
| Chicken Club | 1 sandwich | 620 | 288 | 32 | 7 | 95 | 1280 | 48 | 5 | 35 |
| Classic Veggie | 1 sandwich | 450 | 135 | 15 | 7 | 35 | 1180 | 60 | 7 | 22 |
| Ham & Cheese | 1 sandwich | 380 | 90 | 10 | 4.5 | 50 | 1680 | 49 | 1 | 24 |

| | SERVING SIZE | CAL | CAL FAT | TOT FAT (G) | SAT FAT (G) | CHOL (MG) | SOD (MG) | CARB (G) | FIBER (G) | PROT (G) |
|---|---|---|---|---|---|---|---|---|---|---|
| Hamburger | 1 sandwich | 460 | 180 | 20 | 7 | 65 | 1120 | 48 | 5 | 24 |
| Italian | 1 sandwich | 530 | 234 | 26 | 8 | 65 | 1630 | 50 | 2 | 27 |
| Meatball | 1 sandwich | 670 | 306 | 34 | 13 | 75 | 2260 | 66 | 10 | 28 |
| Pastrami & Cheese | 1 sandwich | 610 | 306 | 34 | 14 | 120 | 1880 | 47 | 5 | 34 |
| Pepperoni | 1 sandwich | 600 | 306 | 34 | 11 | 70 | 1830 | 47 | 7 | 29 |
| Roast Beef | 1 sandwich | 320 | 45 | 5 | 1.5 | 50 | 990 | 46 | 4 | 26 |
| Salami & Cheese | 1 sandwich | 570 | 297 | 33 | 11 | 75 | 1750 | 45 | 4 | 27 |
| Steak & Cheese | 1 sandwich | 590 | 216 | 24 | 11 | 115 | 1650 | 52 | 5 | 42 |
| Tuna | 1 sandwich | 700 | 432 | 48 | 8 | 60 | 900 | 45 | 1 | 22 |
| Turkey | 1 sandwich | 330 | 27 | 3 | 0 | 55 | 540 | 45 | 4 | 30 |
| **WRAPS** | | | | | | | | | | |
| BLT & Cheese | 1 wrap | 590 | 270 | 30 | 13 | 45 | 1620 | 55 | 5 | 24 |
| Cheeseburger | 1 wrap | 600 | 279 | 31 | 12 | 80 | 1530 | 52 | 3 | 28 |
| Chicken Caesar Salad | 1 wrap | 830 | 432 | 48 | 11 | 100 | 2260 | 65 | 6 | 41 |
| Classic Veggie | 1 wrap | 520 | 198 | 22 | 9 | 35 | 1250 | 61 | 6 | 22 |
| Grilled Chicken | 1 wrap | 440 | 117 | 13 | 3 | 65 | 1010 | 50 | 3 | 30 |
| Hamburger | 1 wrap | 600 | 279 | 31 | 11 | 80 | 1240 | 50 | 3 | 28 |
| Meatball | 1 wrap | 760 | 369 | 41 | 15 | 75 | 2370 | 70 | 9 | 28 |
| Pastrami | 1 wrap | 700 | 369 | 41 | 16 | 120 | 1980 | 52 | 3 | 34 |
| Pepperoni | 1 wrap | 560 | 270 | 30 | 9 | 50 | 1420 | 50 | 4 | 23 |
| Roast Beef | 1 wrap | 410 | 108 | 12 | 3.5 | 50 | 1100 | 50 | 3 | 26 |
| Salami & Cheese | 1 wrap | 640 | 342 | 38 | 12 | 70 | 1790 | 49 | 3 | 27 |
| Steak & Cheese | 1 wrap | 660 | 279 | 31 | 13 | 115 | 1720 | 53 | 3 | 42 |
| Tuna | 1 wrap | 780 | 495 | 55 | 10 | 60 | 1010 | 49 | 3 | 22 |
| Turkey | 1 wrap | 410 | 90 | 10 | 2 | 55 | 640 | 49 | 3 | 31 |

## Daily Grill
### BREAKFAST

| | SERVING SIZE | CAL | CAL FAT | TOT FAT (G) | SAT FAT (G) | CHOL (MG) | SOD (MG) | CARB (G) | FIBER (G) | PROT (G) |
|---|---|---|---|---|---|---|---|---|---|---|
| Belgian Waffle | as served | 1096 | n/a | n/a | 28 | n/a | 1697 | 133 | n/a | n/a |
| Buttermilk Pancakes | as served | 656 | n/a | n/a | 1 | n/a | 1886 | 111 | n/a | n/a |
| Croissant | as served | 395 | n/a | n/a | 13 | n/a | 263 | 45 | n/a | n/a |
| Egg White Omelet | 1 omelet | 666 | n/a | n/a | 15 | n/a | 567 | 33 | n/a | n/a |
| French Toast | as served | 657 | n/a | n/a | 4 | n/a | 930 | 96 | n/a | n/a |
| Protein Scramble w/Country Sausage | as served | 1021 | n/a | n/a | 30 | n/a | 1814 | 24 | n/a | n/a |
| **BURGERS, SANDWICHES, & WRAPS** | | | | | | | | | | |
| BLT | 1 entrée | 734 | n/a | n/a | 10 | n/a | 1968 | 77 | n/a | n/a |

| | SERVING SIZE | CAL | CAL FAT | TOT FAT (G) | SAT FAT (G) | CHOL (MG) | SOD (MG) | CARB (G) | FIBER (G) | PROT (G) |
|---|---|---|---|---|---|---|---|---|---|---|
| Charbroiled Chicken Breast | 1 entrée | 626 | n/a | n/a | 7 | n/a | 790 | 75 | n/a | n/a |
| Chicken Burger | 1 entrée | 869 | n/a | n/a | 13 | n/a | 1618 | 81 | n/a | n/a |
| Classic Hamburger | 1 burger | 1787 | n/a | n/a | 33 | n/a | 2829 | 137 | n/a | n/a |
| Crispy Chicken | 1 entrée | 718 | n/a | n/a | 6 | n/a | 713 | 73 | n/a | n/a |
| Hamburger | 1 burger | 899 | n/a | n/a | 17 | n/a | 1096 | 77 | n/a | n/a |
| Original Beef Dip | 1 entrée | 593 | n/a | n/a | n/a | n/a | 1540 | 87 | n/a | n/a |
| Reuben | 1 entrée | 1028 | n/a | n/a | 23 | n/a | 4196 | 75 | n/a | n/a |
| Santa Fe Chicken Wrap | 1 entrée | 981 | n/a | n/a | 11 | n/a | 1680 | 103 | n/a | n/a |
| Tuna Salad | 1 entrée | 754 | n/a | n/a | 6 | n/a | 1369 | 78 | n/a | n/a |

## ENTRÉES & ENTRÉE SALADS

| | SERVING SIZE | CAL | CAL FAT | TOT FAT (G) | SAT FAT (G) | CHOL (MG) | SOD (MG) | CARB (G) | FIBER (G) | PROT (G) |
|---|---|---|---|---|---|---|---|---|---|---|
| Angel Hair Pasta Pomodoro | 1 entrée | 835 | n/a | n/a | 3 | n/a | 1794 | 108 | n/a | n/a |
| Bow Tie Pasta w/Salmon & Chardonnay Dill Sauce | 1 entrée | 1650 | n/a | n/a | 48 | n/a | 2458 | 101 | n/a | n/a |
| Charbroiled Rib Eye, 16 oz | 1 entrée | 1628 | n/a | n/a | 33 | n/a | 1265 | 54 | n/a | n/a |
| Charbroiled Skirt Steak | 1 entrée | 1022 | n/a | n/a | 18 | n/a | 2414 | 61 | n/a | n/a |
| Chicken Caesar Salad | 1 salad | 1258 | n/a | n/a | 23 | n/a | 1269 | 23 | n/a | n/a |
| Chinese Chicken Salad | 1 salad | 1357 | n/a | n/a | 9 | n/a | 1682 | 145 | n/a | n/a |
| Fillet Mignon w/3 Grilled Shrimp, 8 oz | 1 entrée | 685 | n/a | n/a | 18 | n/a | 1105 | 12 | n/a | n/a |
| Fish & Chips | 1 entrée | 1300 | n/a | n/a | 13 | n/a | 1714 | 151 | n/a | n/a |
| Iceberg Wedge | 1 salad | 1006 | n/a | n/a | 21 | n/a | 1493 | 10 | n/a | n/a |
| Loaded Mac & Cheese | 1 entrée | 1519 | n/a | n/a | 33 | n/a | 2578 | 150 | n/a | n/a |
| Meatloaf, Dinner | 1 entrée | 1414 | n/a | n/a | 36 | n/a | 2584 | 77 | n/a | n/a |
| New York Pepper Steak | 1 entrée | 1422 | n/a | n/a | 30 | n/a | 1785 | 65 | n/a | n/a |
| New York Strip Steak, 12 oz | 1 entrée | 1164 | n/a | n/a | 31 | n/a | 948 | 47 | n/a | n/a |
| Parmesan Crusted Chicken Caesar Salad | 1 salad | 1791 | n/a | n/a | 35 | n/a | 1672 | 38 | n/a | n/a |
| Prime Rib, 16 oz | 1 entrée | 2435 | n/a | n/a | 79 | n/a | 3235 | 124 | n/a | n/a |
| Southern Fried Chicken Salad | 1 salad | 1395 | n/a | n/a | 15 | n/a | 1667 | 77 | n/a | n/a |

## SIDES

| | SERVING SIZE | CAL | CAL FAT | TOT FAT (G) | SAT FAT (G) | CHOL (MG) | SOD (MG) | CARB (G) | FIBER (G) | PROT (G) |
|---|---|---|---|---|---|---|---|---|---|---|
| Garlic Mashed Potatoes | as served | 507 | n/a | n/a | 18 | n/a | 800 | 54 | n/a | n/a |
| Macaroni & Cheese | as served | 839 | n/a | n/a | 20 | n/a | 893 | 97 | n/a | n/a |
| Onion Rings | as served | 573 | n/a | n/a | 2 | n/a | 967 | 103 | n/a | n/a |
| Spinach Mashed Potatoes | as served | 349 | n/a | n/a | 12 | n/a | 613 | 38 | n/a | n/a |

## Dairy Queen
### BREAKFAST

| | SERVING SIZE | CAL | CAL FAT | TOT FAT (G) | SAT FAT (G) | CHOL (MG) | SOD (MG) | CARB (G) | FIBER (G) | PROT (G) |
|---|---|---|---|---|---|---|---|---|---|---|
| Bacon Biscuit Sandwich | 1 sandwich | 480 | 280 | 31 | 8 | 185 | 1210 | 37 | 0 | 15 |

# restaurants

| | SERVING SIZE | CAL | CAL FAT | TOT FAT (G) | SAT FAT (G) | CHOL (MG) | SOD (MG) | CARB (G) | FIBER (G) | PROT (G) |
|---|---|---|---|---|---|---|---|---|---|---|
| Biscuits & Gravy | 1 entrée | 820 | 420 | 47 | 13 | 15 | 2590 | 87 | 0 | 13 |
| Country Platter w/Bacon | 1 entrée | 1070 | 590 | 66 | 16 | 360 | 2500 | 92 | 2 | 30 |
| Ham Biscuit Sandwich | 1 sandwich | 460 | 250 | 28 | 7 | 180 | 1420 | 38 | 0 | 16 |
| Pancake Platter w/Bacon | 1 entrée | 400 | 110 | 13 | 3.5 | 20 | 1030 | 57 | 3 | 14 |
| Sausage Biscuit Sandwich | 1 sandwich | 540 | 330 | 37 | 10 | 195 | 1180 | 37 | 0 | 15 |
| Ultimate Breakfast Burrito | 1 burrito | 660 | 330 | 36 | 12 | 210 | 1180 | 59 | 5 | 22 |
| **BURGERS** | | | | | | | | | | |
| GrillBurger, 1/2 lb | 1 burger | 720 | 360 | 40 | 15 | 105 | 1240 | 42 | 2 | 42 |
| GrillBurger, Flame Thrower, 1/2 lb | 1 burger | 1060 | 680 | 75 | 26 | 165 | 1980 | 41 | 2 | 54 |
| Original Bacon Double Cheeseburger | 1 burger | 730 | 370 | 41 | 21 | 150 | 1550 | 35 | 1 | 41 |
| Original Cheeseburger | 1 burger | 400 | 160 | 18 | 9 | 65 | 920 | 34 | 1 | 19 |
| Original Double Cheeseburger | 1 burger | 640 | 310 | 34 | 18 | 125 | 1230 | 34 | 1 | 34 |
| **ENTRÉES** | | | | | | | | | | |
| All-Beef Chili Dog | 1 hot dog | 290 | 150 | 17 | 6 | 35 | 930 | 24 | 1 | 11 |
| All-Beef Foot-Long Hot Dog | 1 sandwich | 560 | 310 | 35 | 14 | 65 | 1600 | 39 | 2 | 20 |
| Barbeque Beef Sandwich | 1 sandwich | 270 | 40 | 4.5 | 1 | 30 | 830 | 43 | 1 | 16 |
| Barbeque Pork Sandwich | 1 sandwich | 340 | 100 | 12 | 1.5 | 55 | 840 | 41 | 1 | 18 |
| Corn Dog | 1 entrée | 460 | 170 | 19 | 5 | 80 | 970 | 56 | 1 | 17 |
| Crispy Chicken Salad | 1 salad | 460 | 170 | 19 | 6 | 70 | 1230 | 31 | 6 | 29 |
| Crispy Chicken Sandwich | 1 entrée | 560 | 250 | 28 | 3.5 | 35 | 980 | 48 | 3 | 20 |
| Crispy Chicken Wrap | 1 entrée | 290 | 140 | 16 | 3 | 30 | 620 | 17 | 2 | 11 |
| Crispy Fish Sandwich w/Cheese | 1 sandwich | 480 | 200 | 22 | 5 | 40 | 1390 | 52 | 2 | 18 |
| Crispy FlameThrower Chicken Wrap | 1 wrap | 310 | 170 | 19 | 4 | 35 | 620 | 17 | 2 | 11 |
| Deluxe Cheeseburger | 1 burger | 400 | 160 | 18 | 9 | 45 | 930 | 35 | 1 | 20 |
| Deluxe Hamburger | 1 burger | 350 | 130 | 14 | 7 | 50 | 680 | 34 | 1 | 17 |
| Grilled Chicken Salad | 1 salad | 280 | 100 | 11 | 5 | 75 | 890 | 14 | 4 | 31 |
| Grilled Chicken Sandwich | 1 sandwich | 370 | 150 | 16 | 2.5 | 55 | 780 | 32 | 1 | 24 |
| Grilled Chicken Wrap | 1 wrap | 200 | 110 | 12 | 3 | 35 | 450 | 9 | 1 | 12 |
| Iron Grilled Classic Club Sandwich | 1 sandwich | 580 | 260 | 29 | 9 | 80 | 1750 | 43 | 2 | 32 |
| Iron Grilled Supreme BLT Sandwich | 1 sandwich | 590 | 300 | 33 | 9 | 75 | 1560 | 42 | 2 | 26 |
| Iron Grilled Veggie Quesadilla Basket | 1 entrée | 1020 | 440 | 49 | 19 | 55 | 2470 | 114 | 9 | 26 |
| Mushroom Swiss GrillBurger | 1 burger | 620 | 340 | 37 | 12 | 75 | 910 | 39 | 2 | 29 |
| Popcorn Shrimp Basket | 1 entrée | 990 | 440 | 49 | 26 | 125 | 3630 | 115 | 8 | 18 |
| Pork Tenderloin Sandwich | 1 sandwich | 610 | 310 | 35 | 6 | 35 | 1330 | 58 | 3 | 19 |
| Shredded Chicken Sandwich | 1 sandwich | 290 | 60 | 7 | 1.5 | 75 | 560 | 30 | 1 | 30 |
| Side Salad | 1 salad | 45 | 0 | 0 | 0 | 0 | 50 | 11 | 3 | 2 |
| Spicy Chili, Bowl | 1 soup | 710 | 210 | 24 | 10 | 85 | 3900 | 81 | 3 | 44 |

| | SERVING SIZE | CAL | CAL FAT | TOT FAT (G) | SAT FAT (G) | CHOL (MG) | SOD (MG) | CARB (G) | FIBER (G) | PROT (G) |
|---|---|---|---|---|---|---|---|---|---|---|
| **TREATS & ICE CREAM** | | | | | | | | | | |
| Arctic Rush, All Flavors, Medium | as served | 310 | 0 | 0 | 0 | 0 | 0 | 63 | 0 | 0 |
| Banana Split | as served | 520 | 120 | 13 | 10 | 30 | 160 | 94 | 3 | 9 |
| Blizzard, Banana Cream Pie, Small | 10 oz | 580 | 200 | 22 | 13 | 60 | 290 | 84 | 0 | 11 |
| Blizzard, Banana Split, Small | 10 oz | 440 | 120 | 13 | 9 | 45 | 190 | 71 | 0 | 11 |
| Blizzard, Butterfinger, Small | 10 oz | 470 | 150 | 16 | 10 | 40 | 220 | 71 | 0 | 11 |
| Blizzard, Chocolate Chip, Small | 10 oz | 590 | 270 | 29 | 12 | 45 | 190 | 70 | 1 | 11 |
| Blizzard, Cookie Dough, Small | 10 oz | 710 | 240 | 27 | 14 | 55 | 350 | 103 | 1 | 13 |
| Blizzard, Heath, Small | 10 oz | 600 | 230 | 25 | 16 | 50 | 310 | 84 | 1 | 11 |
| Blizzard, M&M's Chocolate Candy, Small | 10 oz | 660 | 200 | 22 | 14 | 55 | 230 | 101 | 1 | 13 |
| Blizzard, Oreo Cookies, Small | 10 oz | 550 | 180 | 20 | 10 | 40 | 410 | 81 | 1 | 12 |
| Cheesecake Pieces | as served | 100 | 60 | 6 | 3.5 | 25 | 80 | 10 | 0 | 2 |
| Chewy Baked Brownie Pieces | as served | 130 | 60 | 6 | 1.5 | 20 | 130 | 17 | 0 | 2 |
| Choco Chunks | as served | 150 | 90 | 10 | 8 | 0 | 0 | 17 | 1 | 1 |
| Cookie Dough Pieces | as served | 130 | 50 | 6 | 1.5 | 5 | 70 | 18 | 0 | 1 |
| French Vanilla MooLatte | 16 fl oz | 560 | 160 | 18 | 14 | 35 | 160 | 88 | 0 | 8 |
| Peanut Butter Topping | as served | 180 | 130 | 15 | 2 | 0 | 170 | 8 | 1 | 3 |
| Shake, Banana, Medium | 19 oz | 620 | 170 | 19 | 12 | 65 | 280 | 96 | 2 | 19 |
| Shake, Cherry, Medium | 19 oz | 690 | 190 | 21 | 13 | 70 | 330 | 106 | 0 | 18 |
| Shake, Chocolate, Medium | 19 oz | 790 | 190 | 21 | 13 | 70 | 350 | 130 | 0 | 18 |
| Shake, Hot Fudge, Medium | 19 oz | 850 | 270 | 30 | 22 | 70 | 420 | 123 | 0 | 20 |
| **Davanni's** | | | | | | | | | | |
| **HOT HOAGIES** | | | | | | | | | | |
| BLT | 1/2 sandwich | 644 | 396 | 44 | n/a | 69 | 1320 | 40 | 1 | 25 |
| Chicken Parmigiana | 1/2 sandwich | 487 | 162 | 18 | n/a | 97 | 1090 | 41 | 1 | 39 |
| Ham | 1/2 sandwich | 461 | 225 | 25 | n/a | 49 | 1122 | 39 | 1 | 23 |
| Italian Sausage | 1/2 sandwich | 621 | 342 | 38 | n/a | 72 | 1655 | 46 | 3 | 24 |
| Meatball | 1/2 sandwich | 564 | 297 | 33 | n/a | 19 | 1298 | 49 | 2 | 25 |
| Pizza | 1/2 sandwich | 414 | 171 | 19 | n/a | 54 | 972 | 40 | 2 | 18 |
| Roast Beef | 1/2 sandwich | 468 | 225 | 25 | n/a | 53 | 882 | 39 | 1 | 25 |
| Salami | 1/2 sandwich | 621 | 387 | 43 | n/a | 93 | 1402 | 39 | 1 | 23 |
| Tuna Melt | 1/2 sandwich | 1091 | 720 | 80 | n/a | 47 | 1172 | 74 | 11 | 32 |
| Turkey | 1/2 sandwich | 455 | 216 | 24 | n/a | 46 | 1022 | 39 | 1 | 25 |
| Veggie | 1/2 sandwich | 445 | 216 | 24 | n/a | 23 | 669 | 43 | 2 | 14 |
| **PASTA** | | | | | | | | | | |
| Chicken Florentine | 1 entrée | 584 | 216 | 24 | n/a | 72 | 1213 | 56 | 1 | 28 |
| Lasagna | 1 entrée | 671 | 387 | 43 | n/a | 89 | 1679 | 50 | 4 | 6 |

# restaurants

| | SERVING SIZE | CAL | CAL FAT | TOT FAT (G) | SAT FAT (G) | CHOL (MG) | SOD (MG) | CARB (G) | FIBER (G) | PROT (G) |
|---|---|---|---|---|---|---|---|---|---|---|
| Penne, Plain | 1 entrée | 428 | 133 | 15 | 6 | 20 | 685 | 53 | 1 | 18 |
| **PIZZA** | | | | | | | | | | |
| Calzone, Cheese | 1 calzone | 811 | 387 | 43 | n/a | 51 | 1163 | 79 | 5 | 28 |
| Calzone, Chicken & Tomato | 1 calzone | 858 | 396 | 44 | n/a | 71 | 1321 | 81 | 5 | 36 |
| Calzone, Pepperoni & Sausage | 1 calzone | 959 | 504 | 56 | n/a | 83 | 1676 | 80 | 5 | 35 |
| Cheese, Traditional Crust | 1 slice | 184 | 45 | 5 | n/a | 10 | 375 | 28 | 1 | 8 |
| Chicken & Roma Tomato, Thin Crust | 1 slice | 162 | 45 | 5 | 2 | 20 | 369 | 19 | 1 | 10 |
| Chicken & Roma Tomato, Traditional Crust | 1 slice | 208 | 45 | 5 | n/a | 20 | 455 | 29 | 1 | 12 |
| Chicken Florentine, Traditional Crust | 1 slice | 303 | 139 | 14 | n/a | 30 | 542 | 31 | 2 | 14 |
| Five Meat, Traditional Crust | 1 slice | 527 | 270 | 30 | n/a | 124 | 1887 | 30 | 1 | 31 |
| The Works, Traditional Crust | 1 slice | 269 | 108 | 12 | n/a | 29 | 637 | 29 | 1 | 12 |
| Veggie, Traditional Crust | 1 slice | 226 | 63 | 7 | n/a | 15 | 524 | 29 | 1 | 10 |
| **SALAD** | | | | | | | | | | |
| Caesar | 1 salad | 223 | 90 | 10 | n/a | 20 | 1137 | 13 | 2 | 11 |
| Chicken Cobb | 1 salad | 393 | 180 | 20 | n/a | 286 | 1299 | 7 | 2 | 39 |
| Garden | 1 salad | 226 | 108 | 12 | n/a | 20 | 229 | 19 | 4 | 11 |
| Spinach w/Chicken | 1 salad | 558 | 270 | 30 | n/a | 113 | 1436 | 37 | 7 | 37 |
| **SIDES** | | | | | | | | | | |
| Breadsticks | 1 breadstick | 134 | 36 | 4 | n/a | 3 | 123 | 21 | 3 | 5 |
| **Dave & Buster's** | | | | | | | | | | |
| **APPETIZERS** | | | | | | | | | | |
| Bar Burgers & Wings Platter | as served | 2672 | 1719 | 191 | 11 | 110 | 3431 | 102 | 9 | 127 |
| Cheddar Cheese Sauce | 2 oz | 100 | 72 | 8 | 4 | 15 | 500 | 4 | 0 | 3 |
| Cheesesticks | 8 pieces | 845 | 684 | 76 | 23 | 53 | 1600 | 228 | 9 | 49 |
| Crispy Buffalo Chicken Bites | as served | 777 | 684 | 76 | 2 | 163 | 2016 | 9 | 2 | 38 |
| D & B Appetizer Trio, Small | as served | 2115 | 1647 | 183 | 19 | 74 | 3529 | 105 | 9 | 56 |
| Grilled Chicken Nachos | as served | 1470 | 981 | 109 | 13 | 48 | 2395 | 60 | 14 | 64 |
| Grilled Chicken Quesadillas Appetizers | as served | 1620 | 684 | 76 | 24 | 34 | 4415 | 144 | 14 | 90 |
| Potato Skins | 6 pieces | 2620 | 1593 | 177 | 14 | 38 | 5978 | 176 | 10 | 20 |
| Spinach Dip | 6 oz | 491 | 369 | 41 | 7 | 158 | 1945 | 15 | 6 | 20 |
| **BURGERS & SANDWICHES** | | | | | | | | | | |
| Bar Burgers (4) w/Seasoned French Fries | 1 entrée | 930 | 552 | 58 | 17 | 60 | 1183 | 87 | 8 | 27 |
| BBQ Pork Sliders | 1 entrée | 1483 | 585 | 65 | 19 | 153 | 1697 | 173 | 9 | 51 |
| Black Jack BBQ Cheeseburger | 1 burger | 1101 | 567 | 63 | 22 | 110 | 1285 | 99 | 7 | 41 |
| BLT Turkey Burger | 1 burger | 734 | 405 | 45 | 70 | 166 | 966 | 47 | 6 | 37 |
| Buffalo Chicken Wrapper | 1 wrap | 1071 | 450 | 50 | 3 | 114 | 3179 | 104 | 10 | 46 |

| | SERVING SIZE | CAL | CAL FAT | TOT FAT (G) | SAT FAT (G) | CHOL (MG) | SOD (MG) | CARB (G) | FIBER (G) | PROT (G) |
|---|---|---|---|---|---|---|---|---|---|---|
| Buster's Cheeseburger w/Bacon | 1 burger | 1170 | 576 | 64 | 24 | 60 | 1359 | 85 | 7 | 27 |
| California Bar Burgers (4 ea.) | 1 burger | 1031 | 495 | 55 | 11 | 51 | 1200 | 92 | 8 | 27 |
| Dave's Double Cheeseburger | 1 burger | 1620 | 738 | 82 | 39 | 132 | 2630 | 100 | 7 | 54 |
| Double Stack Chicken Parmesan | 1 sandwich | 1141 | 396 | 44 | 20 | 125 | 2415 | 50 | 5 | 49 |
| Grilled Chicken & Cheddar | 1 sandwich | 1432 | 693 | 77 | 11 | 128 | 1682 | 113 | 6 | 57 |
| Grilled Roast Beef | 1 sandwich | 1308 | 630 | 70 | 15 | 109 | 2211 | 120 | 6 | 43 |
| Roasted Turkey Avocado BLT | 1 sandwich | 1550 | 855 | 95 | 15 | 23 | 3559 | 119 | 9 | 41 |
| **ENTRÉES** | | | | | | | | | | |
| Baked Mac & Cheese Alfredo | 1 entrée | 1391 | 837 | 93 | 20 | 413 | 3945 | 116 | 8 | 67 |
| Black Jack BBQ Chicken/Ribs—35 oz | 1 entrée | 2829 | 1728 | 192 | 75 | 770 | 1640 | 89 | 10 | 175 |
| Blackened Chicken Pasta | 1 entrée | 1600 | 567 | 63 | 5 | 299 | 1677 | 54 | 6 | 49 |
| Cajun Shrimp Alfredo | 1 entrée | 1211 | 729 | 81 | 7 | 311 | 3198 | 89 | 9 | 49 |
| Chargrilled Sirloin & Shrimp (Fried) | 1 entrée | 1276 | 603 | 67 | 43 | 390 | 1600 | 59 | 3 | 82 |
| Chargrilled Strip Steak | 1 entrée | 1705 | 666 | 74 | 39 | 350 | 1224 | 88 | 10 | 99 |
| Chicken Monte Carlo | 1 entrée | 722 | 234 | 26 | 7 | 288 | 769 | 12 | 5 | 90 |
| Chicken Pesto Pasta | 1 entrée | 1382 | 765 | 85 | 6 | 333 | 1991 | 80 | 6 | 59 |
| Dave's Pu Pu Platter | 1 entrée | 1476 | 1089 | 121 | 7 | 251 | 4154 | 79 | 4 | 79 |
| Fire-Grilled Atlantic Salmon | 1 entrée | 715 | 315 | 35 | 7 | 185 | 630 | 29 | 3 | 45 |
| Fired Grilled Salmon | 1 entrée | 680 | 306 | 34 | 12 | 144 | 518 | 32 | 7 | 56 |
| Fish & Chips | 1 entrée | 1319 | 576 | 64 | 9 | 66 | 1667 | 101 | 7 | 20 |
| Flatbread Pizza Margherita | 1 entrée | 664 | 657 | 73 | 3 | 94 | 1766 | 48 | 2 | 40 |
| Fried Shrimp Platter | 1 entrée | 1369 | 603 | 67 | 12 | 286 | 2686 | 159 | 6 | 32 |
| Grilled Chipotle Chicken | 1 entrée | 1102 | 576 | 64 | 6 | 386 | 951 | 35 | 5 | 94 |
| Mountain O' Nachos | 1 entrée | 1232 | 675 | 75 | 5 | 78 | 5351 | 75 | 17 | 30 |
| Parmesan Chicken Alfredo | 1 entrée | 1989 | 891 | 99 | 10 | 423 | 1389 | 111 | 8 | 59 |
| Parmesan Chicken Marinara | 1 entrée | 1311 | 657 | 73 | 5 | 232 | 2213 | 91 | 11 | 82 |
| Peppercorn Strip Steak | 1 entrée | 1855 | 909 | 101 | 26 | 454 | 2741 | 113 | 10 | 97 |
| Soft Taco Platter | 1 entrée | 1194 | 927 | 103 | 6 | 101 | 3559 | 49 | 8 | 25 |
| Teriyaki Sirloin Steak | 1 entrée | 1478 | 540 | 60 | 23 | 213 | 1212 | 88 | 10 | 74 |
| Thai Chicken Dippers | 1 entrée | 1476 | 1089 | 121 | 7 | 251 | 4154 | 79 | 4 | 79 |
| THE MAC & Cheese | 1 entrée | 1443 | 918 | 102 | 28 | 342 | 4557 | 136 | 8 | 62 |
| Toasted Ravioli | 1 entrée | 1012 | 801 | 89 | 23 | 64 | 1612 | 128 | 6 | 36 |
| Wing Master Platter | 1 entrée | 1550 | 855 | 95 | 25 | 133 | 2559 | 119 | 9 | 41 |
| **SIDES** | | | | | | | | | | |
| Crispy Frazzled Onions | as served | 540 | 279 | 31 | 15 | 28 | 842 | 62 | 8 | 7 |
| Seasoned French Fries | as served | 520 | 279 | 31 | 6 | 0 | 260 | 53 | 5 | 5 |
| Sweet Potato French Fries | as served | 450 | 180 | 20 | 2 | 0 | 150 | 25 | 3 | 3 |

| | SERVING SIZE | CAL | CAL FAT | TOT FAT (G) | SAT FAT (G) | CHOL (MG) | SOD (MG) | CARB (G) | FIBER (G) | PROT (G) |
|---|---|---|---|---|---|---|---|---|---|---|
| **SOUPS & SALADS** | | | | | | | | | | |
| Apple Pecan Salad | 1 salad | 188 | 243 | 27 | 0 | 4 | 493 | 17 | 2 | 6 |
| Broccoli Cheese Soup | 4 oz | 160 | 81 | 9 | 6 | 11 | 760 | 12 | 2 | 7 |
| Chicken Tortilla Soup | 4 oz | 211 | 54 | 6 | 1 | 9 | 821 | 14 | 4 | 9 |
| Grilled Chicken Caesar Salad | 1 salad | 345 | 54 | 6 | 1 | 65 | 720 | 20 | 3 | 40 |
| Honey Mustard Spinach Salad | 1 salad | 522 | 306 | 34 | 3 | 9 | 890 | 41 | 7 | 41 |
| House Salad | 1 salad | 30 | 0 | 0 | 0 | 0 | 11 | 4 | 1 | 1 |
| Parmesan Crusted Chicken Caesar Salad | 1 salad | 599 | 81 | 9 | 5 | 35 | 811 | 14 | 3 | 23 |

## Del Taco

### BURGERS

| | SERVING SIZE | CAL | CAL FAT | TOT FAT (G) | SAT FAT (G) | CHOL (MG) | SOD (MG) | CARB (G) | FIBER (G) | PROT (G) |
|---|---|---|---|---|---|---|---|---|---|---|
| Bacon Double Del Cheeseburger | 1 burger | 720 | 430 | 48 | 18 | 125 | 1270 | 40 | 1 | 31 |
| Cheeseburger | 1 burger | 430 | 200 | 22 | 9 | 60 | 990 | 40 | 1 | 18 |
| Double Del Cheeseburger | 1 burger | 560 | 310 | 35 | 12 | 85 | 960 | 35 | 4 | 26 |
| Hamburger | 1 burger | 360 | 140 | 16 | 5 | 40 | 560 | 39 | 1 | 14 |
| Triple Del Cheeseburger | 1 burger | 950 | 600 | 66 | 27 | 185 | 1660 | 40 | 1 | 44 |

### BURRITOS, TACOS, & QUESADILLAS

| | SERVING SIZE | CAL | CAL FAT | TOT FAT (G) | SAT FAT (G) | CHOL (MG) | SOD (MG) | CARB (G) | FIBER (G) | PROT (G) |
|---|---|---|---|---|---|---|---|---|---|---|
| Big Fat Crispy Chicken Taco | 1 taco | 400 | 170 | 19 | 4 | 25 | 850 | 45 | 2 | 16 |
| Big Fat Crispy Ranch Chicken Taco | 1 taco | 430 | 190 | 21 | 5 | 30 | 910 | 46 | 2 | 16 |
| Big Fat Steak Taco | 1 taco | 390 | 170 | 18 | 6 | 40 | 790 | 33 | 1 | 15 |
| Breakfast Del Carbon Taco | 1 taco | 140 | 40 | 5 | 1 | 135 | 170 | 18 | 1 | 7 |
| Cheddar Quesadilla | as served | 480 | 220 | 25 | 16 | 85 | 840 | 36 | 2 | 23 |
| Chicken Cheddar Quesadilla | as served | 570 | 260 | 29 | 16 | 130 | 1180 | 38 | 2 | 34 |
| Crispy Fish Taco | 1 taco | 300 | 150 | 17 | 2 | 25 | 320 | 29 | 3 | 8 |
| Del Beef Burrito | 1 burrito | 470 | 170 | 19 | 8 | 85 | 1060 | 24 | 2 | 29 |
| Del Classic Chicken Burrito | 1 burrito | 475 | 280 | 31 | 7 | 75 | 870 | 23 | 1 | 18 |
| Del Combo Burrito | 1 burrito | 475 | 130 | 14 | 6 | 50 | 1980 | 47 | 10 | 26 |
| Regular Taco | 1 taco | 130 | 70 | 7 | 3 | 20 | 180 | 9 | 1 | 7 |
| Santa Fe Chicken Soft Taco | 1 taco | 240 | 110 | 12 | 3 | 40 | 450 | 21 | 2 | 12 |
| Shredded Beef Combo Burrito | 1 burrito | 500 | 180 | 20 | 6 | 55 | 2010 | 47 | 9 | 28 |
| Soft Taco | 1 taco | 150 | 60 | 6 | 3 | 20 | 330 | 15 | 2 | 8 |
| Steak & Egg Burrito | 1 burrito | 520 | 210 | 23 | 9 | 355 | 1100 | 22 | 1 | 25 |
| Veggie Works Burrito | 1 burrito | 620 | 130 | 14 | 6 | 30 | 2200 | 83 | 9 | 18 |

### FRIES & SIDES

| | SERVING SIZE | CAL | CAL FAT | TOT FAT (G) | SAT FAT (G) | CHOL (MG) | SOD (MG) | CARB (G) | FIBER (G) | PROT (G) |
|---|---|---|---|---|---|---|---|---|---|---|
| Bean & Cheese Cup | as served | 320 | 35 | 4 | 2 | 10 | 2460 | 52 | 18 | 19 |
| Chili Cheese Fries | as served | 550 | 290 | 32 | 10 | 50 | 930 | 42 | 5 | 16 |
| Del Nachos | as served | 440 | 200 | 23 | 5 | 5 | 1140 | 45 | 7 | 10 |

| | SERVING SIZE | CAL | CAL FAT | TOT FAT (G) | SAT FAT (G) | CHOL (MG) | SOD (MG) | CARB (G) | FIBER (G) | PROT (G) |
|---|---|---|---|---|---|---|---|---|---|---|
| Deluxe Taco Salad | as served | 845 | 420 | 47 | 17 | 90 | 2470 | 69 | 14 | 34 |
| Hash Brown Sticks | 5 pieces | 210 | 140 | 15 | 2 | 0 | 180 | 18 | 0 | 0 |
| Jalapeno Rings | as served | 260 | 140 | 15 | 2 | 0 | 820 | 31 | 5 | 3 |
| Medium Fries | as served | 360 | 180 | 21 | 3 | 0 | 440 | 40 | 4 | 4 |

## Denny's
### APPETIZERS
| | | | | | | | | | | |
|---|---|---|---|---|---|---|---|---|---|---|
| Chicken Strips w/Buffalo Sauce | 1 order | 730 | n/a | 32 | .5 | 115 | 2940 | 53 | 1 | 57 |
| Chicken Wings w/Buffalo Sauce | 1 order | 300 | n/a | 21 | 5 | 125 | 1940 | 5 | 2 | 20 |
| Fried Shrimp w/Buffalo Sauce | 1 order | 380 | n/a | 17 | 3.5 | 125 | 2690 | 37 | 4 | 17 |
| Mozzarella Cheese Sticks | 1 order | 750 | n/a | 40 | 17 | 185 | 2270 | 195 | 1 | 16 |
| Sampler | 1 order | 1390 | n/a | 71 | 6 | 80 | 3710 | 139 | 6 | 53 |
| Smothered Cheese Fries | 1 order | 840 | n/a | 50 | 17 | 70 | 1070 | 74 | 7 | 24 |

### BREAKFAST
| | | | | | | | | | | |
|---|---|---|---|---|---|---|---|---|---|---|
| All-American Slam | 1 entrée | 820 | n/a | 69 | 26 | 780 | 1520 | 5 | 1 | 42 |
| Bacon Avocado Burrito | 1 entrée | 1010 | n/a | 59 | 15 | 275 | 2210 | 91 | 8 | 29 |
| Buttermilk Pancakes | 2 items | 340 | n/a | 4 | .5 | 0 | 1180 | 68 | 2 | 2 |
| Buttermilk Pancakes | 1 entrée | 510 | n/a | 6 | 0 | 0 | 1770 | 102 | 3 | 12 |
| Fabulous French Toast Platter | 1 entrée | 1010 | n/a | 52 | 16 | 560 | 2000 | 93 | 5 | 43 |
| French Toast Slam | 1 entrée | 940 | n/a | 53 | 17 | 855 | 1820 | 68 | 4 | 47 |
| Grand Slamwich w/o Hashbrowns | 1 entrée | 1320 | n/a | 90 | 42 | 550 | 3070 | 71 | 3 | 52 |
| Ham & Cheddar Omelette | 1 entrée | 590 | n/a | 44 | 17 | 755 | 1330 | 4 | 0 | 40 |
| Heartland Scramble | 1 entrée | 1150 | n/a | 66 | 20 | 530 | 2800 | 97 | 7 | 40 |
| Hearty Wheat Pancakes | 2 items | 460 | n/a | 2 | 0 | 20 | 1420 | 96 | 12 | 15 |
| Lumber Jack Slam | 1 entrée | 850 | n/a | 46 | 15 | 560 | 2770 | 60 | 3 | 45 |
| Meat Lover's Scramble | 1 entrée | 1130 | n/a | 66 | 29 | 570 | 3180 | 80 | 6 | 51 |
| Moons Over My Hammy | 1 entrée | 780 | n/a | 42 | 16 | 540 | 2580 | 50 | 2 | 46 |
| Southwestern Sizzlin' Skillet | 1 entrée | 990 | n/a | 61 | 21 | 545 | 2140 | 71 | 6 | 35 |
| Southwestern Steak Burrito | 1 entrée | 910 | n/a | 52 | 14 | 285 | 1970 | 76 | 5 | 33 |
| T-Bone Steak & Eggs | 1 entrée | 780 | n/a | 36 | 19 | 605 | 1210 | 4 | 0 | 110 |
| Ultimate Omelette | 1 entrée | 670 | n/a | 54 | 18 | 730 | 1170 | 8 | 2 | 36 |
| Veggie & Cheese Omelette | 1 entrée | 500 | n/a | 37 | 12 | 740 | 940 | 10 | 2 | 29 |

### BURGERS & SANDWICHES
| | | | | | | | | | | |
|---|---|---|---|---|---|---|---|---|---|---|
| Cheesy Three Pack | 1 sandwich | 1930 | n/a | 111 | 21 | 185 | 4120 | 164 | 8 | 73 |
| Chicken Ranch Melt | 1 sandwich | 800 | n/a | 30 | 9 | 110 | 2540 | 80 | 4 | 49 |
| Chicken Sandwich-Grilled w/Dressing | 1 sandwich | 880 | n/a | 51 | 9 | 100 | 1940 | 64 | 3 | 36 |
| Classic Burger w/o Cheese | 1 burger | 790 | n/a | 40 | 14 | 165 | 1010 | 50 | 3 | 55 |
| Fit Fare Boca Burger w/Fruit | 1 burger | 470 | n/a | 11 | 3 | 10 | 1460 | 71 | 11 | 28 |

# restaurants

| | SERVING SIZE | CAL | CAL FAT | TOT FAT (G) | SAT FAT (G) | CHOL (MG) | SOD (MG) | CARB (G) | FIBER (G) | PROT (G) |
|---|---|---|---|---|---|---|---|---|---|---|
| Fit Fare Chicken Sandwich w/Fruit | 1 sandwich | 450 | n/a | 6 | 1 | 70 | 1380 | 62 | 4 | 21 |
| Grand Slamwich w/o Side | 1 burger | 1320 | n/a | 90 | 42 | 550 | 3070 | 71 | 3 | 52 |
| Mushroom Swiss Burger | 1 burger | 910 | n/a | 49 | 18 | 190 | 1710 | 55 | 4 | 61 |
| Prime Rib Philly Melt | 1 burger | 730 | n/a | 43 | 12 | 75 | 1820 | 53 | 4 | 35 |
| Slamburger | 1 burger | 990 | n/a | 54 | 19 | 390 | 1460 | 59 | 2 | 64 |
| Smoked Chicken Melt | 1 sandwich | 950 | n/a | 55 | 14 | 105 | 1820 | 72 | 3 | 38 |
| Smokin' Q Three Pack | 1 sandwich | 2020 | n/a | 110 | 22 | 205 | 3570 | 185 | 9 | 79 |
| Spicy Buffalo Chicken Melt | 1 sandwich | 870 | n/a | 41 | 10 | 95 | 3820 | 82 | 5 | 45 |
| **ENTRÉES** | | | | | | | | | | |
| Chicken Strips | 1 entrée | 560 | n/a | 24 | 0 | 90 | 1300 | 41 | 0 | 45 |
| Country Fried Steak w/Gravy | 1 entrée | 1000 | n/a | 65 | 22 | 75 | 2590 | 54 | 6 | 51 |
| Fit Fare Grilled Chicken | 1 entrée | 380 | n/a | 10 | 2 | 135 | 1280 | 12 | 2 | 57 |
| Fit Fare Grilled Tilapia | 1 entrée | 600 | n/a | 11 | 3 | 110 | 1560 | 66 | 3 | 58 |
| Grilled Chicken | 1 entrée | 280 | n/a | 4 | 1 | 135 | 1190 | 4 | 0 | 55 |
| Grilled Chicken Sizzlin' Skillet Dinner | 1 entrée | 770 | n/a | 34 | 12 | 100 | 2020 | 72 | 5 | 41 |
| Grilled Shrimp Skewers | 1 entrée | 370 | n/a | 10 | 2 | 270 | 1140 | 39 | 2 | 32 |
| Homestyle Meatloaf & Gravy | 1 entrée | 600 | n/a | 46 | 17 | 200 | 1880 | 14 | 0 | 33 |
| Mushroom Swiss Chopped Steak | 1 entrée | 940 | n/a | 66 | 24 | 245 | 1710 | 13 | 1 | 69 |
| Prime Rib Sizzlin' Skillet Dinner | 1 entrée | 900 | n/a | 42 | 17 | 125 | 2480 | 77 | 5 | 49 |
| Sweet & Tangy BBQ Chicken | 1 entrée | 650 | n/a | 11 | 3 | 155 | 2290 | 108 | 3 | 62 |
| T-Bone Steak | 1 entrée | 640 | n/a | 42 | 14 | 135 | 740 | 0 | 0 | 59 |
| **SOUPS, SALADS, & SIDES** | | | | | | | | | | |
| Breaded Shrimp | as served | 190 | n/a | 8 | 2 | 70 | 750 | 20 | 2 | 9 |
| Broccoli & Cheddar Soup | 12 oz | 374 | n/a | 29 | 19 | 69 | 1568 | 16 | 4 | 10 |
| Chicken Deluxe Salad-Chicken Strips | as served | 590 | n/a | 29 | 5 | 90 | 1180 | 44 | 4 | 42 |
| Chicken Deluxe Salad-Grilled Chicken | as served | 290 | n/a | 10 | 5 | 90 | 770 | 15 | 4 | 36 |
| Chicken Noodle Soup | 12 oz | 166 | n/a | 4 | 2 | 48 | 1304 | 19 | 1 | 12 |
| Cranberry-Pecan Chicken Salad (no dressing) | as served | 250 | n/a | 8 | 3 | 85 | 830 | 11 | 1 | 32 |
| Fit-Fare Grilled Chicken Breast | as served | 290 | n/a | 10 | 5 | 90 | 770 | 15 | 4 | 36 |
| Grilled Shrimp Skewer | as served | 90 | n/a | 3.5 | 1 | 135 | 160 | 0 | 0 | 14 |
| Prime Rib & Bleu Salad (no dressing) | as served | 270 | n/a | 16 | 6 | 70 | 930 | 6 | 1 | 24 |
| Ranchero Mashed Potatoes | as served | 140 | n/a | 6 | 2 | 20 | 460 | 50 | 1 | 3 |
| Seasoned Fries | as served | 510 | n/a | 33 | 6 | 0 | 1010 | 48 | 5 | 6 |
| Smoked Cheddar Mashed Potatoes | as served | 120 | n/a | 5 | 2 | 20 | 380 | 49 | 1 | 3 |
| Vegetable Beef Soup | 12 oz | 124 | n/a | 1 | 0 | 21 | 1457 | 18 | 3 | 10 |

# Domino's
## PASTA & SALADS

| | SERVING SIZE | CAL | CAL FAT | TOT FAT (G) | SAT FAT (G) | CHOL (MG) | SOD (MG) | CARB (G) | FIBER (G) | PROT (G) |
|---|---|---|---|---|---|---|---|---|---|---|
| Garden Fresh Salad | 1/2 salad | 70 | 35 | 3.5 | 2.5 | 10 | 80 | 5 | 2 | 4 |
| Grilled Chicken Caesar Salad | 1/2 salad | 90 | 30 | 3.5 | 1.5 | 20 | 290 | 5 | 2 | 9 |
| Pasta in a Breadbowl, Chicken Alfredo | 1/2 bowl | 700 | 230 | 26 | 11 | 50 | 1040 | 93 | 3 | 25 |
| Pasta in a Breadbowl, Chicken Carbonara | 1/2 bowl | 740 | 260 | 28 | 12 | 55 | 1110 | 94 | 3 | 28 |
| Pasta in a Breadbowl, Italian Sausage Marinara | 1/2 bowl | 730 | 240 | 27 | 10 | 35 | 1380 | 97 | 4 | 26 |
| Pasta in a Breadbowl, Mac-N-Cheese | 1/2 bowl | 730 | 250 | 28 | 14 | 55 | 1390 | 95 | 3 | 27 |
| Pasta in a Breadbowl, Pasta Primavera | 1/2 bowl | 670 | 220 | 24 | 11 | 35 | 880 | 94 | 4 | 20 |
| Pasta in a Dish, Chicken Alfredo | 1 bowl | 600 | 260 | 29 | 16 | 100 | 1080 | 58 | 2 | 27 |
| Pasta in a Dish, Italian Sausage Marinara | 1 bowl | 670 | 280 | 32 | 15 | 65 | 1760 | 66 | 5 | 28 |
| Pasta in a Dish, Pasta Primavera | 1 bowl | 540 | 240 | 27 | 16 | 65 | 770 | 59 | 3 | 16 |
| **PIZZA, MEDIUM 12"** | | | | | | | | | | |
| America's Favorite Feast, Deep Dish | 1 slice | 280 | 130 | 14 | 5.5 | 25 | 730 | 29 | 4 | 10 |
| America's Favorite Feast, Hand Tossed | 1 slice | 250 | 105 | 12 | 5 | 25 | 630 | 27 | 2 | 10 |
| America's Favorite Feast, Thin Crust | 1 slice | 420 | 230 | 26 | 10 | 50 | 1000 | 30 | 2 | 16 |
| Buffalo Chicken, Deep Dish | 1 slice | 300 | 150 | 17 | 7 | 35 | 790 | 26 | 3 | 13 |
| Buffalo Chicken, Hand Tossed | 1 slice | 260 | 120 | 14 | 6.5 | 35 | 660 | 24 | 1 | 13 |
| Buffalo Chicken, Thin Crust | 1 slice | 380 | 200 | 22 | 10 | 60 | 1020 | 26 | 1 | 18 |
| Cali Chicken Bacon Ranch, Deep Dish | 1 slice | 360 | 200 | 22 | 7 | 40 | 780 | 27 | 3 | 14 |
| Cali Chicken Bacon Ranch, Hand Tossed | 1 slice | 320 | 165 | 18 | 6.5 | 40 | 660 | 25 | 1 | 14 |
| Cali Chicken Bacon Ranch, Thin Crust | 1 slice | 490 | 290 | 33 | 11 | 70 | 990 | 28 | 2 | 21 |
| Deep Dish Cheese | 1 slice | 260 | 110 | 12 | 5 | 25 | 630 | 29 | 3 | 10 |
| ExtravaganZZa Feast, Deep Dish | 1 slice | 320 | 150 | 16 | 7 | 35 | 870 | 30 | 4 | 13 |
| ExtravaganZZa Feast, Hand Tossed | 1 slice | 290 | 125 | 14 | 6.5 | 35 | 770 | 28 | 2 | 13 |
| ExtravaganZZa Feast, Thin Crust | 1 slice | 480 | 260 | 30 | 12 | 70 | 1280 | 32 | 3 | 21 |
| Fiery Hawaiian (Hot Sauce), Deep Dish | 1 slice | 290 | 140 | 15 | 5.5 | 25 | 890 | 30 | 4 | 12 |
| Fiery Hawaiian (Hot Sauce), Hand Tossed | 1 slice | 250 | 105 | 11 | 5 | 25 | 760 | 27 | 2 | 12 |
| Fiery Hawaiian (Hot Sauce), Thin Crust | 1 slice | 390 | 190 | 22 | 9 | 55 | 1240 | 32 | 2 | 17 |
| Hand Tossed Cheese | 1 slice | 210 | 72 | 8 | 3.5 | 20 | 460 | 25 | 1 | 25 |
| Honolulu Hawaiian, Deep Dish | 1 slice | 290 | 140 | 15 | 5.5 | 25 | 710 | 29 | 4 | 12 |
| Honolulu Hawaiian, Hand Tossed | 1 slice | 250 | 105 | 11 | 5 | 25 | 580 | 26 | 2 | 12 |
| Honolulu Hawaiian, Thin Crust | 1 slice | 390 | 190 | 22 | 9 | 55 | 890 | 31 | 2 | 17 |
| MeatZZa Feast, Deep Dish | 1 slice | 310 | 150 | 16 | 6 | 35 | 860 | 29 | 4 | 12 |
| MeatZZa Feast, Hand Tossed | 1 slice | 280 | 125 | 14 | 5.5 | 35 | 760 | 27 | 2 | 12 |
| MeatZZa Feast, Thin Crust | 1 slice | 470 | 260 | 29 | 12 | 70 | 1260 | 31 | 2 | 21 |

# restaurants

| | SERVING SIZE | CAL | CAL FAT | TOT FAT (G) | SAT FAT (G) | CHOL (MG) | SOD (MG) | CARB (G) | FIBER (G) | PROT (G) |
|---|---|---|---|---|---|---|---|---|---|---|
| Memphis BBQ Chicken, Deep Dish | 1 slice | 300 | 130 | 15 | 6 | 30 | 630 | 30 | 3 | 13 |
| Memphis BBQ Chicken, Hand Tossed | 1 slice | 260 | 100 | 12 | 5.5 | 30 | 500 | 28 | 1 | 13 |
| Memphis BBQ Chicken, Thin Crust | 1 slice | 370 | 170 | 19 | 8 | 55 | 690 | 33 | 2 | 17 |
| Pacific Veggie, Deep Dish | 1 slice | 270 | 120 | 14 | 5 | 20 | 590 | 28 | 4 | 10 |
| Pacific Veggie, Hand Tossed | 1 slice | 230 | 85 | 10 | 4.5 | 20 | 460 | 25 | 2 | 10 |
| Pacific Veggie, Thin Crust | 1 slice | 340 | 170 | 19 | 8 | 40 | 650 | 29 | 2 | 14 |
| Philly Cheese Steak, Deep Dish | 1 slice | 300 | 140 | 16 | 6.5 | 30 | 660 | 26 | 3 | 11 |
| Philly Cheese Steak, Hand Tossed | 1 slice | 260 | 105 | 12 | 6 | 30 | 540 | 24 | 1 | 11 |
| Philly Cheese Steak, Thin Crust | 1 slice | 360 | 190 | 21 | 10 | 55 | 740 | 26 | 1 | 16 |
| Thin Crust Cheese | 1 slice | 330 | 150 | 18 | 7 | 40 | 660 | 30 | 3 | 14 |
| Ultimate Pepperoni Feast, Deep Dish | 1 slice | 290 | 140 | 15 | 6 | 30 | 750 | 27 | 3 | 11 |
| Ultimate Pepperoni Feast, Hand Tossed | 1 slice | 260 | 115 | 13 | 5.5 | 30 | 650 | 25 | 1 | 11 |
| Ultimate Pepperoni Feast, Thin Crust | 1 slice | 430 | 240 | 27 | 11 | 60 | 1020 | 28 | 2 | 18 |
| **SANDWICHES** | | | | | | | | | | |
| Buffalo Chicken w/Blue Cheese | 1 sandwich | 830 | 370 | 41 | 16 | 115 | 2690 | 74 | 3 | 42 |
| Chicken Bacon Ranch | 1 sandwich | 870 | 400 | 45 | 16 | 125 | 2380 | 72 | 2 | 45 |
| Chicken Parm | 1 sandwich | 750 | 270 | 30 | 16 | 120 | 2200 | 73 | 3 | 47 |
| Italian | 1 sandwich | 820 | 370 | 41 | 20 | 130 | 2700 | 70 | 3 | 41 |
| Mediterranean Veggie | 1 sandwich | 680 | 260 | 29 | 1 | 85 | 2050 | 72 | 4 | 32 |
| Philly Cheese Steak | 1 sandwich | 690 | 250 | 28 | 15 | 105 | 2120 | 70 | 3 | 39 |
| Sweet & Spicy Chicken Habanera | 1 sandwich | 800 | 290 | 32 | 17 | 125 | 2170 | 83 | 3 | 46 |
| **SIDES** | | | | | | | | | | |
| Barbeque Buffalo Wings | 2 pieces | 230 | 130 | 14 | 3.5 | 50 | 410 | 6 | 0 | 17 |
| Breadsticks | 1 piece | 110 | 60 | 6 | 1.5 | 0 | 100 | 11 | 0 | 6 |
| Buffalo Chicken Kickers | 2 pieces | 100 | 40 | 4.5 | 1 | 20 | 280 | 7 | 1 | 9 |
| Cheesy Bread | 1 piece | 120 | 60 | 6 | 2 | 5 | 140 | 11 | 0 | 4 |
| Cinna Stix | 1 piece | 120 | 60 | 6 | 1 | 0 | 85 | 14 | 1 | 2 |
| Hot Buffalo Wings | 2 pieces | 200 | 120 | 14 | 3.5 | 50 | 690 | 2 | 0 | 16 |
| **Don Pablo's** | | | | | | | | | | |
| **APPETIZERS** | | | | | | | | | | |
| Don's Boneless Wings | 3 wings | 623 | 502 | 48 | 8 | 52 | 2473 | 28 | 3 | 21 |
| Flautas | 2 flautas | 188 | 133 | 12 | 2 | 26 | 382 | 13 | 2 | 9 |
| Taquitos | 2 taquitos | 209 | 171 | 15 | 7 | 29 | 424 | 9 | 1 | 8 |
| The Don's Sampler | 1/4 item | 497 | 263 | 29 | 14 | 7 | 940 | 35 | 3 | 25 |
| **BURRITOS, ENCHILADAS, & TACOS** | | | | | | | | | | |
| Cheese Enchilada | 1 entrée | 530 | 265 | 29 | 16 | 73 | 1335 | 41 | 5 | 27 |

| | SERVING SIZE | CAL | CAL FAT | TOT FAT (G) | SAT FAT (G) | CHOL (MG) | SOD (MG) | CARB (G) | FIBER (G) | PROT (G) |
|---|---|---|---|---|---|---|---|---|---|---|
| Chicken Burrito | 1 burrito | 1181 | 522 | 58 | 26 | 128 | 2411 | 105 | 11 | 60 |
| Crispy Taco-Beef | 1 taco | 260 | 119 | 13 | 6 | 51 | 406 | 16 | 3 | 18 |
| Crispy Taco-Chicken | 1 taco | 211 | 88 | 10 | 4 | 32 | 583 | 16 | 2 | 15 |
| Soft Taco-Beef | 1 taco | 326 | 145 | 16 | 7 | 51 | 622 | 24 | 2 | 20 |
| Soft Taco-Chicken | 1 taco | 277 | 114 | 13 | 6 | 32 | 800 | 24 | 2 | 16 |
| Spicy Beef & Bean Burrito | 1 burrito | 1285 | 615 | 68 | 30 | 185 | 2000 | 97 | 12 | 69 |
| Three Beef Enchiladas | 1 entrée | 900 | 463 | 49 | 19 | 191 | 2131 | 46 | 5 | 66 |
| Three Chicken Enchiladas | 1 entrée | 814 | 453 | 48 | 23 | 126 | 1700 | 55 | 3 | 42 |
| **CHIMICHANGA** | | | | | | | | | | |
| Chicken | 1 chimichanga | 1110 | 709 | 61 | 21 | 94 | 2209 | 91 | 8 | 49 |
| **ENTRÉES** | | | | | | | | | | |
| Chicken Stix | 1 entrée | 978 | 719 | 66 | 11 | 68 | 2622 | 80 | 4 | 26 |
| Chicken Tenders | 1 entrée | 1007 | 649 | 51 | 10 | 106 | 3144 | 109 | 8 | 33 |
| Corn Dog | 1 entrée | 832 | 347 | 39 | 9 | 20 | 3114 | 107 | 9 | 18 |
| Dogs in a Blanket | 1 entrée | 613 | 239 | 27 | 6 | 0 | 2323 | 83 | 6 | 12 |
| Grilled Chicken Entrée | 1 entrée | 877 | 229 | 25 | 5 | 110 | 3292 | 113 | 3 | 49 |
| Rio Grande Ribs | 1 entrée | 1568 | 949 | 105 | 29 | 222 | 6001 | 116 | 13 | 73 |
| **FAJITAS & FAJITA COMBOS** | | | | | | | | | | |
| Chicken Fajita & Enchilada Combo | 1 entrée | 604 | 257 | 28 | 8 | 76 | 1619 | 60 | 4 | 30 |
| Classic Combo w/Steak & Chicken | 1 entrée | 627 | 281 | 31 | 8 | 96 | 1263 | 47 | 3 | 44 |
| The Ultimate Tex-Mex Combo-Chicken | 1 entrée | 892 | 570 | 63 | 16 | 130 | 2590 | 55 | 4 | 45 |
| **QUESADILLAS, SMALL** | | | | | | | | | | |
| Cheese Quesadilla | 2 pieces | 497 | 316 | 35 | 18 | 66 | 732 | 27 | 2 | 19 |
| Grilled Steak Quesadilla | 2 pieces | 431 | 240 | 27 | 13 | 60 | 699 | 27 | 1 | 21 |
| Mesquite-Grilled Chicken Quesadilla | 2 pieces | 413 | 228 | 25 | 12 | 50 | 706 | 31 | 1 | 16 |
| **RELLANOS** | | | | | | | | | | |
| Beef | as served | 391 | 148 | 17 | 6 | 77 | 1754 | 38 | 4 | 22 |
| Cheese | as served | 498 | 255 | 28 | 15 | 100 | 1799 | 37 | 3 | 25 |
| Chicken | as served | 343 | 118 | 13 | 4 | 58 | 1931 | 39 | 3 | 19 |
| **SALADS & SIDES** | | | | | | | | | | |
| Caesar | 1 salad | 1047 | 614 | 68 | 12 | 39 | 1264 | 89 | 11 | 20 |
| Charra Beans | 4 oz | 192 | 30 | 3 | 1 | 0 | 599 | 31 | 8 | 10 |
| Chile Mashed Potatoes | 4 oz | 182 | 104 | 12 | 4 | 10 | 604 | 16 | 2 | 4 |
| Chicken Nachos | as served | 754 | 401 | 43 | 23 | 151 | 1306 | 43 | 6 | 49 |
| French Fries | 7 oz | 345 | 89 | 10 | 0 | 45 | 708 | 60 | 6 | 6 |
| Refritos | 5 oz | 214 | 60 | 7 | 2 | 7 | 614 | 27 | 7 | 11 |
| Taco Salad w/Beef | 1 salad | 1029 | 560 | 62 | 28 | 191 | 2181 | 50 | 16 | 69 |

# restaurants

| | SERVING SIZE | CAL | CAL FAT | TOT FAT (G) | SAT FAT (G) | CHOL (MG) | SOD (MG) | CARB (G) | FIBER (G) | PROT (G) |
|---|---|---|---|---|---|---|---|---|---|---|
| Taco Salad w/Chicken | 1 salad | 884 | 467 | 52 | 23 | 133 | 2714 | 51 | 14 | 58 |
| Tortilla Salad | 1 salad | 131 | 42 | 5 | 3 | 14 | 58 | 17 | 4 | 6 |

## Donato's
### PIZZA

| | SERVING SIZE | CAL | CAL FAT | TOT FAT (G) | SAT FAT (G) | CHOL (MG) | SOD (MG) | CARB (G) | FIBER (G) | PROT (G) |
|---|---|---|---|---|---|---|---|---|---|---|
| Founder's Favorite, Bakery Style | 2 slices | 760 | 297 | 33 | n/a | n/a | n/a | 76 | 4 | 40 |
| Founder's Favorite, Hand Tossed | 2 slices | 678 | 279 | 31 | n/a | n/a | n/a | 66 | 5 | 30 |
| Founder's Favorite, Thicker Crust | 1/4 pizza | 780 | 378 | 36 | n/a | n/a | n/a | 70 | 4 | 44 |
| Founder's Favorite, Thin Crust | 1/4 pizza | 702 | 342 | 38 | n/a | n/a | n/a | 52 | 2 | 39 |
| Pepperoni, Bakery Style | 2 slices | 700 | 252 | 28 | n/a | n/a | n/a | 75 | 5 | 35 |
| Pepperoni, Hand Tossed | 2 slices | 499 | 243 | 27 | n/a | n/a | n/a | 65 | 5 | 23 |
| Pepperoni, Thicker Crust | 1/4 pizza | 710 | 351 | 32 | n/a | n/a | n/a | 69 | 4 | 37 |
| Pepperoni, Thin Crust | 1/4 pizza | 627 | 306 | 34 | n/a | n/a | n/a | 50 | 2 | 32 |
| Serious Cheese, Bakery Style | 2 slices | 690 | 243 | 27 | n/a | n/a | n/a | 75 | 5 | 36 |
| Serious Cheese, Hand Tossed | 2 slices | 597 | 225 | 25 | n/a | n/a | n/a | 65 | 5 | 27 |
| Serious Cheese, Thicker Crust | 1/4 pizza | 798 | 342 | 38 | n/a | n/a | n/a | 77 | 4 | 40 |
| Serious Cheese, Thin Crust | 1/4 pizza | 710 | 306 | 31 | n/a | n/a | n/a | 69 | 5 | 38 |
| Vegy, Bakery Style | 2 slices | 650 | 117 | 22 | n/a | n/a | n/a | 80 | 4 | 16 |
| Vegy, Hand Tossed | 2 slices | 650 | 198 | 22 | n/a | n/a | n/a | 80 | 7 | 32 |
| Vegy, Thicker Crust | 1/4 pizza | 630 | 261 | 23 | n/a | n/a | n/a | 75 | 6 | 32 |
| Vegy, Thin Crust | 1/4 pizza | 544 | 216 | 24 | n/a | n/a | n/a | 57 | 4 | 26 |

### SALADS & SIDES

| | | | | | | | | | | |
|---|---|---|---|---|---|---|---|---|---|---|
| BBQ Buffalo Wings | 5 wings | 595 | 387 | 43 | n/a | n/a | n/a | 10 | 0 | 34 |
| Breadsticks w/Nacho Cheese Sauce | 2 pieces | 398 | 198 | 22 | n/a | n/a | n/a | 39 | 2 | 13 |
| Buffalo Wings | 5 wings | 552 | 387 | 43 | n/a | n/a | n/a | 10 | 0 | 34 |
| Chicken Breast Strips | 2 pieces | 125 | 36 | 4 | n/a | n/a | n/a | 12 | 0 | 11 |
| Chicken Harvest Salad | 1 salad | 540 | 288 | 32 | n/a | n/a | n/a | 32 | 6 | 32 |
| French Fries-Wedge Side Portion | as served | 261 | 117 | 13 | n/a | n/a | n/a | 34 | 6 | 4 |
| Garlic Bread-3 Cheese | 2 pieces | 174 | 81 | 9 | n/a | n/a | n/a | 16 | 1 | 8 |
| Italian Chef Salad | 1 salad | 290 | 180 | 20 | n/a | n/a | n/a | 8 | 3 | 19 |

### STROMBOLI

| | | | | | | | | | | |
|---|---|---|---|---|---|---|---|---|---|---|
| Cheese | 1 stromboli | 693 | 279 | 31 | n/a | n/a | n/a | 66 | 5 | 35 |
| Pepperoni | 1 stromboli | 716 | 306 | 34 | n/a | n/a | n/a | 67 | 5 | 34 |
| Vegy | 1 stromboli | 606 | 216 | 24 | n/a | n/a | n/a | 69 | 5 | 27 |

### SUBS

| | | | | | | | | | | |
|---|---|---|---|---|---|---|---|---|---|---|
| Big Don Italian, White Bread | 1 sub | 717 | 306 | 34 | n/a | n/a | n/a | 68 | 3 | 35 |
| Buffalo Chicken Sub, White Bread | 1 sub | 720 | 315 | 35 | n/a | n/a | n/a | 64 | 3 | 39 |
| Chicken Bacon Cheddar, White Bread | 1 sub | 818 | 333 | 37 | n/a | n/a | n/a | 68 | 3 | 48 |

| | SERVING SIZE | CAL | CAL FAT | TOT FAT (G) | SAT FAT (G) | CHOL (MG) | SOD (MG) | CARB (G) | FIBER (G) | PROT (G) |
|---|---|---|---|---|---|---|---|---|---|---|
| Fresh Vegy, White Bread | 1 sub | 540 | 171 | 19 | n/a | n/a | n/a | 71 | 5 | 22 |
| Meatball, White Bread | 1 sub | 1119 | 567 | 63 | n/a | n/a | n/a | 78 | 8 | 60 |
| Turkey Club, White Bread | 1 sub | 743 | 270 | 30 | n/a | n/a | n/a | 66 | 3 | 49 |

## Dunkin' Donuts
### BAGELS & CREAM CHEESE

| | SERVING SIZE | CAL | CAL FAT | TOT FAT (G) | SAT FAT (G) | CHOL (MG) | SOD (MG) | CARB (G) | FIBER (G) | PROT (G) |
|---|---|---|---|---|---|---|---|---|---|---|
| Blueberry Bagel | 1 bagel | 330 | 25 | 3 | 1 | 0 | 620 | 65 | 5 | 11 |
| Cinnamon Raisin Bagel | 1 bagel | 330 | 30 | 3.5 | .5 | 0 | 450 | 65 | 5 | 11 |
| Everything Bagel | 1 bagel | 350 | 40 | 4.5 | .5 | 0 | 660 | 66 | 5 | 13 |
| Multigrain Bagel | 1 bagel | 390 | 70 | 8 | .5 | 0 | 560 | 65 | 9 | 14 |
| Plain Bagel | 1 bagel | 230 | 25 | 2.5 | .5 | 0 | 660 | 63 | 5 | 11 |
| Poppy Seed Bagel | 1 bagel | 350 | 50 | 6 | .5 | 0 | 660 | 64 | 5 | 13 |
| Reduced Fat Plain Cream Cheese | 1-1/2 oz | 100 | 70 | 8 | 5 | 25 | 250 | 5 | 0 | 4 |
| Reduced Fat Strawberry Cream Cheese | 1-1/2 oz | 150 | 90 | 10 | 6 | 30 | 200 | 15 | 0 | 2 |
| Wheat Bagel | 1 bagel | 320 | 30 | 3.5 | 0 | 0 | 550 | 61 | 5 | 12 |

### BAKERY

| | SERVING SIZE | CAL | CAL FAT | TOT FAT (G) | SAT FAT (G) | CHOL (MG) | SOD (MG) | CARB (G) | FIBER (G) | PROT (G) |
|---|---|---|---|---|---|---|---|---|---|---|
| Bavarian Kreme Donut | 1 doughnut | 250 | 110 | 12 | 5 | 0 | 330 | 31 | 1 | 3 |
| Blueberry Muffin | 1 muffin | 480 | 140 | 15 | 1.5 | 15 | 470 | 81 | 2 | 6 |
| Boston Kreme Donut | 1 doughnut | 280 | 110 | 12 | 5 | 0 | 350 | 38 | 1 | 3 |
| Chocolate Frosted Donut | 1 doughnut | 230 | 90 | 10 | 4 | 0 | 330 | 32 | 1 | 3 |
| Chocolate Glazed Cake Donut | 1 doughnut | 280 | 140 | 15 | 7 | 0 | 400 | 33 | 1 | 3 |
| Chocolate Kreme Filled Donut | 1 doughnut | 310 | 140 | 16 | 7 | 0 | 340 | 37 | 1 | 4 |
| Corn Muffin | 1 muffin | 490 | 140 | 16 | 1.5 | 20 | 820 | 80 | 1 | 6 |
| Double Chocolate Cake Donut | 1 doughnut | 290 | 150 | 16 | 7 | 0 | 410 | 34 | 1 | 3 |
| Éclair | 1 pastry | 350 | 120 | 14 | 5 | 0 | 460 | 53 | 1 | 4 |
| Glazed Cake Donut | 1 doughnut | 320 | 160 | 18 | 8 | 25 | 310 | 37 | 1 | 3 |
| Jelly Filled Donut | 1 doughnut | 260 | 100 | 11 | 5 | 0 | 330 | 36 | 1 | 3 |
| Jelly Filled Munchkin | 1 piece | 60 | 20 | 2.5 | 1 | 0 | 65 | 8 | 0 | 1 |
| Old Fashioned Cake Donut | 1 doughnut | 280 | 160 | 18 | 8 | 25 | 310 | 27 | 1 | 3 |
| Plain Cake Munchkin | 1 piece | 50 | 30 | 3 | 1.5 | 5 | 60 | 5 | 0 | 1 |
| Plain Croissant | 1 croissant | 310 | 150 | 16 | 7 | 0 | 350 | 35 | 1 | 7 |
| Powdered Cake Donut | 1 doughnut | 300 | 160 | 18 | 8 | 25 | 310 | 30 | 1 | 3 |
| Powdered Cake Munchkin | 1 piece | 60 | 30 | 3.5 | 1.5 | 5 | 60 | 6 | 0 | 1 |
| Reduced Fat Blueberry Muffin | 1 muffin | 430 | 80 | 9 | 1 | 15 | 650 | 80 | 2 | 6 |
| Vanilla Kreme Filled Donut | 1 doughnut | 320 | 160 | 17 | 8 | 0 | 340 | 37 | 1 | 3 |

### BEVERAGES, MEDIUM

| | SERVING SIZE | CAL | CAL FAT | TOT FAT (G) | SAT FAT (G) | CHOL (MG) | SOD (MG) | CARB (G) | FIBER (G) | PROT (G) |
|---|---|---|---|---|---|---|---|---|---|---|
| Coffee Coolatta w/Milk | 24 fl oz | 360 | 50 | 6 | 3.5 | 25 | 130 | 75 | 0 | 6 |
| Coffee w/Skim Milk & Splenda | 14 fl oz | 30 | 0 | 0 | 0 | 0 | 35 | 6 | 0 | 2 |

# restaurants

| | SERVING SIZE | CAL | CAL FAT | TOT FAT (G) | SAT FAT (G) | CHOL (MG) | SOD (MG) | CARB (G) | FIBER (G) | PROT (G) |
|---|---|---|---|---|---|---|---|---|---|---|
| Freshly Brewed Sweetened Iced Tea | 16 fl oz | 80 | 0 | 0 | 0 | 0 | 0 | 20 | 0 | 0 |
| Freshly Brewed Unsweetened Iced Tea | 16 fl oz | 5 | 0 | 0 | 0 | 0 | 0 | 1 | 0 | 0 |
| Iced Coffee w/Skim Milk & Splenda | 24 fl oz | 40 | 0 | 0 | 0 | 0 | 35 | 8 | 0 | 3 |
| Iced Dunkin' Dark Roast Coffee w/Cream & Sugar | 24 fl oz | 190 | 80 | 9 | 5 | 30 | 30 | 30 | 0 | 2 |
| Iced Latte Lite | 24 fl oz | 120 | 0 | 0 | 0 | 5 | 170 | 19 | 0 | 10 |
| Iced Mocha Raspberry Latte | 24 fl oz | 340 | 80 | 9 | 6 | 35 | 160 | 54 | 2 | 10 |
| Iced Mocha Spice Latte | 24 fl oz | 330 | 80 | 9 | 6 | 35 | 140 | 53 | 2 | 10 |
| Latte Lite | 16 fl oz | 120 | 0 | 0 | 0 | 5 | 170 | 19 | 0 | 10 |
| Mocha Coffee w/Cream | 14 fl oz | 260 | 80 | 9 | 6 | 30 | 45 | 41 | 2 | 3 |
| Mocha Raspberry Latte | 16 fl oz | 340 | 80 | 9 | 6 | 35 | 160 | 54 | 2 | 10 |
| Mocha Spice Latte | 16 fl oz | 330 | 80 | 9 | 6 | 35 | 140 | 53 | 2 | 10 |
| Peach Flavored Iced Tea | 16 fl oz | 15 | 0 | 0 | 0 | 0 | 0 | 2 | 0 | 0 |
| Peach Flavored Sweetened Iced Tea | 16 fl oz | 90 | 0 | 0 | 0 | 0 | 0 | 21 | 0 | 0 |
| Strawberry Fruit Coolatta | 24 fl oz | 440 | 0 | 0 | 0 | 0 | 60 | 108 | 0 | 1 |
| Tropicana Orange Coolatta | 24 fl oz | 330 | 0 | 0 | 0 | 0 | 55 | 79 | 0 | 2 |
| Vanilla Bean Coolatta | 24 fl oz | 650 | 80 | 9 | 5 | 30 | 260 | 136 | 0 | 4 |
| Vanilla Chai | 14 fl oz | 330 | 80 | 9 | 8 | 10 | 170 | 53 | 0 | 11 |
| **BREAKFAST** | | | | | | | | | | |
| Bacon, Egg, & Cheese on English Muffin | 1 sandwich | 360 | 140 | 16 | 6 | 195 | 1020 | 34 | 2 | 18 |
| Bacon, Egg White, & Cheese on English Muffin | 1 sandwich | 310 | 70 | 8 | 4 | 15 | 1030 | 34 | 2 | 19 |
| Egg & Cheese on English Muffin | 1 sandwich | 320 | 120 | 13 | 5 | 195 | 840 | 34 | 2 | 15 |
| Egg White & Cheese on English Muffin | 1 sandwich | 270 | 45 | 5 | 3 | 10 | 850 | 34 | 2 | 16 |
| Egg White Turkey Sausage Flatbread | 1 sandwich | 290 | 70 | 8 | 3 | 20 | 600 | 34 | 3 | 21 |
| Egg White Veggie Flatbread | 1 sandwich | 330 | 110 | 12 | 5 | 25 | 820 | 35 | 4 | 20 |
| Ham, Egg & Cheese on English Muffin | 1 sandwich | 360 | 140 | 15 | 6 | 215 | 1140 | 35 | 2 | 21 |
| Sausage, Egg &Cheese on English Muffin | 1 sandwich | 490 | 250 | 28 | 10 | 240 | 1240 | 35 | 2 | 22 |
| **Edo Japan** | | | | | | | | | | |
| **BENTO BOXES** | | | | | | | | | | |
| Beef Yakisoba w/o Teriyaki Sauce | 30 oz | 830 | 270 | 30 | 8 | 100 | 1580 | 102 | 3 | 43 |
| Chicken & Beef w/o Teriyaki Sauce | 20 oz | 880 | 234 | 26 | 7 | 120 | 1260 | 120 | 4 | 40 |
| Sukiyaki Beef w/o Teriyaki Sauce | 20 oz | 900 | 252 | 28 | 8 | 100 | 1240 | 120 | 4 | 39 |
| Teriyaki Chicken w/o Teriyaki Sauce | 21 oz | 870 | 216 | 24 | 6 | 135 | 1280 | 120 | 4 | 41 |
| **EXTRAS** | | | | | | | | | | |
| California Roll | 8 oz | 430 | 153 | 17 | 2.5 | 55 | 490 | 61 | 1 | 9 |
| Vegetable Spring Roll | 1-1/2 oz | 120 | 54 | 6 | 1.5 | 0 | 310 | 14 | 2 | 3 |

| | SERVING SIZE | CAL | CAL FAT | TOT FAT (G) | SAT FAT (G) | CHOL (MG) | SOD (MG) | CARB (G) | FIBER (G) | PROT (G) |
|---|---|---|---|---|---|---|---|---|---|---|
| **SOUP** | | | | | | | | | | |
| Beef Udon | 34 oz | 580 | 153 | 17 | 7 | 65 | 3370 | 72 | 7 | 34 |
| Chicken Udon | 34 oz | 550 | 117 | 13 | 4 | 105 | 3440 | 72 | 7 | 36 |
| Vegetable Udon | 32 oz | 370 | 13.5 | 1.5 | 1 | 0 | 3250 | 77 | 9 | 13 |
| **TERIYAKI DISHES** | | | | | | | | | | |
| Beef Yakisoba w/o Sauce | 15 oz | 540 | 162 | 18 | 6 | 65 | 1150 | 62 | 2 | 36 |
| Chicken & Beef w/o Sauce | 15 oz | 590 | 126 | 14 | 4.5 | 85 | 830 | 80 | 3 | 32 |
| Sukiyaki Beef & Shrimp w/o Sauce | 17 oz | 690 | 171 | 19 | 6 | 150 | 1170 | 82 | 3 | 43 |
| Sukiyaki Beef w/o Sauce | 15 oz | 610 | 144 | 16 | 6 | 65 | 810 | 80 | 3 | 32 |

## Einstein Bros Bagels

| | SERVING SIZE | CAL | CAL FAT | TOT FAT (G) | SAT FAT (G) | CHOL (MG) | SOD (MG) | CARB (G) | FIBER (G) | PROT (G) |
|---|---|---|---|---|---|---|---|---|---|---|
| **BAGELS** | | | | | | | | | | |
| Everything | 1 bagel | 280 | 15 | 2 | 0 | 0 | 650 | 58 | 2 | 10 |
| Plain | 1 bagel | 250 | 10 | 1 | 0 | 0 | 460 | 54 | 2 | 9 |
| Power | 1 bagel | 310 | 45 | 5 | .5 | 0 | 280 | 61 | 4 | 11 |
| Sesame Dip'd | 1 bagel | 270 | 25 | 3 | 0 | 0 | 460 | 54 | 2 | 10 |
| **BREAKFAST** | | | | | | | | | | |
| Egg Way, Plain | 1 sandwich | 510 | 180 | 20 | 9 | 395 | 810 | 57 | 2 | 29 |
| Lox & Bagel | 1 bagel | 490 | 190 | 21 | 11 | 50 | 950 | 61 | 3 | 24 |
| Santa Fe Wrap | 1 wrap | 680 | 310 | 34 | 13 | 435 | 1260 | 60 | 7 | 34 |
| **SALADS** | | | | | | | | | | |
| Asiago Chicken Caesar | 1 salad | 720 | 510 | 56 | 12 | 130 | 1960 | 22 | 4 | 37 |
| Bros Bistro | 1 salad | 810 | 610 | 68 | 11 | 25 | 500 | 36 | 7 | 14 |
| Chicken Chipotle | 1 salad | 700 | 360 | 41 | 9 | 95 | 1960 | 52 | 10 | 34 |
| **SANDWICHES & WRAPS** | | | | | | | | | | |
| Chicken Caesar Wrap | 1 wrap | 750 | 380 | 42 | 12 | 120 | 1570 | 59 | 7 | 36 |
| Chicken Salad Wrap | 1 wrap | 1010 | 740 | 82 | 13 | 70 | 780 | 55 | 7 | 14 |
| Deli Tuna Salad Sandwich | 1 sandwich | 320 | 90 | 10 | 1.5 | 25 | 360 | 43 | 3 | 24 |
| Deli Turkey Sandwich | 1 sandwich | 370 | 100 | 11 | 4.5 | 55 | 950 | 41 | 3 | 31 |
| Tasty Turkey on Asiago Bagel Sandwich | 1 sandwich | 560 | 180 | 20 | 12 | 95 | 1460 | 66 | 3 | 36 |
| Veg Out on Sesame Seed Bagel Sandwich | 1 sandwich | 460 | 180 | 19 | 6 | 25 | 740 | 64 | 4 | 12 |
| **WHIPPED CREAM CHEESE** | | | | | | | | | | |
| Plain | 2 tbsp | 70 | 60 | 7 | 4.5 | 20 | 65 | 1 | 0 | 1 |
| Reduced Fat Blueberry | 2 tbsp | 70 | 45 | 5 | 3.5 | 15 | 50 | 6 | 0 | 1 |
| Reduced Fat Plain | 2 tbsp | 60 | 45 | 5 | 3.5 | 15 | 100 | 2 | 0 | 1 |

## El Pollo Loco

| | SERVING SIZE | CAL | CAL FAT | TOT FAT (G) | SAT FAT (G) | CHOL (MG) | SOD (MG) | CARB (G) | FIBER (G) | PROT (G) |
|---|---|---|---|---|---|---|---|---|---|---|
| **BOWLS & SALADS** | | | | | | | | | | |
| Chicken Caesar Bowl | 1 bowl | 490 | 200 | 22 | 4.5 | 85 | 2520 | 44 | 2 | 28 |

# restaurants

| | SERVING SIZE | CAL | CAL FAT | TOT FAT (G) | SAT FAT (G) | CHOL (MG) | SOD (MG) | CARB (G) | FIBER (G) | PROT (G) |
|---|---|---|---|---|---|---|---|---|---|---|
| Chicken Caesar Salad No Dressing | 1 salad | 230 | 70 | 7 | 2 | 75 | 517 | 18 | 3 | 35 |
| Chicken Tostada Salad No Dressing | 1 salad | 899 | 380 | 42 | 12 | 100 | 1489 | 86 | 7 | 40 |
| Chicken Tostada Salad No Dressing, No Shell | 1 salad | 410 | 110 | 13 | 6 | 100 | 1310 | 39 | 5 | 33 |
| Garden Salad, No Dressing, No Tortilla Strips, Sm. | 1 salad | 35 | 15 | 1.5 | .5 | 5 | 170 | 4 | 1 | 2 |
| Loco Salad w/Creamy Cilantro Dressing | 3 oz | 170 | 130 | 14 | 3 | 10 | 210 | 7 | 1 | 3 |
| Original Pollo Bowl | 1 bowl | 690 | 90 | 10 | 2 | 70 | 1870 | 106 | 12 | 40 |
| Ultimate Pollo Bowl | 1 bowl | 1050 | 300 | 34 | 14 | 200 | 2500 | 110 | 13 | 71 |
| **BURRITOS & TACOS** | | | | | | | | | | |
| BRC Burrito | 7-1/2 oz | 440 | 110 | 12 | 4.5 | 15 | 1000 | 68 | 6 | 15 |
| Chicken Soft Taco | 5-1/2 oz | 260 | 110 | 12 | 6 | 70 | 580 | 18 | 2 | 16 |
| Classic Chicken Burrito | 10 oz | 550 | 150 | 17 | 6 | 95 | 1350 | 69 | 6 | 31 |
| Crunchy Chicken Taco | 3-1/2 oz | 190 | 70 | 8 | 2.5 | 20 | 480 | 16 | 2 | 12 |
| Twice Grilled Burrito | 15 oz | 840 | 350 | 39 | 18 | 215 | 2000 | 56 | 6 | 66 |
| Ultimate Grilled Burrito | 14 oz | 710 | 200 | 23 | 9 | 100 | 1690 | 86 | 8 | 39 |
| **CHICKEN** | | | | | | | | | | |
| Chicken Breast | 4-3/10 oz | 220 | 80 | 9 | 2.5 | 140 | 620 | 0 | 0 | 36 |
| Chicken Breast, Skinless | 4 oz | 180 | 35 | 3.5 | 1 | 110 | 620 | 0 | 0 | 35 |
| Chopped Breast Meat | 3 oz | 100 | 15 | 1.5 | .5 | 70 | 290 | 0 | 0 | 21 |
| Leg | 1-1/2 oz | 90 | 35 | 4 | 1 | 70 | 560 | 0 | 0 | 12 |
| Thigh | 1 thigh | 220 | 130 | 15 | 4.5 | 180 | 170 | 0 | 0 | 21 |
| Wing | 1 wing | 90 | 45 | 5 | 1.5 | 60 | 320 | 0 | 0 | 11 |
| **EXTRAS** | | | | | | | | | | |
| Cheese Quesadilla | 4-1/2 oz | 420 | 210 | 23 | 13 | 60 | 810 | 35 | 2 | 19 |
| Chicken Taquito w/Avocado Salsa | 1 oz | 230 | 110 | 12 | 2.5 | 25 | 590 | 20 | 5 | 10 |
| Chips & Guacamole | 2-3/5 oz | 250 | 130 | 14 | 2 | 0 | 350 | 26 | 6 | 3 |
| Churros, two | 2 oz | 300 | 170 | 18 | 4.5 | 25 | 210 | 32 | 2 | 3 |
| Grilled Chicken Nachos | 13 oz | 810 | 360 | 40 | 14 | 105 | 1990 | 70 | 10 | 39 |
| Grilled Chicken Tortilla Roll No Sauce | 6 oz | 390 | 140 | 16 | 6 | 95 | 1050 | 37 | 3 | 26 |
| Mashed Potatoes | 5 oz | 110 | 15 | 1.5 | .5 | 0 | 400 | 23 | 1 | 2 |
| Pinto Beans | 6 oz | 200 | 35 | 4 | .5 | 0 | 370 | 29 | 4 | 11 |
| Refried Beans w/Cheese | 6 oz | 270 | 60 | 7 | 1.5 | 10 | 730 | 36 | 10 | 14 |
| Spanish Rice | 6 oz | 220 | 20 | 2 | 0 | 0 | 650 | 45 | 8 | 4 |
| Taco al Carbon | 3 oz | 150 | 45 | 5 | 1.5 | 40 | 290 | 17 | 1 | 11 |

## Famous Dave's

| | SERVING SIZE | CAL | CAL FAT | TOT FAT (G) | SAT FAT (G) | CHOL (MG) | SOD (MG) | CARB (G) | FIBER (G) | PROT (G) |
|---|---|---|---|---|---|---|---|---|---|---|
| Char-Grilled Chicken Sandwich | 1 sandwich | 410 | 63 | 7 | 1.5 | 110 | 950 | 43 | 3 | 48 |
| BBQ Pork Salad (Lunch Portion) | as served | 410 | 189 | 21 | 7 | 60 | 1490 | 39 | 4 | 19 |

| | SERVING SIZE | CAL | CAL FAT | TOT FAT (G) | SAT FAT (G) | CHOL (MG) | SOD (MG) | CARB (G) | FIBER (G) | PROT (G) |
|---|---|---|---|---|---|---|---|---|---|---|
| Sassy BBQ Chicken Salad Lunch Portion | as served | 380 | 180 | 20 | 7 | 65 | 1440 | 35 | 4 | 20 |
| Sweet & Sassy Grilled Salmon Fillet | as served | 450 | 234 | 26 | 5 | 120 | 1130 | 11 | <1 | 43 |

## Fatburger
### BURGERS & SANDWICHES

| | | | | | | | | | | |
|---|---|---|---|---|---|---|---|---|---|---|
| Bacon & Egg | 1 sandwich | 350 | 144 | 16 | 5 | 230 | 970 | 37 | 1 | 18 |
| Crispy Chicken | 1 sandwich | 560 | 243 | 27 | 5 | 60 | 1540 | 53 | 2 | 26 |
| Fatburger, 5.3 oz | 1 burger | 590 | 279 | 31 | 9 | 105 | 1190 | 46 | 2 | 33 |
| Kingburger, 8 oz | 1 burger | 850 | 369 | 41 | 13 | 150 | 1490 | 69 | 4 | 50 |
| Sausage & Egg | 1 sandwich | 780 | 477 | 53 | 21 | 305 | 1810 | 47 | 1 | 27 |
| Spicy Chicken | 1 sandwich | 520 | 189 | 21 | 6 | 60 | 2160 | 58 | 2 | 26 |
| Turkeyburger | 1 burger | 480 | 189 | 21 | 4.5 | 80 | 1270 | 50 | 3 | 26 |
| Veggieburger | 1 burger | 510 | 180 | 20 | 4.5 | 20 | 1560 | 60 | 11 | 33 |

### HOT DOGS

| | | | | | | | | | | |
|---|---|---|---|---|---|---|---|---|---|---|
| Chili Cheese | 1 hot dog | 480 | 243 | 27 | 11 | 80 | 1150 | 35 | 2 | 24 |
| Regular | 1 hot dog | 320 | 135 | 15 | 6 | 40 | 780 | 32 | 1 | 13 |

### SALADS & SIDES

| | | | | | | | | | | |
|---|---|---|---|---|---|---|---|---|---|---|
| Chili Cheese Fat Fries | as served | 590 | 297 | 33 | 11 | 50 | 590 | 53 | 6 | 21 |
| Chili Fat Fries | as served | 480 | 216 | 24 | 6 | 20 | 410 | 52 | 6 | 14 |
| Fat Fries | as served | 380 | 162 | 18 | 4 | 0 | 40 | 47 | 5 | 6 |
| Onion Rings | as served | 540 | 261 | 29 | 6 | 5 | 490 | 64 | 4 | 7 |
| Wedge w/Chicken, no dressing | 1 salad | 210 | 54 | 6 | 1.5 | 80 | 610 | 8 | 2 | 33 |
| Wedge, no dressing | 1 salad | 60 | 31.5 | 3.5 | 1.5 | 10 | 140 | 5 | 2 | 5 |

## Fazoli's
### ENTRÉES

| | | | | | | | | | | |
|---|---|---|---|---|---|---|---|---|---|---|
| Baked Spaghetti | 1 entrée | 640 | 190 | 22 | 12 | 75 | 1340 | 80 | 7 | 29 |
| Cheesy Baked Ziti | 1 entrée | 670 | 240 | 27 | 15 | 90 | 1630 | 71 | 7 | 34 |
| Chicken Parmigiano | 1 entrée | 1000 | 350 | 39 | 15 | 125 | 2550 | 108 | 8 | 51 |
| Rigatoni Romano | 1 entrée | 880 | 390 | 44 | 20 | 125 | 2510 | 76 | 7 | 44 |
| Tortellini Robusto | 1 entrée | 1020 | 450 | 50 | 28 | 210 | 2580 | 80 | 5 | 59 |
| Twice Baked Lasagna | 1 entrée | 700 | 350 | 39 | 20 | 115 | 2420 | 47 | 6 | 41 |

### FRESH MADE PASTA

| | | | | | | | | | | |
|---|---|---|---|---|---|---|---|---|---|---|
| Chicken Carbonara | 1 entrée | 800 | 250 | 27 | 13 | 110 | 1790 | 88 | 4 | 42 |
| Fettucine w/Alfredo | 1 entrée | 800 | 240 | 26 | 15 | 75 | 1480 | 108 | 5 | 26 |
| Ravioli w/Meat Sauce | 1 entrée | 570 | 190 | 21 | 10 | 95 | 1530 | 70 | 8 | 27 |
| Spaghetti or Penne w/Meat Sauce | 1 entrée | 680 | 100 | 12 | 3.5 | 20 | 1640 | 113 | 10 | 28 |
| Tortellini & Sun-Dried Tomato Rustico | 1 entrée | 850 | 420 | 46 | 15 | 85 | 1380 | 81 | 6 | 30 |

# restaurants

| | SERVING SIZE | CAL | CAL FAT | TOT FAT (G) | SAT FAT (G) | CHOL (MG) | SOD (MG) | CARB (G) | FIBER (G) | PROT (G) |
|---|---|---|---|---|---|---|---|---|---|---|
| **PIZZA** | | | | | | | | | | |
| Margherita Pizza | 5 oz | 330 | 140 | 15 | 6 | 30 | 710 | 33 | 2 | 14 |
| Pepperoni Classico Pizza | 4 oz | 300 | 110 | 13 | 6 | 30 | 810 | 32 | 2 | 14 |
| Supremo Pizza | 5 oz | 320 | 130 | 14 | 6 | 35 | 870 | 33 | 2 | 15 |
| **SALADS** | | | | | | | | | | |
| Chicken & Pasta Caesar Salad | 1 salad | 470 | 130 | 15 | 5 | 80 | 1620 | 38 | 3 | 37 |
| Crispy Chicken BLT Salad | 1 salad | 480 | 230 | 26 | 7 | 75 | 1430 | 31 | 4 | 32 |
| Grilled Chicken Artichoke Salad | 1 salad | 240 | 40 | 4.5 | 2.5 | 70 | 910 | 11 | 4 | 32 |

## Finagle
### BAGELS & CREAM CHEESE

| | SERVING SIZE | CAL | CAL FAT | TOT FAT (G) | SAT FAT (G) | CHOL (MG) | SOD (MG) | CARB (G) | FIBER (G) | PROT (G) |
|---|---|---|---|---|---|---|---|---|---|---|
| 100% Whole Wheat | 1 bagel | 320 | 36 | 4 | 1 | 0 | 444 | 62 | 6 | 14 |
| Cinnamon Raisin | 1 bagel | 300 | 10 | 1 | 0 | 0 | 350 | 67 | 5 | 8 |
| Everything | 1 bagel | 310 | 30 | 3 | 1 | 0 | 420 | 62 | 5 | 9 |
| Harvest Vegetable Cream Cheese | 2 tbsp | 90 | 80 | 9 | 6 | 25 | 105 | 2 | 0 | 2 |
| Light Harvest Vegetable Cream Cheese | 2 tbsp | 60 | 50 | 6 | 3 | 15 | 120 | 1 | 0 | 2 |
| Light Plain Cream Cheese | 2 tbsp | 60 | 50 | 6 | 4 | 20 | 120 | <1 | 0 | 3 |
| Original Plain Cream Cheese | 2 tbsp | 90 | 80 | 9 | 6 | 30 | 75 | <1 | 0 | 2 |
| Plain | 1 bagel | 290 | 10 | 1 | 0 | 0 | 410 | 63 | 4 | 8 |
| Poppy | 1 bagel | 310 | 35 | 4 | 1 | 0 | 409 | 60 | 4 | 11 |
| Strawberry Cream Cheese | 2 tbsp | 90 | 70 | 8 | 5 | 25 | 90 | 4 | 0 | 1 |
| Sesame | 1 bagel | 310 | 40 | 4.5 | 1.5 | 0 | 380 | 60 | 5 | 10 |
| **SOUPS, CHOWDERS, & SALADS** | | | | | | | | | | |
| Beef Chili | 1/2 bowl | 270 | 120 | 13 | 5 | 45 | 700 | 22 | 6 | 17 |
| Boston Clam Chowder | 1/2 bowl | 320 | 180 | 20 | 12 | 70 | 590 | 25 | <1 | 18 |
| Caesar Salad w/o Dressing or Croutons | 1 salad | 200 | 110 | 12 | 7 | 30 | 730 | 6 | 3 | 18 |
| Cobb Salad w/o Dressing or Croutons | 1 salad | 380 | 250 | 28 | 11 | 285 | 970 | 10 | 4 | 23 |
| Chicken Soup | 1/2 bowl | 90 | 20 | 2 | .5 | 30 | 940 | 6 | <1 | 11 |
| Garden Salad w/o Dressing or Croutons | 1 salad | 50 | 5 | .5 | 0 | 0 | 35 | 11 | 4 | 2 |

## Firehouse Subs
### SOUPS & CHILI

| | SERVING SIZE | CAL | CAL FAT | TOT FAT (G) | SAT FAT (G) | CHOL (MG) | SOD (MG) | CARB (G) | FIBER (G) | PROT (G) |
|---|---|---|---|---|---|---|---|---|---|---|
| Broccoli Cheese Soup | as served | 300 | 170 | 19 | 12 | 65 | 1060 | 17 | 2 | 16 |
| Chicken Noodle Soup | as served | 160 | 70 | 8 | 2 | 15 | 1130 | 17 | 1 | 5 |
| Chili | as served | 340 | 153 | 17 | 6 | 50 | 960 | 25 | 6 | 20 |
| **SUBS (on white)** | | | | | | | | | | |
| Beef Brisket, Medium | 1 sub | 890 | 520 | 59 | 19 | 105 | 1690 | 64 | 2 | 30 |

| | SERVING SIZE | CAL | CAL FAT | TOT FAT (G) | SAT FAT (G) | CHOL (MG) | SOD (MG) | CARB (G) | FIBER (G) | PROT (G) |
|---|---|---|---|---|---|---|---|---|---|---|
| Chicken, Medium | 1 sub | 690 | 340 | 38 | 9 | 100 | 1750 | 55 | 3 | 37 |
| Chicken Salad, Medium | 1 sub | 820 | 440 | 48 | 10 | 85 | 1370 | 60 | 4 | 34 |
| Club, Medium | 1 sub | 780 | 380 | 42 | 11 | 90 | 1910 | 64 | 3 | 40 |
| Corned Beef, Medium | 1 sub | 730 | 380 | 42 | 11 | 90 | 2290 | 54 | 3 | 35 |
| Engine Company, Medium | 1 sub | 700 | 330 | 36 | 9 | 85 | 1750 | 57 | 4 | 36 |
| Engineer, Medium | 1 sub | 690 | 320 | 35 | 8 | 65 | 1910 | 61 | 3 | 39 |
| Ham, Medium | 1 sub | 730 | 330 | 36 | 9 | 80 | 1630 | 70 | 3 | 37 |
| Hero, Medium | 1 sub | 770 | 340 | 37 | 14 | 100 | 2170 | 64 | 3 | 48 |
| Hook & Ladder, Medium | 1 sub | 700 | 330 | 36 | 21 | 80 | 1660 | 64 | 3 | 35 |
| Italian, Medium | 1 sub | 910 | 530 | 57 | 31 | 105 | 2430 | 64 | 3 | 38 |
| Meatball, Medium | 1 sub | 820 | 440 | 50 | 15 | 15 | 1910 | 60 | 4 | 37 |
| Pastrami, Medium | 1 sub | 690 | 340 | 37 | 0 | 80 | 2110 | 56 | 3 | 33 |
| Roast Beef, Medium | 1 sub | 710 | 330 | 36 | 21 | 90 | 1820 | 54 | 3 | 39 |
| Steak, Medium | 1 sub | 770 | 420 | 68 | 17 | 90 | 1720 | 56 | 3 | 38 |
| Steamer, Medium | 1 sub | 720 | 390 | 79 | 31 | 85 | 2360 | 51 | 2 | 33 |
| Sweet/Spicy MB, Medium | 1 sub | 880 | 440 | 120 | 21 | 95 | 2380 | 76 | 4 | 37 |
| Tuna, Medium | 1 sub | 1000 | 620 | 76 | 18 | 70 | 1610 | 67 | 4 | 36 |
| Turkey Bacon Ranch, Medium | 1 sub | 840 | 440 | 52 | 12 | 85 | 2240 | 59 | 3 | 42 |
| Turkey, Medium | 1 sub | 670 | 310 | 64 | 17 | 60 | 1850 | 58 | 3 | 37 |
| Veggie, Medium | 1 sub | 720 | 410 | 84 | 29 | 60 | 1520 | 60 | 4 | 25 |

## Five Guys
### BURGERS

| | SERVING SIZE | CAL | CAL FAT | TOT FAT (G) | SAT FAT (G) | CHOL (MG) | SOD (MG) | CARB (G) | FIBER (G) | PROT (G) |
|---|---|---|---|---|---|---|---|---|---|---|
| Bacon Burger | 1 burger | 780 | 460 | 50 | 22.5 | 140 | 690 | 39 | 2 | 43 |
| Bacon Cheeseburger | 1 burger | 920 | 560 | 62 | 29.5 | 180 | 1310 | 40 | 2 | 51 |
| Cheeseburger | 1 burger | 840 | 500 | 55 | 26.5 | 165 | 1050 | 40 | 2 | 47 |
| Hamburger | 1 burger | 700 | 400 | 43 | 19.5 | 125 | 430 | 39 | 2 | 39 |
| Little Bacon Burger | 1 burger | 560 | 300 | 33 | 14.5 | 80 | 640 | 39 | 2 | 27 |
| Little Bacon Cheeseburger | 1 burger | 630 | 350 | 39 | 18 | 100 | 950 | 39.5 | 2 | 31 |
| Little Cheeseburger | 1 burger | 550 | 290 | 32 | 15 | 85 | 690 | 39.5 | 2 | 27 |
| Little Hamburger | 1 burger | 480 | 240 | 26 | 11.5 | 65 | 380 | 39 | 2 | 23 |

### DOGS & SANDWICHES

| | SERVING SIZE | CAL | CAL FAT | TOT FAT (G) | SAT FAT (G) | CHOL (MG) | SOD (MG) | CARB (G) | FIBER (G) | PROT (G) |
|---|---|---|---|---|---|---|---|---|---|---|
| Bacon Dog | 1 dog | 625 | 375 | 42 | 18.5 | 76 | 1390 | 40 | 2 | 22 |
| Cheese Dog | 1 dog | 615 | 365 | 41 | 19 | 81 | 1440 | 40.5 | 2 | 22 |
| Grilled Cheese | 1 sandwich | 470 | 230 | 26 | 9 | 35 | 715 | 41 | 2.5 | 11 |
| Hot Dog | 1 dog | 545 | 315 | 35 | 15.5 | 61 | 1130 | 40 | 2 | 18 |
| Veggie Sandwich | 1 sandwich | 440 | 140 | 15 | 6 | 25 | 1040 | 60 | 2 | 16 |

| | SERVING SIZE | CAL | CAL FAT | TOT FAT (G) | SAT FAT (G) | CHOL (MG) | SOD (MG) | CARB (G) | FIBER (G) | PROT (G) |
|---|---|---|---|---|---|---|---|---|---|---|
| **FRIES** | | | | | | | | | | |
| Fries (1/2 regular order) | as served | 310 | 130 | 15 | 3 | n/a | 45 | 39 | 3 | 5 |
| **Freshens** | | | | | | | | | | |
| **FRUIT CLASSIC** | | | | | | | | | | |
| **SMOOTHIES** | | | | | | | | | | |
| Citrus Mango | 1 smoothie | 490 | 61 | 7 | 4.5 | 10 | 60 | 108 | 1 | 2 |
| Jamaican Jammer | 1 smoothie | 350 | 0 | 0 | 0 | 0 | 180 | 77 | 2 | 12 |
| Mango Beach Low Cal. (No Sugar Added) | 1 smoothie | 80 | 0 | 0 | 0 | 0 | 16 | 49 | 2 | 1 |
| Maui Mango | 1 smoothie | 290 | 2 | 0 | 0 | 0 | 20 | 74 | 2 | 1 |
| Orange Sunrise | 1 smoothie | 360 | 26 | 3 | 1.5 | 10 | 45 | 82 | 2 | 3 |
| Raspberry Passion Fruit Low Cal. (No Sugar Added) | 1 smoothie | 80 | 3 | 0 | 0 | 0 | 20 | 50 | 2 | 1 |
| Strawberry Oasis Low Cal. (No Sugar Added) | 1 smoothie | 70 | 0 | 0 | 0 | 0 | 10 | 50 | 1 | 0 |
| Strawberry Shooter | 1 smoothie | 250 | 0 | 0 | 0 | 0 | 10 | 64 | 1 | 0 |
| **NATURE'S ENERGY** | | | | | | | | | | |
| **SMOOTHIES** | | | | | | | | | | |
| Acai | 1 smoothie | 288 | 0 | 0 | 0 | 0 | 16 | 73 | 2 | 1 |
| Tart Berry | 1 smoothie | 320 | 2 | 0 | 0 | 0 | 10 | 82 | 2 | 1 |
| **CONES** | | | | | | | | | | |
| Chocolate Cake | 1 cone | 210 | 4.5 | 0.5 | 0 | 5 | 120 | 40 | 1 | 6 |
| Vanilla Cake | 1 cone | 200 | 0 | 0 | 0 | 5 | 120 | 40 | 0 | 5 |
| Vanilla Waffle | 1 cone | 300 | 13.5 | 1.5 | 0 | 5 | 160 | 62 | 1 | 8 |
| **FAT-FREE FROZEN** | | | | | | | | | | |
| **YOGURT** | | | | | | | | | | |
| Chocolate | 9 oz | 330 | 9 | 1 | 0 | 10 | 190 | 62 | 2 | 10 |
| Tart | 9 oz | 300 | 9 | 1 | 0 | 5 | 190 | 62 | 0 | 13 |
| Vanilla | 9 oz | 300 | 9 | 1 | 0 | 5 | 190 | 62 | 0 | 9 |
| **FRO-YO BLASTS** | | | | | | | | | | |
| Cookie Dough | 1 blast | 570 | 63 | 7 | 2.5 | 5 | 320 | 112 | 1 | 12 |
| Oreo Overload | 1 blast | 430 | 31.5 | 3.5 | 1 | 5 | 370 | 83 | 1 | 12 |
| Peach Cobbler | 1 blast | 460 | 36 | 4 | 1 | 20 | 240 | 88 | 2 | 13 |
| Strawberry Shortcake | 1 blast | 470 | 18 | 2 | 1 | 20 | 240 | 95 | 1 | 11 |
| **INDULGENT SHAKES** | | | | | | | | | | |
| Chocolate | 1 shake | 530 | 36 | 4 | 2.5 | 20 | 320 | 103 | 0 | 15 |
| Strawberry | 1 shake | 500 | 22.5 | 2.5 | 1 | 10 | 290 | 94 | 1 | 15 |
| Vanilla | 1 shake | 490 | 36 | 4 | 2.5 | 20 | 280 | 99 | 0 | 15 |

| | SERVING SIZE | CAL | CAL FAT | TOT FAT (G) | SAT FAT (G) | CHOL (MG) | SOD (MG) | CARB (G) | FIBER (G) | PROT (G) |
|---|---|---|---|---|---|---|---|---|---|---|

## Friendly's
### APPETIZERS

| | | | | | | | | | | |
|---|---|---|---|---|---|---|---|---|---|---|
| Chicken Quesadilla | as served | 570 | 320 | 35 | 18 | 100 | 1340 | 29 | 3 | 35 |
| Jumbo Fronions | as served | 1430 | 810 | 90 | 13 | 30 | 2970 | 140 | 7 | 14 |
| Kickin Buffalo Chicken Strips | as served | 1090 | 800 | 88 | 21 | 140 | 2740 | 39 | 4 | 35 |
| Loaded Waffle Fries | as served | 1650 | 1000 | 112 | 28 | 100 | 4720 | 123 | 9 | 31 |
| Mini Mozzarella Cheese Sticks | as served | 680 | 360 | 40 | 14 | 60 | 1870 | 55 | 3 | 23 |
| Munchie Mania Cheeseburger Sliders | as served | 500 | 190 | 21 | 7 | 50 | 1440 | 57 | 6 | 20 |
| Munchie Mania Chicken Sandwich Sliders | as served | 740 | 370 | 42 | 9 | 60 | 1210 | 69 | 7 | 23 |

### BURGERS, SANDWICHES, & WRAPS

| | | | | | | | | | | |
|---|---|---|---|---|---|---|---|---|---|---|
| All American Burger | 1 burger | 1190 | 610 | 68 | 19 | 120 | 1170 | 103 | 8 | 43 |
| BBQ Fronion Burgers | 1 burger | 1560 | 820 | 91 | 30 | 160 | 2020 | 134 | 8 | 55 |
| Buffalo Chicken Wrap | 1 wrap | 1510 | 840 | 94 | 19 | 130 | 2640 | 123 | 9 | 42 |
| Cheddar Jack Chicken Supermelt | 1 sandwich | 1070 | 440 | 49 | 18 | 140 | 2270 | 98 | 6 | 56 |
| Crispy Chicken Caesar Wrap | 1 wrap | 1500 | 840 | 94 | 18 | 160 | 2300 | 123 | 9 | 43 |
| Crispy Chicken Wrap | 1 wrap | 1140 | 490 | 54 | 8 | 60 | 1610 | 132 | 10 | 31 |
| Deluxe Cheese Burgermelt "Set-Up" | as served | 1180 | 670 | 75 | 25 | 140 | 1310 | 83 | 7 | 44 |
| Fishamajig | as served | 970 | 450 | 51 | 14 | 70 | 1520 | 99 | 7 | 30 |
| Grilled Cheese | as served | 790 | 330 | 37 | 12 | 30 | 1280 | 96 | 6 | 20 |
| Grilled Chicken Deluxe | as served | 1000 | 410 | 45 | 9 | 90 | 1810 | 108 | 8 | 43 |
| Grilled Chicken Pesto Supermelt | 1 sandwich | 1360 | 740 | 82 | 26 | 160 | 2060 | 98 | 6 | 59 |
| Honey BBQ Chicken Supermelt | 1 sandwich | 1400 | 680 | 75 | 22 | 110 | 2160 | 134 | 8 | 49 |
| Kickin Buffalo Chicken Supermelt | 1 sandwich | 1430 | 780 | 86 | 25 | 100 | 2520 | 118 | 7 | 45 |
| Mushroom Swiss Bacon Burger | 1 burger | 1570 | 900 | 100 | 33 | 190 | 2040 | 109 | 7 | 61 |
| Reuben Supermelt | 1 sandwich | 1130 | 500 | 56 | 18 | 100 | 2910 | 105 | 6 | 54 |
| Soft Pretzel Bacon Burger | 1 burger | 1420 | 710 | 79 | 29 | 190 | 1360 | 119 | 7 | 58 |
| Steak 'n Mushroom Supermelt | 1 sandwich | 1150 | 550 | 61 | 19 | 90 | 2120 | 108 | 7 | 44 |
| Swiss Patty Burgermelt | as served | 1360 | 700 | 78 | 27 | 150 | 1220 | 110 | 8 | 56 |
| Tuna Roll | as served | 920 | 520 | 57 | 10 | 60 | 1080 | 73 | 6 | 28 |
| Tuna Supermelt | 1 sandwich | 1140 | 590 | 66 | 15 | 80 | 1700 | 98 | 7 | 39 |
| Turkey Club Supermelt | 1 sandwich | 990 | 410 | 46 | 14 | 90 | 2290 | 53 | 3 | 45 |
| Ultimate Bacon Cheese Burger | 1 burger | 1400 | 770 | 86 | 29 | 170 | 2040 | 103 | 7 | 55 |
| Ultimate Grilled Cheese Burgermelt | as served | 1500 | 870 | 97 | 38 | 180 | 2090 | 101 | 9 | 54 |
| Vermonter Burger | 1 burger | 1420 | 780 | 87 | 32 | 190 | 1530 | 102 | 7 | 59 |
| Zesty Queso Burgermelt | as served | 1380 | 710 | 79 | 26 | 140 | 2410 | 117 | 7 | 53 |

| | SERVING SIZE | CAL | CAL FAT | TOT FAT (G) | SAT FAT (G) | CHOL (MG) | SOD (MG) | CARB (G) | FIBER (G) | PROT (G) |
|---|---|---|---|---|---|---|---|---|---|---|
| **DESSERT BEVERAGES** | | | | | | | | | | |
| Double Thick Milkshake—Chocolate | 1 milkshake | 700 | 290 | 32 | 21 | 110 | 300 | 85 | 1 | 21 |
| Double Thick Milkshake—Coffee | 1 milkshake | 770 | 290 | 32 | 18 | 110 | 270 | 107 | 0 | 15 |
| Orange Slammer | 1 slammer | 600 | 40 | 4 | 3 | 20 | 80 | 138 | 0 | 3 |
| Oreo Mocha Crunch Signature Milk Shake | 1 milkshake | 1090 | 440 | 49 | 32 | 120 | 450 | 146 | 3 | 19 |
| Original Fribble—Strawberry | 1 fribble | 630 | 170 | 19 | 12 | 60 | 460 | 103 | 0 | 16 |
| Original Fribble—Vanilla | 1 fribble | 620 | 170 | 19 | 12 | 60 | 360 | 100 | 0 | 16 |
| Watermelon Slammer | 1 fribble | 450 | 40 | 4 | 3 | 20 | 80 | 100 | 0 | 3 |
| **ENTRÉES** | | | | | | | | | | |
| 2+2 Chicken Strips w/BBQ Sauce | 1 entrée | 410 | 170 | 19 | 3 | 50 | 960 | 39 | 2 | 19 |
| 2+2 Chicken Strips w/Honey Mustard Sauce | 1 entrée | 510 | 310 | 34 | 5 | 60 | 760 | 31 | 2 | 19 |
| 2+2 Kickin' Buffalo Chicken Strips | 1 entrée | 690 | 510 | 57 | 8 | 90 | 1490 | 22 | 2 | 22 |
| 2+2 Sirloin Steak Tips | 1 entrée | 410 | 150 | 16 | 5 | 90 | 2320 | 31 | 5 | 35 |
| Chicken Fajita Quesadillas | as served | 1540 | 820 | 91 | 42 | 210 | 3870 | 106 | 7 | 74 |
| Chicken Quesadilla | as served | 530 | 740 | 36 | 16 | 90 | 940 | 31 | 7 | 20 |
| Chicken Strips Basket 6 Strips w/o Sauce | 1 entrée | 1030 | 520 | 58 | 8 | 90 | 1330 | 93 | 8 | 37 |
| Clamboat Basket | 1 entrée | 1710 | 920 | 102 | 15 | 90 | 3340 | 170 | 11 | 28 |
| Create Your Own Chicken Strips—6 Strips | 1 entrée | 1750 | 1010 | 112 | 16 | 150 | 2920 | 144 | 8 | 41 |
| Friendly Frank | 1 entrée | 750 | 400 | 44 | 13 | 30 | 1070 | 73 | 5 | 15 |
| Honey BBQ Chicken Strips—6 Strips | 1 entrée | 1670 | 720 | 81 | 12 | 120 | 2430 | 195 | 9 | 45 |
| Kickin' Buffalo Chicken Strips—6 Strips | 1 entrée | 1640 | 1040 | 115 | 14 | 160 | 3040 | 104 | 9 | 46 |
| New England Fish 'N Chips | 1 entrée | 1150 | 630 | 70 | 10 | 80 | 2120 | 106 | 9 | 25 |
| Shrimp Basket | 1 entrée | 1090 | 540 | 60 | 7 | 180 | 3290 | 110 | 9 | 27 |
| Sirloin Steak Tips | 1 entrée | 1140 | 460 | 51 | 19 | 200 | 3350 | 92 | 13 | 77 |
| **ICE CREAMS, SHERBETS, & YOGURTS** | | | | | | | | | | |
| No Sugar Added Vanilla Ice Cream | 1 scoop | 100 | 60 | 7 | 5 | 30 | 25 | 11 | 3 | 2 |
| Non Fat Yogurt (average of all flavors) | 1 scoop | 85 | 0 | 0 | 0 | 0 | 50 | 18 | 0 | 3 |
| Regular Ice Cream (average of all flavors) | 1 scoop | 130 | 61 | 7 | 4 | 22 | 45 | 15 | 1 | 2 |
| Sherbet (average of all flavors) | 1 scoop | 80 | 10 | 1 | 1 | 3 | 15 | 17 | 0 | 1 |
| **SMOOTHIES & SUNDAES** | | | | | | | | | | |
| Butterfinger Sundae | 1 sundae | 830 | 320 | 36 | 23 | 90 | 370 | 117 | 2 | 9 |
| Caramel Cone Crunch Sundae | 1 sundae | 690 | 290 | 32 | 20 | 90 | 280 | 91 | 3 | 10 |
| Caramel Fudge Brownie Sundae | 1 sundae | 1410 | 600 | 66 | 40 | 230 | 620 | 186 | 2 | 19 |
| Cookie Jar Sundae | 1 sundae | 750 | 320 | 36 | 22 | 90 | 290 | 98 | 3 | 11 |
| Forbidden Fudge Brownie | 1 sundae | 940 | 360 | 41 | n/a | 130 | 340 | 131 | 4 | 13 |
| Happy Ending Hot Fudge Sundae | 1 sundae | 330 | 150 | 17 | 11 | 60 | 110 | 40 | 1 | 5 |

| | SERVING SIZE | CAL | CAL FAT | TOT FAT (G) | SAT FAT (G) | CHOL (MG) | SOD (MG) | CARB (G) | FIBER (G) | PROT (G) |
|---|---|---|---|---|---|---|---|---|---|---|
| Jim Dandy w/Topping | 1 sundae | 1090 | 420 | 47 | 27 | 150 | 156 | 157 | 2 | 14 |
| Kit Kat Sundae | 1 sundae | 740 | 340 | 37 | 25 | 90 | 210 | 91 | 1 | 10 |
| Nuts Over Caramel Lava Cake Sundae | 1 sundae | 1370 | 500 | 56 | 24 | 140 | 970 | 197 | 5 | 21 |
| Pineapple Smoothie | as served | 590 | 40 | 4 | 2 | 20 | 290 | 122 | 1 | 16 |
| Reese's Peanut Butter Cup 3 Scoop | 1 sundae | 890 | 470 | 52 | 50 | 90 | 380 | 90 | 7 | 17 |
| Reese's Pieces 3 Scoop | 1 sundae | 930 | 480 | 53 | 26 | 90 | 360 | 95 | 4 | 18 |
| Royal Banana Split | 1 sundae | 880 | 320 | 35 | 20 | 110 | 200 | 132 | 2 | 10 |
| Strawberry Banana Smoothie | as served | 520 | 40 | 4 | 2 | 20 | 290 | 105 | 2 | 17 |
| Strawberry Shortcake Sundae | 1 sundae | 580 | 240 | 27 | 16 | 110 | 190 | 79 | 2 | 8 |
| **SOUPS SALADS** | | | | | | | | | | |
| Apple Walnut Chicken | 1 salad | 390 | 160 | 18 | 7 | 110 | 1140 | 22 | 5 | 38 |
| Asian Chicken | 1 salad | 490 | 180 | 20 | 3 | 80 | 1200 | 41 | 6 | 36 |
| Broccoli Cheddar Soup | 1 cup | 200 | 110 | 13 | 7 | 40 | 780 | 14 | 1 | 7 |
| Chicken Caesar | 1 salad | 1030 | 760 | 84 | 16 | 220 | 2010 | 32 | 3 | 47 |
| Chili | 1 cup | 270 | 150 | 16 | 6 | 40 | 910 | 18 | 3 | 14 |
| Chunky Chicken Noodle Soup | 1 cup | 280 | 90 | 10 | 3 | 70 | 1970 | 31 | 2 | 20 |
| Crispy Caesar | 1 salad | 1140 | 840 | 93 | 20 | 230 | 2160 | 40 | 4 | 53 |
| Homestyle Clam Chowder | 1 cup | 270 | 160 | 18 | 10 | 60 | 890 | 17 | 1 | 11 |
| Kickin Buffalo Chicken | 1 salad | 710 | 420 | 47 | 9 | 90 | 1370 | 42 | 7 | 29 |
| Minestrone Soup | 1 cup | 90 | 10 | 1 | 0 | 0 | 620 | 15 | 2 | 4 |
| Southwest Chipotle Chicken | 1 salad | 550 | 200 | 22 | 3 | 80 | 1440 | 50 | 8 | 37 |
| Steak & Bleu Cheese | 1 salad | 640 | 300 | 64 | 11 | 120 | 1240 | 41 | 8 | 44 |

## Golden Corral
### BREAKFAST BUFFET

| | | | | | | | | | | |
|---|---|---|---|---|---|---|---|---|---|---|
| Bacon & Cheese Quiche | 1 slice | 290 | 190 | 21 | 8 | 100 | 730 | 15 | 1 | 10 |
| Cheese Grits | 1/2 cup | 170 | 80 | 9 | 4 | 20 | 310 | 16 | 0 | 7 |
| Hash Brown Casserole | 1/2 cup | 130 | 45 | 5 | 2.5 | 10 | 530 | 14 | 1 | 5 |
| Mini Bacon & Cheese Tart | 1 piece | 250 | 160 | 18 | 6 | 65 | 600 | 15 | 0 | 7 |
| Mini Cin-a-Gold Rolls | 1 piece | 230 | 80 | 9 | 2.5 | 15 | 210 | 35 | 1 | 3 |
| Spinach Quiche | 1 slice | 239 | 150 | 17 | 5 | 65 | 480 | 15 | 0 | 5 |
| **HOT BUFFET** | | | | | | | | | | |
| Awesome Pot Roast | 3 oz | 100 | 40 | 4.5 | 2 | 35 | 200 | 5 | 1 | 10 |
| Baby Back Ribs | 1 piece | 190 | 140 | 15 | 6 | 50 | 280 | 2 | 0 | 10 |
| BBQ Chicken (Leg Quarter) | 1 piece | 490 | 200 | 22 | 9 | 205 | 1080 | 21 | 2 | 50 |
| Boneless BBQ Pork Ribs | 2 pieces | 240 | 130 | 14 | 5 | 65 | 420 | 7 | 0 | 19 |
| Buffalo Wings | 3 pieces | 210 | 140 | 15 | 4 | 70 | 200 | 1 | 1 | 17 |
| Cheese Pizza | 1 slice | 170 | 60 | 7 | 3 | 15 | 360 | 21 | 1 | 8 |

# restaurants

| | SERVING SIZE | CAL | CAL FAT | TOT FAT (G) | SAT FAT (G) | CHOL (MG) | SOD (MG) | CARB (G) | FIBER (G) | PROT (G) |
|---|---|---|---|---|---|---|---|---|---|---|
| Chipotle Chicken Tenders | 1 piece | 130 | 35 | 4 | .5 | 30 | 310 | 9 | 0 | 12 |
| Country Breaded Wings | 3 pieces | 310 | 200 | 22 | 6 | 75 | 400 | 7 | 0 | 19 |
| Golden Delicious Shrimp | 6 pieces | 210 | 80 | 9 | 1.5 | 55 | 330 | 23 | 1 | 9 |
| Grilled BBQ Wings | 3 pieces | 210 | 130 | 14 | 4 | 65 | 180 | 3 | 0 | 16 |
| Ham & Cheese Bistro Melt | 1 piece | 320 | 160 | 18 | 6 | 45 | 1000 | 22 | 1 | 15 |
| Homemade Italian Meatballs | 2 pieces | 140 | 90 | 16 | 5 | 55 | 590 | 9 | 1 | 12 |
| Macaroni & Cheese | 1/2 cup | 190 | 80 | 9 | 3.5 | 15 | 450 | 19 | 1 | 9 |
| Meatloaf | 1 slice | 220 | 100 | 11 | 4.5 | 105 | 600 | 12 | 4 | 18 |
| Pepperoni Pizza | 1 slice | 210 | 90 | 10 | 4.5 | 25 | 500 | 21 | 1 | 10 |
| Philly Steak Sandwich | 1 piece | 380 | 190 | 21 | 6 | 60 | 780 | 24 | 1 | 21 |
| Popcorn Shrimp | 15 pieces | 130 | 60 | 6 | 1 | 30 | 490 | 14 | 1 | 5 |
| Sweet Potato Casserole | 1/2 cup | 190 | 30 | 3.5 | 1 | 5 | 50 | 37 | 2 | 2 |
| Turkey & Bacon Bistro Melt | 1 melt | 300 | 160 | 18 | 7 | 55 | 680 | 8 | 0 | 21 |
| **SOUPS & SALADS** | | | | | | | | | | |
| Chicken Noodle Soup | 1 cup | 80 | 10 | 1.5 | 0 | 20 | 900 | 12 | 0 | 6 |
| Chicken Salad | 1/2 cup | 240 | 180 | 20 | 3 | 115 | 370 | 3 | 0 | 12 |
| Clam Chowder | 1 cup | 160 | 50 | 5 | 2.5 | 15 | 730 | 18 | 1 | 8 |
| Egg Salad | 1/2 cup | 200 | 150 | 17 | 3.5 | 290 | 280 | 3 | 0 | 8 |
| Macaroni Salad | 1/2 cup | 280 | 200 | 22 | 3 | 20 | 280 | 19 | 2 | 2 |
| Timberline Chili | 1 cup | 230 | 80 | 9 | 3 | 40 | 890 | 26 | 8 | 15 |

## Good Times
### BURGERS & SANDWICHES

| | SERVING SIZE | CAL | CAL FAT | TOT FAT (G) | SAT FAT (G) | CHOL (MG) | SOD (MG) | CARB (G) | FIBER (G) | PROT (G) |
|---|---|---|---|---|---|---|---|---|---|---|
| Bacon Cheeseburger | 1 burger | 550 | 279 | 31 | 11 | 85 | 1420 | 37 | 1 | 32 |
| BBQ Burger | 1 burger | 400 | 126 | 14 | 4.5 | 55 | 910 | 46 | 1 | 22 |
| Big Daddy Bacon Cheeseburger | 1 burger | 960 | 558 | 62 | 22 | 170 | 2550 | 40 | 1 | 60 |
| Buffalo Chicken Sandwich | 1 sandwich | 570 | 288 | 32 | 4 | 55 | 1740 | 47 | 2 | 26 |
| Crispy Chicken Sandwich | 1 sandwich | 490 | 207 | 23 | 3.5 | 50 | 1160 | 46 | 2 | 25 |
| Double Good Time | 1 burger | 690 | 351 | 39 | 15 | 140 | 1280 | 39 | 1 | 43 |
| Double Mushroom Swiss Burger | 1 burger | 610 | 297 | 33 | 12 | 125 | 1030 | 39 | 2 | 42 |
| Mammoth Burger | 1 burger | 870 | 450 | 50 | 21 | 205 | 1620 | 39 | 1 | 63 |
| Mighty Deluxe Cheeseburger | 1 burger | 460 | 207 | 23 | 8 | 75 | 960 | 39 | 1 | 24 |
| Oven Roasted Chicken Sandwich | 1 sandwich | 420 | 180 | 20 | 3 | 60 | 1100 | 40 | 2 | 21 |
| Ranch Burger | 1 burger | 480 | 243 | 27 | 6 | 65 | 740 | 38 | 1 | 22 |
| **GLACIERS, SHAKES, & SUNDAES** | | | | | | | | | | |
| Cherry Glacier | 16.7 oz | 300 | 0 | 0 | 0 | 0 | 30 | 73 | 0 | 0 |
| Chocolate Shake, small | 16 oz | 760 | 270 | 30 | 17 | 135 | 300 | 116 | 0 | 16 |

| | SERVING SIZE | CAL | CAL FAT | TOT FAT (G) | SAT FAT (G) | CHOL (MG) | SOD (MG) | CARB (G) | FIBER (G) | PROT (G) |
|---|---|---|---|---|---|---|---|---|---|---|
| Hot Fudge Peak Sundae | 1 sundae | 490 | 234 | 26 | 12 | 60 | 330 | 57 | 2 | 9 |
| Lemon Glacier | 16.7 oz | 250 | 0 | 0 | 0 | 0 | 20 | 61 | 0 | 0 |
| Raspberry Avalanche Sundae | 1 sundae | 300 | 117 | 13 | 8 | 60 | 125 | 41 | 1 | 5 |
| Strawberry Shake, small | 16 oz | 780 | 270 | 30 | 17 | 110 | 270 | 120 | 0 | 13 |
| Strawberry Shortcake Sundae | 1 sundae | 400 | 162 | 18 | 9 | 80 | 200 | 54 | 1 | 6 |
| Turtle Sundae | 1 sundae | 600 | 306 | 34 | 13 | 90 | 210 | 66 | 2 | 9 |
| Vanilla Shake, small | 16 oz | 740 | 297 | 33 | 18 | 110 | 280 | 105 | 0 | 14 |
| Watermelon Glacier | 16.7 oz | 300 | 0 | 0 | 0 | 0 | 30 | 72 | 0 | 0 |
| **FROZEN CUSTARD & SPOONBENDERS** | | | | | | | | | | |
| Build-A-Bender Spoonbender, 1 topping | 16 oz | 740 | 351 | 39 | 22 | 195 | 340 | 84 | 0 | 15 |
| Butter Pecan | 1 scoop | 500 | 315 | 35 | 12 | 85 | 190 | 40 | 2 | 10 |
| Butterfinger | 1 scoop | 460 | 234 | 26 | 12 | 80 | 250 | 48 | 0 | 10 |
| Caramel Toffee Spoonbender | 16 oz | 1190 | 513 | 57 | 27 | 295 | 610 | 150 | 2 | 19 |
| Chocolate Chocolate Chip | 1 scoop | 500 | 243 | 27 | 18 | 85 | 220 | 61 | 2 | 8 |
| Chocolate Malt Whopper | 1 scoop | 460 | 180 | 20 | 13 | 80 | 290 | 62 | 1 | 9 |
| Cookies 'N Cream Spoonbender | 16 oz | 1030 | 432 | 48 | 24 | 195 | 620 | 135 | 2 | 17 |
| Deluxe Toffee | 1 scoop | 510 | 243 | 27 | 14 | 95 | 450 | 58 | 0 | 7 |
| Mocha Cappucino Spoonbender | 16 oz | 1310 | 558 | 62 | 42 | 200 | 370 | 178 | 2 | 18 |
| Mudd Pie Sundae | 1 scoop | 610 | 243 | 27 | 14 | 65 | 410 | 82 | 2 | 6 |
| New York Cheesecake | 1 scoop | 400 | 189 | 21 | 12 | 105 | 300 | 46 | 0 | 7 |
| Orangesicle | 1 scoop | 330 | 162 | 18 | 10 | 90 | 160 | 37 | 0 | 7 |
| Oreo Mint | 1 scoop | 410 | 180 | 20 | 11 | 90 | 320 | 49 | 0 | 8 |
| Peanut Butter Cup | 1 scoop | 510 | 270 | 30 | 13 | 85 | 290 | 51 | 1 | 11 |
| Pumpkin | 1 scoop | 320 | 153 | 17 | 10 | 85 | 150 | 36 | 0 | 6 |
| Raspberry Torte Spoonbender | 16 oz | 1090 | 468 | 52 | 27 | 195 | 620 | 141 | 3 | 18 |
| Strawberries & Cream | 1 scoop | 310 | 135 | 15 | 8 | 75 | 130 | 39 | 0 | 6 |
| Strawberry Cheesecake Spoonbender | 16 oz | 1070 | 423 | 47 | 27 | 230 | 690 | 144 | 2 | 17 |
| Turtle Crunch | 1 scoop | 660 | 369 | 41 | 20 | 80 | 190 | 67 | 3 | 9 |
| Turtle Spoonbender | 16 oz | 1320 | 711 | 79 | 28 | 195 | 460 | 137 | 5 | 19 |
| Vanilla custard | 1 scoop | 330 | 162 | 18 | 10 | 90 | 160 | 37 | 0 | 7 |
| **SIDES** | | | | | | | | | | |
| Wild Fries, small | 5 oz | 450 | 234 | 26 | 10 | 0 | 560 | 48 | 5 | 5 |

## Great Steak & Potato
### BREAKFAST SANDWICHES

| | SERVING SIZE | CAL | CAL FAT | TOT FAT (G) | SAT FAT (G) | CHOL (MG) | SOD (MG) | CARB (G) | FIBER (G) | PROT (G) |
|---|---|---|---|---|---|---|---|---|---|---|
| Bacon, Egg & Cheese | 1 sandwich | 600 | 320 | 36 | 11 | 440 | 1300 | 39 | 2 | 29 |
| Egg & Cheese | 1 sandwich | 500 | 260 | 29 | 9 | 425 | 890 | 39 | 2 | 23 |

# restaurants

| | SERVING SIZE | CAL | CAL FAT | TOT FAT (G) | SAT FAT (G) | CHOL (MG) | SOD (MG) | CARB (G) | FIBER (G) | PROT (G) |
|---|---|---|---|---|---|---|---|---|---|---|
| Ham, Egg & Cheese | 1 sandwich | 570 | 290 | 32 | 10 | 450 | 1540 | 42 | 2 | 31 |
| Sausage, Egg & Cheese | 1 sandwich | 700 | 420 | 47 | 15 | 465 | 1300 | 39 | 2 | 30 |
| **BURGERS** | | | | | | | | | | |
| Cheeseburger | 1 burger | 640 | 310 | 35 | 12 | 105 | 730 | 41 | 3 | 40 |
| Hamburger | 1 burger | 590 | 270 | 30 | 9 | 105 | 480 | 40 | 3 | 37 |
| Philly Burger | 1 burger | 530 | 250 | 28 | 9 | 80 | 500 | 39 | 4 | 31 |
| **CONDIMENTS, SAUCES, & TOPPINGS** | | | | | | | | | | |
| Buffalo | 1 oz | 10 | 3 | 0 | 0 | 0 | 855 | 2 | 0 | 0 |
| Cheese, Philly Wiz, Cheese | 1 oz | 80 | 50 | 6 | 4 | 20 | 460 | 2 | 0 | 4 |
| Tzatziki | 1 oz | 50 | 40 | 4 | 4 | 0 | 80 | 2 | 0 | 0 |
| **FRIES** | | | | | | | | | | |
| Cheese Fries | as served | 490 | 240 | 27 | 9 | 30 | 1600 | 51 | 5 | 12 |
| Chili | as served | 440 | 220 | 24 | 14 | 85 | 1480 | 34 | 19 | 27 |
| Coney Island Fry | as served | 570 | 270 | 30 | 10 | 45 | 2030 | 61 | 12 | 18 |
| Great Fry | as served | 440 | 180 | 20 | 3 | 0 | 1130 | 60 | 7 | 7 |
| King Fry | as served | 630 | 350 | 39 | 14 | 70 | 1970 | 52 | 5 | 20 |
| Potato Skins | as served | 390 | 230 | 26 | 12 | 65 | 1070 | 24 | 2 | 17 |
| **THE GREAT POTATO** | | | | | | | | | | |
| Chicken | 1 potato | 500 | 200 | 22 | 11 | 100 | 1310 | 37 | 4 | 32 |
| Ham | 1 potato | 420 | 150 | 16 | 10 | 95 | 2360 | 43 | 4 | 29 |
| King | 1 potato | 490 | 260 | 29 | 16 | 95 | 740 | 31 | 3 | 26 |
| Steak | 1 potato | 520 | 240 | 26 | 11 | 105 | 1250 | 37 | 4 | 35 |
| Turkey | 1 potato | 390 | 120 | 13 | 8 | 85 | 1810 | 39 | 4 | 31 |
| **GREAT STEAK SANDWICHES 7" & WRAPS** | | | | | | | | | | |
| Bacon Cheddar Cheesesteak | 1 sandwich | 720 | 280 | 32 | 12 | 105 | 1930 | 62 | 5 | 45 |
| Buffalo Chicken Philly | 1 sandwich | 660 | 220 | 24 | 10 | 60 | 2420 | 65 | 5 | 37 |
| Chicagoland Cheesesteak | 1 sandwich | 680 | 260 | 29 | 11 | 85 | 2480 | 63 | 5 | 43 |
| Chicken Philly Slider | 1 sandwich | 300 | 110 | 13 | 6 | 50 | 880 | 24 | 2 | 19 |
| Great Steak Cheesesteak | 1 sandwich | 740 | 330 | 37 | 9 | 95 | 1270 | 62 | 5 | 41 |
| Great Steak Cheesesteak Wrap | 1 wrap | 820 | 380 | 43 | 11 | 95 | 1400 | 67 | 5 | 40 |
| Gyro | 1 sandwich | 580 | 270 | 30 | 10 | 60 | 1550 | 52 | 5 | 29 |
| Ham Delight | 1 sandwich | 710 | 300 | 33 | 10 | 85 | 2190 | 71 | 5 | 36 |
| Ham Explosion | 1 sandwich | 710 | 300 | 34 | 10 | 85 | 2200 | 70 | 6 | 37 |
| Kansas City (BBQ) Cheesesteak | 1 sandwich | 680 | 230 | 26 | 10 | 65 | 1740 | 71 | 5 | 40 |
| Original Chicken Philly | 1 sandwich | 620 | 190 | 22 | 9 | 85 | 1670 | 62 | 5 | 37 |

| | SERVING SIZE | CAL | CAL FAT | TOT FAT (G) | SAT FAT (G) | CHOL (MG) | SOD (MG) | CARB (G) | FIBER (G) | PROT (G) |
|---|---|---|---|---|---|---|---|---|---|---|
| Original Chicken Philly Wrap | 1 wrap | 700 | 250 | 28 | 11 | 85 | 1800 | 67 | 4 | 36 |
| Original Philly Cheesesteak | 1 sandwich | 650 | 230 | 26 | 10 | 95 | 2570 | 62 | 5 | 40 |
| Pastrami | 1 sandwich | 790 | 370 | 41 | 16 | 110 | 1850 | 65 | 5 | 43 |
| Reuben | 1 sandwich | 690 | 290 | 33 | 11 | 95 | 2550 | 61 | 5 | 37 |
| Steak Philly Slider | 1 sandwich | 310 | 130 | 15 | 6 | 55 | 850 | 24 | 2 | 20 |
| Super Steak Cheesesteak | 1 sandwich | 750 | 330 | 37 | 9 | 95 | 1270 | 64 | 6 | 42 |
| Super Steak Cheesesteak Wrap | 1 wrap | 930 | 480 | 54 | 13 | 105 | 1500 | 69 | 5 | 41 |
| Teriyaki Chicken Philly | 1 sandwich | 740 | 290 | 32 | 9 | 85 | 2280 | 65 | 5 | 40 |
| Turkey Philly | 1 sandwich | 670 | 270 | 30 | 8 | 75 | 1650 | 64 | 5 | 38 |
| Ultimate Chicken Philly | 1 sandwich | 730 | 300 | 33 | 11 | 65 | 1590 | 64 | 6 | 38 |
| Ultimate Chicken Philly Wrap | 1 sandwich | 810 | 350 | 39 | 13 | 65 | 1720 | 69 | 5 | 36 |
| Veggie Delight | 1 sandwich | 510 | 170 | 19 | 6 | 20 | 950 | 64 | 5 | 18 |
| Wisconsin Inside-Out | 1 sandwich | 560 | 240 | 27 | 12 | 20 | 1360 | 57 | 4 | 24 |

**SALADS**

| | SERVING SIZE | CAL | CAL FAT | TOT FAT (G) | SAT FAT (G) | CHOL (MG) | SOD (MG) | CARB (G) | FIBER (G) | PROT (G) |
|---|---|---|---|---|---|---|---|---|---|---|
| Chef | 1 salad | 260 | 100 | 11 | 6 | 70 | 1320 | 15 | 4 | 28 |
| Garden | 1 salad | 60 | 5 | 1 | 0 | 0 | 40 | 13 | 5 | 3 |
| Grilled Chicken | 1 salad | 380 | 160 | 18 | 8 | 80 | 460 | 18 | 5 | 31 |
| Grilled Steak | 1 salad | 400 | 200 | 23 | 7 | 85 | 590 | 18 | 5 | 33 |
| Grilled Turkey | 1 salad | 330 | 150 | 17 | 6 | 65 | 970 | 20 | 5 | 30 |
| Side | 1 salad | 30 | 5 | 0 | 0 | 0 | 20 | 6 | 2 | 2 |

# Hardee's
## BREAKFAST

| | SERVING SIZE | CAL | CAL FAT | TOT FAT (G) | SAT FAT (G) | CHOL (MG) | SOD (MG) | CARB (G) | FIBER (G) | PROT (G) |
|---|---|---|---|---|---|---|---|---|---|---|
| Bacon, Egg & Cheese Biscuit | 1 biscuit | 530 | 320 | 36 | 11 | 195 | 1390 | 36 | 0 | 15 |
| Big Country Breakfast Platter—Bacon | as served | 910 | 430 | 48 | 12 | 385 | 2210 | 91 | 4 | 27 |
| Country Ham Biscuit | 1 biscuit | 440 | 240 | 26 | 6 | 35 | 1710 | 36 | 0 | 14 |
| Country Potatoes, Medium | as served | 200 | 110 | 12 | 2.5 | 0 | 710 | 30 | 4 | 6 |
| Country Steak Biscuit | 1 biscuit | 590 | 360 | 40 | 10 | 25 | 1290 | 43 | 1 | 13 |
| Frisco Breakfast Sandwich | 1 sandwich | 400 | 160 | 18 | 7 | 215 | 1250 | 39 | 2 | 20 |
| Ham, Egg & Cheese Biscuit | 1 biscuit | 540 | 300 | 33 | 10 | 220 | 1830 | 36 | 0 | 23 |
| Loaded Biscuit 'N' Gravy Breakfast Bowl | as served | 740 | 460 | 52 | 14 | 220 | 1920 | 49 | 1 | 20 |
| Loaded Breakfast Burrito | 1 burrito | 760 | 440 | 49 | 21 | 445 | 1700 | 39 | 1 | 39 |
| Loaded Omelet Biscuit | 1 biscuit | 610 | 380 | 42 | 14 | 220 | 1540 | 36 | 0 | 20 |
| Low Carb Breakfast Bowl | as served | 620 | 450 | 50 | 21 | 325 | 1380 | 6 | 2 | 36 |
| Made From Scratch Biscuit | 1 biscuit | 370 | 210 | 23 | 5 | 0 | 890 | 35 | 0 | 5 |
| Monster Biscuit | 1 biscuit | 770 | 500 | 55 | 18 | 250 | 2310 | 37 | 0 | 29 |
| Pancakes | 3 pancakes | 300 | 45 | 5 | 1 | 25 | 830 | 55 | 2 | 8 |
| Sausage Biscuit | 1 biscuit | 530 | 340 | 38 | 10 | 30 | 1240 | 36 | 0 | 11 |

# restaurants

| | SERVING SIZE | CAL | CAL FAT | TOT FAT (G) | SAT FAT (G) | CHOL (MG) | SOD (MG) | CARB (G) | FIBER (G) | PROT (G) |
|---|---|---|---|---|---|---|---|---|---|---|
| **FRIED CHICKEN** | | | | | | | | | | |
| Breast | 1 piece | 370 | 130 | 15 | 4 | 75 | 1190 | 29 | 0 | 29 |
| Leg | 1 piece | 170 | 60 | 7 | 2 | 45 | 570 | 15 | 0 | 13 |
| Thigh | 1 piece | 330 | 130 | 15 | 4 | 60 | 1000 | 30 | 0 | 19 |
| Wing | 1 piece | 200 | 70 | 8 | 2 | 30 | 740 | 23 | 0 | 10 |
| **FRIES** | | | | | | | | | | |
| Crispy Curls—Medium | as served | 410 | 180 | 20 | 5 | 0 | 1020 | 52 | 4 | 5 |
| Natural-Cut French Fries—Medium | as served | 430 | 170 | 19 | 4 | 5 | 960 | 60 | 4 | 5 |
| **THICKBURGERS & SANDWICHES** | | | | | | | | | | |
| 1/3 lb Low Carb Thickburger | 1 burger | 420 | 280 | 32 | 12 | 115 | 1010 | 5 | 2 | 30 |
| 1/3 lb Original Thickburger | 1 burger | 770 | 430 | 48 | 16 | 95 | 1560 | 53 | 4 | 35 |
| Chicken Strips | 5 strips | 610 | 390 | 43 | 9 | 50 | 1030 | 32 | 3 | 23 |
| BBQ Chicken Fillet Sandwich | 1 sandwich | 710 | 350 | 38 | 7 | 55 | 1610 | 62 | 5 | 33 |
| Jumbo Chili Dog | 1 hot dog | 400 | 240 | 26 | 9 | 55 | 1170 | 25 | 1 | 16 |
| Little Thickburger | 1 burger | 570 | 350 | 39 | 12 | 80 | 1140 | 35 | 3 | 24 |
| Low Carb Charbroiled Chicken Club Sandwich | 1 sandwich | 360 | 200 | 23 | 7 | 75 | 1290 | 14 | 1 | 24 |
| Regular Roast Beef | 1 sandwich | 310 | 130 | 15 | 5 | 40 | 840 | 28 | 1 | 17 |
| Six Dollar Thickburger | 1 burger | 930 | 530 | 59 | 21 | 130 | 1960 | 57 | 4 | 46 |
| Spicy Chicken Sandwich | 1 sandwich | 440 | 180 | 21 | 5 | 50 | 1140 | 41 | 3 | 11 |

## Hot Dog on a Stick
### HOT DOGS

| | SERVING SIZE | CAL | CAL FAT | TOT FAT (G) | SAT FAT (G) | CHOL (MG) | SOD (MG) | CARB (G) | FIBER (G) | PROT (G) |
|---|---|---|---|---|---|---|---|---|---|---|
| American Cheese on a Stick | 1 hot dog | 270 | n/a | 14 | 7 | 60 | 900 | 26 | 1 | 10 |
| Beef Hot Dog on a Bun | 1 hot dog | 460 | n/a | 29 | 11 | 60 | 1440 | 37 | 2 | 14 |
| Pepperjack Cheese on a Stick | 1 hot dog | 260 | n/a | 13 | 6 | 50 | 850 | 25 | 2 | 9 |
| Turkey | 1 hot dog | 240 | n/a | 11 | 2.5 | 60 | 610 | 28 | 1 | 9 |
| Veggie Dog On A Stick | 1 hot dog | 250 | n/a | 5 | 1 | 20 | 930 | 35 | 2 | 16 |
| **SIDES & PLATTERS** | | | | | | | | | | |
| Fish & Zucchini Platter | 1 serving | 560 | n/a | 37 | 6 | 79 | 718 | 42 | 1 | 20 |
| Fish Platter | 1 serving | 320 | n/a | 21 | 3.5 | 45 | 410 | 24 | 1 | 11 |
| French Fries | 1 serving | 390 | n/a | 15 | 2.5 | 0 | 70 | 60 | 4 | 5 |
| Funnel Cake Sticks | 1 serving | 220 | n/a | 9 | 2 | 25 | 170 | 31 | 1 | 2 |
| Zucchini Platter | 1 serving | 780 | n/a | 68 | 11 | 0 | 700 | 35 | 5 | 6 |

## Houlihan's
### APPETIZERS & SMALL PLATES

| | SERVING SIZE | CAL | CAL FAT | TOT FAT (G) | SAT FAT (G) | CHOL (MG) | SOD (MG) | CARB (G) | FIBER (G) | PROT (G) |
|---|---|---|---|---|---|---|---|---|---|---|
| Blackened Chicken Quesadilla | as served | 1126 | 666 | 74 | 35 | n/a | 2271 | 64 | 8 | 49 |

| | SERVING SIZE | CAL | CAL FAT | TOT FAT (G) | SAT FAT (G) | CHOL (MG) | SOD (MG) | CARB (G) | FIBER (G) | PROT (G) |
|---|---|---|---|---|---|---|---|---|---|---|
| Bruschetta & Shrimp | as served | 1325 | 864 | 96 | 24 | n/a | 822 | 66 | 5 | 52 |
| Calamari | as served | 428 | 144 | 16 | 2 | n/a | 1018 | 34 | 2 | 32 |
| Cheese Burger Slider, Single | as served | 379 | 207 | 23 | 9 | n/a | 435 | 20 | 1 | 22 |
| Chicken Fingers, Buffalo Style | as served | 763 | 297 | 33 | 6 | n/a | 2263 | 54 | 6 | 59 |
| Chicken Wings, Thai Chile Style | as served | 1116 | 504 | 56 | 9 | n/a | 4979 | 105 | 1 | 48 |
| Chipotle Chicken Nachos | as served | 2285 | 1314 | 146 | 65 | n/a | 4320 | 127 | 11 | 101 |
| Disco Fries | as served | 592 | 297 | 33 | 15 | n/a | 1015 | 44 | 4 | 21 |
| Flatbread, BBQ Chicken | as served | 348 | 117 | 13 | 6 | n/a | 766 | 39 | 1 | 18 |
| Flatbread, Wild Mushroom & Arugula | as served | 383 | 189 | 21 | 9 | n/a | 732 | 32 | 2 | 14 |
| Goat Cheese & Artichoke Poppers | as served | 520 | 288 | 32 | 12 | n/a | 1264 | 41 | 3 | 19 |
| Grilled Chinese Dumpling Kabobs | as served | 547 | 342 | 38 | 14 | n/a | 1525 | 16 | 1 | 31 |
| Grilled Shrimp Azteca | as served | 306 | 153 | 17 | 6 | n/a | 442 | 18 | 3 | 19 |
| Grilled Vegetable Pizza | as served | 744 | 360 | 40 | 15 | n/a | 1354 | 65 | 6 | 32 |
| Jumbo Stuffed Shrooms | as served | 1193 | 567 | 63 | 26 | n/a | 1609 | 124 | 6 | 33 |
| Lettuce Wraps | as served | 538 | 153 | 17 | 4 | n/a | 1865 | 71 | 4 | 25 |
| Mini Spinach Dip & Tortilla Chips | as served | 675 | 270 | 30 | 15 | n/a | 660 | 77 | 5 | 14 |
| Miniature Burger Threesome | as served | 1142 | 612 | 68 | 27 | n/a | 1471 | 87 | 4 | 45 |
| Parmesan Frites | as served | 330 | 126 | 14 | 3 | n/a | 466 | 42 | 4 | 4 |
| Seared Rare Tuna Wontons | as served | 351 | 162 | 18 | 2 | n/a | 777 | 27 | 1 | 20 |
| Shrimp Po' Boy Slider, Single | as served | 213 | 72 | 8 | 3 | n/a | 344 | 25 | 1 | 9 |
| Smoked Pork Flatbread | as served | 466 | 261 | 29 | 9 | n/a | 648 | 31 | 2 | 20 |
| Spinach Dip w/Lavosh Crackers | as served | 1359 | 639 | 71 | 38 | n/a | 2480 | 137 | 3 | 44 |
| Steamed Mussels w/Andouille | as served | 634 | 333 | 37 | 13 | n/a | 2116 | 38 | 5 | 33 |
| Tandoori Chicken Skewer | as served | 156 | 36 | 4 | 0 | n/a | 152 | 2 | 1 | 30 |
| Vietnamese Spring Eggrolls | as served | 207 | 9 | 1 | 0 | n/a | 307 | 30 | 1 | 13 |
| **ENTRÉES** | | | | | | | | | | |
| 4 Jumbo Fried Shrimp | 2 pieces | 246 | 63 | 7 | 2 | n/a | 451 | 19 | 1 | 25 |
| Atlantic Salmon, Mustard Encrusted | 1 entrée | 1158 | 765 | 85 | 31 | n/a | 1513 | 36 | 3 | 47 |
| BBQ Veggie Melt | 1 entrée | 707 | 342 | 38 | 13 | n/a | 1194 | 63 | 8 | 26 |
| Chicken Fettuccine Alfredo | 1 entrée | 1413 | 612 | 68 | 36 | n/a | 1693 | 110 | 5 | 80 |
| Chicken Finger Platter | 1 entrée | 1241 | 477 | 53 | 9 | n/a | 2227 | 101 | 9 | 83 |
| Chicken Parmesan | 1 entrée | 1384 | 468 | 52 | 18 | n/a | 2035 | 149 | 8 | 74 |
| Chipotle Smoked Chicken Enchiladas | 1 entrée | 1211 | 603 | 67 | 31 | n/a | 2492 | 94 | 12 | 56 |
| Full Slab of Ribs | 1 entrée | 1475 | 666 | 74 | 21 | n/a | 4841 | 144 | 6 | 59 |
| Grilled Rosemary Chicken | 1 entrée | 718 | 333 | 37 | 17 | n/a | 1781 | 39 | 8 | 54 |
| Herb Grilled Chicken | 1 entrée | 489 | 162 | 18 | 5 | n/a | 791 | 27 | 3 | 51 |
| Huge Panko Battered Shrimp | 1 entrée | 961 | 387 | 43 | 7 | n/a | 2061 | 94 | 7 | 49 |

# restaurants

| | SERVING SIZE | CAL | CAL FAT | TOT FAT (G) | SAT FAT (G) | CHOL (MG) | SOD (MG) | CARB (G) | FIBER (G) | PROT (G) |
|---|---|---|---|---|---|---|---|---|---|---|
| Lobster Tail Add-On for Steaks | 1 entrée | 112 | 0 | 0 | 0 | n/a | 168 | 0 | 0 | 27 |
| Meatloaf #9 | 1 entrée | 1141 | 639 | 71 | 38 | n/a | 2811 | 70 | 9 | 48 |
| Seared Scallops w/Asparagus Risotto | 1 entrée | 591 | 288 | 32 | 7 | n/a | 1512 | 31 | 3 | 44 |
| Shrimp Scampi | 1 entrée | 1205 | 621 | 69 | 32 | n/a | 1390 | 94 | 5 | 44 |
| Sizzling Fajitas, Combo | 1 entrée | 1262 | 486 | 54 | 23 | n/a | 3060 | 117 | 13 | 74 |
| Stir Fry, Chicken | 1 entrée | 1056 | 261 | 29 | 6 | n/a | 2127 | 151 | 7 | 45 |
| Stuffed Chicken Breast | 1 entrée | 1081 | 540 | 60 | 26 | n/a | 2572 | 74 | 10 | 57 |
| Tuscany Lemon Chicken Pasta | 1 entrée | 1608 | 747 | 83 | 40 | n/a | 1834 | 112 | 6 | 77 |
| **ENTRÉE SALADS** | | | | | | | | | | |
| Buffalo Bleu | 1 salad | 1435 | 927 | 103 | 27 | n/a | 3069 | 63 | 11 | 64 |
| Chicken Asian Chop Chop | 1 salad | 999 | 459 | 51 | 9 | n/a | 2297 | 99 | 10 | 33 |
| Chicken Caesar | 1 salad | 1333 | 882 | 98 | 21 | n/a | 2081 | 43 | 6 | 60 |
| Fire Grilled BBQ Salmon | 1 salad | 1182 | 549 | 61 | 9 | n/a | 1719 | 103 | 12 | 53 |
| Heartland Fried Chicken | 1 salad | 1337 | 783 | 87 | 21 | n/a | 2266 | 79 | 10 | 61 |
| Heartland Grilled Chicken | 1 salad | 1014 | 693 | 77 | 19 | n/a | 1535 | 27 | 7 | 55 |
| Large House Salad, w/Bleu Cheese, No Dressing | 1 salad | 384 | 198 | 22 | 10 | n/a | 685 | 33 | 4 | 14 |
| Mandarin Chicken | 1 salad | 1015 | 351 | 39 | 6 | n/a | 2089 | 114 | 8 | 48 |
| Prime Steak & Wedge | 1 salad | 1370 | 1026 | 114 | 36 | n/a | 2145 | 35 | 7 | 53 |
| Seared Ahi Tuna | 1 salad | 1074 | 603 | 67 | 17 | n/a | 1092 | 77 | 8 | 36 |
| Tuscan White Bean | 1 salad | 644 | 360 | 40 | 10 | n/a | 992 | 56 | 12 | 18 |
| **SANDWICHES** | | | | | | | | | | |
| Brentwood Chicken Sandwich | 1 sandwich | 907 | 423 | 47 | 14 | n/a | 1794 | 53 | 3 | 65 |
| Buffalo Chicken | 1 sandwich | 762 | 225 | 25 | 6 | n/a | 1311 | 83 | 4 | 49 |
| Cheddar Roast Beef Sandwich | 1 sandwich | 698 | 306 | 34 | 9 | n/a | 1412 | 47 | 3 | 50 |
| Cheesy Royale Yum Yum Burger | 1 burger | 1108 | 648 | 72 | 25 | n/a | 2664 | 58 | 3 | 58 |
| French Dip | 1 sandwich | 962 | 342 | 38 | 14 | n/a | 2926 | 67 | 2 | 89 |
| Low Carb Burger w/Cauli Mash & Vegetables | 1 burger | 846 | 522 | 58 | 27 | n/a | 1782 | 20 | 8 | 57 |
| Rueben | 1 sandwich | 1081 | 621 | 69 | 24 | n/a | 3367 | 66 | 7 | 44 |
| Southwest Grilled Chicken Wrap | 1 wrap | 839 | 513 | 57 | 13 | n/a | 1493 | 47 | 5 | 35 |
| Spicy Fritos Burger | 1 burger | 1171 | 657 | 73 | 24 | n/a | 1909 | 68 | 5 | 56 |
| Veggie Club | 1 sandwich | 570 | 252 | 28 | 11 | n/a | 894 | 56 | 11 | 25 |
| Whole Grain Club | 1 sandwich | 540 | 225 | 25 | 9 | n/a | 2115 | 41 | 2 | 38 |

# Hungry Howies
## BREAD

| | SERVING SIZE | CAL | CAL FAT | TOT FAT (G) | SAT FAT (G) | CHOL (MG) | SOD (MG) | CARB (G) | FIBER (G) | PROT (G) |
|---|---|---|---|---|---|---|---|---|---|---|
| Cajun Bread | 1/4 of bread | 300 | 78 | 8.7 | 1.9 | 2 | 239 | 46 | 1 | 9 |
| Cinnamon Bread | 1/4 of bread | 313 | 78 | 8.7 | 1.9 | 2 | 239 | 59 | 1.2 | 9 |

| | SERVING SIZE | CAL | CAL FAT | TOT FAT (G) | SAT FAT (G) | CHOL (MG) | SOD (MG) | CARB (G) | FIBER (G) | PROT (G) |
|---|---|---|---|---|---|---|---|---|---|---|
| Howie Bread | 1/4 of bread | 300 | 78 | 8.7 | 1.9 | 2 | 239 | 46 | 1 | 9.4 |
| Three Cheeser Bread | 1/4 of bread | 370 | 123 | 13.7 | 4.9 | 17 | 384 | 47.1 | 1 | 14.7 |

## PIZZA

| | SERVING SIZE | CAL | CAL FAT | TOT FAT (G) | SAT FAT (G) | CHOL (MG) | SOD (MG) | CARB (G) | FIBER (G) | PROT (G) |
|---|---|---|---|---|---|---|---|---|---|---|
| Cheese, Large Thin Crust | 1 slice | 124 | 50 | 5.6 | 3.2 | 13 | 323 | 10.6 | .6 | 8 |
| Cheese, Medium | 1 slice | 191 | 41 | 5.7 | n/a | 11.2 | 437 | 23.2 | 0.9 | 11 |
| Cheese, Small | 1 slice | 161 | 32 | 3.6 | 3.2 | 10.6 | 370 | 20 | 9.6 | 8 |
| Cheese, X-Large | 1 slice | 395 | 84 | 9.3 | 5.9 | 25.1 | 882 | 41.9 | 2.1 | 23.2 |

## SALADS, LARGE

| | SERVING SIZE | CAL | CAL FAT | TOT FAT (G) | SAT FAT (G) | CHOL (MG) | SOD (MG) | CARB (G) | FIBER (G) | PROT (G) |
|---|---|---|---|---|---|---|---|---|---|---|
| Antipasto | 1/4 salad | 101 | 60 | 6.7 | 3.4 | 24 | 477 | 2.8 | 1.4 | 7.8 |
| Chef Salad | 1/4 salad | 99 | 54 | 6 | 3 | 24 | 341 | 3.6 | 1.6 | 8.1 |
| Garden Salad | 1/4 salad | 17 | 3 | 0.3 | 0 | 0 | 9 | 2.9 | 1.5 | 1 |
| Greek Salad | 1/4 salad | 109 | 60 | 6.7 | 4.3 | 25 | 501 | 7.1 | 1.8 | 5.6 |

## SUBS

| | SERVING SIZE | CAL | CAL FAT | TOT FAT (G) | SAT FAT (G) | CHOL (MG) | SOD (MG) | CARB (G) | FIBER (G) | PROT (G) |
|---|---|---|---|---|---|---|---|---|---|---|
| Deluxe Italian | 1/2 sandwich | 506 | 166 | 18 | 8.4 | 44 | 1005 | 61.2 | 1.8 | 24.3 |
| Pizza | 1/2 sandwich | 689 | 305 | 33.9 | 14.3 | 86 | 1722 | 66.7 | 2.7 | 29.7 |
| Steak & Cheese | 1/2 sandwich | 491 | 131 | 14.6 | 6.7 | 47 | 914 | 63.7 | 2 | 26.5 |
| Turkey Club | 1/2 sandwich | 556 | 137 | 15.2 | 7.7 | 42 | 1065 | 63.2 | 1.8 | 41.8 |
| Vegetarian | 1/2 sandwich | 530 | 185 | 20.5 | 10.7 | 39 | 895 | 64.4 | 3 | 22 |

## WINGS

| | SERVING SIZE | CAL | CAL FAT | TOT FAT (G) | SAT FAT (G) | CHOL (MG) | SOD (MG) | CARB (G) | FIBER (G) | PROT (G) |
|---|---|---|---|---|---|---|---|---|---|---|
| Boneless Wings | 3 pieces | 145 | 45 | 5 | 1 | 30 | 520 | 12 | 0 | 13 |
| Howie Wings | 5 pieces | 180 | 117 | 13 | 3.5 | 60 | 760 | 0 | 0 | 14 |

# IHOP
## APPETIZERS

| | SERVING SIZE | CAL | CAL FAT | TOT FAT (G) | SAT FAT (G) | CHOL (MG) | SOD (MG) | CARB (G) | FIBER (G) | PROT (G) |
|---|---|---|---|---|---|---|---|---|---|---|
| Chicken Fajita Quesadilla | 1 order | 1060 | 510 | 57 | 29 | 220 | 2410 | 70 | 5 | 69 |
| Crispy Chicken Strips & Fries | 1 order | 1230 | 600 | 67 | 12 | 85 | 1330 | 117 | 9 | 41 |
| Monster Mozzarella Sticks | 1 order | 770 | 340 | 38 | 16 | 70 | 2680 | 68 | 7 | 39 |
| Onion Rings | 1 order | 1250 | 620 | 69 | 12 | 0 | 1110 | 140 | 7 | 17 |
| Sampler | 1 order | 1780 | 890 | 99 | 23 | 115 | 3120 | 163 | 12 | 60 |
| Seasoned Fries | 1 order | 590 | 220 | 24 | 5 | 0 | 980 | 87 | 9 | 6 |
| Wings | 1 order | 680 | 390 | 44 | 11 | 265 | 1960 | 15 | <1 | 57 |

## BREAKFAST COMBOS

| | SERVING SIZE | CAL | CAL FAT | TOT FAT (G) | SAT FAT (G) | CHOL (MG) | SOD (MG) | CARB (G) | FIBER (G) | PROT (G) |
|---|---|---|---|---|---|---|---|---|---|---|
| Belgian Waffle Plain | 1 entrée | 360 | 140 | 15 | 8 | 95 | 520 | 47 | 2 | 8 |
| Big Country Breakfast | 1 entrée | 1790 | 970 | 110 | 46 | 785 | 3910 | 156 | 10 | 48 |
| Big Two-Egg Breakfast | 1 entrée | 880 | 450 | 50 | 15 | 490 | 1870 | 80 | 6 | 28 |
| Biscuits & Gravy Combo, Country Gravy | 1 entrée | 1420 | 860 | 95 | 34 | 485 | 3080 | 99 | 5 | 39 |
| Breakfast Sampler | 1 entrée | 1180 | 660 | 74 | 23 | 560 | 3160 | 82 | 6 | 49 |
| Chicken Fried Chicken & Egg, Country Gravy | 1 entrée | 1240 | 620 | 69 | 19 | 545 | 2950 | 105 | 9 | 57 |

# restaurants

| | SERVING SIZE | CAL | CAL FAT | TOT FAT (G) | SAT FAT (G) | CHOL (MG) | SOD (MG) | CARB (G) | FIBER (G) | PROT (G) |
|---|---|---|---|---|---|---|---|---|---|---|
| Chorizo & Eggs | 1 entrée | 1400 | 730 | 82 | 25 | 770 | 3160 | 111 | 8 | 55 |
| Classic Skillets | 1 entrée | 1460 | 870 | 97 | 37 | 565 | 2740 | 102 | 8 | 48 |
| Corned Beef Hash & Eggs | 1 entrée | 1110 | 550 | 61 | 23 | 770 | 2970 | 91 | 6 | 51 |
| Country Chicken Fried Steak & Eggs, Country Gravy | 1 entrée | 1570 | 780 | 87 | 26 | 555 | 3710 | 139 | 11 | 57 |
| Eggs Benedict | 1 entrée | 1020 | 510 | 57 | 22 | 530 | 3140 | 80 | 6 | 43 |
| Huevos Rancheros | 1 entrée | 1110 | 580 | 65 | 23 | 705 | 1810 | 83 | 11 | 50 |
| Sirloin Tip & Eggs | 1 entrée | 1350 | 680 | 76 | 22 | 580 | 3050 | 99 | 8 | 69 |
| Smokehouse Combo | 1 entrée | 1340 | 810 | 91 | 29 | 580 | 3180 | 84 | 6 | 47 |
| South of the Border Burrito | 1 entrée | 1380 | 660 | 74 | 29 | 550 | 3330 | 130 | 10 | 50 |
| Split Decision Breakfast | 1 entrée | 1170 | 660 | 75 | 28 | 705 | 2280 | 80 | 6 | 46 |
| T-bone Steak & Eggs | 1 entrée | 1250 | 610 | 68 | 26 | 850 | 2840 | 74 | 4 | 86 |
| Thick Cut Bone-In Ham & Eggs | 1 entrée | 1170 | 540 | 61 | 19 | 620 | 4310 | 88 | 6 | 70 |
| **CREPES & BLINTZES** | | | | | | | | | | |
| Bacon & Cheddar Crepes, Stuffed | 1 crepe | 1130 | 740 | 82 | 37 | 705 | 1500 | 43 | 2 | 54 |
| Cheese Blintzes | 1 blintz | 1000 | 620 | 69 | 30 | 335 | 1260 | 66 | 4 | 27 |
| Nutella Crepes | 1 crepe | 910 | 440 | 48 | 13 | 205 | 620 | 109 | 7 | 16 |
| Strawberry Banana Danish Fruit Crepes | 1 crepe | 1000 | 600 | 67 | 26 | 590 | 1150 | 68 | 4 | 35 |
| **FRENCH TOAST** | | | | | | | | | | |
| Cinnamon Swirl French Toast Combo | 1 entrée | 1210 | 670 | 75 | 25 | 540 | 1370 | 102 | 8 | 33 |
| CINN-A-STACK French Toast | 1 entrée | 1110 | 460 | 51 | 14 | 480 | 1190 | 109 | 6 | 29 |
| Create Your Own Viva La French Toast Combo | 1 entrée | 1170 | 640 | 71 | 20 | 760 | 1530 | 93 | 9 | 40 |
| Original French Toast | 1 entrée | 920 | 450 | 50 | 15 | 480 | 1100 | 88 | 8 | 31 |
| Strawberry Banana French Toast | 1 entrée | 1060 | 400 | 45 | 12 | 460 | 1050 | 135 | 11 | 32 |
| Stuffed French Toast, Combo | 1 entrée | 950 | 470 | 52 | 14 | 475 | 1150 | 92 | 5 | 28 |
| Stuffed French Toast, Full Order | 1 entrée | 900 | 350 | 39 | 17 | 90 | 740 | 120 | 4 | 18 |
| **HEARTY DINNER FAVORITES** | | | | | | | | | | |
| Chicken Fried Chicken, Country Gravy | 1 entrée | 690 | 290 | 33 | 11 | 75 | 2160 | 74 | 5 | 29 |
| Country Chicken Fried Steak, Country Gravy | 1 entrée | 830 | 340 | 38 | 14 | 80 | 2300 | 82 | 7 | 39 |
| Crispy Chicken Strips | 1 entrée | 1010 | 500 | 56 | 14 | 105 | 1680 | 89 | 9 | 40 |
| French Onion Pot Roast | 1 entrée | 790 | 340 | 39 | 15 | 130 | 2770 | 73 | 3 | 42 |
| Grilled Liver | 1 entrée | 810 | 340 | 39 | 13 | 575 | 1370 | 63 | 4 | 59 |
| Grilled Tilapia Hollandaise | 1 entrée | 810 | 410 | 46 | 13 | 120 | 1890 | 46 | 8 | 51 |
| Thick-cut Bone-In Ham Dinner | 1 entrée | 680 | 220 | 25 | 10 | 150 | 3580 | 73 | 4 | 48 |
| Mediterranean Lemon Chicken | 1 entrée | 780 | 370 | 41 | 13 | 180 | 1350 | 44 | 7 | 57 |
| Savory Pork Chops | 1 entrée | 620 | 210 | 23 | 6 | 100 | 890 | 41 | 7 | 61 |

| | SERVING SIZE | CAL | CAL FAT | TOT FAT (G) | SAT FAT (G) | CHOL (MG) | SOD (MG) | CARB (G) | FIBER (G) | PROT (G) |
|---|---|---|---|---|---|---|---|---|---|---|
| Simple & Fit, Grilled Balsamic-Glazed Chicken | 1 entrée | 440 | 200 | 22 | 4 | 90 | 940 | 25 | 8 | 39 |
| Simple & Fit, Grilled Tilapia | 1 entrée | 490 | 200 | 23 | 4 | 90 | 1270 | 27 | 8 | 49 |
| Sirloin Steak Tips Dinner | 1 entrée | 800 | 360 | 40 | 13 | 110 | 2250 | 69 | 4 | 46 |
| Smoked Sausage | 1 entrée | 830 | 570 | 64 | 22 | 110 | 2650 | 40 | 6 | 25 |
| Top Sirloin Steak | 1 entrée | 810 | 340 | 38 | 15 | 150 | 2100 | 48 | 9 | 66 |
| **OMELETS** | | | | | | | | | | |
| Avocado, Bacon, & Cheese | 1 omelet | 840 | 590 | 65 | 26 | 830 | 1080 | 17 | 5 | 49 |
| Bacon Temptation | 1 omelet | 980 | 680 | 75 | 30 | 880 | 1900 | 17 | 2 | 62 |
| Corned Beef Hash & Cheese | 1 omelet | 990 | 650 | 72 | 31 | 860 | 1860 | 30 | 4 | 57 |
| Country | 1 omelet | 1140 | 720 | 80 | 31 | 870 | 2060 | 50 | 6 | 58 |
| Create Your Own, Plain | 1 omelet | 440 | 290 | 32 | 9 | 755 | 500 | 10 | 2 | 28 |
| Create Your Own, Plain w/Egg Substitute | 1 omelet | 140 | 40 | 4 | 0 | 10 | 320 | 2 | 0 | 23 |
| Garden | 1 omelet | 840 | 600 | 66 | 26 | 815 | 890 | 18 | 4 | 45 |
| Spinach & Mushroom | 1 omelet | 910 | 640 | 71 | 26 | 815 | 1580 | 23 | 5 | 45 |
| **PANCAKES & COMBOS** | | | | | | | | | | |
| CINN-A-STACK | 4 pancakes | 890 | 200 | 23 | 8 | 70 | 1700 | 106 | 4 | 14 |
| Double Blueberry | 3 pancakes | 640 | 120 | 13 | 5 | 60 | 1630 | 117 | 9 | 14 |
| Original Buttermilk | 3 pancakes | 490 | 160 | 18 | 8 | 80 | 1610 | 69 | 4 | 13 |
| Pancake Platter | 1 entrée | 490 | 160 | 18 | 8 | 80 | 1610 | 69 | 4 | 13 |
| Pick-A-Pancake Combo, Double Blueberry | 1 entrée | 1020 | 410 | 45 | 12 | 470 | 1890 | 124 | 10 | 29 |
| Pick-A-Pancake, Original Buttermilk | 1 entrée | 880 | 450 | 50 | 15 | 490 | 1870 | 80 | 6 | 28 |
| Three Eggs & Pancakes w/Hash Browns | 1 entrée | 1130 | 550 | 62 | 18 | 725 | 2480 | 104 | 8 | 40 |
| Two x Two x Two | 1 entrée | 560 | 270 | 31 | 11 | 490 | 1280 | 49 | 3 | 25 |
| **SANDWICHES & BURGERS** | | | | | | | | | | |
| Bacon Cheeseburger w/Beef Patty | 1 burger | 820 | 480 | 54 | 27 | 170 | 1200 | 40 | 3 | 48 |
| Chicken Clubhouse Super Stacker | 1 burger | 1180 | 720 | 81 | 33 | 200 | 2690 | 55 | 4 | 53 |
| Double BLT | 1 sandwich | 660 | 400 | 45 | 10 | 60 | 1460 | 39 | 2 | 23 |
| Ham & Egg Melt | 1 sandwich | 1090 | 510 | 58 | 30 | 580 | 2390 | 78 | 3 | 64 |
| Monster Bacon 'N Beef Cheeseburger | 1 burger | 1160 | 700 | 85 | 42 | 275 | 1410 | 41 | 3 | 74 |
| Patty Melt | 1 sandwich | 940 | 590 | 67 | 31 | 175 | 1500 | 44 | 5 | 43 |
| Philly Cheese Steak Stacker | 1 sandwich | 820 | 380 | 43 | 18 | 130 | 2300 | 56 | 3 | 47 |
| Pot Roast Melt | 1 sandwich | 1050 | 490 | 55 | 30 | 175 | 2350 | 83 | 3 | 57 |
| Turkey & Bacon Club Sandwich | 1 sandwich | 720 | 350 | 39 | 10 | 95 | 2030 | 49 | 2 | 40 |
| Tuscan Chicken Griller | 1 sandwich | 900 | 500 | 56 | 19 | 140 | 2270 | 54 | 7 | 47 |
| **SIMPLE & FIT BREAKFAST** | | | | | | | | | | |
| Blueberry Harvest Grain'N Nut Combo | 1 entrée | 560 | 210 | 23 | 4 | 60 | 1040 | 64 | 8 | 25 |
| Seasonal Fresh Fruit Crepes | 1 entrée | 590 | 210 | 24 | 5 | 135 | 430 | 84 | 7 | 12 |

# restaurants

| | SERVING SIZE | CAL | CAL FAT | TOT FAT (G) | SAT FAT (G) | CHOL (MG) | SOD (MG) | CARB (G) | FIBER (G) | PROT (G) |
|---|---|---|---|---|---|---|---|---|---|---|
| Simply Chicken Sandwich w/Fresh Fruit | 1 sandwich | 470 | 80 | 9 | 3 | 95 | 980 | 59 | 5 | 42 |
| Spinach, Mushroom, & Tomato Omelet w/Fresh Fruit | 1 entrée | 330 | 110 | 12 | 5 | 25 | 690 | 30 | 5 | 28 |
| Turkey Bacon Omelet w/Fresh Fruit | 1 entrée | 420 | 190 | 21 | 10 | 75 | 730 | 24 | 2 | 36 |
| Two Egg Breakfast | 1 entrée | 350 | 70 | 8 | 2 | 30 | 710 | 48 | 7 | 25 |
| Two x Two x Two | 1 entrée | 400 | 110 | 12 | 3 | 70 | 1450 | 48 | 3 | 25 |
| Veggie Omelet w/Fresh Fruit | 1 entrée | 320 | 90 | 10 | 1 | 10 | 420 | 40 | 8 | 21 |
| Whole Wheat French Toast Combo | 1 entrée | 490 | 140 | 15 | 4 | 220 | 930 | 56 | 5 | 33 |
| **SOUPS, SALADS, & SIDES** | | | | | | | | | | |
| Chicken & Spinach Salad | 1 salad | 1600 | 1060 | 118 | 32 | 350 | 2340 | 72 | 7 | 63 |
| Chicken Fajita Salad | 1 salad | 870 | 470 | 52 | 22 | 160 | 1600 | 54 | 7 | 52 |
| Crispy Chicken Salad w/Fried Chicken | 1 salad | 1450 | 850 | 94 | 26 | 375 | 2110 | 93 | 10 | 63 |
| Grilled Chicken Caesar Salad | 1 salad | 960 | 650 | 72 | 15 | 130 | 2140 | 39 | 6 | 42 |
| House Salad | 1 salad | 90 | 25 | 3 | 0 | 0 | 170 | 15 | 3 | 3 |
| Loaded Potato & Bacon Soup | 1 soup | 430 | 260 | 29 | 17 | 85 | 1310 | 30 | 1 | 13 |
| Soup of the Day, Chicken Noodle Soup | as served | 170 | 45 | 5 | 2 | 35 | 1110 | 18 | 1 | 12 |
| Soup of the Day, New England Clam Chowder | as served | 460 | 300 | 34 | 19 | 115 | 1060 | 25 | 1 | 13 |
| **In-N-Out Burger** | | | | | | | | | | |
| Cheeseburger w/Onion | 1 burger | 480 | 240 | 27 | 10 | 60 | 1000 | 39 | 3 | 22 |
| Double-Double w/Onion | 1 burger | 670 | 370 | 41 | 18 | 120 | 1440 | 39 | 3 | 37 |
| French Fries | as served | 395 | 160 | 18 | 5 | 0 | 245 | 54 | 2 | 7 |
| Hamburger w/Onion | 1 burger | 390 | 170 | 19 | 5 | 40 | 650 | 27 | 3 | 16 |
| **Jack in the Box** **BURGERS, SANDWICHES, & MORE** | | | | | | | | | | |
| Bacon Ultimate Cheeseburger | 1 burger | 940 | 590 | 66 | 27 | 125 | 1840 | 45 | 2 | 41 |
| Big Cheeseburger | 1 burger | 610 | 340 | 38 | 15 | 65 | 1110 | 44 | 2 | 26 |
| Chicken Sandwich | 1 sandwich | 440 | 210 | 23 | 4 | 35 | 910 | 42 | 2 | 15 |
| Chicken Teriyaki Bowl | 1 bowl | 690 | 50 | 6 | 1 | 40 | 1700 | 133 | 5 | 27 |
| Crispy Chicken Strips | 4 pieces | 560 | 220 | 24 | 3 | 60 | 1580 | 53 | 3 | 33 |
| Fish Sandwich | as served | 470 | 160 | 18 | 2 | 25 | 1030 | 59 | 3 | 18 |
| Grilled Chicken Strips | 4 pieces | 240 | 50 | 6 | 1 | 115 | 1060 | 5 | 0 | 43 |
| Hamburger Deluxe | 1 burger | 360 | 170 | 19 | 6 | 40 | 580 | 33 | 2 | 15 |
| Jack's Spicy Chicken | 1 sandwich | 570 | 230 | 25 | 4 | 55 | 950 | 60 | 3 | 28 |
| Jumbo Jack | 1 burger | 540 | 290 | 32 | 11 | 45 | 850 | 45 | 2 | 16 |
| Junior Bacon Cheeseburger | 1 burger | 420 | 210 | 24 | 8 | 50 | 960 | 32 | 1 | 18 |
| Sirloin Cheeseburger | 1 burger | 900 | 540 | 60 | 19 | 140 | 1870 | 52 | 3 | 40 |

| | SERVING SIZE | CAL | CAL FAT | TOT FAT (G) | SAT FAT (G) | CHOL (MG) | SOD (MG) | CARB (G) | FIBER (G) | PROT (G) |
|---|---|---|---|---|---|---|---|---|---|---|
| Sirloin Swiss & Grilled Onion Burger | 1 burger | 880 | 530 | 59 | 18 | 140 | 1550 | 52 | 3 | 40 |
| Sourdough Grilled Chicken Club | 1 sandwich | 550 | 260 | 29 | 7 | 90 | 1490 | 38 | 3 | 37 |
| Sourdough Jack | 1 burger | 680 | 420 | 46 | 17 | 70 | 1220 | 40 | 3 | 27 |
| Sourdough Steak Melt | 1 burger | 650 | 340 | 38 | 13 | 95 | 1300 | 37 | 3 | 37 |
| Sourdough Ultimate Cheeseburger | 1 burger | 900 | 600 | 67 | 27 | 115 | 1430 | 38 | 3 | 37 |
| Steak Teriyaki Bowl | 1 bowl | 750 | 100 | 11 | 3 | 45 | 1450 | 133 | 5 | 31 |
| Turkey Bacon & Cheddar Grilled Sandwich | 1 sandwich | 650 | 270 | 30 | 11 | 95 | 2130 | 54 | 5 | 39 |
| Ultimate Cheeseburger | 1 burger | 870 | 550 | 61 | 26 | 115 | 1490 | 44 | 2 | 36 |
| **SALADS** | | | | | | | | | | |
| Chicken Club w/Crispy Chicken Strips | 1 salad | 510 | 240 | 27 | 8 | 65 | 700 | 34 | 5 | 23 |
| Grilled Chicken | 1 salad | 240 | 70 | 8 | 3.5 | 70 | 650 | 15 | 5 | 28 |
| Southwest Chicken w/Crispy Chicken Strips | 1 salad | 500 | 210 | 23 | 7 | 55 | 1260 | 53 | 8 | 29 |
| **SIDES** | | | | | | | | | | |
| Bacon Cheddar Potato Wedges | as served | 710 | 400 | 45 | 12 | 45 | 910 | 58 | 5 | 20 |
| Egg Roll | 1 piece | 150 | 70 | 7 | 1.5 | 5 | 320 | 15 | 2 | 5 |
| French Fries, Medium | as served | 410 | 170 | 19 | 1.5 | 0 | 750 | 56 | 4 | 5 |
| Mozzarella Cheese Sticks | 3 pieces | 280 | 150 | 16 | 6 | 25 | 590 | 22 | 2 | 12 |
| Onion Rings | as served | 450 | 250 | 28 | 2 | 0 | 620 | 45 | 3 | 6 |
| Seasoned Curly Fries, Medium | as served | 430 | 220 | 25 | 2 | 0 | 940 | 46 | 4 | 5 |
| Stuffed Jalapenos | 3 pieces | 220 | 110 | 12 | 4.5 | 15 | 730 | 21 | 1 | 6 |

## Jamba Juice
### FOOD

| | SERVING SIZE | CAL | CAL FAT | TOT FAT (G) | SAT FAT (G) | CHOL (MG) | SOD (MG) | CARB (G) | FIBER (G) | PROT (G) |
|---|---|---|---|---|---|---|---|---|---|---|
| Apple Cinnamon Pretzel | 1 pretzel | 380 | 36 | 4 | 0 | 0 | 250 | 76 | 4 | 11 |
| Cheddar Tomato Twist | 1 twist | 240 | 40.5 | 4.5 | 1.5 | 5 | 430 | 41 | 2 | 8 |
| Omega-3 Chocolate Brownie Cookie | 1 cookie | 150 | 31.5 | 3.5 | 1 | 0 | 15 | 30 | 2 | 3 |
| Omega-3 Oatmeal Cookie | 1 cookie | 150 | 54 | 6 | 1.5 | 5 | 85 | 26 | 3 | 2 |
| Orange Dark Chocolate Chip Scone | 1 scone | 380 | 135 | 15 | 3 | 55 | 65 | 57 | 2 | 6 |
| Plain Oatmeal w/Brown Sugar | as served | 220 | 31.5 | 3.5 | 1 | 0 | 20 | 44 | 5 | 9 |
| Sourdough Parmesan Pretzel | 1 pretzel | 410 | 90 | 10 | 2 | 5 | 640 | 67 | 3 | 14 |

### SMOOTHIES & JUICES

| | SERVING SIZE | CAL | CAL FAT | TOT FAT (G) | SAT FAT (G) | CHOL (MG) | SOD (MG) | CARB (G) | FIBER (G) | PROT (G) |
|---|---|---|---|---|---|---|---|---|---|---|
| Acai Super Antioxidant | 24 fl oz | 380 | 54 | 6 | 2 | 5 | 55 | 77 | 5 | 5 |
| Aloha Pineapple Power | 24 fl oz | 410 | 13.5 | 1.5 | .5 | 5 | 55 | 97 | 4 | 6 |
| Banana Berry | 24 fl oz | 400 | 13.5 | 1.5 | 0.5 | 5 | 90 | 94 | 4 | 4 |
| Berry Fulfilling | 24 fl oz | 230 | 9 | 1 | 0 | 5 | 240 | 51 | 6 | 7 |
| Blackberry Bliss | 24 fl oz | 340 | 13.5 | 1.5 | 0 | 0 | 35 | 82 | 6 | 2 |
| Caribbean Passion | 24 fl oz | 360 | 13.5 | 1.5 | 0.5 | 5 | 50 | 82 | 3 | 3 |
| Chill-icious Chai | 24 fl oz | 440 | 0 | 0 | 0 | 5 | 340 | 92 | 0 | 13 |

| | SERVING SIZE | CAL | CAL FAT | TOT FAT (G) | SAT FAT (G) | CHOL (MG) | SOD (MG) | CARB (G) | FIBER (G) | PROT (G) |
|---|---|---|---|---|---|---|---|---|---|---|
| Mango-a-go-go Original | 24 fl oz | 400 | 13.5 | 1.5 | 0.5 | 5 | 45 | 94 | 3 | 3 |
| Matcha Green Tea Blast Original | 24 fl oz | 420 | 0 | 0 | 0 | 0 | 230 | 90 | 1 | 10 |
| Mega Mango Original | 24 fl oz | 320 | 9 | 1 | 0 | 0 | 10 | 80 | 5 | 3 |
| Mocha Mojo Original | 24 fl oz | 510 | 13.5 | 1.5 | 1 | 5 | 330 | 107 | 1 | 13 |
| Peanut Butter Moo'd Original | 24 fl oz | 770 | 180 | 20 | 4.5 | 10 | 490 | 125 | 4 | 20 |
| Pomegranate Tea Infusion Original | 24 fl oz | 240 | 0 | 0 | 0 | 0 | 30 | 59 | 1 | 1 |
| Prickly Pear Tea Infusion Original | 24 fl oz | 230 | 0 | 0 | 0 | 0 | 30 | 56 | 2 | 1 |
| Protein Berry Workout Original | 24 fl oz | 370 | 4.5 | 0.5 | 0 | 5 | 150 | 72 | 4 | 20 |
| Pumpkin Smash Original | 24 fl oz | 550 | 4.5 | 0.5 | 0 | 5 | 460 | 118 | 2 | 14 |
| Razzmatazz Original | 24 fl oz | 390 | 13.5 | 1.5 | 1 | 5 | 55 | 91 | 4 | 3 |
| Strawberries Wild Original | 24 fl oz | 370 | 0 | 0 | 0 | 5 | 140 | 87 | 3 | 5 |
| Strawberry Surf Rider Original | 24 fl oz | 430 | 13.5 | 1.5 | 0.5 | 5 | 10 | 103 | 4 | 3 |
| Strawberry Whirl Original | 24 fl oz | 300 | 4.5 | 0.5 | 0 | 0 | 25 | 75 | 6 | 2 |
| Wheatgrass Shot | 1 fl oz | 5 | 0 | 0 | n/a | 0 | 0 | 1 | 0 | 1 |

## Johnny Rockets
### APPETIZERS

| | SERVING SIZE | CAL | CAL FAT | TOT FAT (G) | SAT FAT (G) | CHOL (MG) | SOD (MG) | CARB (G) | FIBER (G) | PROT (G) |
|---|---|---|---|---|---|---|---|---|---|---|
| American Fries | as served | 550 | 200 | 22 | 4 | n/a | 50 | 78 | n/a | n/a |
| Chilli Fries | as served | 1010 | 550 | 62 | 21 | n/a | 1020 | 85 | n/a | n/a |
| Mini Chili Dogs | 3 dogs | 1470 | 930 | 105 | 48 | n/a | 3600 | 78 | n/a | n/a |
| Mini Hot Dogs | 3 dogs | 690 | 330 | 36 | 14 | n/a | 2040 | 66 | n/a | n/a |
| Onion Rings | as served | 790 | 320 | 36 | 6 | n/a | 2010 | 80 | n/a | n/a |
| Rocket Wings | as served | 640 | 320 | 36 | 7 | n/a | 2600 | 26 | n/a | n/a |
| Sliders, Traditional | 3 sliders | 750 | 390 | 42 | 12 | n/a | 1170 | 63 | n/a | n/a |

### BURGERS & SANDWICHES

| | SERVING SIZE | CAL | CAL FAT | TOT FAT (G) | SAT FAT (G) | CHOL (MG) | SOD (MG) | CARB (G) | FIBER (G) | PROT (G) |
|---|---|---|---|---|---|---|---|---|---|---|
| #12 Hamburger | 1 burger | 900 | 530 | 59 | 18 | n/a | 1370 | 55 | n/a | n/a |
| Bacon Cheddar Single Hamburger | 1 burger | 860 | 480 | 53 | 18 | n/a | 1220 | 42 | n/a | n/a |
| Chicken Club Sandwich | 1 burger | 930 | 460 | 51 | 10 | n/a | 1860 | 58 | n/a | n/a |
| Original Hamburger | 1 burger | 820 | 480 | 53 | 14 | n/a | 1270 | 52 | n/a | n/a |
| Patty Melt Hamburger | 1 burger | 690 | 330 | 37 | 17 | n/a | 1090 | 49 | n/a | n/a |
| Rocket Single Hamburger | 1 burger | 710 | 390 | 44 | 15 | n/a | 770 | 45 | n/a | n/a |
| Tuna Melt | 1 sandwich | 900 | 390 | 62 | 17 | n/a | 1448 | 40 | n/a | n/a |
| Tuna Salad Sandwich | 1 sandwich | 800 | 450 | 50 | 8 | n/a | 1010 | 41 | n/a | n/a |

### SALADS

| | SERVING SIZE | CAL | CAL FAT | TOT FAT (G) | SAT FAT (G) | CHOL (MG) | SOD (MG) | CARB (G) | FIBER (G) | PROT (G) |
|---|---|---|---|---|---|---|---|---|---|---|
| Caesar Salad | 1 salad | 481 | 323 | 35 | 6 | n/a | 1052 | 15 | n/a | n/a |
| Chicken Club Salad (w/Chicken Tenders) | 1 salad | 620 | 340 | 37 | 15 | n/a | 1740 | 27 | n/a | n/a |
| Garden Salad | 1 salad | 240 | 130 | 14 | 8 | n/a | 360 | 12 | n/a | n/a |
| Grilled Chicken Caesar Salad | 1 salad | 343 | 290 | 31 | 5 | n/a | 687 | 13 | n/a | n/a |

## KFC

| | SERVING SIZE | CAL | CAL. FAT | TOT FAT (G) | SAT FAT (G) | CHOL (MG) | SOD (MG) | CARB (G) | FIBER (G) | PROT (G) |
|---|---|---|---|---|---|---|---|---|---|---|
| **CHICKEN** | | | | | | | | | | |
| Crispy Strips | 2 pieces | 230 | 70 | 7 | 2.5 | 50 | 850 | 18 | 2 | 22 |
| Extra Crispy—Thigh | 1 piece | 340 | 220 | 24 | 5 | 80 | 780 | 10 | 0 | 20 |
| Extra Crispy—Breast | 1 piece | 510 | 290 | 33 | 7 | 110 | 1010 | 16 | 0 | 39 |
| Extra Crispy—Drumstick | 1 piece | 150 | 90 | 10 | 2 | 55 | 360 | 5 | 0 | 12 |
| Extra Crispy—Whole Wing | 1 piece | 190 | 110 | 13 | 2.5 | 55 | 410 | 6 | 0 | 12 |
| Grilled—Breast | 1 piece | 210 | 70 | 8 | 2.5 | 105 | 460 | 0 | 0 | 34 |
| Grilled—Drumstick | 1 piece | 80 | 35 | 4 | 1 | 55 | 230 | 0 | 0 | 11 |
| Grilled—Thigh | 1 piece | 160 | 100 | 11 | 3 | 85 | 420 | 0 | 0 | 16 |
| Grilled—Whole Wing | 1 piece | 80 | 45 | 5 | 1.5 | 40 | 250 | 1 | 0 | 9 |
| Grilled Filet | 1 piece | 140 | 25 | 3 | 1 | 70 | 560 | 1 | 0 | 26 |
| Individual Sized Popcorn Chicken | as served | 400 | 230 | 26 | 4.5 | 60 | 1160 | 22 | 3 | 21 |
| Original Recipe—Breast | 1 piece | 320 | 130 | 15 | 3.5 | 110 | 710 | 4 | 0 | 12 |
| Original Recipe—Breast w/o skin or breading | 1 piece | 150 | 25 | 2.5 | .5 | 85 | 430 | 0 | 0 | 31 |
| Original Recipe—Drumstick | 1 piece | 120 | 60 | 7 | 1.5 | 50 | 340 | 3 | 0 | 12 |
| Original Recipe—Thigh | 1 piece | 220 | 130 | 15 | 4 | 80 | 620 | 5 | 0 | 18 |
| Original Recipe—Whole Wing | 1 piece | 140 | 70 | 8 | 2 | 50 | 390 | 4 | 0 | 12 |
| Original Recipe Filet | 1 piece | 170 | 60 | 7 | 1.5 | 55 | 360 | 4 | 1 | 23 |
| Wings—Fiery Buffalo | 1 wing | 80 | 45 | 5 | 1 | 20 | 230 | 4 | 1 | 4 |
| Wings—Fiery Grilled | 1 wing | 70 | 35 | 4 | 1 | 35 | 210 | 0 | 0 | 8 |
| Wings—Honey BBQ | 1 wing | 80 | 45 | 5 | 1 | 20 | 170 | 5 | 1 | 4 |
| **SANDWICHES & WRAPS** | | | | | | | | | | |
| Crispy Twister w/Crispy Strip w/o Sauce | 1 sandwich | 460 | 110 | 13 | 4.5 | 50 | 1480 | 58 | 4 | 29 |
| Grilled Filet Sandwich w/o Sauce | 1 sandwich | 290 | 40 | 4.5 | 1.5 | 70 | 720 | 32 | 2 | 32 |
| Grilled Twister w/o Sauce | 1 sandwich | 370 | 80 | 8 | 3 | 70 | 1180 | 41 | 2 | 33 |
| Honey BBQ Sandwich | 1 sandwich | 320 | 35 | 3.5 | 1 | 70 | 770 | 47 | 3 | 24 |
| Mini Melt | 1 sandwich | 250 | 60 | 7 | 3 | 45 | 690 | 31 | 2 | 15 |
| Original Recipe Filet Sandwich | 1 sandwich | 480 | 210 | 23 | 4 | 60 | 1160 | 42 | 3 | 26 |
| Snacker w/Crispy Strip | 1 sandwich | 290 | 100 | 11 | 2.5 | 30 | 730 | 33 | 3 | 15 |
| **SIDES** | | | | | | | | | | |
| Biscuit | as served | 180 | 70 | 8 | 6 | 0 | 530 | 23 | 1 | 4 |
| Cole Slaw | as served | 180 | 100 | 11 | 1.5 | 0 | 160 | 19 | 2 | 1 |
| Cornbread Muffin | as served | 210 | 80 | 9 | 1.5 | 35 | 240 | 28 | 1 | 3 |
| Macaroni & Cheese | as served | 180 | 80 | 9 | 3 | 5 | 880 | 20 | 2 | 6 |
| Mashed Potatoes w/o Gravy | as served | 90 | 25 | 3 | .5 | 0 | 320 | 15 | 1 | 2 |
| Potato Wedges | as served | 260 | 110 | 13 | 2.5 | 0 | 740 | 33 | 3 | 4 |

| | SERVING SIZE | CAL | CAL FAT | TOT FAT (G) | SAT FAT (G) | CHOL (MG) | SOD (MG) | CARB (G) | FIBER (G) | PROT (G) |
|---|---|---|---|---|---|---|---|---|---|---|
| **Krispy Kreme** | | | | | | | | | | |
| Chocolate Enrobed Doughnut Holes | 4 pieces | 270 | 150 | 17 | 8 | 15 | 210 | 27 | 2 | 3 |
| Chocolate Iced Glazed Cruller | 1 cruller | 280 | 130 | 15 | 3.5 | 15 | 240 | 35 | <1 | 2 |
| Chocolate Iced Glazed Doughnut | 1 doughnut | 250 | 110 | 12 | 3 | 5 | 100 | 33 | <1 | 3 |
| Chocolate Mini Cake | 1 cake | 270 | 160 | 17 | 9 | 10 | 240 | 26 | 3 | 3 |
| Cinnamon Bun | 1 bun | 260 | 140 | 16 | 4 | 5 | 125 | 28 | <1 | 3 |
| Cinnamon Twist | 1 twist | 230 | 90 | 9 | 2.5 | 5 | 85 | 33 | 1 | 3 |
| Glazed Doughnut | 1 doughnut | 200 | 110 | 12 | 3 | 5 | 95 | 22 | <1 | 2 |
| Glazed Cherry Filled Doughnut | 1 doughnut | 290 | 130 | 14 | 4 | n/a | 160 | 36 | 5 | 5 |
| Glazed Cruller | 1 cruller | 240 | 130 | 14 | 3.5 | 15 | 240 | 26 | <1 | 2 |
| Glazed Devil's Food Old Fashioned Cake | 1 doughnut | 340 | 160 | 18 | 4.5 | 20 | 310 | 42 | <1 | 3 |
| Glazed Doughnut Holes | 4 pieces | 220 | 120 | 13 | 3 | 10 | 170 | 25 | 1 | 2 |
| Glazed Mini Crullers | 3 pieces | 230 | 90 | 10 | 3 | 10 | 190 | 32 | 1 | 2 |
| Glazed Twist | 1 twist | 210 | 80 | 9 | 2.5 | 5 | 80 | 28 | <1 | 3 |
| Honey Bun | 1 bun | 410 | 220 | 24 | 6 | 10 | 170 | 44 | 1 | 5 |
| Old Fashioned Sour Cream Cake Doughnut | 1 doughnut | 280 | 100 | 11 | 2.5 | 20 | 210 | 41 | 0 | 3 |
| Plain Mini Cake | 1 cake | 250 | 130 | 14 | 4 | 15 | 370 | 27 | 1 | 4 |
| Powdered Sugar Cake Doughnut | 1 doughnut | 260 | 120 | 13 | 3 | 20 | 320 | 33 | <1 | 3 |
| Powdered Sugar Doughnut Holes | 4 pieces | 220 | 120 | 13 | 4 | 10 | 170 | 23 | 2 | 2 |
| Powdered Sugar Mini Cake | 1 cake | 210 | 90 | 10 | 2.5 | n/a | 230 | 26 | <1 | 2 |
| Sugar Doughnut | 1 doughnut | 200 | 110 | 12 | 3 | 5 | 95 | 21 | 0 | 2 |
| Traditional Cake Doughnut | 1 doughnut | 220 | 120 | 13 | 3 | 20 | 320 | 25 | <1 | 3 |
| Traditional Cake-Chocolate Iced Doughnut | 1 doughnut | 270 | 120 | 13 | 3 | 20 | 320 | 36 | <1 | 3 |
| **Krystal** | | | | | | | | | | |
| **BREAKFAST** | | | | | | | | | | |
| Bacon Breakfast Toast Sandwich | 1 sandwich | 330 | 150 | 16 | 7 | 210 | 960 | 26 | 1 | 15 |
| Bacon Egg & Cheese Biscuit | 1 sandwich | 440 | 220 | 24 | 9 | 210 | 1460 | 34 | 0 | 15 |
| Big Stack Breakfast Plate | 1 entrée | 780 | 460 | 51 | 17 | 445 | 1240 | 45 | 1 | 27 |
| Chik Biscuit | 1 sandwich | 400 | 160 | 18 | 6 | 25 | 1240 | 43 | 1 | 15 |
| Express Breakfast Plate | 1 entrée | 550 | 260 | 29 | 9 | 385 | 980 | 51 | 2 | 22 |
| Original Scrambler | 1 scrambler | 420 | 240 | 26 | 10 | 280 | 1270 | 27 | 1 | 17 |
| Pancake Scrambler | 1 scrambler | 380 | 220 | 25 | 8 | 275 | 530 | 23 | 1 | 15 |
| Sausage Gravy Scrambler | 1 scrambler | 630 | 370 | 41 | 13 | 275 | 1650 | 46 | 0 | 17 |
| Sunrise | 1 sandwich | 200 | 100 | 11 | 4 | 115 | 620 | 16 | 1 | 11 |
| **BURGERS** | | | | | | | | | | |
| Double Big Angus Bacon Cheeseburger | 1 burger | 850 | 530 | 59 | 22 | 120 | 1580 | 48 | 3 | 32 |
| Krystal Cheeseburger | 1 burger | 160 | 70 | 8 | 4 | 20 | 470 | 20 | 1 | 7 |

| | SERVING SIZE | CAL | CAL FAT | TOT FAT (G) | SAT FAT (G) | CHOL (MG) | SOD (MG) | CARB (G) | FIBER (G) | PROT (G) |
|---|---|---|---|---|---|---|---|---|---|---|
| Krystal Double Burger | 1 burger | 350 | 150 | 17 | 8 | 45 | 860 | 34 | 2 | 15 |
| Krystal Famous Burger | 1 burger | 130 | 50 | 6 | 2.5 | 15 | 330 | 20 | 1 | 6 |
| Original Big Angus Burger | 1 burger | 550 | 320 | 35 | 10 | 50 | 770 | 46 | 3 | 17 |
| **CHIKS & CHIK'N** | | | | | | | | | | |
| Chik | 1 sandwich | 300 | 140 | 16 | 4 | 35 | 800 | 27 | 2 | 14 |
| Chik Club | 1 sandwich | 320 | 140 | 16 | 6 | 40 | 970 | 29 | 2 | 16 |
| **PUPS** | | | | | | | | | | |
| Chili | 1 hot dog | 170 | 90 | 10 | 4 | 20 | 470 | 16 | 1 | 7 |
| Plain | 1 hot dog | 150 | 80 | 8 | 3.5 | 20 | 450 | 15 | 1 | 6 |
| **SIDES** | | | | | | | | | | |
| Chili Cheese Fries | as served | 570 | 270 | 29 | 15 | 55 | 340 | 62 | 7 | 15 |
| Kryspers | as served | 150 | 60 | 7 | 3.5 | 5 | 270 | 19 | 2 | 1 |
| Small Fries | as served | 180 | 70 | 7 | 3.5 | 5 | 40 | 27 | 3 | 2 |

## LaRosa's Pizzeria

| **APPETIZERS** | | | | | | | | | | |
|---|---|---|---|---|---|---|---|---|---|---|
| Antipasto for One | 1 salad | 317 | n/a | 21 | 10 | 68 | 1285 | 12 | 3 | 19 |
| Baked Onion Soup | as served | 304 | n/a | 16 | 5 | 17 | 3252 | 28 | .5 | 13 |
| Barbecue Wings | 1 wing | 105 | n/a | 6 | 2 | 47 | 358 | 4 | <1 | 9 |
| Boneless Wings—BBQ | 1 wing | 75 | n/a | 3 | 1 | 7 | 312 | 8 | <1 | 4 |
| Breadsticks | 5 sticks | 998 | n/a | 13 | 3 | 0 | 2826 | 190 | 5 | 35 |
| Cheesy Flatbread | 1/4 item | 354 | n/a | 22 | 8 | 24 | 675 | 26 | 1 | 13 |
| Chicken Tenders | as served | 541 | n/a | 31 | 6 | 75 | 1000 | 30 | 0 | 35 |
| Four Taste Sampler | as served | 1569 | n/a | 99 | 26 | 323 | 3975 | 82 | 3 | 83 |
| French Fry Basket | as served | 533 | n/a | 32 | 6 | 0 | 933 | 70 | 7 | 7 |
| Grilled Chicken Salad | 1 salad | 296 | n/a | 12 | 4 | 100 | 1177 | 11 | 3 | 35 |
| Mozzarella Cheese Sticks | as served | 636 | n/a | 43 | 17 | 60 | 1320 | 36 | 0 | 18 |
| Onion Twists—Regular | as served | 462 | n/a | 27 | 5 | 0 | 415 | 48 | 2 | 7 |
| **CALZONES** | | | | | | | | | | |
| 3 Meat & 3 Cheese | 1 calzone | 1080 | n/a | 55 | 24 | 120 | 2330 | 102 | 5 | 46 |
| Cheese & Pepperoni | 1 calzone | 960 | n/a | 45 | 21 | 100 | 1970 | 101 | 5 | 39 |
| **HOAGY** | | | | | | | | | | |
| Meatball | 1 sandwich | 689 | n/a | 26 | 9 | 113 | 1839 | 77 | 4 | 36 |
| Original Steak | 1 sandwich | 727 | n/a | 35 | 15 | 85 | 1015 | 65 | 3 | 39 |
| Turkey | 1 sandwich | 418 | n/a | 2 | 1 | 40 | 1586 | 66 | 3 | 15 |
| **PASTA ENTRÉES** | | | | | | | | | | |
| Lasagna w/Meat Sauce | 1 entrée | 735 | n/a | 38 | 18 | 128 | 2301 | 61 | 7 | 40 |
| Meat Ravioli | 1 entrée | 621 | n/a | 22 | 6 | 110 | 1276 | 102 | 8 | 30 |

| | SERVING SIZE | CAL | CAL FAT | TOT FAT (G) | SAT FAT (G) | CHOL (MG) | SOD (MG) | CARB (G) | FIBER (G) | PROT (G) |
|---|---|---|---|---|---|---|---|---|---|---|
| Spaghetti & Meatballs | 1 entrée | 870 | n/a | 28 | 7 | 85 | 1988 | 119 | 11 | 35 |
| Spaghetti or Ziti w/Alfredo Sauce | 1 entrée | 976 | n/a | 50 | 28 | 129 | 1546 | 104 | 4 | 24 |
| **PIZZA, MEDIUM** | | | | | | | | | | |
| Traditional Crust Double Pepperoni | 1 slice | 280 | n/a | 16 | 8 | 40 | 500 | 20 | 1 | 13 |
| Traditional Crust Cheese | 1 slice | 200 | n/a | 10 | 5 | 20 | 300 | 19 | 1 | 9 |
| Traditional Crust Big 4 Veggie | 1 slice | 198 | n/a | 8 | 4 | 18 | 344 | 21 | 2 | 10 |
| Hand Tossed Double Pepperoni | 1 slice | 298 | n/a | 14 | 6 | 34 | 764 | 29 | 1 | 14 |
| Hand Tossed Big 4 Veggie | 1 slice | 238 | n/a | 7 | 4 | 18 | 521 | 30 | 2 | 12 |
| Pan Crust Double Pepperoni | 1 slice | 370 | n/a | 22 | 9 | 40 | 620 | 30 | 1 | 14 |
| Pan Crust Cheese | 1 slice | 300 | n/a | 16 | 6 | 20 | 420 | 30 | 1 | 10 |
| Pan Crust Big 4 Veggie | 1 slice | 235 | n/a | 7 | 3 | 18 | 644 | 30 | 2 | 11 |

## Little Caesars
### PIZZA

| | SERVING SIZE | CAL | CAL FAT | TOT FAT (G) | SAT FAT (G) | CHOL (MG) | SOD (MG) | CARB (G) | FIBER (G) | PROT (G) |
|---|---|---|---|---|---|---|---|---|---|---|
| 3 Meat Treat Pizza | 1 slice | 340 | 150 | 17 | 7 | 35 | 730 | 32 | 2 | 16 |
| 14" Round Hot-N-Ready Pizza, Just Cheese | 1 slice | 250 | 80 | 9 | 4 | 20 | 440 | 32 | 1 | 12 |
| 14" Round Hot-N-Ready Pizza, Pepperoni | 1 slice | 280 | 100 | 11 | 5 | 25 | 560 | 32 | 2 | 14 |
| Deep Dish Pizza, Pepperoni | 1 slice | 360 | 140 | 16 | 6 | 25 | 640 | 38 | 2 | 16 |
| Deep Dish Pizza, Just Cheese | 1 slice | 320 | 120 | 13 | 5 | 20 | 510 | 38 | 2 | 14 |
| Baby Pan!Pan! Pizza, Cheese & Pepperoni | 1 pizza | 360 | 130 | 18 | 7 | 35 | 520 | 33 | 2 | 15 |
| Baby Pan!Pan! Pizza, Just Cheese | 1 pizza | 320 | 140 | 15 | 6 | 25 | 500 | 33 | 1 | 14 |
| Ultimate Supreme Pizza | 1 slice | 310 | 120 | 13 | 6 | 25 | 640 | 33 | 2 | 15 |
| Vegetarian Pizza | 1 slice | 270 | 90 | 10 | 4.5 | 20 | 530 | 32 | 2 | 13 |
| **SIDES** | | | | | | | | | | |
| Crazy Bread | 1 stick | 100 | 25 | 3 | .5 | 0 | 150 | 15 | 1 | 3 |
| Italian Cheese Bread | 1 slice | 130 | 60 | 6 | 2.5 | 10 | 240 | 13 | 1 | 6 |
| Pepperoni Cheese Bread | 1 slice | 150 | 70 | 8 | 3 | 15 | 280 | 13 | 1 | 7 |
| Wings, Barbecue | 1 wing | 70 | 35 | 4 | 1 | 20 | 220 | 3 | 0 | 4 |
| Wings, Hot | 1 wing | 50 | 35 | 4 | 1 | 20 | 350 | 0 | 0 | 4 |
| Wings, Mild | 1 wing | 50 | 35 | 4 | 1 | 20 | 250 | 0 | 0 | 4 |
| Wings, Oven Roasted | 1 wing | 50 | 35 | 3.5 | 1 | 20 | 150 | 0 | 0 | 4 |

## Long John Silver's
### FISH & SEAFOOD

| | SERVING SIZE | CAL | CAL FAT | TOT FAT (G) | SAT FAT (G) | CHOL (MG) | SOD (MG) | CARB (G) | FIBER (G) | PROT (G) |
|---|---|---|---|---|---|---|---|---|---|---|
| Battered Fish | 1 piece | 260 | 140 | 16 | 4 | 35 | 790 | 17 | 0 | 12 |
| Battered Shrimp | 3 pieces | 130 | 80 | 9 | 2.5 | 45 | 480 | 8 | 0 | 5 |
| Crispy Breaded Whitefish | 1 piece | 190 | 90 | 10 | 2.5 | 20 | 540 | 17 | 1 | 9 |
| Grilled Pacific Salmon | 2 pieces | 150 | 45 | 5 | 1 | 50 | 440 | 2 | 0 | 24 |

| | SERVING SIZE | CAL | CAL FAT | TOT FAT (G) | SAT FAT (G) | CHOL (MG) | SOD (MG) | CARB (G) | FIBER (G) | PROT (G) |
|---|---|---|---|---|---|---|---|---|---|---|
| Grilled Tilapia | 1 piece | 110 | 20 | 2.5 | 1 | 55 | 250 | 1 | 0 | 22 |
| Langostino Lobster Stuffed Crab Cakes | 1 piece | 170 | 80 | 9 | 2 | 30 | 390 | 16 | 1 | 6 |
| Shrimp Scampi | 8 pieces | 200 | 120 | 13 | 2.5 | 135 | 650 | 3 | 0 | 17 |
| **SANDWICHES & PLANKS** | | | | | | | | | | |
| Chicken Plank | 1 piece | 140 | 70 | 8 | 2 | 20 | 480 | 9 | 0 | 8 |
| Chicken Sandwich | 1 sandwich | 440 | 270 | 30 | 6 | 50 | 1350 | 47 | 4 | 22 |
| Fish Sandwich | 1 sandwich | 470 | 210 | 23 | 5 | 40 | 1180 | 49 | 3 | 18 |
| Ultimate Fish Sandwich | 1 sandwich | 530 | 240 | 27 | 8 | 55 | 1500 | 50 | 3 | 21 |
| **SIDES** | | | | | | | | | | |
| Breaded Mozzarella Sticks | 3 pieces | 150 | 80 | 9 | 3.5 | 10 | 350 | 13 | 1 | 5 |
| Breadstick | 1 stick | 170 | 30 | 3.5 | 1 | 0 | 290 | 29 | 1 | 6 |
| Broccoli Cheese Bites | 5 pieces | 230 | 110 | 12 | 4.5 | 15 | 550 | 25 | 2 | 5 |
| Fries | 3 oz | 230 | 90 | 10 | 2.5 | 0 | 350 | 33 | 3 | 3 |
| Hushpuppy | 1 piece | 60 | 20 | 2.5 | .5 | 0 | 200 | 9 | 1 | 1 |
| Jalapeño Cheddar Bites | 5 pieces | 240 | 120 | 14 | 5 | 15 | 730 | 23 | 2 | 6 |
| Jalapeño Peppers | 1 whole | 15 | 0 | 0 | 0 | 0 | 190 | 2 | 0 | 1 |
| Rice | 5 oz | 180 | 10 | 1 | .5 | 0 | 470 | 37 | 2 | 4 |
| Vegetable Medley | 4 oz | 50 | 15 | 2 | .5 | 0 | 360 | 8 | 3 | 1 |
| **Manchu Wok** | | | | | | | | | | |
| BBQ Pork | 1 entrée | 240 | 100 | 11 | 2.5 | 70 | 730 | 16 | 0 | 22 |
| Beef & Broccoli | 1 entrée | 180 | 120 | 13 | 2.5 | 20 | 710 | 12 | 2 | 7 |
| Chicken w/Snow Peas | 1 entrée | 140 | 80 | 9 | 1.5 | 20 | 710 | 11 | 2 | 7 |
| General Tso's Chicken | 1 entrée | 360 | 190 | 21 | 3.5 | 50 | 880 | 31 | 1 | 14 |
| Mixed Vegetables | 1 entrée | 130 | 90 | 10 | 1.5 | 0 | 510 | 11 | 3 | 2 |
| Orange Chicken | 1 entrée | 400 | 190 | 21 | 3.5 | 55 | 700 | 42 | 1 | 15 |
| Seafood Rangoon | 1 entrée | 300 | 190 | 21 | 7 | 35 | 240 | 20 | 1 | 4 |
| Sesame Chicken | 1 entrée | 370 | 130 | 14 | 3 | 55 | 940 | 46 | 0 | 15 |
| Spicy Beef | 1 entrée | 180 | 130 | 14 | 3 | 10 | 560 | 10 | 1 | 7 |
| Spicy Chicken | 1 entrée | 150 | 80 | 9 | 1.5 | 25 | 640 | 10 | 1 | 8 |
| Sweet & Sour Pork | 1 entrée | 360 | 170 | 19 | 3.5 | 35 | 470 | 37 | 0 | 14 |
| Sweet & Sour Chicken Tenders | 1 entrée | 340 | 160 | 18 | 3 | 100 | 170 | 17 | 0 | 28 |
| Vegetable Egg Roll | 1 entrée | 150 | 50 | 6 | 1 | 5 | 380 | 20 | 1 | 4 |
| **Maui Tacos** | | | | | | | | | | |
| **BOWLS & SALADS** | | | | | | | | | | |
| Bowl, Steak Napili | 1 bowl | 550 | 171 | 19 | 6 | 60 | 1360 | 56 | 10 | 39 |
| Bowl, Vegetarian | 1 bowl | 390 | 72 | 8 | 1 | 0 | 1655 | 64 | 16 | 16 |
| Salad, Taco (Beef) | 1 bowl | 1130 | 612 | 68 | 27 | 145 | 1930 | 80 | 15 | 51 |

# restaurants

| | SERVING SIZE | CAL | CAL FAT | TOT FAT (G) | SAT FAT (G) | CHOL (MG) | SOD (MG) | CARB (G) | FIBER (G) | PROT (G) |
|---|---|---|---|---|---|---|---|---|---|---|
| **BURRITOS & MAUI TACOS** | | | | | | | | | | |
| Chicken Maui Taco | 1 taco | 525 | 225 | 25 | 11.5 | 90 | 750 | 45 | 9 | 31 |
| Fish Maui Taco | 1 taco | 620 | 369 | 41 | 6.5 | 55 | 695 | 46 | 10 | 19 |
| Lahaina (Chicken) | 1 burrito | 780 | 306 | 34 | 11 | 100 | 1960 | 79 | 6 | 37 |
| Lahaina (Steak) | 1 burrito | 840 | 342 | 38 | 13 | 110 | 1970 | 79 | 6 | 42 |
| Vegetarian Maui Taco | 1 taco | 400 | 171 | 19 | 10 | 50 | 1070 | 36 | 7 | 20 |
| **ENCHILADAS & QUESADILLAS** | | | | | | | | | | |
| Chicken Enchilada | 1 item | 320 | 153 | 17 | 7 | 60 | 530 | 23 | 1 | 19 |
| Chicken Quesadilla | 1 item | 870 | 486 | 54 | 26 | 155 | 1620 | 53 | 5 | 42 |
| **Max & Erma's** | | | | | | | | | | |
| **ENTRÉES** | | | | | | | | | | |
| Black Bean Roll-Ups | 1 roll up | 577 | 90 | 10 | 2.4 | 14 | 1203 | 95.3 | 10.2 | 28.5 |
| Black Bean Veggie Burger | 1 burger | 649 | 252 | 28 | 4.3 | 20 | 1495 | 79.1 | 9.3 | 32.7 |
| Caribbean Chicken, Lunch Portion | 1 entrée | 536 | 180 | 20 | 8.3 | 97 | 1151 | 59.4 | 2.9 | 28.2 |
| **SALADS** | | | | | | | | | | |
| Baby Greens | 1 salad | 119 | 99 | 11 | 1.1 | 0 | 259 | 6.1 | 2 | 1.2 |
| Hula Bowl w/Fat-Free Honey Mustard | 1 salad | 583 | 86.4 | 9.6 | 1.5 | 112 | 1345 | 78 | 5.5 | 47.6 |
| **Mazzio's** | | | | | | | | | | |
| **DIPPIN' ZONE** | | | | | | | | | | |
| Breadsticks w/o Sauce | as served | 150 | 27 | 3 | 0.7 | 0.6 | 353 | 26 | 1 | 5 |
| Cheese Dippers w/o Sauce | as served | 405 | 153 | 18 | 5 | 20 | 639 | 47 | 2 | 13 |
| Garlic Toast w/o Sauce | as served | 160 | 90 | 10 | 2 | n/a | 280 | 15 | 1 | 3 |
| Mozzarella Sticks w/o Sauce | as served | 181 | 108 | 12 | 5 | 11 | 369 | 10 | n/a | 9 |
| **HOT SANDWICHES** | | | | | | | | | | |
| Chicken Bacon & Swiss on a Hoagie | 1 sandwich | 1362 | 648 | 72 | 19 | 147 | 2391 | 120 | 6 | 60 |
| Ham & Cheddar on a Hoagie | 1 sandwich | 1088 | 441 | 50 | 14 | 95 | 3260 | 119 | 5 | 49 |
| Sub on Focaccia | 1 sandwich | 768 | 441 | 49 | 15 | 100 | 2790 | 45 | 1 | 37 |
| Sub on a Hoagie | 1 sandwich | 1109 | 468 | 52 | 16 | 100 | 3290 | 117 | 5 | 49 |
| Turkey & Swiss on a Hoagie | 1 sandwich | 1059 | 360 | 40 | 12 | 106 | 2750 | 118 | 5 | 53 |
| Tuscan Smash on a Hoagie | 1 sandwich | 986 | 324 | 36 | 9 | 90 | 2723 | 117 | 5 | 46 |
| **PIZZA, MEDIUM** | | | | | | | | | | |
| Average Deep Pan Pricebuster | 1 slice | 365 | 162 | 18 | 5 | 27 | 760 | 38 | 2 | 12 |
| Average Deep Pan Specialty | 1 slice | 380 | 171 | 19 | 9 | 31 | 865 | 39 | 2 | 14 |
| Average French Bread | 1 pizza | 515 | 180 | 20 | 8 | 31 | 1640 | 60 | 3 | 24 |
| Average Original Crust One Topping | 1 slice | 250 | 85.5 | 9.5 | 4 | 75 | 607 | 25 | 2 | 11 |
| Average Original Crust Specialty | 1 slice | 280 | 108 | 12 | 5 | 30 | 700 | 31 | 2 | 12 |

| | SERVING SIZE | CAL | CAL FAT | TOT FAT (G) | SAT FAT (G) | CHOL (MG) | SOD (MG) | CARB (G) | FIBER (G) | PROT (G) |
|---|---|---|---|---|---|---|---|---|---|---|
| Average Price Buster | 1 slice | 210 | 99 | 11 | 4 | 26 | 585 | 18 | 1 | 10 |
| Average Specialty | 1 slice | 230 | 117 | 13 | 5 | 30 | 690 | 19 | 1.5 | 11 |
| Average Thin Crust One Topping | 1 slice | 179 | 72 | 8 | 3 | 25 | 572 | 18 | 1 | 10 |
| **SIGNATURE PASTAS** | | | | | | | | | | |
| Fettuccine Alfredo | 1 entrée | 1061 | 504 | 56 | 33 | 187 | 1055 | 107 | 4 | 33 |
| Greek Pasta | 1 entrée | 1456 | 846 | 94 | 19 | 51 | 2582 | 107 | 6 | 41 |
| Lasagna w/Marinara | 1 entrée | 704 | 270 | 30 | 13 | 185 | 3426 | 73 | 8 | 38 |
| Spaghetti w/Marinara | 1 entrée | 641 | 72 | 8 | 2 | 4 | 1689 | 120 | 8 | 22 |

## McDonald's
### BREAKFAST

| | SERVING SIZE | CAL | CAL FAT | TOT FAT (G) | SAT FAT (G) | CHOL (MG) | SOD (MG) | CARB (G) | FIBER (G) | PROT (G) |
|---|---|---|---|---|---|---|---|---|---|---|
| Bacon Egg & Cheese Biscuit, Regular | 1 sandwich | 420 | 210 | 23 | 12 | 235 | 1160 | 37 | 2 | 15 |
| Bacon Egg & Cheese McGriddle | 1 sandwich | 420 | 160 | 18 | 8 | 240 | 1110 | 48 | 2 | 15 |
| Big Breakfast w/Hotcakes Regular | 1 entrée | 1090 | 510 | 56 | 19 | 575 | 2150 | 111 | 6 | 36 |
| Biscuit Regular | 1 biscuit | 260 | 110 | 12 | 7 | 0 | 740 | 33 | 2 | 5 |
| Egg McMuffin | 1 sandwich | 300 | 110 | 12 | 5 | 260 | 820 | 30 | 2 | 18 |
| Fruit 'n Yogurt Parfait | 1 parfait | 160 | 20 | 2 | 1 | 5 | 85 | 31 | 1 | 4 |
| Hash Brown | 1 item | 150 | 80 | 9 | 1.5 | 0 | 310 | 15 | 2 | 1 |
| Hotcakes (w/o Syrup & Margarine) | 1 entrée | 350 | 80 | 9 | 2 | 20 | 590 | 60 | 3 | 8 |
| McSkillet Burrito w/Sausage | 1 burrito | 610 | 320 | 36 | 14 | 410 | 1390 | 44 | 3 | 27 |
| Sausage Biscuit Regular | 1 entrée | 430 | 240 | 27 | 12 | 30 | 1080 | 34 | 2 | 11 |
| Sausage Burrito | 1 burrito | 300 | 140 | 16 | 7 | 115 | 830 | 26 | 1 | 12 |
| Sausage Egg & Cheese McGriddles | 1 sandwich | 560 | 290 | 32 | 12 | 265 | 1360 | 48 | 2 | 20 |
| Sausage McGriddles | 1 sandwich | 420 | 200 | 22 | 8 | 35 | 1030 | 44 | 2 | 11 |
| Sausage McMuffin | 1 sandwich | 370 | 200 | 22 | 8 | 45 | 850 | 29 | 2 | 14 |
| Southern Style Chicken Biscuit Regular | 1 biscuit | 410 | 180 | 20 | 8 | 30 | 1180 | 41 | 2 | 17 |
| **BURGERS & SANDWICHES** | | | | | | | | | | |
| Angus Bacon & Cheese | 1 burger | 790 | 350 | 39 | 17 | 145 | 2070 | 63 | 4 | 45 |
| Angus Bacon & Cheese Snack Wrap | 1 burger | 390 | 190 | 21 | 9 | 75 | 1080 | 28 | 1 | 21 |
| Angus Deluxe | 1 burger | 750 | 350 | 39 | 16 | 135 | 1700 | 61 | 4 | 40 |
| Angus Deluxe Snack Wrap | 1 burger | 410 | 220 | 25 | 10 | 75 | 990 | 27 | 2 | 20 |
| Angus Mushroom & Swiss | 1 burger | 770 | 360 | 40 | 17 | 135 | 1170 | 59 | 4 | 44 |
| Angus Mushroom & Swiss Snack Wrap | 1 burger | 430 | 230 | 26 | 10 | 75 | 730 | 27 | 2 | 22 |
| Big Mac | 1 burger | 540 | 260 | 29 | 10 | 75 | 1040 | 45 | 3 | 25 |
| Big N' Tasty | 1 burger | 460 | 220 | 24 | 8 | 70 | 720 | 37 | 3 | 24 |
| Cheeseburger | 1 burger | 300 | 110 | 12 | 6 | 40 | 750 | 33 | 2 | 15 |
| Chipotle BBQ Snack Wrap, Crispy | 1 wrap | 330 | 140 | 15 | 4.5 | 30 | 810 | 35 | 1 | 14 |
| Double Cheeseburger | 1 burger | 440 | 210 | 23 | 11 | 80 | 1150 | 34 | 2 | 25 |

# restaurants

| | SERVING SIZE | CAL | CAL FAT | TOT FAT (G) | SAT FAT (G) | CHOL (MG) | SOD (MG) | CARB (G) | FIBER (G) | PROT (G) |
|---|---|---|---|---|---|---|---|---|---|---|
| Filet-O-Fish | 1 sandwich | 380 | 170 | 18 | 3.5 | 40 | 640 | 38 | 2 | 15 |
| Hamburger | 1 burger | 250 | 80 | 9 | 3.5 | 25 | 520 | 31 | 2 | 12 |
| Honey Mustard Snack Wrap, Crispy | 1 wrap | 330 | 140 | 16 | 4.5 | 30 | 780 | 34 | 1 | 14 |
| Mac Snack Wrap | 1 sandwich | 330 | 170 | 19 | 7 | 45 | 690 | 26 | 1 | 15 |
| McChicken | 1 sandwich | 360 | 150 | 16 | 3 | 35 | 830 | 40 | 2 | 14 |
| McDouble | 1 sandwich | 390 | 170 | 19 | 8 | 65 | 920 | 33 | 2 | 22 |
| McRib | 1 sandwich | 500 | 240 | 26 | 10 | 70 | 980 | 44 | 3 | 22 |
| Premium Crispy Chicken Classic | 1 sandwich | 530 | 180 | 20 | 3.5 | 50 | 1150 | 59 | 3 | 28 |
| Premium Crispy Chicken Club | 1 sandwich | 630 | 250 | 28 | 7 | 75 | 1360 | 60 | 4 | 35 |
| Premium Crispy Chicken Ranch BLT | 1 sandwich | 580 | 200 | 23 | 4.5 | 65 | 1400 | 62 | 3 | 31 |
| Quarter Pounder | 1 burger | 410 | 170 | 19 | 7 | 65 | 730 | 37 | 2 | 24 |
| Ranch Snack Wrap, Crispy | 1 wrap | 340 | 150 | 17 | 4.5 | 30 | 810 | 33 | 1 | 14 |
| Ranch Snack Wrap, Grilled | 1 wrap | 270 | 90 | 10 | 4 | 45 | 830 | 26 | 1 | 18 |
| Southern Style Crispy Chicken | 1 sandwich | 400 | 150 | 17 | 3 | 45 | 1030 | 39 | 1 | 24 |
| **CHICKEN** | | | | | | | | | | |
| McNugget 4 pc | 4 nuggets | 190 | 100 | 12 | 2 | 30 | 400 | 11 | 0 | 10 |
| Selects Premium Breast Strips, 3 pc | 3 strips | 400 | 210 | 24 | 3.5 | 50 | 1010 | 23 | 0 | 23 |
| **FRENCH FRIES** | | | | | | | | | | |
| Large | as served | 500 | 220 | 25 | 3.5 | 0 | 350 | 63 | 6 | 6 |
| Medium | as served | 380 | 170 | 19 | 2.5 | 0 | 270 | 48 | 5 | 4 |
| Small | as served | 230 | 100 | 11 | 1.5 | 0 | 160 | 29 | 3 | 3 |
| **SALADS** | | | | | | | | | | |
| Premium Bacon Ranch w/o Chicken | 1 salad | 140 | 70 | 7 | 3.5 | 25 | 300 | 10 | 3 | 9 |
| Premium Caesar w/Crispy Chicken | 1 salad | 330 | 150 | 17 | 4.5 | 60 | 840 | 20 | 3 | 26 |
| Premium Caesar w/Grilled Chicken | 1 salad | 220 | 60 | 6 | 3 | 75 | 890 | 12 | 3 | 30 |
| Premium Southwest w/o Chicken | 1 salad | 140 | 40 | 4.5 | 2 | 10 | 150 | 20 | 6 | 6 |

## Miami Subs

### 6″ SUBS

| | SERVING SIZE | CAL | CAL FAT | TOT FAT (G) | SAT FAT (G) | CHOL (MG) | SOD (MG) | CARB (G) | FIBER (G) | PROT (G) |
|---|---|---|---|---|---|---|---|---|---|---|
| Cheesesteak—Original | 1 sub | 409 | 99 | 11 | 7 | 77 | 925 | 45 | 0.8 | 31 |
| Ham & Cheese | 1 sub | 452 | 162 | 18 | 5 | 59 | 2051 | 49 | 1.5 | 23 |
| Italian Deli | 1 sub | 516 | 225 | 25 | 8 | 69 | 2151 | 49 | 1.5 | 24 |
| Meatball Sub | 1 sub | 491 | 198 | 22 | 9 | 76 | 1319 | 49 | 4 | 28 |
| Turkey Sub | 1 sub | 484 | 171 | 19 | 5 | 69 | 2009 | 51 | 1.5 | 29 |
| **DELUXE BURGERS** | | | | | | | | | | |
| Bacon Cheeseburger | 1 burger | 919 | 630 | 70 | 23 | 61 | 963 | 32 | 1 | 34 |
| Burger | 1 burger | 784 | 531 | 59 | 17 | 30 | 532 | 31 | 1 | 28 |
| Cheeseburger | 1 burger | 859 | 585 | 65 | 21 | 47 | 736 | 32 | 1 | 31 |

| | SERVING SIZE | CAL | CAL FAT | TOT FAT (G) | SAT FAT (G) | CHOL (MG) | SOD (MG) | CARB (G) | FIBER (G) | PROT (G) |
|---|---|---|---|---|---|---|---|---|---|---|
| **GYROS** | | | | | | | | | | |
| Chicken Pita | 1 gyro | 392 | 117 | 13 | 3 | 75 | 546 | 34 | 5 | 34 |
| Gyros Pita | 1 gyro | 662 | 351 | 39 | 27 | 84 | 1998 | 47 | 5 | 32 |
| **SALADS & SIDES** | | | | | | | | | | |
| Caesar—Includes Dressing | 1 salad | 459 | 306 | 34 | 6.2 | 14 | 1089 | 26 | 4.2 | 12 |
| Chicken Caesar—Includes Dressing | 1 salad | 609 | 351 | 39 | 7.2 | 74 | 1929 | 28 | 4.2 | 35 |
| Chicken Club | 1 salad | 490 | 225 | 25 | 10.4 | 210 | 1433 | 23 | 4.9 | 42 |
| Miami Greek | 1 salad | 284 | 135 | 15 | 5.11 | 123 | 906 | 24 | 5.4 | 14 |
| Mozzarella Sticks | as served | 757 | 513 | 57 | 16 | 60 | 1607 | 34 | 1.4 | 25 |
| Onion rings | as served | 869 | 612 | 68 | 9.8 | 0 | 895 | 56 | 2.4 | 4.8 |
| Spicy Fries—Regular | as served | 533 | 351 | 39 | 9.8 | 18.6 | 575 | 39 | 3.7 | 3.7 |

## Mimi's Café

### BREADS

| | SERVING SIZE | CAL | CAL FAT | TOT FAT (G) | SAT FAT (G) | CHOL (MG) | SOD (MG) | CARB (G) | FIBER (G) | PROT (G) |
|---|---|---|---|---|---|---|---|---|---|---|
| Blueberry Toast, Dry | 2 slices | 380 | 81 | 9 | 3 | 0 | 600 | 68 | 2 | 10 |
| Famous Carrot Raisin Nut Loaf | 1 slice | 151 | 78 | 9 | 1 | 21 | 170 | 17 | 1 | 2 |
| Seasonal Bread Loaf | 1 slice | 151 | 78 | 9 | 1 | 21 | 170 | 17 | 1 | 2 |
| **BREAKFAST SANDWICHES, WRAPS, & BURRITOS** | | | | | | | | | | |
| Ciabatta Breakfast Sandwich | 1 sandwich | 944 | 478 | 53 | 19 | 309 | 2681 | 77 | 3 | 43 |
| Crab Cake Florentine | 1 entrée | 1290 | 933 | 104 | 31 | 652 | 1850 | 50 | 1 | 40 |
| Crepes Brie Cheese Lorraine | 1 entrée | 552 | 369 | 41 | 19 | 527 | 1005 | 21 | 1 | 30 |
| Eggs Benedict | 1 entrée | 808 | 503 | 56 | 27 | 602 | 2778 | 36 | 0 | 43 |
| Eggs Florentine | 1 entrée | 691 | 451 | 50 | 25 | 533 | 1330 | 36 | 1 | 28 |
| Flatbread Breakfast Wrap | 1 wrap | 865 | 467 | 52 | 18 | 522 | 2271 | 54 | 9 | 48 |
| Quiche Lorraine | 1 entrée | 748 | 432 | 48 | 17 | 267 | 1266 | 49 | 4 | 30 |
| Santa Fe Breakfast Wrap | 1 wrap | 720 | 301 | 32 | 12 | 669 | 865 | 69 | 6 | 41 |
| **EGG COMBO PLATES** | | | | | | | | | | |
| Country Fried Steak & Eggs | 1 entrée | 464 | 235 | 26 | 7 | 472 | 541 | 30 | 1 | 31 |
| Smoked Bacon or Sausage & Eggs | 1 entrée | 293 | 194 | 22 | 7 | 453 | 941 | 1 | 0 | 23 |
| Smoked Ham & Eggs | 1 entrée | 344 | 195 | 22 | 7 | 506 | 2100 | 2 | 0 | 34 |
| **FRENCH TOAST & PANCAKES** | | | | | | | | | | |
| Belgian Waffle Breakfast | 1 entrée | 394 | 153 | 17 | 10 | 138 | 470 | 50 | 2 | 10 |
| Blueberry Stuffed French Toast Breakfast | 1 entrée | 576 | 176 | 20 | 9 | 31 | 686 | 93 | 6 | 13 |
| Buttermilk Pancake Breakfast | 1 entrée | 954 | 315 | 35 | 11 | 127 | 1970 | 139 | 3 | 23 |
| French Toast Breakfast | 1 entrée | 472 | 136 | 15 | 6 | 239 | 880 | 71 | 0 | 16 |

# restaurants

| | SERVING SIZE | CAL | CAL FAT | TOT FAT (G) | SAT FAT (G) | CHOL (MG) | SOD (MG) | CARB (G) | FIBER (G) | PROT (G) |
|---|---|---|---|---|---|---|---|---|---|---|
| **QUICHES** | | | | | | | | | | |
| Cheddar & Broccoli Quiche | 1 entrée | 699 | 413 | 46 | 17 | 258 | 915 | 49 | 5 | 23 |
| Asparagus & Brie Quiche | 1 entrée | 712 | 417 | 46 | 16 | 263 | 1162 | 49 | 5 | 26 |
| **OMELETS** | | | | | | | | | | |
| Asparagus | 1 omelet | 577 | 416 | 47 | 20 | 702 | 818 | 10 | 3 | 33 |
| Avocado BLT | 1 omelet | 553 | 384 | 43 | 17 | 692 | 749 | 9 | 4 | 37 |

## Moe's Southwest Grill
### DINNERS

| | SERVING SIZE | CAL | CAL FAT | TOT FAT (G) | SAT FAT (G) | CHOL (MG) | SOD (MG) | CARB (G) | FIBER (G) | PROT (G) |
|---|---|---|---|---|---|---|---|---|---|---|
| Bowl of Chicken Enchilada soup | 1 bowl | 360 | 190 | 21 | 9 | 75 | 1730 | 26 | 5 | 18 |
| Bowl of Chicken Enchilada soup w/chips | 1 bowl | 1020 | 430 | 47 | 13 | 75 | 1940 | 122 | 11 | 28 |
| Burrito, Art Vandalay Junior Vegetarian | 1 item | 423 | 139 | 15 | 7.1 | 30 | 768 | 54 | 7 | 16 |
| Burrito, Art Vandalay Vegetarian | 1 item | 775 | 263 | 30 | 13.8 | 60 | 1446 | 97 | 14 | 29 |
| Burrito, Homewrecker, Chicken | 1 item | 935 | 317 | 39 | 16.8 | 129 | 1686 | 95 | 20 | 41 |
| Burrito, Homewrecker Junior, Chicken | 1 item | 503 | 179 | 21 | 8.9 | 65 | 888 | 51 | 8 | 28 |
| Burrito, Triple Lindy Junior | 1 item | 458 | 173 | 20 | 9.5 | 58 | 1143 | 48 | 7 | 20 |
| Close Talker, Chicken & Crispy Salad Bowl | 1 salad | 844 | 405 | 46 | 13 | 99 | 1438 | 61 | 13 | 45 |
| Fajita, Alfredo Garcia, Chicken | 1 entrée | 965 | 390 | 45 | 19 | 198 | 1587 | 79 | 7 | 73 |
| Fajita, Fat Sam, Chicken | 1 entrée | 1108 | 514 | 59 | 24.6 | 228 | 1828 | 71 | 9 | 75 |
| Quesadilla, John Coctosan, Chicken | 1 item | 770 | 337 | 41 | 20.3 | 159 | 2763 | 52 | 11 | 53 |
| Quesadilla, Super Kingpin Vegetarian | 1 item | 495 | 268 | 32 | 17.3 | 90 | 823 | 36 | 2 | 21 |
| Salad, Personal Trainer Vegetarian | 1 salad | 685 | 345 | 39 | 10 | 30 | 1198 | 61 | 13 | 21 |
| Taco, Overachiever, Chicken | 1 taco | 428 | 164 | 17 | 7.9 | 65 | 801 | 40 | 7 | 26 |
| Taco, Unanimous Decision Vegetarian | 1 taco | 333 | 122 | 13 | 6.4 | 25 | 677 | 40 | 7 | 14 |
| **SIDES, ADD ONS, & EXTRAS** | | | | | | | | | | |
| Bowl of Pico de Gallo & Chips | 1 order | 750 | 240 | 26 | 4 | 9 | 1530 | 114 | 12 | 60 |
| Bowl of Queso & Chips | 1 order | 1580 | 940 | 103 | 51 | 225 | 3740 | 126 | 7 | 46 |
| Burrito Joey Bag of Donuts | 1 serving | 784 | 210 | 24 | 10 | 99 | 1443 | 91 | 11 | 50 |
| Pork | as served | 135 | 60 | 6 | 1.5 | 60 | 510 | 0 | 0 | 18 |
| Salad Crispy Bowl | as served | 350 | 200 | 23 | 4.5 | 0 | 520 | 33 | 2 | 5 |
| Salad Crispy Whole Grain Bowl | as served | 370 | 200 | 23 | 4.5 | 0 | 380 | 36 | 6 | 6 |

## Mrs. Fields
### BROWNIES

| | SERVING SIZE | CAL | CAL FAT | TOT FAT (G) | SAT FAT (G) | CHOL (MG) | SOD (MG) | CARB (G) | FIBER (G) | PROT (G) |
|---|---|---|---|---|---|---|---|---|---|---|
| Bites, Double Fudge | 3 bites | 200 | 90 | 10 | 5 | 45 | 75 | 27 | 1 | 2 |
| Butterscotch Blondie | 1 item | 260 | 90 | 10 | 6 | 50 | 20 | 38 | 0 | 3 |
| Double Fudge | 1 item | 260 | 120 | 13 | 8 | 60 | 95 | 34 | 1 | 3 |
| Walnut Fudge | 1 item | 270 | 140 | 15 | 7 | 55 | 95 | 32 | 2 | 3 |

| | SERVING SIZE | CAL | CAL FAT | TOT FAT (G) | SAT FAT (G) | CHOL (MG) | SOD (MG) | CARB (G) | FIBER (G) | PROT (G) |
|---|---|---|---|---|---|---|---|---|---|---|
| **COOKIES** | | | | | | | | | | |
| Bite-Size Nibblers, Semi-Sweet Chocolate | 3 cookies | 170 | 70 | 8 | 3.5 | 10 | 140 | 23 | 1 | 2 |
| Butter | 1 cookie | 200 | 80 | 8 | 3.5 | 20 | 180 | 29 | <1 | 2 |
| Cinnamon Sugar | 1 cookie | 210 | 80 | 8 | 3.5 | 20 | 210 | 31 | 0 | 2 |
| Oatmeal, Raisins & Walnuts | 1 cookie | 200 | 80 | 9 | 3 | 15 | 180 | 27 | 1 | 3 |
| Peanut Butter | 1 cookie | 200 | 100 | 12 | 4 | 20 | 210 | 24 | 1 | 4 |
| Triple Chocolate | 1 cookie | 210 | 90 | 10 | 6 | 15 | 170 | 28 | 1 | 2 |
| **MUFFINS** | | | | | | | | | | |
| Blueberry | 1 muffin | 190 | 80 | 9 | 2.5 | 25 | 280 | 24 | 1 | 3 |
| Chocolate Chip | 1 muffin | 200 | 90 | 10 | 3 | 25 | 270 | 26 | 1 | 3 |
| Raspberry | 1 muffin | 190 | 80 | 9 | 2.5 | 25 | 280 | 24 | 1 | 3 |

## Nathan's

### BURGERS & SANDWICHES

| | SERVING SIZE | CAL | CAL FAT | TOT FAT (G) | SAT FAT (G) | CHOL (MG) | SOD (MG) | CARB (G) | FIBER (G) | PROT (G) |
|---|---|---|---|---|---|---|---|---|---|---|
| Bacon Cheeseburger | 1 burger | 783 | 454 | 50 | 20 | 136 | 1365 | 45 | 2 | 36 |
| Cheesesteak Supreme | 1 sandwich | 880 | 396 | 45 | 20 | 151 | 1625 | 76 | 3 | 46 |
| Chicken Cheesesteak Supreme | 1 sandwich | 601 | 162 | 19 | 9 | 79 | 1719 | 70 | 3 | 40 |
| Chicken Tender Pita | 1 sandwich | 823 | 469 | 52 | 8 | 40 | 1462 | 66 | 5 | 22 |
| Double Burger w/Cheese | 1 burger | 1178 | 766 | 84 | 32 | 235 | 1299 | 45 | 2 | 57 |
| Hamburger w/Cheese | 1 burger | 705 | 395 | 43 | 16 | 117 | 1071 | 45 | 2 | 33 |
| Krispy Southwest Chipotle Wrap | 1 sandwich | 750 | 350 | 39 | 13 | 100 | 1160 | 62 | 1 | 68 |
| Supercheese Burger | 1 burger | 987 | 651 | 72 | 23 | 149 | 1349 | 47 | 3 | 35 |
| **CHICKEN** | | | | | | | | | | |
| Grilled Platter | as served | 839 | 504 | 56 | 9 | 59 | 1134 | 58 | 7 | 24 |
| Tender Platter | as served | 1245 | 822 | 90 | 14 | 44 | 1352 | 80 | 10 | 26 |
| Tenders | as served | 526 | 347 | 39 | 6 | 30 | 900 | 24 | 3 | 21 |
| Wings | 10 wings | 800 | 467 | 53 | 13 | 167 | 1300 | 23 | 0 | 53 |
| **HOT DOG** | | | | | | | | | | |
| Cheese Dog & Roll | 1 hot dog | 390 | 220 | 25 | 8 | 35 | 1440 | 30 | 1 | 12 |
| Chilidog & Roll | 1 hot dog | 400 | 210 | 23 | 6 | 50 | 1000 | 33 | 2 | 16 |
| Corn Dog on a Stick | 1 hot dog | 380 | 190 | 21 | 5 | 15 | 730 | 39 | 1 | 7 |
| Hot Dog & Roll | 1 hot dog | 297 | 163 | 18 | 7 | 34 | 692 | 24 | 1 | 11 |
| Pretzel Dog | 1 hot dog | 390 | 150 | 16 | 6 | 25 | 970 | 49 | 1 | 12 |
| **SIDES** | | | | | | | | | | |
| King-Size Pretzel | as served | 180 | 10 | 1 | 0 | 0 | 940 | 38 | 1 | 6 |
| Mozzarella Sticks—3pc | as served | 390 | 253 | 28 | 8 | 32 | 941 | 20 | 1 | 14 |
| Onion Rings—Small | as served | 544 | 392 | 44 | 6 | 0 | 580 | 36 | 1 | 3 |
| Regular Cheese Fries | as served | 564 | 376 | 42 | 7 | 0 | 785 | 41 | 4 | 5 |

## Ninety Nine

| | SERVING SIZE | CAL | CAL FAT | TOT FAT (G) | SAT FAT (G) | CHOL (MG) | SOD (MG) | CARB (G) | FIBER (G) | PROT (G) |
|---|---|---|---|---|---|---|---|---|---|---|
| **ENTRÉES** | | | | | | | | | | |
| Baby Back Ribs | 1 entrée | 2030 | 540 | 59 | 24 | 285 | 11320 | 239 | 11 | 133 |
| Baja Crab Cakes | 1 entrée | 1050 | 860 | 96 | 28 | 305 | 2020 | 20 | 5 | 29 |
| Balsamic Grilled Chicken | 1 entrée | 620 | 200 | 22 | 4 | 195 | 630 | 29 | 0 | 72 |
| Chicken Marsala | 1 entrée | 1110 | 510 | 57 | 18 | 215 | 1650 | 70 | 4 | 75 |
| Country Fried Chicken | 1 entrée | 990 | 400 | 45 | 16 | 95 | 2490 | 100 | 3 | 45 |
| Filet Mignon | 1 entrée | 420 | 200 | 23 | 12 | 130 | 610 | 1 | 0 | 47 |
| Fish & Chips | 1 entrée | 1790 | 680 | 124 | 13 | 165 | 4130 | 60 | 3 | 51 |
| Grilled Double BBQ Turkey Tips | 1 entrée | 810 | 190 | 21 | 11 | 195 | 2890 | 73 | 1 | 76 |
| Honey BBQ Boneless Wings | 1 entrée | 1240 | 690 | 77 | 11 | 160 | 3220 | 75 | 3 | 63 |
| King Tips 24 oz. | 1 entrée | 1630 | 430 | 120 | 18 | 345 | 2190 | 4 | 2 | 149 |
| Original Crispy Chicken Tenders | 1 entrée | 1130 | 670 | 75 | 13 | 155 | 6620 | 54 | 2 | 60 |
| Sirloin Tips & Chicken Tenders | 1 entrée | 1430 | 330 | 91 | 10 | 200 | 5070 | 37 | 2 | 87 |
| **SANDWICHES & STEAKBURGERS** | | | | | | | | | | |
| All Star Steakburger | 1 burger | 1190 | 730 | 81 | 27 | 205 | 2260 | 55 | 2 | 56 |
| Bacon & Cheese Steakburger | 1 burger | 940 | 520 | 57 | 23 | 185 | 1700 | 46 | 2 | 55 |
| Chicken Parmigiana Sandwich | 1 sandwich | 880 | 320 | 36 | 10 | 90 | 2680 | 92 | 7 | 48 |
| Grilled Chicken Club | 1 sandwich | 1250 | 260 | 67 | 6 | 110 | 2470 | 61 | 2 | 48 |
| Mushroom & Cheese | 1 burger | 950 | 520 | 58 | 23 | 175 | 1530 | 49 | 3 | 53 |
| Steakburger | 1 burger | 810 | 420 | 47 | 18 | 160 | 1260 | 45 | 2 | 48 |
| Triple Decker Turkey Club | 1 sandwich | 950 | 330 | 37 | 6 | 115 | 2260 | 107 | 7 | 53 |
| Ultimate Sirloin Steak Sandwich | 1 sandwich | 1040 | 570 | 63 | 18 | 110 | 1980 | 71 | 3 | 46 |
| **SALADS** | | | | | | | | | | |
| Acapulco Shrimp Salad | 1 salad | 740 | 500 | 56 | 16 | 185 | 1890 | 27 | 7 | 33 |
| Chicken Caesar Salad | 1 salad | 900 | 510 | 57 | 11 | 145 | 2320 | 51 | 7 | 55 |
| Fire Grilled SW Cobb Salad | 1 salad | 930 | 530 | 59 | 17 | 360 | 1800 | 31 | 7 | 63 |
| Tropical Chicken Salad | 1 salad | 800 | 380 | 42 | 6 | 115 | 1260 | 59 | 5 | 44 |
| **STARTERS & SIDES** | | | | | | | | | | |
| Boneless Buffalo Wings | as served | 1120 | 670 | 45 | 11 | 160 | 4510 | 44 | 2 | 62 |
| Buffalo Wings Bone-In, Regular | as served | 1310 | 970 | 108 | 22 | 180 | 5640 | 12 | 1 | 56 |
| Chipotle Chicken Quesadilla | as served | 1500 | 940 | 106 | 47 | 210 | 2890 | 78 | 6 | 59 |
| French Fries | as served | 510 | 300 | 34 | 6 | 0 | 1280 | 48 | 5 | 5 |
| Southwest Egg Rolls, Small Plate | as served | 800 | 520 | 58 | 12 | 30 | 1580 | 54 | 5 | 12 |
| Spinach & Artichoke Dip | as served | 850 | 530 | 59 | 21 | 75 | 2470 | 67 | 3 | 21 |
| Sweet Potato Fries | as served | 550 | 320 | 36 | 6 | 0 | 540 | 50 | 8 | 5 |

## Nothing But Noodles
### ENTRÉES

| | SERVING SIZE | CAL | CAL FAT | TOT FAT (G) | SAT FAT (G) | CHOL (MG) | SOD (MG) | CARB (G) | FIBER (G) | PROT (G) |
|---|---|---|---|---|---|---|---|---|---|---|
| Beef Stroganoff | as served | 508 | 278 | 31 | 14 | 122 | 1499 | 33 | 2 | 26 |
| Buttery Noodles | as served | 651 | 393 | 44 | 26 | 178 | 1538 | 46 | 2 | 19 |
| Fettucini Alfredo | as served | 723 | 505 | 56 | 35 | 175 | 1053 | 36 | 2 | 20 |
| General Tso's Chicken | as served | 760 | 390 | 44 | 5 | 50 | 1538 | 69 | 1 | 24 |
| Kung Pao Chicken | as served | 935 | 460 | 51 | 6 | 50 | 460 | 89 | 5 | 31 |
| Margherita Pasta | as served | 474 | 281 | 31 | 5 | 5 | 2153 | 36 | 3 | 9 |
| Santa Fe Pasta | as served | 705 | 481 | 54 | 29 | 140 | 1714 | 40 | 3 | 18 |
| Sesame Lo Mein | as served | 411 | 101 | 11 | 2 | 7 | 1737 | 64 | 4 | 5 |
| Shrimp Pesto Florentine | as served | 308 | 224 | 25 | 12 | 154 | 357 | 5 | 2 | 16 |
| Spicy Cajun Pasta | as served | 660 | 445 | 50 | 29 | 148 | 1517 | 44 | 4 | 9 |
| Spicy Japanese Noodles | as served | 419 | 69 | 8 | 1 | 0 | 1453 | 74 | 4 | 10 |
| Southwest Chipolte | as served | 713 | 521 | 58 | 32 | 156 | 1822 | 41 | 4 | 11 |
| Thai Peanut | as served | 568 | 181 | 20 | 5 | 0 | 1638 | 89 | 5 | 11 |
| Thai Peanut Sauce Stir Fry | as served | 595 | 245 | 27 | 5 | 50 | 885 | 59 | 3 | 29 |
| Three Cheese Macaroni | as served | 446 | 184 | 21 | 12 | 115 | 392 | 45 | 2 | 20 |

### STARTERS & SOUP

| | SERVING SIZE | CAL | CAL FAT | TOT FAT (G) | SAT FAT (G) | CHOL (MG) | SOD (MG) | CARB (G) | FIBER (G) | PROT (G) |
|---|---|---|---|---|---|---|---|---|---|---|
| Fresh Mozzarella | as served | 767 | 241 | 27 | 10 | 50 | 488 | 134 | 1 | 20 |
| Garlic Breadsticks | as served | 106 | 39 | 4 | 1 | 0 | 214 | 28 | 1 | 2 |
| Mozzarella Cheese Bread | as served | 633 | 153 | 17 | 8 | 40 | 1314 | 86 | 3 | 33 |

## O'Charley's
### BURGERS & SANDWICHES

| | SERVING SIZE | CAL | CAL FAT | TOT FAT (G) | SAT FAT (G) | CHOL (MG) | SOD (MG) | CARB (G) | FIBER (G) | PROT (G) |
|---|---|---|---|---|---|---|---|---|---|---|
| Better Cheddar Bacon Burger | 1 burger | 990 | 520 | 57 | 23 | 180 | 1710 | 55 | 3 | 59 |
| Classic Burger | 1 burger | 740 | 340 | 37 | 12 | 130 | 1180 | 54 | 3 | 44 |
| Philly Burger | 1 burger | 1230 | 690 | 77 | 22 | 190 | 2580 | 71 | 4 | 61 |
| Prime Rib Philly Sandwich | 1 sandwich | 980 | 510 | 56 | 14 | 95 | 2540 | 82 | 5 | 41 |
| Roast Beef Sandwich | 1 sandwich | 880 | 430 | 47 | 14 | 95 | 2660 | 74 | 4 | 42 |
| Wild West Burger | 1 burger | 1210 | 710 | 79 | 23 | 170 | 1860 | 67 | 4 | 53 |

### ENTRÉES

| | SERVING SIZE | CAL | CAL FAT | TOT FAT (G) | SAT FAT (G) | CHOL (MG) | SOD (MG) | CARB (G) | FIBER (G) | PROT (G) |
|---|---|---|---|---|---|---|---|---|---|---|
| 12 Spice Chicken Pasta | 1 entrée | 1390 | 690 | 77 | 35 | 230 | 1760 | 103 | 7 | 64 |
| Grilled Top Sirloin | 7 oz | 430 | 250 | 28 | 9 | 95 | 920 | 1 | 0 | 43 |
| Baked Penne Italiano | 1 entrée | 1700 | 890 | 99 | 41 | 195 | 3350 | 142 | 7 | 54 |
| Bayou Shrimp Pasta | 1 entrée | 1640 | 780 | 87 | 32 | 170 | 3420 | 155 | 8 | 59 |
| Boneless Buffalo O'Tenders | 1 entrée | 880 | 590 | 66 | 12 | 115 | 3500 | 27 | 2 | 46 |
| Cedar Planked Salmon | 1 entrée | 530 | 280 | 32 | 6 | 160 | 940 | 2 | 1 | 57 |
| Chicken Parmesan Pasta | 1 entrée | 1500 | 690 | 77 | 18 | 110 | 3980 | 138 | 7 | 65 |

# restaurants

| | SERVING SIZE | CAL | CAL FAT | TOT FAT (G) | SAT FAT (G) | CHOL (MG) | SOD (MG) | CARB (G) | FIBER (G) | PROT (G) |
|---|---|---|---|---|---|---|---|---|---|---|
| Chicken Tenders & Naked Twisted Chips w/o Sauce | 1 entrée | 1150 | 540 | 60 | 11 | 90 | 3170 | 110 | 9 | 55 |
| Filet Mignon | 1 entrée | 450 | 250 | 28 | 9 | 140 | 910 | 0 | 0 | 47 |
| Grilled Atlantic Salmon w/Chipotle | 1 entrée | 610 | 290 | 33 | 7 | 160 | 500 | 17 | 1 | 57 |
| Half Rack Baby Back Ribs | 1 entrée | 740 | 430 | 48 | 17 | 185 | 2630 | 38 | 2 | 39 |
| Hand Battered Fish n' Chips | 1 entrée | 1140 | 750 | 85 | 16 | 120 | 2040 | 43 | 3 | 52 |
| Sicilian Meatballs & Linguini | 1 entrée | 1250 | 620 | 69 | 25 | 140 | 3390 | 103 | 6 | 56 |
| Southwestern Chicken Quesadilla | 1 entrée | 1060 | 540 | 60 | 28 | 195 | 2690 | 64 | 4 | 63 |
| Teriyaki Sesame Chicken | 1 entrée | 1030 | 220 | 25 | 4.5 | 80 | 3740 | 151 | 5 | 46 |
| **SALADS (no dressing)** | | | | | | | | | | |
| A La Carte House | 1 salad | 140 | 50 | 6 | 2.5 | 15 | 300 | 16 | 2 | 6 |
| Original Southern Fried Chicken | 1 salad | 900 | 370 | 42 | 12 | 130 | 3130 | 74 | 6 | 60 |
| Pecan Chicken Tende | 1 salad | 1020 | 530 | 60 | 11 | 95 | 2020 | 81 | 10 | 46 |
| **SIDES** | | | | | | | | | | |
| Authentic Spinach & Artichoke Dip | as served | 780 | 390 | 44 | 13 | 45 | 1530 | 86 | 6 | 14 |
| Beer Battered Onion Rings | as served | 380 | 230 | 26 | 5 | 0 | 660 | 32 | 1 | 3 |
| French Fries | as served | 390 | 220 | 24 | 5 | 0 | 760 | 40 | 3 | 4 |
| Loaded Baked Potato | as served | 480 | 250 | 29 | 10 | 25 | 570 | 54 | 6 | 12 |
| Overloaded Potato Skins | as served | 1260 | 880 | 98 | 43 | 195 | 1980 | 43 | 0 | 56 |
| Southwestern Cheese Dip & Chips | as served | 820 | 400 | 45 | 18 | 85 | 1630 | 84 | 4 | 24 |
| Southwestern Twisted Chips | as served | 1280 | 790 | 89 | 26 | 85 | 2140 | 111 | 12 | 31 |
| Spicy Jack Cheese Wedges | as served | 880 | 540 | 60 | 25 | 140 | 2540 | 55 | 0 | 29 |
| Three Cheese Shrimp Dip | as served | 870 | 440 | 49 | 16 | 200 | 1540 | 86 | 10 | 32 |
| **Olive Garden** | | | | | | | | | | |
| **APPETIZERS** | | | | | | | | | | |
| Breadstick w/Garlic-Butter Spread | 1 stick | 150 | 18 | 2 | 0 | n/a | 400 | 28 | 2 | n/a |
| Calamari Sampler | as served | 440 | 243 | 27 | 2.5 | n/a | 1160 | 32 | 0 | n/a |
| Chicken Alfredo Pizza | 1 pizza | 1180 | 360 | 40 | 17 | n/a | 3330 | 144 | 11 | n/a |
| Chicken Fingers Sampler | as served | 330 | 144 | 16 | 1.5 | n/a | 930 | 22 | 0 | n/a |
| Fried Mozzarella Sampler | as served | 370 | 198 | 22 | 9 | n/a | 800 | 26 | 2 | n/a |
| Fried Zucchini Sampler | as served | 370 | 180 | 20 | 1.5 | n/a | 630 | 42 | 4 | n/a |
| Garden-Fresh Salad w/o Dressing | 1 salad | 120 | 31.5 | 3.5 | 0.5 | n/a | 550 | 17 | 3 | n/a |
| Grilled Chicken Caeser Salad | 1 salad | 850 | 576 | 64 | 13 | n/a | 1880 | 14 | 4 | n/a |
| Grilled Chicken Flatbread Appetizer | as served | 760 | 396 | 44 | 15 | n/a | 1500 | 47 | 5 | n/a |
| Grilled Chicken Spiedini Appetizer | as served | 460 | 117 | 13 | 2.5 | n/a | 1180 | 26 | 7 | n/a |
| Herb-Grilled Salmon Appetizer | as served | 510 | 234 | 26 | 6 | n/a | 760 | 5 | 2 | n/a |
| Lasagna Fritta Appetizer | as served | 1030 | 567 | 63 | 21 | n/a | 1590 | 82 | 9 | n/a |

| | SERVING SIZE | CAL | CAL FAT | TOT FAT (G) | SAT FAT (G) | CHOL (MG) | SOD (MG) | CARB (G) | FIBER (G) | PROT (G) |
|---|---|---|---|---|---|---|---|---|---|---|
| Mussels di Napoli | as served | 180 | 72 | 8 | 4 | n/a | 1770 | 13 | 0 | n/a |
| Pasta e Fagioli Appetizer | as served | 130 | 22.5 | 2.5 | 1 | n/a | 680 | 17 | 6 | n/a |
| Sicilian Scampi Appetizer | as served | 500 | 198 | 22 | 10 | n/a | 1850 | 43 | 7 | n/a |
| Smoked Mozzarella Fonduta Appetizer | as served | 940 | 432 | 48 | 28 | n/a | 1940 | 72 | 7 | n/a |
| Stuffed Mushrooms Appetizer Sampler | as served | 280 | 171 | 19 | 5 | n/a | 720 | 15 | 3 | n/a |
| Toasted Beef & Pork Ravioli Appetizer Sampler | as served | 360 | 144 | 16 | 2.5 | n/a | 780 | 39 | 2 | n/a |
| Zuppa Toscana Appetizer | as served | 170 | 36 | 4 | 2 | n/a | 960 | 24 | 2 | n/a |
| **ENTRÉES** | | | | | | | | | | |
| Capellini di Mare | 1 entrée | 650 | 162 | 18 | 5 | n/a | 1830 | 82 | 7 | n/a |
| Chianti Braised Short Ribs | 1 entrée | 1060 | 522 | 58 | 26 | n/a | 2970 | 71 | 17 | n/a |
| Chicken & Shrimp Carbonara | 1 entrée | 1440 | 792 | 88 | 38 | n/a | 3000 | 80 | 9 | n/a |
| Chicken Alfredo | 1 entrée | 1440 | 738 | 82 | 48 | n/a | 2070 | 103 | 5 | n/a |
| Parmesan Crusted Bistecca | 1 entrée | 690 | 315 | 35 | 19 | n/a | 1480 | 40 | 7 | n/a |
| Parmesan Crusted Tilapia | 1 entrée | 590 | 225 | 25 | 10 | n/a | 910 | 42 | 6 | n/a |
| Pork Milanese | 1 entrée | 1510 | 783 | 87 | 37 | n/a | 3100 | 118 | 11 | n/a |
| Steak Gorgonzola Alfredo | 1 entrée | 1310 | 657 | 73 | 41 | n/a | 2190 | 82 | 9 | n/a |
| Stuffed Chicken Marsala | 1 entrée | 800 | 324 | 36 | 16 | n/a | 2830 | 40 | 6 | n/a |

## Orange Julius
### FRUIT DRINKS

| | SERVING SIZE | CAL | CAL FAT | TOT FAT (G) | SAT FAT (G) | CHOL (MG) | SOD (MG) | CARB (G) | FIBER (G) | PROT (G) |
|---|---|---|---|---|---|---|---|---|---|---|
| Bananarilla | 16 fl oz | 320 | 60 | 7 | 6 | 5 | 70 | 65 | 5 | 3 |
| Cranberry Banana Julius | 16 fl oz | 140 | 5 | .5 | 0 | 0 | 20 | 35 | 3 | 1 |
| Mango Julius | 16 fl oz | 150 | 5 | .5 | 0 | 0 | 20 | 38 | 1 | 1 |
| Original Orange Julius | 16 fl oz | 130 | 5 | .5 | 0 | 0 | 20 | 33 | 0 | 1 |
| Peach Julius | 16 fl oz | 140 | 5 | 0 | 0 | 0 | 20 | 34 | 1 | 1 |
| Piña Colada | 16 fl oz | 260 | 60 | 7 | 6 | 5 | 75 | 52 | 2 | 2 |
| Pineapple Julius | 16 fl oz | 120 | 5 | 0 | 0 | 0 | 25 | 31 | 1 | 0 |
| Pomegranate Julius | 16 fl oz | 160 | 5 | .5 | 0 | 0 | 25 | 40 | 1 | 1 |
| Raspberry Julius | 16 fl oz | 200 | 5 | 1 | 0 | 0 | 20 | 51 | 3 | 1 |
| Strawberry Banana | 16 fl oz | 300 | 60 | 7 | 6 | 5 | 65 | 60 | 4 | 3 |
| Tripleberry | 16 fl oz | 310 | 60 | 7 | 6 | 5 | 65 | 63 | 4 | 2 |
| Tropical | 16 fl oz | 350 | 60 | 7 | 6 | 5 | 70 | 71 | 4 | 3 |

### SMOOTHIES

| | SERVING SIZE | CAL | CAL FAT | TOT FAT (G) | SAT FAT (G) | CHOL (MG) | SOD (MG) | CARB (G) | FIBER (G) | PROT (G) |
|---|---|---|---|---|---|---|---|---|---|---|
| 3-Berry Blast | 20 fl oz | 460 | 5 | 0 | 0 | 5 | 150 | 108 | 6 | 8 |
| Berry Banana Squeeze | 20 fl oz | 270 | 0 | 0 | 0 | 0 | 10 | 70 | 4 | 1 |
| Berry Lemon Lively | 20 fl oz | 440 | 5 | 0 | 0 | 5 | 150 | 106 | 5 | 8 |
| Blackberry Storm | 20 fl oz | 680 | 140 | 15 | 13 | 15 | 290 | 128 | 6 | 12 |

# restaurants

| | SERVING SIZE | CAL | CAL FAT | TOT FAT (G) | SAT FAT (G) | CHOL (MG) | SOD (MG) | CARB (G) | FIBER (G) | PROT (G) |
|---|---|---|---|---|---|---|---|---|---|---|
| Blackberry Toner | 20 fl oz | 410 | 5 | 0 | 0 | 5 | 150 | 94 | 4 | 8 |
| Cocoa Latte Swirl | 20 fl oz | 960 | 210 | 23 | 19 | 20 | 870 | 156 | 5 | 34 |
| Cranberry Orange Chill/Tart 'N' Berry | 20 fl oz | 410 | 20 | 2.5 | 1 | 5 | 55 | 99 | 7 | 2 |
| Mango Passion | 20 fl oz | 370 | 0 | 0 | 0 | 5 | 170 | 86 | 1 | 7 |
| Orange Swirl | 20 fl oz | 540 | 110 | 12 | 10 | 15 | 150 | 103 | 3 | 4 |
| Peach White Tea | 20 fl oz | 320 | 5 | 0 | 0 | 5 | 140 | 75 | 1 | 7 |
| Peaches & Cream | 20 fl oz | 360 | 0 | 0 | 0 | 5 | 170 | 83 | 2 | 8 |
| Pomegranate & Berries | 20 fl oz | 400 | 0 | 0 | 0 | 5 | 150 | 92 | 3 | 7 |
| Raspberry Crème | 20 fl oz | 650 | 140 | 15 | 13 | 15 | 290 | 118 | 5 | 12 |
| Raspberry White Tea | 20 fl oz | 410 | 10 | 1 | 0 | 5 | 140 | 97 | 5 | 7 |
| Strawberry Sensation | 20 fl oz | 430 | 0 | 0 | 0 | 5 | 160 | 100 | 2 | 7 |
| Strawberry Xtreme | 20 fl oz | 390 | 0 | 0 | 0 | 5 | 160 | 89 | 2 | 8 |
| Tropical Tango | 20 fl oz | 380 | 0 | 0 | 0 | 0 | 120 | 92 | 3 | 1 |
| Tropi-Colada | 20 fl oz | 530 | 90 | 10 | 9 | 10 | 260 | 99 | 3 | 11 |

## Outback Steakhouse
### APPETIZERS

| | | | | | | | | | | |
|---|---|---|---|---|---|---|---|---|---|---|
| Aussie Cheese Fries—Regular | 1/6 order | 356 | 226 | 25 | 12 | 41 | 390 | 23 | 3 | 10 |
| Bloomin' Onion | 1/6 order | 259 | 124 | 14 | 5 | 15 | 918 | 31 | 4 | 5 |
| Grilled Shrimp on the Barbie | 1 order | 315 | 186 | 21 | 8 | 190 | 657 | 6 | 1 | 26 |
| Kookaburra Wings—Mild | 1/4 order | 328 | 209 | 23 | 7 | 91 | 897 | 7 | 1 | 22 |
| Seared Ahi Tuna—Regular | 1/4 order | 120 | 65 | 7 | 1 | 13 | 594 | 4 | 1 | 8 |

### BURGERS & SANDWICHES

| | | | | | | | | | | |
|---|---|---|---|---|---|---|---|---|---|---|
| Bacon Cheese Burger | 1 burger | 1272 | 855 | 95 | 38 | 279 | 2308 | 44 | 3 | 58 |
| Bloomin' Burger | 1 burger | 1221 | 697 | 77 | 30 | 249 | 2831 | 76 | 7 | 56 |
| Grilled Chicken & Swiss Sandwich | 1 sandwich | 750 | 354 | 39 | 13 | 163 | 1372 | 50 | 3 | 48 |
| Outbacker Burger | 1 burger | 810 | 459 | 51 | 20 | 197 | 1291 | 43 | 4 | 43 |
| Roasted Filet Sandwich | 1 sandwich | 814 | 234 | 26 | 9 | 87 | 3374 | 88 | 4 | 55 |

### ENTRÉES

| | | | | | | | | | | |
|---|---|---|---|---|---|---|---|---|---|---|
| Atlantic Salmon | as served | 525 | 306 | 34 | 11 | 115 | 754 | 12 | 4 | 42 |
| Baby Back Ribs—Half Rack | as served | 834 | 513 | 57 | 23 | 217 | 1633 | 22 | 0 | 58 |
| Chargrilled Ribeye | 10 oz | 787 | 565 | 63 | 26 | 193 | 2389 | 2 | 0 | 50 |
| Filet & Shrimp Scampi | as served | 615 | 335 | 37 | 20 | 204 | 2290 | 17 | 3 | 52 |
| Grilled Chicken on the Barbie | as served | 525 | 182 | 20 | 9 | 190 | 959 | 11 | 0 | 70 |
| Lobster Tails | as served | 640 | 430 | 48 | 30 | 283 | 1179 | 6 | 2 | 47 |
| Melbourne, The | 20 oz | 1009 | 520 | 58 | 23 | 342 | 904 | 1 | 0 | 114 |
| New Zealand Rack of Lamb | as served | 1303 | 1012 | 112 | 58 | 306 | 1473 | 5 | 1 | 61 |
| Prime Rib | 8 oz | 537 | 404 | 45 | 19 | 123 | 888 | 2 | 0 | 29 |

| | SERVING SIZE | CAL | CAL FAT | TOT FAT (G) | SAT FAT (G) | CHOL (MG) | SOD (MG) | CARB (G) | FIBER (G) | PROT (G) |
|---|---|---|---|---|---|---|---|---|---|---|
| Ribeye | 10 oz | 882 | 668 | 74 | 33 | 224 | 626 | 1 | 0 | 50 |
| Ribs & Alice Springs Chicken | as served | 1220 | 799 | 89 | 37 | 302 | 1952 | 16 | 1 | 88 |
| Special Steak | 6 oz | 332 | 174 | 19 | 10 | 110 | 562 | 1 | 0 | 37 |
| Special Steak & Grilled Shrimp on the Barbie | 6 oz | 549 | 311 | 35 | 15 | 207 | 1128 | 7 | 2 | 51 |
| Sweet Glazed Roasted Pork Tenderloin | as served | 385 | 110 | 12 | 6 | 122 | 462 | 32 | 1 | 37 |
| Teriyaki Marinated Sirloin | 9 oz | 418 | 105 | 12 | 4 | 118 | 1815 | 17 | 0 | 57 |
| Victoria's Filet | 6 oz | 518 | 374 | 42 | 19 | 140 | 551 | 1 | 0 | 34 |
| **SALADS** | | | | | | | | | | |
| Blue Cheese Pecan Chopped | 1 salad | 523 | 327 | 36 | 9 | 34 | 892 | 35 | 6 | 13 |
| Caesar | 1 salad | 329 | 238 | 26 | 9 | 8 | 745 | 16 | 3 | 8 |
| Chicken Caesar | 1 salad | 1030 | 584 | 65 | 23 | 203 | 1772 | 26 | 6 | 83 |
| Classic Blue Cheese Wedge Salad | as served | 357 | 215 | 24 | 8 | 38 | 1159 | 26 | 2 | 8 |
| Classic Roasted Filet Wedge | 1 salad | 562 | 267 | 30 | 10 | 95 | 2083 | 27 | 2 | 43 |
| House | 1 salad | 212 | 128 | 14 | 8 | 14 | 339 | 16 | 3 | 7 |
| Shrimp Caesar | 1 salad | 712 | 473 | 53 | 18 | 166 | 1721 | 26 | 6 | 34 |
| **SIDES** | | | | | | | | | | |
| Aussie Fries—Side order | as served | 354 | 172 | 19 | 9 | 10 | 110 | 43 | 5 | 4 |
| Baked Potato—No toppings | as served | 329 | 40 | 4 | 0 | 0 | 2298 | 65 | 7 | 8 |
| Garlic Mashed Potatoes | as served | 367 | 217 | 24 | 11 | 9 | 1197 | 32 | 6 | 7 |
| Potato Wedges | as served | 278 | 132 | 15 | 6 | 14 | 1255 | 33 | 4 | 4 |

## Panda Express
### APPETIZERS

| | SERVING SIZE | CAL | CAL FAT | TOT FAT (G) | SAT FAT (G) | CHOL (MG) | SOD (MG) | CARB (G) | FIBER (G) | PROT (G) |
|---|---|---|---|---|---|---|---|---|---|---|
| Chicken Egg Roll | 1 roll | 200 | 100 | 12 | 4 | 20 | 390 | 16 | 2 | 8 |
| Cream Cheese Rangoon | 3 pieces | 190 | 70 | 8 | 5 | 35 | 180 | 24 | 2 | 5 |
| Hot & Sour Soup | 10-1/2 oz | 90 | 30 | 3.5 | .5 | 65 | 970 | 12 | 1 | 4 |
| Veggie Spring Rolls | 2 rolls | 160 | 60 | 7 | 1 | 0 | 540 | 22 | 4 | 4 |
| **ENTRÉES** | | | | | | | | | | |
| Beijing Beef | 5-1/2 oz | 850 | 450 | 50 | 9 | 75 | 1120 | 67 | 4 | 31 |
| Black Pepper Chicken | 6 oz | 250 | 130 | 14 | 3 | 120 | 980 | 12 | 2 | 19 |
| Broccoli Beef | 5-1/2 oz | 150 | 50 | 6 | 1.5 | 25 | 720 | 12 | 3 | 11 |
| Broccoli Chicken | 5-1/2 oz | 180 | 80 | 9 | 2 | 65 | 630 | 11 | 3 | 13 |
| Chow Mein | 8 oz | 400 | 110 | 12 | 2 | 0 | 1060 | 61 | 8 | 12 |
| Crispy Shrimp | 6 pieces | 260 | 120 | 13 | 2.5 | 60 | 810 | 26 | 1 | 9 |
| Fried Rice | 10 oz | 570 | 160 | 18 | 4 | 130 | 900 | 85 | 8 | 16 |
| Kung Pao Chicken | 6 oz | 300 | 170 | 19 | 3.5 | 110 | 880 | 13 | 2 | 19 |
| Mandarin Chicken | 6 oz | 310 | 150 | 16 | 4 | 115 | 740 | 8 | 0 | 34 |

# restaurants

| | SERVING SIZE | CAL | CAL FAT | TOT FAT (G) | SAT FAT (G) | CHOL (MG) | SOD (MG) | CARB (G) | FIBER (G) | PROT (G) |
|---|---|---|---|---|---|---|---|---|---|---|
| Mongolian Beef | 7 oz | 230 | 100 | 11 | 2.5 | 45 | 1040 | 17 | 3 | 17 |
| Orange Chicken | 5-1/2 oz | 400 | 170 | 20 | 3.5 | 90 | 640 | 42 | 0 | 15 |
| String Bean Chicken | 5 oz | 190 | 90 | 10 | 2 | 75 | 720 | 11 | 2 | 12 |
| Sweet & Sour Chicken | 5-1/2 oz | 400 | 150 | 17 | 3 | 40 | 370 | 46 | 1 | 15 |
| Sweet & Sour Pork | 6 oz | 400 | 210 | 23 | 4.5 | 30 | 360 | 36 | 2 | 13 |
| Thai Cashew Chicken Breast | 5-1/2 oz | 280 | 170 | 19 | 3.5 | 50 | 980 | 21 | 2 | 23 |

## Panera Bread
### BAKED EGG SOUFFLÉS

| | SERVING SIZE | CAL | CAL FAT | TOT FAT (G) | SAT FAT (G) | CHOL (MG) | SOD (MG) | CARB (G) | FIBER (G) | PROT (G) |
|---|---|---|---|---|---|---|---|---|---|---|
| Four Cheese | 1 entrée | 480 | 261 | 29 | 16 | 195 | 700 | 36 | 2 | 16 |
| Ham & Swiss | 1 entrée | 490 | 270 | 30 | 16 | 175 | 800 | 35 | 2 | 20 |

### BAKERY, BAGELS, & BREADS

| | SERVING SIZE | CAL | CAL FAT | TOT FAT (G) | SAT FAT (G) | CHOL (MG) | SOD (MG) | CARB (G) | FIBER (G) | PROT (G) |
|---|---|---|---|---|---|---|---|---|---|---|
| Ciabatta | as served | 460 | 54 | 6 | 1 | 0 | 760 | 84 | 3 | 16 |
| Cinnamon Chip Scone | 1 scone | 600 | 279 | 31 | 19 | 125 | 370 | 73 | 2 | 9 |
| Cinnamon Coffee Crumb Cake | 1 cake | 470 | 225 | 25 | 9 | 105 | 310 | 54 | 1 | 6 |
| Cinnamon Sweet Roll | 1 roll | 620 | 216 | 24 | 14 | 100 | 480 | 89 | 3 | 13 |
| Focaccia | as served | 180 | 40.5 | 4.5 | 0.5 | 0 | 320 | 28 | 1 | 5 |
| French Baguette | as served | 150 | 9 | 1 | 0 | 0 | 370 | 30 | 1 | 5 |
| French Toast Bagel | 1 bagel | 350 | 45 | 5 | 2 | 0 | 620 | 67 | 2 | 9 |
| Honey Wheat Loaf | as served | 170 | 27 | 3 | 1.5 | 0 | 240 | 30 | 2 | 5 |
| Plain Bagel | 1 bagel | 290 | 13.5 | 1.5 | 0 | 0 | 460 | 59 | 6 | 13 |
| Sourdough Soup Bowl | as served | 590 | 22.5 | 2.5 | 0 | 0 | 1210 | 118 | 4 | 21 |
| Whole Grain Bagel | 1 bagel | 340 | 31.5 | 2.5 | 0 | 0 | 400 | 67 | 6 | 13 |
| Wild Blueberry Muffin | 1 muffin | 440 | 153 | 17 | 3 | 60 | 330 | 66 | 2 | 6 |

### HOT PANINI

| | SERVING SIZE | CAL | CAL FAT | TOT FAT (G) | SAT FAT (G) | CHOL (MG) | SOD (MG) | CARB (G) | FIBER (G) | PROT (G) |
|---|---|---|---|---|---|---|---|---|---|---|
| Half Chicken Caesar on Three Cheese | 1/2 panino | 360 | 144 | 16 | 5 | 65 | 640 | 35 | 2 | 22 |
| Half Chipotle Chicken on Artisan French | 1/2 panino | 500 | 252 | 28 | 8 | 75 | 1180 | 36 | 2 | 26 |
| Half Italian Combo on Ciabatta | 1/2 panino | 520 | 207 | 22 | 9 | 80 | 1540 | 47 | 2 | 31 |
| Half Smokehouse Turkey on Three Cheese | 1/2 panino | 360 | 126 | 13 | 6 | 55 | 1270 | 34 | 2 | 26 |
| Half Tomato & Mozzarella on Ciabatta | 1/2 panino | 380 | 135 | 15 | 5 | 40 | 1210 | 45 | 3 | 21 |

### SANDWICHES

| | SERVING SIZE | CAL | CAL FAT | TOT FAT (G) | SAT FAT (G) | CHOL (MG) | SOD (MG) | CARB (G) | FIBER (G) | PROT (G) |
|---|---|---|---|---|---|---|---|---|---|---|
| Bacon, Egg, & Cheese On Ciabatta | 1 sandwich | 510 | 216 | 24 | 10 | 215 | 1060 | 44 | 2 | 28 |
| Egg & Cheese on Ciabatta | 1 sandwich | 380 | 126 | 14 | 6 | 190 | 620 | 43 | 2 | 18 |
| Half Smoked Ham & Swiss on Stone-Milled Rye | 1 sandwich | 290 | 72 | 8 | 4 | 45 | 1130 | 33 | 3 | 22 |
| Half Smoked Turkey Breast on Country | 1 sandwich | 220 | 14 | 1.5 | 0 | 25 | 930 | 35 | 2 | 17 |
| Half Tuna Salad on Honey Wheat | 1 sandwich | 240 | 72 | 8 | 2.5 | 10 | 490 | 33 | 3 | 10 |

| | SERVING SIZE | CAL | CAL FAT | TOT FAT (G) | SAT FAT (G) | CHOL (MG) | SOD (MG) | CARB (G) | FIBER (G) | PROT (G) |
|---|---|---|---|---|---|---|---|---|---|---|
| Sausage, Egg, & Cheese on Ciabatta | 1 sandwich | 540 | 252 | 28 | 11 | 230 | 950 | 44 | 2 | 26 |
| **SOUPS & SALADS** | | | | | | | | | | |
| Broccoli Cheddar Soup | as served | 290 | 144 | 16 | 9 | 30 | 1540 | 24 | 7 | 12 |
| French Onion Soup | as served | 250 | 108 | 11 | 5 | 25 | 2380 | 30 | 3 | 10 |
| Full Chicken Caesar Salad | 1 salad | 510 | 261 | 29 | 9 | 115 | 820 | 29 | 3 | 37 |
| Full Chopped Chicken Cobb Salad | 1 salad | 500 | 324 | 36 | 9 | 140 | 1120 | 11 | 3 | 38 |
| Full Classic Café Salad | 1 salad | 170 | 99 | 11 | 1.5 | 0 | 270 | 18 | 4 | 2 |
| Full Greek Salad | 1 salad | 380 | 306 | 34 | 8 | 20 | 1670 | 14 | 5 | 8 |
| New England Clam Chowder | as served | 450 | 306 | 34 | 20 | 50 | 1190 | 29 | 3 | 8 |

# Papa Gino's
## APPETIZERS, SMALL

| | SERVING SIZE | CAL | CAL FAT | TOT FAT (G) | SAT FAT (G) | CHOL (MG) | SOD (MG) | CARB (G) | FIBER (G) | PROT (G) |
|---|---|---|---|---|---|---|---|---|---|---|
| BBQ Chicken Tenders | as served | 520 | 162 | 18 | 3 | 55 | 1520 | 55 | 2 | 29 |
| Cheese Breadsticks | as served | 1300 | 351 | 39 | 18 | 65 | 3730 | 116 | 4 | 44 |
| Chicken Wings BBQ | as served | 640 | 288 | 32 | 7 | 90 | 2820 | 58 | 2 | 26 |
| Chicken Wings Buffalo | as served | 930 | 684 | 76 | 16 | 135 | 4150 | 33 | 6 | 29 |
| Chicken Wings Plain | as served | 480 | 288 | 32 | 7 | 90 | 1880 | 24 | 2 | 26 |
| Cinnamon Sticks | as served | 620 | 171 | 19 | 8 | 5 | 430 | 100 | 4 | 11 |
| Mozzarella Sticks | as served | 950 | 531 | 59 | 21 | 95 | 2350 | 69 | 3 | 44 |
| **PASTA** | | | | | | | | | | |
| Penne or Spaghetti | 1 entrée | 650 | 99 | 11 | 1.5 | 5 | 1130 | 118 | 3 | 21 |
| Penne Alfredo | 1 entrée | 1660 | 324 | 36 | 22 | 110 | 1210 | 111 | 1 | 29 |
| Penne Alfredo Chicken Broccoli | 1 entrée | 1050 | 378 | 42 | 25 | 170 | 1070 | 116 | 4 | 49 |
| Ravioli | 1 entrée | 590 | 216 | 24 | 12 | 25 | 1360 | 71 | 3 | 24 |
| **PIZZA** | | | | | | | | | | |
| Rustic Pizza, Buffalo Chicken | 1 slice | 220 | 81 | 9 | 4 | 20 | 690 | 23 | 2 | 11 |
| Rustic Pizza, Cheese | 1 slice | 200 | 81 | 9 | 4 | 10 | 490 | 23 | 1 | 8 |
| Rustic Pizza, Chicken & Roasted Garlic | 1 slice | 240 | 90 | 10 | 4.5 | 25 | 550 | 25 | 1 | 12 |
| Rustic Pizza, Hawaiian | 1 slice | 220 | 81 | 9 | 4 | 15 | 540 | 26 | 1 | 8 |
| Rustic Pizza, Pepperoni | 1 slice | 240 | 108 | 12 | 5 | 25 | 610 | 24 | 1 | 10 |
| Rustic Pizza, Super Veggie | 1 slice | 230 | 81 | 9 | 4.5 | 15 | 530 | 26 | 2 | 9 |
| Rustic Pizza, The Works | 1 slice | 250 | 117 | 13 | 5 | 25 | 580 | 24 | 2 | 10 |
| Thick Crust, BBQ Chicken | 1 slice | 470 | 81 | 9 | 5 | 35 | 1430 | 70 | 2 | 23 |
| Thick Crust, Buffalo Chicken | 1 slice | 430 | 90 | 10 | 5 | 35 | 1560 | 61 | 4 | 23 |
| Thick Crust, Cheese | 1 slice | 450 | 117 | 13 | 7 | 30 | 1260 | 62 | 3 | 21 |
| Thick Crust, Pepperoni | 1 slice | 480 | 135 | 15 | 7 | 35 | 1340 | 64 | 3 | 21 |
| Thick Crust, Super Veggie | 1 slice | 430 | 90 | 10 | 5 | 20 | 1180 | 66 | 4 | 19 |
| Thick Crust, The Works | 1 slice | 500 | 153 | 17 | 8 | 40 | 1350 | 64 | 4 | 23 |

# restaurants

| | SERVING SIZE | CAL | CAL FAT | TOT FAT (G) | SAT FAT (G) | CHOL (MG) | SOD (MG) | CARB (G) | FIBER (G) | PROT (G) |
|---|---|---|---|---|---|---|---|---|---|---|
| Small Thin Crust Pizza, BBQ Chicken | 1 slice | 210 | 41 | 5 | 2.5 | 15 | 640 | 31 | 1 | 10 |
| Small Thin Crust Pizza, Buffalo Chicken | 1 slice | 180 | 41 | 5 | 2.5 | 15 | 580 | 23 | 1 | 10 |
| Small Thin Crust Pizza, Cheese | 1 slice | 160 | 36 | 4 | 2 | 10 | 420 | 24 | 1 | 7 |
| Small Thin Crust Pizza, Pepperoni | 1 slice | 200 | 72 | 8 | 3.5 | 20 | 560 | 24 | 1 | 9 |
| Small Thin Crust Pizza, Super Veggie | 1 slice | 180 | 45 | 5 | 2.5 | 10 | 480 | 27 | 2 | 8 |
| Large Thin Crust Pizza, BBQ Chicken | 1 slice | 270 | 63 | 7 | 3.5 | 25 | 800 | 38 | 1 | 14 |
| Large Thin Crust Pizza, Buffalo Chicken | 1 slice | 240 | 63 | 7 | 3.5 | 25 | 900 | 31 | 2 | 14 |
| Large Thin Crust Pizza, Pepperoni | 1 slice | 270 | 99 | 11 | 5 | 25 | 740 | 31 | 1 | 12 |
| Large Thin Crust Pizza, Super Veggie | 1 slice | 240 | 63 | 7 | 3.5 | 15 | 620 | 35 | 2 | 11 |
| Large Thin Crust Pizza, The Works | 1 slice | 300 | 108 | 12 | 6 | 30 | 740 | 33 | 2 | 14 |
| **SUB SANDWICHES, SMALL** | | | | | | | | | | |
| BLT | 1 sub | 1010 | 315 | 35 | 13 | 55 | 4080 | 71 | 3 | 29 |
| Chicken Cutlet | 1 sub | 930 | 342 | 38 | 6 | 70 | 1910 | 105 | 3 | 39 |
| Italian | 1 sub | 1260 | 567 | 63 | 27 | 195 | 3810 | 105 | 5 | 66 |
| Meatball | 1 sub | 1210 | 495 | 55 | 23 | 140 | 3180 | 120 | 4 | 56 |
| Steak | 1 sub | 630 | 225 | 25 | 9 | 95 | 780 | 65 | 2 | 34 |
| Tuna | 1 sub | 740 | 351 | 39 | 6 | 60 | 1150 | 67 | 3 | 30 |
| Turkey | 1 sub | 650 | 54 | 5 | 1 | 60 | 1970 | 100 | 3 | 50 |
| Vegetarian | 1 sub | 710 | 135 | 15 | 7 | 35 | 1670 | 112 | 7 | 33 |
| **Papa Johns** | | | | | | | | | | |
| **PIZZA** | | | | | | | | | | |
| 8" Pepperoni | 1 slice | 210 | 80 | 9 | 3.5 | 15 | 560 | 25 | 1 | 8 |
| 10" BBQ Chicken & Bacon | 1 slice | 230 | 70 | 8 | 3 | 25 | 680 | 30 | 1 | 10 |
| 10" Cheese | 1 slice | 180 | 50 | 6 | 2.5 | 15 | 440 | 25 | 1 | 7 |
| 10" Garden Fresh | 1 slice | 140 | 40 | 4.5 | 2 | 10 | 350 | 20 | 1 | 5 |
| 10" Hawaiian BBQ Chicken | 1 slice | 240 | 70 | 8 | 3 | 25 | 680 | 31 | 1 | 10 |
| 10" Pepperoni | 1 slice | 220 | 90 | 9 | 4 | 20 | 580 | 25 | 1 | 8 |
| 10" Sausage | 1 slice | 220 | 90 | 10 | 4 | 20 | 550 | 25 | 1 | 8 |
| 10" Spicy Italian | 1 slice | 240 | 100 | 11 | 4.5 | 20 | 610 | 25 | 1 | 9 |
| 10" Spinach Alfredo | 1 slice | 190 | 70 | 8 | 4 | 20 | 430 | 24 | 1 | 7 |
| 10" The Meats | 1 slice | 250 | 110 | 12 | 4.5 | 25 | 700 | 25 | 1 | 10 |
| 10" The Works | 1 slice | 220 | 80 | 9 | 3.5 | 20 | 620 | 26 | 1 | 9 |
| 10" Tuscan Six Cheese | 1 slice | 220 | 80 | 9 | 4 | 20 | 540 | 26 | 1 | 10 |
| 12" BBQ Chicken & Bacon | 1 slice | 250 | 80 | 8 | 3.5 | 25 | 730 | 32 | 1 | 11 |
| 12" Cheese | 1 slice | 210 | 70 | 8 | 3.5 | 20 | 530 | 26 | 1 | 8 |
| 12" Garden Fresh | 1 slice | 200 | 60 | 7 | 3 | 15 | 500 | 27 | 2 | 8 |
| 12" Hawaiian BBQ Chicken | 1 slice | 240 | 70 | 8 | 3 | 25 | 730 | 33 | 1 | 11 |

| | SERVING SIZE | CAL | CAL FAT | TOT FAT (G) | SAT FAT (G) | CHOL (MG) | SOD (MG) | CARB (G) | FIBER (G) | PROT (G) |
|---|---|---|---|---|---|---|---|---|---|---|
| 12" Pepperoni | 1 slice | 230 | 90 | 10 | 4 | 20 | 610 | 26 | 1 | 9 |
| 12" Sausage | 1 slice | 240 | 100 | 11 | 4.5 | 20 | 600 | 26 | 1 | 8 |
| 12" Spicy Italian | 1 slice | 270 | 120 | 13 | 5 | 25 | 690 | 27 | 1 | 10 |
| 12" Spinach Alfredo | 1 slice | 210 | 70 | 8 | 4 | 20 | 470 | 25 | 1 | 8 |
| 12" The Meats | 1 slice | 250 | 100 | 12 | 5 | 25 | 710 | 26 | 1 | 11 |
| 12" The Works | 1 slice | 230 | 80 | 9 | 4 | 20 | 650 | 27 | 1 | 9 |
| 12" Tuscan Six Cheese | 1 slice | 230 | 80 | 9 | 4.5 | 25 | 580 | 26 | 1 | 10 |
| **SIDES** | | | | | | | | | | |
| Breadsticks | 2 sticks | 290 | 40 | 4.5 | .5 | 0 | 540 | 54 | 2 | 8 |
| Buffalo Wings | as served | 170 | 110 | 13 | 3 | 50 | 1070 | 3 | 0 | 12 |
| Cheesesticks | 4 sticks | 370 | 150 | 16 | 7 | 35 | 860 | 41 | 2 | 14 |
| Chickenstrips | 2 strips | 130 | 40 | 4.5 | .5 | 25 | 430 | 10 | 0 | 12 |

# Peet's Coffee & Tea
## BAKERY

| | SERVING SIZE | CAL | CAL FAT | TOT FAT (G) | SAT FAT (G) | CHOL (MG) | SOD (MG) | CARB (G) | FIBER (G) | PROT (G) |
|---|---|---|---|---|---|---|---|---|---|---|
| Bagel | 1 bagel | 275 | 6 | 1 | 0 | 0 | 430 | 58 | 2 | 8 |
| Blueberry Muffin | 1 muffin | 480 | 180 | 21 | 9 | 100 | 530 | 65 | 2 | 8 |
| Carrot Cake w/Cream Cheese Frosting | 1 cake | 440 | 190 | 21 | 4 | 60 | 230 | 58 | 1 | 4 |
| Chocolate Chip Cookie | 1 cookie | 410 | 180 | 20 | 9 | 50 | 280 | 50 | 4 | 5 |
| Devil's Food Cupcake | as served | 500 | 220 | 25 | 10 | 55 | 330 | 68 | 1 | 4 |
| Fudge Brownie | as served | 390 | 180 | 20 | 10 | 105 | 80 | 50 | 4 | 5 |
| Low Fat Banana Blueberry Muffin | 1 muffin | 290 | 50 | 3 | 1 | 0 | 300 | 54 | 2 | 4 |
| Low Fat Brownie | as served | 360 | 45 | 6 | 2 | 36 | 270 | 73 | 6 | 4 |
| Peanut Butter Cookie | 1 cookie | 430 | 210 | 23 | 9 | 55 | 260 | 52 | 2 | 9 |
| Reduced Fat Carrot Ginger Muffin | 1 muffin | 350 | 60 | 6 | .5 | 0 | 330 | 69 | 3 | 7 |
| Sugar Cookie | 1 cookie | 290 | 90 | 12 | 7 | 55 | 150 | 40 | 1 | 4 |
| **BLENDED FREDDOS** | | | | | | | | | | |
| Berry Pomegranate, Standard | 16 fl oz | 207 | 0 | 0 | 0 | 0 | 131 | 53 | 1 | 0 |
| Caffe Extra Bold, Reduced Fat Milk | 16 fl oz | 229 | 27 | 3 | 2 | 10 | 200 | 48 | 1 | 5 |
| Caffe, Reduced Fat Milk | 16 fl oz | 229 | 27 | 3 | 2 | 10 | 200 | 48 | 1 | 5 |
| Chai, Reduced Fat Milk | 16 fl oz | 331 | 36 | 4 | 2 | 15 | 231 | 67 | 0 | 8 |
| Chocolate & Caramel Swirl, Reduced Fat Milk | 16 fl oz | 394 | 27 | 3 | 2 | 10 | 245 | 84 | 2 | 8 |
| Dark Chocolate. Caramel Mocha, Reduced Fat Milk | 16 fl oz | 402 | 45 | 5 | 3 | 10 | 203 | 83 | 2 | 8 |
| Madagascar Vanilla, Reduced Fat Milk | 16 fl oz | 306 | 27 | 3 | 2 | 10 | 186 | 67 | 0 | 5 |
| Mango Tea, 2% Milk | 16 fl oz | 301 | 36 | 4 | 2 | 15 | 226 | 61 | 1 | 8 |
| Mocha, Reduced Fat Milk | 16 fl oz | 251 | 27 | 3 | 2 | 10 | 196 | 51 | 1 | 6 |

| | SERVING SIZE | CAL | CAL FAT | TOT FAT (G) | SAT FAT (G) | CHOL (MG) | SOD (MG) | CARB (G) | FIBER (G) | PROT (G) |
|---|---|---|---|---|---|---|---|---|---|---|
| **BREWED COFFEE** | | | | | | | | | | |
| Caffe au Lait, Reduced Fat Milk | 16 fl oz | 70 | 27 | 3 | 2 | 21 | 70 | 7 | 0 | 5 |
| **ESPRESSO BEVERAGES** | | | | | | | | | | |
| **(reduced fat milk)** | | | | | | | | | | |
| Caffe Latte | 16 fl oz | 211 | 72 | 8 | 5 | 33 | 228 | 21 | 0 | 16 |
| Caffe Mocha | 16 fl oz | 300 | 72 | 8 | 5 | 30 | 230 | 40 | 2 | 16 |
| Caffe Vanilla Latte | 16 fl oz | 310 | 72 | 8 | 5 | 30 | 210 | 46 | 0 | 15 |
| Cappuccino | 16 fl oz | 130 | 45 | 5 | 3 | 20 | 140 | 13 | 0 | 10 |
| Caramel Caffe Latte | 16 fl oz | 381 | 72 | 8 | 4 | 29 | 254 | 61 | 0 | 17 |
| Latte Macchiato | 16 fl oz | 211 | 72 | 8 | 5 | 33 | 228 | 21 | 0 | 16 |
| **ICED COFFEES** | | | | | | | | | | |
| **(reduced fat milk)** | | | | | | | | | | |
| Caffe Latte | 16 fl oz | 175 | 54 | 6 | 4 | 25 | 175 | 18 | 0 | 3 |
| Caffe Latte w/Vanilla | 16 fl oz | 275 | 54 | 6 | 4 | 25 | 175 | 43 | 0 | 11 |
| Caffe Mocha | 16 fl oz | 248 | 54 | 6 | 3 | 23 | 178 | 35 | 2 | 13 |
| Cappuccino | 16 fl oz | 158 | 54 | 6 | 3 | 23 | 158 | 16 | 0 | 11 |
| Caramel Latte | 16 fl oz | 338 | 54 | 6 | 3 | 23 | 210 | 56 | 0 | 14 |
| **TEAS** | | | | | | | | | | |
| Hibiscus Breeze Iced Tea Cooler | 16 fl oz | 98 | 0 | 0 | 0 | 0 | 5 | 25 | 0 | 0 |
| Iced Masala Chai Latte, Reduced Fat Milk | 16 fl oz | 213 | 36 | 4 | 3 | 18 | 133 | 34 | 0 | 9 |
| Jasmine Lime Iced Tea Cooler | 16 fl oz | 127 | 0 | 0 | 0 | 0 | 7 | 32 | 0 | 0 |
| Masala Chai Latte, Reduced Fat Milk | 16 fl oz | 213 | 36 | 4 | 3 | 18 | 133 | 34 | 0 | 9 |

## Pei Wei Asian Diner
### FRIED RICE

| | SERVING SIZE | CAL | CAL FAT | TOT FAT (G) | SAT FAT (G) | CHOL (MG) | SOD (MG) | CARB (G) | FIBER (G) | PROT (G) |
|---|---|---|---|---|---|---|---|---|---|---|
| Beef | 1 entrée | 520 | 144 | 16 | 4 | n/a | 1380 | 68 | 3 | 24 |
| Chicken | 1 entrée | 500 | 108 | 12 | 2.5 | n/a | 1210 | 66 | 2 | 29 |
| Shrimp | 1 entrée | 460 | 99 | 11 | 2.5 | n/a | 1330 | 65 | 2 | 23 |
| Vegetables & Tofu | 1 entrée | 530 | 144 | 16 | 3 | n/a | 1360 | 72 | 6 | 22 |
| **NOODLES** | | | | | | | | | | |
| Beef Lo Mein | 1 entrée | 540 | 180 | 20 | 4.5 | n/a | 1260 | 68 | 5 | 25 |
| Chicken Lo Mein | 1 entrée | 560 | 180 | 20 | 3.5 | n/a | 1170 | 67 | 5 | 30 |
| Egg Noodles | 1 entrée | 220 | 27 | 3 | .5 | n/a | 10 | 39 | 2 | 7 |
| Rice Noodles | 1 entrée | 270 | 0 | 0 | 0 | n/a | 10 | 67 | 0 | 0 |
| **SALADS** | | | | | | | | | | |
| Asian Chopped Chicken, w/o dressing | 1 salad | 170 | 36 | 4 | 1 | n/a | 160 | 12 | 2 | 22 |
| Spicy Chicken, w/o dressing | 1 salad | 505 | 171 | 19 | 3 | n/a | 1210 | 60 | 5 | 23 |
| Vietnamese Chicken Rolls w/o sauce | 3 rolls | 160 | 54 | 6 | 0.5 | n/a | 430 | 18 | 1 | 9 |

| | SERVING SIZE | CAL | CAL FAT | TOT FAT (G) | SAT FAT (G) | CHOL (MG) | SOD (MG) | CARB (G) | FIBER (G) | PROT (G) |
|---|---|---|---|---|---|---|---|---|---|---|
| **SMALL PLATES & SOUPS** | | | | | | | | | | |
| Crispy Potstickers w/o sauce | 2 items | 150 | 72 | 8 | 2.5 | n/a | 310 | 12 | 1 | 7 |
| Hot & Sour Soup, Cup | 6 oz | 190 | 72 | 8 | 2 | n/a | 1640 | 12 | 2 | 16 |
| Pork Egg Rolls w/o sauce | 1 egg roll | 180 | 63 | 7 | 2.5 | n/a | 1360 | 19 | 2 | 8 |
| Thai Wonton Soup, Cup | 6 oz | 110 | 54 | 6 | 2 | n/a | 1030 | 5 | 1 | 10 |
| **SWEET & SOUR** | | | | | | | | | | |
| Beef | 1 entrée | 290 | 72 | 8 | 2.5 | n/a | 660 | 39 | 2 | 17 |
| Chicken | 1 entrée | 360 | 90 | 10 | 2 | n/a | 690 | 48 | 5 | 22 |

## Pepe's Mexican Restaurants
### TACOS & BURRITOS

| | SERVING SIZE | CAL | CAL FAT | TOT FAT (G) | SAT FAT (G) | CHOL (MG) | SOD (MG) | CARB (G) | FIBER (G) | PROT (G) |
|---|---|---|---|---|---|---|---|---|---|---|
| Beef & Bean Suizo Burrito | 1 burrito | 640 | 310 | 34 | 14 | 70 | 1170 | 55 | 10 | 30 |
| Beef, Crisp Shell | 1 taco | 210 | 100 | 11 | 4.5 | 30 | 400 | 16 | 3 | 12 |
| Beef, Soft Corn Shell | 1 taco | 250 | 90 | 10 | 4 | 30 | 440 | 28 | 4 | 13 |
| Beef, Soft Flour Shell | 1 taco | 250 | 100 | 11 | 4.5 | 30 | 520 | 24 | 3 | 13 |
| Chicken & Bean Suizo Burrito | 1 burrito | 610 | 280 | 31 | 13 | 80 | 1140 | 54 | 9 | 30 |
| Chicken, Crisp Shell | 1 taco | 190 | 80 | 9 | 3 | 35 | 380 | 15 | 2 | 12 |
| Chicken, Soft Corn Shell | 1 taco | 230 | 70 | 8 | 35 | 35 | 420 | 27 | 4 | 13 |
| Chicken, Soft Flour Shell | 1 taco | 230 | 80 | 9 | 3 | 35 | 500 | 23 | 2 | 14 |
| Pork & Bean Suizo Burrito | 1 burrito | 600 | 260 | 29 | 12 | 70 | 1150 | 54 | 10 | 32 |
| **TOSTADAS & FLAUTAS** | | | | | | | | | | |
| Beef & Bean Suiza | 1 tostada | 440 | 260 | 29 | 11 | 55 | 750 | 26 | 4 | 19 |
| Beef Flautas w/Cheese & Sauce | 1 flauta | 190 | 110 | 12 | 3 | 25 | 300 | 11 | 2 | 10 |
| Chicken & Bean Suiza | 1 tostada | 410 | 240 | 26 | 10 | 60 | 740 | 25 | 4 | 19 |
| Chicken Flautas w/Cheese & Sauce | 1 flauta | 230 | 120 | 13 | 2 | 10 | 250 | 17 | 2 | 11 |
| Pork & Bean Suiza | 1 tostada | 410 | 230 | 25 | 9 | 55 | 740 | 26 | 4 | 20 |
| **SALADS** | | | | | | | | | | |
| Beef Taco w/4 oz Salsa—No Shell | 1 salad | 330 | 170 | 19 | 9 | 60 | 1300 | 20 | 6 | 22 |
| Chicken Taco w/4 oz Salsa—No Shell | 1 salad | 300 | 140 | 16 | 7 | 70 | 1270 | 19 | 6 | 22 |
| Pork Taco w/4 oz Salsa—No Shell | 1 salad | 290 | 120 | 13 | 7 | 55 | 1280 | 19 | 6 | 24 |

## Perkins
### APPETIZERS

| | SERVING SIZE | CAL | CAL FAT | TOT FAT (G) | SAT FAT (G) | CHOL (MG) | SOD (MG) | CARB (G) | FIBER (G) | PROT (G) |
|---|---|---|---|---|---|---|---|---|---|---|
| Buffalo Dippers | 1 entrée | 1090 | 670 | 74 | 13 | 165 | 6010 | 64 | 2 | 46 |
| Chick'n Cheese Quesadilla | 1 entrée | 920 | 430 | 48 | 25 | 165 | 2490 | 67 | 4 | 56 |
| Perkins Sampler Platter | 1 entrée | 1970 | 1120 | 125 | 28 | 210 | 4210 | 150 | 6 | 64 |
| **BREAKFAST** | | | | | | | | | | |
| All American Breakfast | 1 entrée | 990 | 380 | 42 | 11 | 445 | 2690 | 121 | 8 | 33 |

# restaurants

| | SERVING SIZE | CAL | CAL FAT | TOT FAT (G) | SAT FAT (G) | CHOL (MG) | SOD (MG) | CARB (G) | FIBER (G) | PROT (G) |
|---|---|---|---|---|---|---|---|---|---|---|
| Belgian Waffle | 1 entrée | 700 | 300 | 33 | 14 | 125 | 1020 | 92 | 2 | 9 |
| Blueberry Compote | 1 entrée | 210 | 0 | 0 | 0 | 0 | 95 | 53 | 2 | 0 |
| Border Grilled Chicken Omelette | 1 entrée | 400 | 70 | 8 | 2 | 40 | 1290 | 43 | 5 | 38 |
| Classic Eggs & Bacon | 1 entrée | 1420 | 520 | 58 | 16 | 530 | 3920 | 181 | 7 | 44 |
| French Toast Combo | 1 entrée | 910 | 370 | 41 | 12 | 675 | 1280 | 98 | 2 | 38 |
| Short Stack Pancakes | 1 entrée | 730 | 310 | 35 | 11 | 65 | 1500 | 92 | 0 | 12 |
| Smoked Ham Steak | 1 entrée | 260 | 90 | 10 | 2.5 | 100 | 2100 | 9 | 0 | 34 |
| Southern Fried Chicken Biscuit Platter | 1 entrée | 1860 | 780 | 86 | 43 | 555 | 6680 | 196 | 11 | 74 |
| Southern Fried Chicken Scrambler | 1 entrée | 1440 | 620 | 69 | 20 | 560 | 3120 | 158 | 6 | 47 |
| Steak & Eggs | 1 entrée | 1490 | 480 | 54 | 15 | 600 | 3460 | 181 | 7 | 71 |
| **ENTRÉES** | | | | | | | | | | |
| Cavatappi Marinara Pasta | 1 entrée | 960 | 490 | 54 | 16 | 5 | 1610 | 96 | 8 | 23 |
| Down Home Meatloaf | 1 entrée | 1040 | 590 | 65 | 26 | 270 | 2530 | 72 | 6 | 41 |
| Grilled Pork Chops | 1 entrée | 1110 | 520 | 58 | 20 | 175 | 2050 | 75 | 9 | 69 |
| Island Tilapia Dinner | 1 entrée | 450 | 50 | 6 | 1.5 | 100 | 1060 | 50 | 5 | 50 |
| Mushroom 'n Swiss Chicken Dinner | 1 entrée | 1130 | 400 | 45 | 15 | 125 | 2320 | 123 | 8 | 58 |
| Roast Beef Dinner | 1 entrée | 780 | 380 | 42 | 17 | 130 | 2210 | 57 | 6 | 41 |
| Top Sirloin Steak Dinner | 1 entrée | 770 | 310 | 34 | 12 | 115 | 470 | 67 | 8 | 50 |
| **SANDWICHES & BURGERS** | | | | | | | | | | |
| Buffalo Wrap | 1 wrap | 1460 | 880 | 98 | 25 | 125 | 5270 | 105 | 6 | 42 |
| Chicken Crisp Melt | 1 sandwich | 1710 | 1000 | 111 | 28 | 165 | 3750 | 128 | 5 | 61 |
| Chipotle Bleu Chicken Sandwich | 1 sandwich | 1210 | 610 | 68 | 15 | 70 | 2890 | 115 | 9 | 39 |
| Country Club Melt | 1 sandwich | 1380 | 760 | 84 | 29 | 155 | 3630 | 95 | 5 | 62 |
| Ham & Turkey BLT Wrap | 1 wrap | 1080 | 620 | 69 | 14 | 80 | 3090 | 89 | 6 | 31 |
| Hamburger | 1 burger | 1060 | 560 | 62 | 18 | 160 | 1220 | 71 | 6 | 56 |
| Kickin Chicken Sandwich | 1 sandwich | 1350 | 670 | 75 | 20 | 115 | 3450 | 118 | 8 | 54 |
| **SOUPS & SALADS** | | | | | | | | | | |
| Broccoli & Cheddar Cheese Soup | 1 cup | 180 | 100 | 12 | 5 | 35 | 930 | 13 | 1 | 6 |
| BLT Chicken Breast Salad | 1 salad | 620 | 320 | 36 | 11 | 130 | 1430 | 25 | 4 | 50 |
| Chef Deluxe Salad | 1 salad | 830 | 490 | 55 | 21 | 370 | 2120 | 27 | 4 | 58 |
| Chicken & Spinach Salad | 1 salad | 960 | 590 | 65 | 14 | 320 | 2210 | 37 | 5 | 56 |
| Homestyle Chicken Noodle Soup | 1 cup | 100 | 25 | 3 | .5 | 35 | 220 | 10 | 1 | 7 |
| Honey Mustard Chicken Crunch Salad | 1 salad | 1240 | 740 | 83 | 21 | 160 | 2510 | 78 | 5 | 50 |
| New England Clam Chowder | 1 cup | 160 | 80 | 9 | 5 | 40 | 710 | 12 | 1 | 9 |
| Vegetable Beef Soup | 1 cup | 100 | 25 | 3 | .5 | 10 | 740 | 12 | 3 | 6 |

# Petro's Chili & Chips

| | SERVING SIZE | CAL | CAL FAT | TOT FAT (G) | SAT FAT (G) | CHOL (MG) | SOD (MG) | CARB (G) | FIBER (G) | PROT (G) |
|---|---|---|---|---|---|---|---|---|---|---|
| Chili & Cheese Hot Dog | 1 hot dog | 347 | 172.8 | 19.2 | 6.8 | 33.5 | 987 | 29 | 1.5 | 13.8 |

| | SERVING SIZE | CAL | CAL FAT | TOT FAT (G) | SAT FAT (G) | CHOL (MG) | SOD (MG) | CARB (G) | FIBER (G) | PROT (G) |
|---|---|---|---|---|---|---|---|---|---|---|
| Loaded Potato | 1 potato | 679 | 297 | 33 | 15 | 56 | 573 | 78 | 9 | 21 |
| Nacho Chips & Queso | as served | 500 | 243 | 27 | 8 | 22 | 896 | 60 | n/a | 11 |
| Pasta Petro, Medium | as served | 627 | 239.4 | 26.6 | 11 | 61.2 | 1260 | 67.6 | 9.5 | 29.7 |
| Pasta Petro Lite, Medium | as served | 494 | 31.5 | 3.5 | .2 | 15 | 1277 | 79.7 | 6.7 | 33.1 |
| Petro Nachos | as served | 880 | 459 | 51 | 21 | 89 | 1805 | 79 | .7 | 34 |
| Petro Lite, Medium | as served | 532 | 144 | 16 | 3 | 33 | 1906 | 66 | 3 | 30 |
| Petro, Original, Medium | as served | 665 | 324 | 36 | 15 | 76 | 1728 | 59 | 3 | 27 |
| Petro, Vegetarian, Medium | as served | 745 | 369 | 41 | 16 | 56 | 1576 | 70 | 3 | 24 |

## P. F. Chang's
### CHICKEN

| | SERVING SIZE | CAL | CAL FAT | TOT FAT (G) | SAT FAT (G) | CHOL (MG) | SOD (MG) | CARB (G) | FIBER (G) | PROT (G) |
|---|---|---|---|---|---|---|---|---|---|---|
| Almond & Cashew Chicken | 1/3 entrée | 373 | 162 | 18 | 3 | n/a | 1960 | 24 | 2 | 29 |
| Kung Pao Chicken | 1/3 entrée | 383 | 207 | 23 | 4 | n/a | 940 | 14 | 2 | 33 |
| Mandarin Chicken | 1/2 entrée | 360 | 135 | 15 | 2 | n/a | 1715 | 29 | 3 | 33 |
| Mu shu Chicken | 1/2 entrée | 285 | 117 | 13 | 3 | n/a | 1540 | 16 | 3 | 26 |
| Sesame Chicken | 1/3 entrée | 343 | 126 | 14 | 2 | n/a | 1020 | 25 | 2 | 30 |
| Sweet & Sour Chicken | 1/3 entrée | 370 | 171 | 19 | 3 | n/a | 367 | 38 | 0 | 12 |

### GLUTEN FREE

| | SERVING SIZE | CAL | CAL FAT | TOT FAT (G) | SAT FAT (G) | CHOL (MG) | SOD (MG) | CARB (G) | FIBER (G) | PROT (G) |
|---|---|---|---|---|---|---|---|---|---|---|
| Beef a la Sichuan | 1/3 entrée | 293 | 99 | 11 | 3 | n/a | 910 | 26 | 1 | 23 |
| Beef w/Broccoli | 1/3 entrée | 290 | 108 | 12 | 3 | n/a | 1300 | 21 | 2 | 24 |
| Cantonese Shrimp | 1/2 entrée | 215 | 90 | 10 | 2 | n/a | 950 | 10 | 2 | 21 |
| Chang's Fried Rice (Combo) | 1/4 entrée | 353 | 117 | 13 | 3 | n/a | 900 | 40 | 1 | 19 |
| Chicken Lettuce Wraps | 1/4 entrée | 158 | 63 | 7 | 1 | n/a | 670 | 15 | 2 | 9 |
| Dali Chicken | 1/3 entrée | 280 | 108 | 12 | 2 | n/a | 370 | 16 | 1 | 27 |
| Egg Drop Soup | 7 oz | 60 | 27 | 3 | 0 | n/a | 640 | 8 | 0 | 1 |
| Ginger Chicken w/Broccoli | 1/3 entrée | 270 | 99 | 11 | 2 | n/a | 990 | 17 | 2 | 28 |
| Hong Kong Beef w/Snow Peas | 1/2 entrée | 335 | 126 | 14 | 3 | n/a | 1480 | 28 | 3 | 25 |
| Salmon Steamed w/Ginger | 1/2 entrée | 220 | 27 | 3 | 1 | n/a | 1160 | 13 | 2 | 32 |
| Singapore Street Noodles | 1/3 entrée | 300 | 63 | 7 | 1 | n/a | 980 | 41 | 3 | 11 |

### NOODLES & RICE

| | SERVING SIZE | CAL | CAL FAT | TOT FAT (G) | SAT FAT (G) | CHOL (MG) | SOD (MG) | CARB (G) | FIBER (G) | PROT (G) |
|---|---|---|---|---|---|---|---|---|---|---|
| Canton Chicken & Mushrooms | 1/2 entrée | 550 | 207 | 23 | 4 | n/a | 1410 | 48 | 3 | 38 |
| Cantonese Chow Fun (Chicken) | 1/2 entrée | 790 | 180 | 20 | 4 | n/a | 1615 | 88 | 5 | 32 |
| Dan Dan Noodles | 1/4 entrée | 270 | 63 | 7 | 1 | n/a | 1388 | 30 | 2 | 13 |
| Double Pan Fried Noodles (Combo) | 1/4 entrée | 455 | 189 | 21 | 2 | n/a | 1923 | 44 | 1 | 16 |
| Garlic Noodles | 1/4 entrée | 178 | 36 | 4 | 1 | n/a | 360 | 31 | 1 | 5 |
| Lo Mein (Combo) | 1/3 entrée | 347 | 126 | 14 | 0 | n/a | 1413 | 23 | 2 | 23 |

### SEAFOOD

| | SERVING SIZE | CAL | CAL FAT | TOT FAT (G) | SAT FAT (G) | CHOL (MG) | SOD (MG) | CARB (G) | FIBER (G) | PROT (G) |
|---|---|---|---|---|---|---|---|---|---|---|
| Kung Pao Scallops | 1/3 entrée | 307 | 180 | 20 | 3 | n/a | 1126 | 17 | 2 | 16 |

| | SERVING SIZE | CAL | CAL FAT | TOT FAT (G) | SAT FAT (G) | CHOL (MG) | SOD (MG) | CARB (G) | FIBER (G) | PROT (G) |
|---|---|---|---|---|---|---|---|---|---|---|
| Kung Pao Shrimp | 1/3 entrée | 280 | 153 | 17 | 3 | n/a | 1083 | 12 | 2 | 21 |
| Lemongrass Prawns w/Garlic Noodles | 1/2 entrée | 485 | 270 | 30 | 10 | n/a | 935 | 32 | 2 | 24 |
| Mahi-Mahi | 1/2 entrée | 420 | 153 | 17 | 8 | n/a | 605 | 42 | 2 | 25 |
| Sichuan from the Sea (Combo) | 1/4 entrée | 215 | 108 | 12 | 2 | n/a | 553 | 14 | 0 | 12 |
| **STARTERS & SMALL PLATES** | | | | | | | | | | |
| Crab Wontons | 6 wontons | 163 | 90 | 10 | 4 | n/a | 303 | 13 | 0 | 5 |
| Egg Rolls | 2 rolls | 174 | 72 | 8 | 1 | n/a | 673 | 22 | 3 | 5 |
| Pan Fried Pork Dumplings | 1 dumpling | 70 | 36 | 4 | 1 | n/a | 125 | 6 | 0 | 4 |
| Spring Rolls | 2 rolls | 156 | 72 | 8 | 1 | n/a | 271 | 17 | 2 | 4 |
| Vegetarian Lettuce Wraps | 1/4 plate | 140 | 63 | 7 | 1 | n/a | 530 | 11 | 2 | 6 |
| **VEGETARIAN** | | | | | | | | | | |
| Buddha's Feast (Steamed) | 1/2 entrée | 55 | 0 | 0 | 0 | n/a | 40 | 11 | 4 | 4 |
| Coconut Curry Vegetables | 1/2 entrée | 510 | 324 | 36 | 12 | n/a | 650 | 26 | 5 | 22 |
| Fried Rice | 1/4 entrée | 190 | 18 | 2 | 0 | n/a | 230 | 38 | 2 | 5 |
| Ma Po Tofu | 1/3 entrée | 350 | 207 | 23 | 5 | n/a | 1060 | 17 | 2 | 20 |
| Stir-Fried Eggplant | 1/4 entrée | 270 | 198 | 22 | 3 | n/a | 760 | 14 | 2 | 2 |
| Vegetable Chow Fun | 1/4 entrée | 250 | 18 | 2 | 0 | n/a | 750 | 46 | 3 | 2 |
| **Pinkberry** **FROZEN YOGURT** | | | | | | | | | | |
| Chocolate | 1/2 cup | 120 | 10 | 1.5 | 1 | <5 | 110 | 23 | 2 | 5 |
| Coconut | 1/2 cup | 140 | 5 | .5 | 0 | <5 | 50 | 30 | 0 | 4 |
| Fruit Parafait | 1 cup | 270 | 50 | 5 | 0 | <5 | 50 | 49 | 2 | 7 |
| Green Tea | 1/2 cup | 110 | 0 | 0 | 0 | 5 | 45 | 25 | 1 | 4 |
| Mango | 1/2 cup | 100 | 0 | 0 | 0 | 5 | 45 | 23 | 0 | 3 |
| Original | 1/2 cup | 100 | 0 | 0 | 0 | 5 | 50 | 21 | 0 | 3 |
| Passionfruit | 1/2 cup | 110 | 0 | 0 | 0 | 0 | 45 | 24 | 0 | 3 |
| Pomegranate | 1/2 cup | 120 | 0 | 0 | 0 | 0 | 40 | 26 | 0 | 3 |
| **SMOOTHIES** | | | | | | | | | | |
| Green Tea | 16 fl oz | 240 | 0 | 0 | 0 | 7 | 151 | 49 | 0 | 9 |
| Original | 16 fl oz | 280 | 0 | 0 | 0 | 10 | 135 | 58 | 2 | 11 |
| **Pizza Hut** **PIZZA** | | | | | | | | | | |
| Average of all 12" Fit 'n Delicious Pizza | 1 slice | 160 | 40 | 4.5 | 1.5 | 20 | 720 | 22 | 1 | 11 |
| 6" Pan Pizza, Cheese Only | 1 pizza | 590 | 210 | 24 | 10 | 55 | 1290 | 69 | 3 | 26 |
| 6" Pan Pizza, Meat Lover's | 1 pizza | 830 | 410 | 46 | 17 | 100 | 2110 | 68 | 3 | 36 |
| 6" Pan Pizza, Pepperoni & Mushroom | 1 pizza | 570 | 200 | 23 | 9 | 45 | 1250 | 68 | 4 | 24 |

| | SERVING SIZE | CAL | CAL FAT | TOT FAT (G) | SAT FAT (G) | CHOL (MG) | SOD (MG) | CARB (G) | FIBER (G) | PROT (G) |
|---|---|---|---|---|---|---|---|---|---|---|
| 9" PANormous Pizza, Cheese Only | 1 pizza | 1100 | 410 | 45 | 19 | 105 | 2400 | 124 | 6 | 48 |
| 9" PANormous Pizza, Meat Lover's | 1 pizza | 1470 | 720 | 80 | 30 | 175 | 3670 | 123 | 6 | 64 |
| 9" PANormous Pizza, Pepperoni | 1 pizza | 1100 | 430 | 48 | 18 | 100 | 2540 | 121 | 6 | 47 |
| 9" PANormous Pizza, Pepperoni & Mushroom | 1 pizza | 1050 | 380 | 42 | 16 | 85 | 2290 | 123 | 7 | 45 |
| Hand Tossed Pizza, Dan's Original | 1 slice | 380 | 160 | 18 | 8 | 40 | 960 | 38 | 2 | 17 |
| Pan Pizza, Dan's Original | 1 slice | 420 | 200 | 22 | 8 | 40 | 880 | 37 | 2 | 17 |
| Stuffed Crust Pizza, Dan's Original | 1 slice | 420 | 190 | 21 | 9 | 50 | 1090 | 39 | 2 | 19 |
| Thin 'N Crispy Pizza, Dan's Original | 1 slice | 320 | 150 | 16 | 7 | 40 | 890 | 29 | 1 | 15 |
| **SIDES** | | | | | | | | | | |
| Fried Cheese Sticks | 4 pieces | 380 | 220 | 24 | 9 | 40 | 1020 | 29 | 2 | 13 |
| Stuffed Pizza Rollers | 1 piece | 230 | 90 | 10 | 4.5 | 25 | 590 | 24 | 1 | 9 |
| Wedge Fries | 1/2 order | 320 | 160 | 18 | 3.5 | 0 | 530 | 35 | 3 | 4 |
| **TUSCANI PASTA** | | | | | | | | | | |
| Bacon Mac N Cheese | 1/2 entrée | 520 | 200 | 22 | 12 | 60 | 1170 | 54 | 4 | 24 |
| Chicken Alfredo | 1/2 entrée | 630 | 300 | 33 | 11 | 70 | 1180 | 56 | 4 | 27 |
| Lasagna | 1/2 entrée | 600 | 300 | 33 | 15 | 100 | 1600 | 43 | 5 | 31 |
| **WINGS** | | | | | | | | | | |
| All American, Bone Out | 2 wings | 150 | 70 | 8 | 1.5 | 20 | 490 | 11 | 1 | 10 |
| All American, Crispy Bone In | 2 wings | 200 | 130 | 14 | 2.5 | 45 | 500 | 8 | 1 | 9 |
| All American, Traditional | 2 wings | 80 | 45 | 5 | 1.5 | 40 | 290 | 0 | 0 | 7 |
| Burnin' Hot Buffalo, Bone Out | 2 wings | 190 | 80 | 8 | 1.5 | 20 | 1000 | 18 | 1 | 10 |
| Burnin' Hot Buffalo, Crispy Bone In | 2 wings | 230 | 130 | 15 | 3 | 45 | 1020 | 16 | 1 | 9 |
| Cajun, Bone Out | 2 wings | 220 | 70 | 8 | 1.5 | 20 | 790 | 21 | 1 | 10 |
| Cajun, Crispy Bone In | 2 wings | 240 | 130 | 14 | 3 | 45 | 810 | 19 | 2 | 10 |
| Honey BBQ, Traditional | 2 wings | 140 | 45 | 5 | 1.5 | 40 | 530 | 16 | 0 | 8 |
| Spicy BBQ, Bone Out | 2 wings | 200 | 70 | 8 | 1.5 | 25 | 940 | 21 | 1 | 10 |
| Spicy BBQ, Traditional | 2 wings | 120 | 45 | 5 | 1.5 | 45 | 750 | 11 | 0 | 8 |

## Pollo Tropical
### DESSERTS

| | SERVING SIZE | CAL | CAL FAT | TOT FAT (G) | SAT FAT (G) | CHOL (MG) | SOD (MG) | CARB (G) | FIBER (G) | PROT (G) |
|---|---|---|---|---|---|---|---|---|---|---|
| Flan | as served | 210 | 81 | 9 | 5 | 90 | 550 | 26 | 1 | 8 |
| Guava Cheesecake | as served | 310 | 153 | 17 | 10 | 50 | 230 | 36 | 1 | 5 |
| Tres Leches | as served | 380 | 81 | 9 | 5 | 70 | 210 | 76 | 0 | 9 |
| Cream Smoothies Average | 1 smoothie | 330 | 72 | 8 | 6 | 20 | 80 | 63 | 0 | 3 |
| **ENTRÉES** | | | | | | | | | | |
| 1/2 Rack Ribs | 1 entrée | 400 | 279 | 31 | 13 | 100 | 680 | 2 | 0 | 29 |
| 1/4 Chicken Dark Meat w/o Skin | 1 entrée | 180 | 81 | 9 | 5 | 105 | 250 | 0 | 0 | 24 |
| 1/4 Chicken White Meat | 1 entrée | 350 | 153 | 17 | 5 | 185 | 770 | 0 | 0 | 47 |

# restaurants

| | SERVING SIZE | CAL | CAL FAT | TOT FAT (G) | SAT FAT (G) | CHOL (MG) | SOD (MG) | CARB (G) | FIBER (G) | PROT (G) |
|---|---|---|---|---|---|---|---|---|---|---|
| Boneless Chicken Breasts | 2 pieces | 230 | 36 | 4 | 1 | 160 | 330 | 0 | 0 | 51 |
| Caribbean Cobb Chicken Salad | 1 salad | 1190 | 495 | 55 | 17 | 240 | 2140 | 72 | 8 | 17 |
| Chicken Caesar Salad | 1 salad | 620 | 360 | 40 | 8 | 195 | 860 | 15 | 4 | 59 |
| Chicken Caesar Wrap | 1 wrap | 370 | 153 | 17 | 3 | 60 | 690 | 30 | 3 | 24 |
| Chicken Fajita | 1 entrée | 1130 | 306 | 34 | 13 | 155 | 2590 | 149 | 15 | 66 |
| Chicken TropiChops w/White Rice, Black Beans | 1 entrée | 530 | 90 | 10 | 2 | 55 | 1460 | 90 | 10 | 31 |
| Churrasco Steak | 1 entrée | 170 | 63 | 7 | 3 | 25 | 740 | 4 | 0 | 19 |
| Cuban Wrap | 1 wrap | 400 | 189 | 21 | 7 | 60 | 1120 | 29 | 3 | 26 |
| Pork TropiChops w/White Rice, Black Beans | 1 entrée | 680 | 198 | 22 | 8 | 70 | 1530 | 92 | 11 | 39 |
| Roast Pork | 1 entrée | 400 | 198 | 22 | 10 | 145 | 320 | 1 | 0 | 48 |
| Ropa Vieja TropiChops | 1 entrée | 600 | 144 | 16 | 4 | 65 | 1990 | 98 | 12 | 28 |
| Steak Fajita | 1 entrée | 1140 | 360 | 40 | 14 | 60 | 3270 | 154 | 17 | 47 |
| Vegetarian Tropichops | 1 entrée | 580 | 108 | 12 | 3 | 0 | 1200 | 110 | 16 | 18 |
| **SIDES** | | | | | | | | | | |
| Caesar Salad, Regular | 1 salad | 210 | 171 | 19 | 4 | 25 | 350 | 7 | 2 | 5 |
| Cheezy Yuca Bites | 6 pieces | 290 | 126 | 14 | 4 | 15 | 770 | 32 | 2 | 6 |
| Curly Fries, Regular | as served | 290 | 144 | 16 | 2 | 0 | 690 | 33 | 5 | 4 |

## Popeye's Louisiana Kitchen

### CHICKEN

| | SERVING SIZE | CAL | CAL FAT | TOT FAT (G) | SAT FAT (G) | CHOL (MG) | SOD (MG) | CARB (G) | FIBER (G) | PROT (G) |
|---|---|---|---|---|---|---|---|---|---|---|
| Cajun Wing Segments | 6 pieces | 595 | 387 | 43 | 15 | 260 | 1274 | 19 | 0 | 34 |
| Chicken Biscuit | as served | 350 | 180 | 20 | 9 | 35 | 930 | 30 | <1 | 13 |
| Chicken Bowl | as served | 570 | 261 | 29 | 10 | 100 | 1600 | 44 | 8 | 35 |
| Chicken Etouffee | as served | 160 | 90 | 10 | 3 | 20 | 870 | 6 | 2 | 12 |
| Chicken Sausage Jambalaya | as served | 220 | 99 | 11 | 3 | 32 | 760 | 20 | 1 | 10 |
| Loaded Chicken Wrap | 1 wrap | 400 | 153 | 17 | 6 | 35 | 1100 | 44 | 4 | 19 |
| Louisiana Travelers Nuggets | 6 pieces | 220 | 108 | 12 | 5 | 40 | 500 | 13 | <1 | 15 |
| Louisiana Travelers Spicy Tenders | 3 pieces | 405 | 153 | 17 | 7 | 84 | 2160 | 30 | 0 | 33 |
| Mild (Skinless, breading removed) Breast | as served | 120 | 18 | 2 | 1 | 120 | 540 | 0 | 0 | 24 |
| Mild (Skinless, breading removed) Strips | 2 pieces | 130 | 22.5 | 2.5 | 1 | 50 | 620 | 3 | 0 | 25 |
| Mild (Skinless, breading removed) Wing | as served | 40 | 13.5 | 1.5 | .5 | 58 | 400 | 0 | <1 | 7 |
| **SANDWICHES** | | | | | | | | | | |
| Crispy Chicken Sandwich | 1 sandwich | 560 | 207 | 23 | 8 | 75 | 1690 | 56 | 3 | 33 |
| Deluxe Mild or Spicy Sandwich w/Mayo | 1 sandwich | 630 | 279 | 31 | 8 | 71 | 1480 | 53 | 3 | 35 |
| Deluxe Mild Sandwich w/o Mayo | 1 sandwich | 480 | 135 | 15 | 6 | 55 | 1290 | 54 | 3 | 33 |
| Po Boy Sandwich | 1 sandwich | 330 | 153 | 17 | 3 | 10 | 560 | 36 | 0 | 8 |

| | SERVING SIZE | CAL | CAL FAT | TOT FAT (G) | SAT FAT (G) | CHOL (MG) | SOD (MG) | CARB (G) | FIBER (G) | PROT (G) |
|---|---|---|---|---|---|---|---|---|---|---|
| **SEAFOOD** | | | | | | | | | | |
| Butterfly Shrimp | 1 entrée | 310 | 171 | 19 | 8 | 90 | 800 | 22 | 2 | 13 |
| Crawfish Etouffee | 1 entrée | 180 | 45 | 5 | 1 | 48 | 640 | 25 | 2 | 7 |
| Popcorn Shrimp | 1 entrée | 280 | 144 | 16 | 6 | 95 | 1110 | 22 | <1 | 12 |
| Sides | | | | | | | | | | |
| French Fries | as served | 310 | 153 | 17 | 7 | 7 | 660 | 35 | 3 | 4 |

## Pretzel Time/ Pretzelmaker

| | SERVING SIZE | CAL | CAL FAT | TOT FAT (G) | SAT FAT (G) | CHOL (MG) | SOD (MG) | CARB (G) | FIBER (G) | PROT (G) |
|---|---|---|---|---|---|---|---|---|---|---|
| Cheddar Cheese Sauce | 1 portion | 80 | 45 | 5 | 3 | 10 | 410 | 4 | 0 | 3 |
| Honey Mustard Sauce | 1 portion | 80 | 0 | 0 | 0 | 0 | 240 | 20 | 0 | 0 |
| Icing | 1 portion | 180 | 0 | 0 | 0 | 0 | 0 | 45 | 0 | 0 |
| Mustard Sauce | 1 portion | 10 | 0 | 0 | 0 | 0 | 125 | 1 | 0 | 0 |
| Salted Pretzel | 1 pretzel | 310 | 35 | 4 | .5 | 0 | 780 | 59 | 2 | 8 |
| Salted Pretzel Bites Plain | 2 pieces | 250 | 10 | 1 | 0 | 0 | 0 | 52 | 2 | 7 |
| Unsalted Pretzel | 1 pretzel | 280 | 10 | 1 | 0 | 0 | 0 | 59 | 2 | 8 |

## Quiznos
### SUBS SANDWICHES (regular)

| | SERVING SIZE | CAL | CAL FAT | TOT FAT (G) | SAT FAT (G) | CHOL (MG) | SOD (MG) | CARB (G) | FIBER (G) | PROT (G) |
|---|---|---|---|---|---|---|---|---|---|---|
| Bourbon Grille Steak w/o Cheese | 1 sandwich | 680 | 200 | 22 | 1.5 | 95 | 1920 | 79 | 3 | 43 |
| California Club w/o Cheese | 1 sandwich | 730 | 300 | 34 | 7 | 70 | 2550 | 69 | 7 | 35 |
| Chicken Carbonara | 1 sandwich | 840 | 375 | 41 | 14 | 100 | 1920 | 63 | 3 | 41 |
| Classic Club w/o Cheese | 1 sandwich | 770 | 370 | 42 | 8.5 | 100 | 2340 | 66 | 4 | 36 |
| Classic Italian w/o Cheese | 1 sandwich | 800 | 410 | 45 | 16.5 | 85 | 2630 | 66 | 4 | 31 |
| Double Cheese Cheesesteak | 1 sandwich | 1040 | 560 | 62 | 8 | 140 | 2105 | 68 | 4 | 54 |
| Ham & Swiss | 1 sandwich | 780 | 380 | 43 | 8 | 90 | 2155 | 66 | 4 | 37 |
| Roast Beef & Cheddar | 1 sandwich | 780 | 380 | 42 | 11 | 90 | 2060 | 67 | 4 | 35 |
| Steakhouse Prime Rib Dip w/o Cheese | 1 sandwich | 780 | 340 | 38 | 4.5 | 110 | 2520 | 66 | 3 | 43 |
| Triple Meat Club w/o Cheese | 1 sandwich | 590 | 210 | 24 | 5 | 50 | 2220 | 68 | 4 | 29 |
| Tuna Melt w/o Cheese | 1 sandwich | 910 | 530 | 59 | 9.5 | 90 | 1220 | 62 | 4 | 37 |
| Turkey & Cheddar | 1 sandwich | 770 | 380 | 43 | 11 | 90 | 2060 | 66 | 4 | 33 |
| Turkey & Ham w/o Cheese | 1 sandwich | 690 | 330 | 36 | 6.5 | 70 | 1860 | 65 | 4 | 29 |
| Veggie w/o Cheese | 1 sandwich | 610 | 280 | 30 | 5 | 5 | 1730 | 65 | 8 | 16 |
| **TOASTED SANDWICHES** | | | | | | | | | | |
| Beef & Bacon Toasty Bullet | 1 sandwich | 360 | 120 | 14 | 3 | 30 | 1170 | 41 | 2 | 17 |
| Bistro Steak Flatbread Sammie w/o Cheese | 1 sandwich | 350 | 175 | 19 | 3.5 | 30 | 960 | 30 | 1 | 13 |
| Chicken, Bacon Ranch Flatbread Sammie | 1 sandwich | 330 | 130 | 15 | 4 | 35 | 770 | 27 | 1 | 16 |
| Pesto Turkey Toasty Bullet | 1 sandwich | 305 | 95 | 10.5 | 1.5 | 15 | 1095 | 42 | 2 | 14 |
| Pesto Turkey Toasty Torpedo | 1 sandwich | 660 | 180 | 19 | 3.5 | 35 | 2240 | 93 | 5 | 29 |

| | SERVING SIZE | CAL | CAL FAT | TOT FAT (G) | SAT FAT (G) | CHOL (MG) | SOD (MG) | CARB (G) | FIBER (G) | PROT (G) |
|---|---|---|---|---|---|---|---|---|---|---|
| Tuna Melt Toasty Bullet w/o Cheese | 1 sandwich | 430 | 220 | 24 | 3.5 | 35 | 605 | 38 | 2 | 13 |
| Tuna Melt Toasty Torpedo w/o Cheese | 1 sandwich | 860 | 400 | 44 | 7 | 60 | 1275 | 88 | 4 | 28 |
| Turkey Club Toasty Bullet w/o Cheese | 1 sandwich | 380 | 160 | 18 | 3.5 | 30 | 1190 | 41 | 2 | 15 |
| Turkey Club Toasty Torpedo w/o Cheese | 1 sandwich | 800 | 300 | 33 | 6.5 | 55 | 2410 | 93 | 5 | 32 |
| Veggie Flatbread Sammie w/o Cheese | 1 sandwich | 280 | 140 | 15 | 2.5 | 15 | 680 | 29 | 3 | 6 |

## Red Lobster
### APPETIZERS

| | SERVING SIZE | CAL | CAL FAT | TOT FAT (G) | SAT FAT (G) | CHOL (MG) | SOD (MG) | CARB (G) | FIBER (G) | PROT (G) |
|---|---|---|---|---|---|---|---|---|---|---|
| Buffalo Chicken Wings | as served | 680 | 351 | 39 | 9 | n/a | 1750 | 0 | n/a | n/a |
| Chicken Breast Strips | as served | 410 | 216 | 24 | 2 | n/a | 1320 | 28 | n/a | n/a |
| Chilled Jumbo Shrimp Cocktail | as served | 120 | 4.5 | 0.5 | 0 | n/a | 580 | 9 | n/a | n/a |
| Clam Strips | as served | 370 | 198 | 22 | 2 | n/a | 820 | 31 | n/a | n/a |
| Crispy Calamari & Vegetables | as served | 760 | 441 | 49 | 6 | n/a | 1530 | 58 | n/a | n/a |
| Fried Crawfish | as served | 1190 | 621 | 69 | 7 | n/a | 2740 | 104 | n/a | n/a |
| Fried Oysters | as served | 590 | 279 | 31 | 3 | n/a | 1220 | 66 | n/a | n/a |
| Hand-Shucked Oysters | 12 oysters | 100 | 22.5 | 2.5 | 1 | n/a | 250 | 7 | n/a | n/a |
| Lobster Nachos | as served | 1090 | 576 | 64 | 19 | n/a | 1680 | 94 | n/a | n/a |
| Mozzarella Cheesesticks | as served | 680 | 351 | 39 | 14 | n/a | 1910 | 49 | n/a | n/a |
| New England Seafood Sampler | as served | 750 | 387 | 42 | 10 | n/a | 2160 | 45 | n/a | n/a |
| Pan-Seared Crab Cakes | as served | 280 | 126 | 14 | 2.5 | n/a | 1110 | 13 | n/a | n/a |

### ENTRÉES

| | SERVING SIZE | CAL | CAL FAT | TOT FAT (G) | SAT FAT (G) | CHOL (MG) | SOD (MG) | CARB (G) | FIBER (G) | PROT (G) |
|---|---|---|---|---|---|---|---|---|---|---|
| Admiral's Feast | 1 entrée | 1280 | 657 | 73 | 6 | n/a | 4300 | 92 | n/a | n/a |
| Broiled Seafood Platter | 1 entrée | 300 | 90 | 10 | 3 | n/a | 1880 | 9 | n/a | n/a |
| Cajun Chicken Linguini Alfredo | 1 entrée | 1260 | 477 | 53 | 19 | n/a | 3110 | 91 | n/a | n/a |
| Center-Cut NY Strip Steak (14oz) | 1 entrée | 590 | 297 | 33 | 14 | n/a | 1420 | 0 | n/a | n/a |
| Coconut Shrimp Bites | 1 entrée | 290 | 162 | 18 | 3 | n/a | 830 | 19 | n/a | n/a |
| Crunchy Popcorn Shrimp | 1 entrée | 560 | 243 | 27 | 2.5 | n/a | 2100 | 51 | n/a | n/a |
| Garlic-Grilled Jumbo Shrimp | 1 entrée | 370 | 81 | 9 | 2 | n/a | 2160 | 40 | n/a | n/a |
| Garlic Shrimp Scampi | 1 entrée | 180 | 99 | 11 | 2 | n/a | 1400 | 0 | n/a | n/a |
| North Pacific King Crab Legs | 1 entrée | 390 | 31.5 | 3.5 | 1 | n/a | 3520 | 2 | n/a | n/a |
| NY Strip & Rock Lobster Tail | 1 entrée | 690 | 315 | 35 | 14 | n/a | 1930 | 0 | n/a | n/a |
| Popcorn Shrimp | 1 entrée | 180 | 81 | 9 | 1 | n/a | 670 | 16 | n/a | n/a |
| Rock Lobster Tail | 1 entrée | 90 | 9 | 1 | 0 | n/a | 490 | 0 | n/a | n/a |
| Scampi | 1 entrée | 130 | 72 | 8 | 1.5 | n/a | 990 | 0 | n/a | n/a |
| Shrimp Linguini Alfredo | 1/2 serving | 550 | 261 | 29 | 10 | n/a | 1580 | 41 | n/a | n/a |
| Steamed Snow Crab Legs | 1 entrée | 80 | 9 | 1 | 0 | n/a | 790 | 0 | n/a | n/a |
| Stuffed Maine Lobster | 1 entrée | 330 | 108 | 12 | 3.5 | n/a | 1090 | 2 | n/a | n/a |
| Wood-Grilled Fresh Salmon | 1 entrée | 210 | 81 | 9 | 2 | n/a | 240 | 0 | n/a | n/a |

| | SERVING SIZE | CAL | CAL FAT | TOT FAT (G) | SAT FAT (G) | CHOL (MG) | SOD (MG) | CARB (G) | FIBER (G) | PROT (G) |
|---|---|---|---|---|---|---|---|---|---|---|
| Wood-Grilled Lobster, Shrimp & Scallops | 1 entrée | 500 | 99 | 11 | 2.5 | n/a | 3220 | 42 | n/a | n/a |
| Wood-Grilled Peppercorn Sirloin | 1 entrée | 280 | 90 | 10 | 4 | n/a | 850 | 0 | n/a | n/a |
| Wood-Grilled Peppercorn Sirloin & Shrimp | 1 entrée | 590 | 198 | 22 | 10 | n/a | 2230 | 30 | n/a | n/a |
| Ultimate Feast | 1 entrée | 600 | 252 | 28 | 3.5 | n/a | 3660 | 25 | n/a | n/a |
| **SIDES** | | | | | | | | | | |
| Caesar Salad | 1 salad | 270 | 189 | 21 | 4.5 | n/a | 560 | 13 | n/a | n/a |
| Cheddar Bay Biscuit | 1 biscuit | 150 | 72 | 8 | 2.5 | n/a | 350 | 16 | n/a | n/a |
| Garden Salad | 1 salad | 90 | 27 | 3 | 0 | n/a | 105 | 13 | n/a | n/a |
| Langostino Lobster Baked Potato | as served | 380 | 198 | 14 | 4.5 | n/a | 1100 | 50 | n/a | n/a |

## Red Mango
### FROZEN YOGURT

| | SERVING SIZE | CAL | CAL FAT | TOT FAT (G) | SAT FAT (G) | CHOL (MG) | SOD (MG) | CARB (G) | FIBER (G) | PROT (G) |
|---|---|---|---|---|---|---|---|---|---|---|
| Madagascar Vanilla Nonfat | 1/2 cup | 100 | 0 | 0 | 0 | 0 | 125 | 21 | 0 | 3 |
| Original Nonfat | 1/2 cup | 90 | 0 | 0 | 0 | 0 | 125 | 20 | 0 | 3 |
| Pomegranate | 1/2 cup | 100 | 0 | 0 | 0 | 0 | 120 | 22 | 0 | 3 |

### SMOOTHIES

| | SERVING SIZE | CAL | CAL FAT | TOT FAT (G) | SAT FAT (G) | CHOL (MG) | SOD (MG) | CARB (G) | FIBER (G) | PROT (G) |
|---|---|---|---|---|---|---|---|---|---|---|
| 4 Berry Blend | 16 fl oz | 220 | 0 | .5 | 0 | 0 | 220 | 53 | 4 | 6 |
| Acai Berry | 16 fl oz | 300 | 15 | 1.5 | 0 | 0 | 180 | 66 | 1 | 5 |
| Citrus Green Tea | 16 fl oz | 260 | 0 | 0 | 0 | 0 | 180 | 60 | 1 | 4 |
| Healthy Bones | 16 fl oz | 230 | 0 | 0 | 0 | 0 | 230 | 55 | 2 | 6 |
| Immunity Boost | 16 fl oz | 280 | 0 | 0 | 0 | 0 | 230 | 62 | 1 | 5 |
| Mandarin Mango | 16 fl oz | 250 | 0 | 0 | 0 | 0 | 230 | 61 | 2 | 6 |
| Pomegranate | 16 fl oz | 280 | 0 | 0 | 0 | 0 | 230 | 68 | 1 | 5 |
| Protein Power | 16 fl oz | 400 | 45 | 5 | 1 | 5 | 320 | 73 | 6 | 20 |
| Raspberry Green Tea | 16 fl oz | 210 | 0 | 0 | 0 | 0 | 230 | 49 | 3 | 6 |
| Revitalizing Energy | 16 fl oz | 280 | 0 | 0 | 0 | 0 | 230 | 62 | 1 | 5 |
| Strawberry Hibiscus Tea | 16 fl oz | 260 | 0 | 0 | 0 | 0 | 180 | 60 | 1 | 4 |
| Tropical Mango | 16 fl oz | 240 | 0 | 0 | 0 | 0 | 220 | 60 | 2 | 6 |

### TEAS & CHILLERS

| | SERVING SIZE | CAL | CAL FAT | TOT FAT (G) | SAT FAT (G) | CHOL (MG) | SOD (MG) | CARB (G) | FIBER (G) | PROT (G) |
|---|---|---|---|---|---|---|---|---|---|---|
| Chiller Lemonade Green Tea | 16 fl oz | 230 | 0 | 0 | 0 | 0 | 180 | 53 | 0 | 4 |
| Chiller Pomegranate Green Tea | 16 fl oz | 200 | 0 | 0 | 0 | 0 | 190 | 49 | 0 | 4 |
| Chiller Vanilla Black Tea | 16 fl oz | 240 | 0 | 0 | 0 | 0 | 180 | 56 | 0 | 4 |
| Lemonade Green Tea | 16 fl oz | 90 | 0 | 0 | 0 | 0 | 0 | 21 | 0 | 0 |
| Pomegranate Green Tea | 16 fl oz | 120 | 0 | 0 | 0 | 0 | 15 | 30 | 0 | 0 |
| Vanilla Black Tea | 16 fl oz | 90 | 0 | 0 | 0 | 0 | 0 | 24 | 0 | 0 |

## Red Robin
### BURGERS

| | SERVING SIZE | CAL | CAL FAT | TOT FAT (G) | SAT FAT (G) | CHOL (MG) | SOD (MG) | CARB (G) | FIBER (G) | PROT (G) |
|---|---|---|---|---|---|---|---|---|---|---|
| A.1. Peppercorn Burger | 1 burger | 1025 | 531 | 59 | n/a | n/a | 2032 | 70 | 3 | 51 |

# restaurants

| | SERVING SIZE | CAL | CAL FAT | TOT FAT (G) | SAT FAT (G) | CHOL (MG) | SOD (MG) | CARB (G) | FIBER (G) | PROT (G) |
|---|---|---|---|---|---|---|---|---|---|---|
| All American Patty Melt | 1 burger | 1315 | 801 | 89 | n/a | n/a | 2064 | 60 | 3 | 48 |
| Bacon Cheeseburger | 1 burger | 1030 | 621 | 69 | n/a | n/a | 1930 | 51 | 3 | 51 |
| Bleu Ribbon Burger | 1 burger | 999 | 513 | 57 | n/a | n/a | 2076 | 70 | 4 | 47 |
| Burnin' Love Burger | 1 burger | 936 | 540 | 60 | n/a | n/a | 2198 | 55 | 3 | 45 |
| Chili Chili Cheeseburger | 1 burger | 923 | 450 | 50 | n/a | n/a | 1610 | 59 | 5 | 55 |
| Garden Burger | 1 burger | 561 | 207 | 23 | n/a | n/a | 1724 | 73 | 6 | 10 |
| Gourmet Cheeseburger | 1 burger | 931 | 540 | 60 | n/a | n/a | 1818 | 53 | 3 | 45 |
| Grilled Turkey Burger | 1 burger | 641 | 333 | 37 | n/a | n/a | 1000 | 50 | 3 | 30 |
| Guacamole Bacon Burger | 1 burger | 1046 | 576 | 64 | n/a | n/a | 1515 | 54 | 4 | 61 |
| Lettuce Wrapped Burger | 1 burger | 422 | 243 | 27 | n/a | n/a | 398 | 8 | 2 | 34 |
| Natural Burger | 1 burger | 569 | 216 | 24 | n/a | n/a | 989 | 51 | 3 | 37 |
| Sautéed 'Shroom Burger | 1 burger | 961 | 504 | 56 | n/a | n/a | 1352 | 58 | 6 | 59 |
| Whiskey River BBQ Burger | 1 burger | 1114 | 612 | 68 | n/a | n/a | 1815 | 72 | 4 | 48 |
| **ENTRÉES** | | | | | | | | | | |
| Buffalo Clucks & Fries | 1 entrée | 1696 | 1089 | 121 | n/a | n/a | 4479 | 100 | 8 | 53 |
| Classic Creamy Mac 'n' Cheese | 1 entrée | 1320 | 657 | 73 | n/a | n/a | 2606 | 91 | 6 | 49 |
| Grilled Chicken alla Caprese | 1 entrée | 646 | 306 | 34 | n/a | n/a | 1309 | 35 | 5 | 54 |
| Steak Sliders Entrée (3 Sliders) | 1 entrée | 795 | 378 | 42 | n/a | n/a | 1723 | 65 | 7 | 40 |
| Triple S Riblet Basket | 1 entrée | 1429 | 765 | 85 | n/a | n/a | 3700 | 59 | 4 | 108 |
| **SALADS** | | | | | | | | | | |
| Apple Harvest Chicken | 1 salad | 812 | 396 | 44 | n/a | n/a | 1769 | 64 | 8 | 45 |
| Crispy Chicken Tender | 1 salad | 1450 | 873 | 97 | n/a | n/a | 2520 | 86 | 7 | 61 |
| Mighty Caesar w/Grilled Chicken | 1 salad | 800 | 423 | 47 | n/a | n/a | 1397 | 43 | 6 | 47 |
| Southwest Grilled Chicken | 1 salad | 888 | 504 | 56 | n/a | n/a | 1979 | 44 | 9 | 49 |
| **SIDES** | | | | | | | | | | |
| Steak Fries | as served | 434 | 162 | 18 | n/a | n/a | 444 | 60 | 4 | 3 |
| **Romano's Macaroni Grill** | | | | | | | | | | |
| **ENTRÉES** | | | | | | | | | | |
| Grilled Specialties Calabrese Strip | 1 entrée | 1050 | n/a | 65 | 24 | n/a | 850 | 37 | 5 | 79 |
| Grilled Specialties Center-Cut Filet | 1 entrée | 710 | n/a | 37 | 16 | n/a | 500 | 29 | 15 | 65 |
| Grilled Specialties Grilled Pork Chops | 1 entrée | 1380 | n/a | 77 | 39 | n/a | 4040 | 96 | 14 | 74 |
| Prime Pork Loin | 1 entrée | 670 | n/a | n/a | 6 | n/a | 1820 | 57 | 0 | 0 |
| Rosemary Spiedini Grilled Chicken | 1 entrée | 360 | n/a | 10 | 2 | n/a | 1150 | 17 | 8 | 51 |
| **NEAPOLITAN PIZZA** | | | | | | | | | | |
| Italian Sausage | as served | 970 | n/a | 39 | 18 | n/a | 2430 | 95 | 8 | 61 |
| Margherita | as served | 720 | n/a | 20 | 11 | n/a | 1490 | 95 | 8 | 40 |

| | SERVING SIZE | CAL | CAL FAT | TOT FAT (G) | SAT FAT (G) | CHOL (MG) | SOD (MG) | CARB (G) | FIBER (G) | PROT (G) |
|---|---|---|---|---|---|---|---|---|---|---|
| Pepperoni | as served | 920 | n/a | 37 | 17 | n/a | 2200 | 102 | 7 | 45 |
| Roasted Vegetali | as served | 800 | n/a | 27 | 13 | n/a | 1550 | 102 | 10 | 39 |
| **PASTA** | | | | | | | | | | |
| Classico Chicken Parmigiana | 1 entrée | 870 | n/a | 39 | 11 | n/a | 1880 | 77 | 10 | 53 |
| Classico Eggplant Parmigiana | 1 entrée | 820 | n/a | 49 | 14 | n/a | 1550 | 67 | 11 | 30 |
| Classico Fettuccine Alfredo | 1 entrée | 780 | n/a | 46 | 27 | n/a | 1130 | 71 | 5 | 20 |
| Classico Lasagna Al Forno | 1 entrée | 760 | n/a | 43 | 21 | n/a | 1160 | 45 | 4 | 49 |
| Classico Mama's Trio | 1 entrée | 1280 | n/a | 67 | 28 | n/a | 3360 | 74 | 12 | 96 |
| Classico Spaghetti Bolognese | 1 entrée | 570 | n/a | 19 | 6 | n/a | 1480 | 72 | 7 | 24 |
| Handcrafted Antonio's Beef Rigatoni | 1 entrée | 770 | n/a | 31 | 10 | n/a | 1320 | 80 | 10 | 43 |
| Handcrafted Capellini Pomodoro | 1 entrée | 390 | n/a | 14 | 2 | n/a | 980 | 55 | 7 | 10 |
| Handcrafted Carmela's Chicken Rigatoni | 1 entrée | 930 | n/a | 54 | 26 | n/a | 950 | 75 | 9 | 36 |
| Handcrafted Chicken Cannelloni | 1 entrée | 600 | n/a | 29 | 15 | n/a | 1410 | 42 | 6 | 42 |
| Handcrafted Mushroom Ravioli | 1 entrée | 790 | n/a | 44 | 19 | n/a | 990 | 70 | 9 | 26 |
| Handcrafted Milano | 1 entrée | 750 | n/a | 24 | 10 | n/a | 1730 | 93 | 7 | 40 |
| Handcrafted Penne Rustica | 1 entrée | 980 | n/a | 38 | 17 | n/a | 2830 | 94 | 13 | 65 |
| Handcrafted Pollo Caprese | 1 entrée | 550 | n/a | 20 | 5 | n/a | 1660 | 45 | 7 | 46 |
| **SALADS** | | | | | | | | | | |
| Caesar | 1 salad | 260 | n/a | 20 | 4 | n/a | 480 | 14 | 2 | 5 |
| Chicken Caesar | 1 salad | 650 | n/a | 42 | 9 | n/a | 1450 | 29 | 5 | 40 |
| Fresh Greens | 1 salad | 320 | n/a | 26 | 5 | n/a | 300 | 20 | 3 | 3 |
| Insalata Blu | 1 salad | 640 | n/a | 55 | 13 | n/a | 1420 | 22 | 6 | 16 |
| Parmesan-Crusted Chicken | 1 salad | 870 | n/a | 57 | 12 | n/a | 1180 | 40 | 5 | 48 |
| Scallops & Spinach | 1 salad | 330 | n/a | 18 | 4 | n/a | 820 | 16 | 8 | 25 |
| Warm Spinach | 1 salad | 330 | n/a | 20 | 7 | n/a | 1810 | 21 | 18 | 8 |
| **Roy Rogers** | | | | | | | | | | |
| **CHICKEN** | | | | | | | | | | |
| Tenders | as served | 629 | n/a | 25 | 5 | 135 | 810 | 45 | n/a | 57 |
| Fried Breast | as served | 370 | n/a | 15 | 4 | 75 | 1190 | 29 | n/a | 29 |
| Fried Leg | as served | 170 | n/a | 7 | 2 | 45 | 570 | 15 | n/a | 13 |
| Fried Thigh | as served | 330 | n/a | 15 | 4 | 60 | 1000 | 30 | n/a | 19 |
| Fried Wing | as served | 200 | n/a | 8 | 2 | 30 | 740 | 23 | n/a | 10 |
| **SANDWICHES** | | | | | | | | | | |
| Bacon Cheeseburger | 1 burger | 520 | n/a | 33 | 18 | 72 | 1620 | 32 | n/a | 24 |
| Double-R-Bar Burger | 1 burger | 733 | n/a | 43 | 17 | 152 | 1722 | 42 | n/a | 44 |
| Gold Rush Chicken Filet | 1 burger | 558 | n/a | 30 | 9 | 35 | 1326 | 51 | n/a | 22 |

| | SERVING SIZE | CAL | CAL FAT | TOT FAT (G) | SAT FAT (G) | CHOL (MG) | SOD (MG) | CARB (G) | FIBER (G) | PROT (G) |
|---|---|---|---|---|---|---|---|---|---|---|
| Grilled Chicken Filet | 1 burger | 413 | n/a | 17 | 3 | 70 | 1325 | 39 | n/a | 31 |
| Hamburger | 1 burger | 343 | n/a | 18 | 9 | 36 | 1160 | 32 | n/a | 17 |
| Quarter Pound Cheeseburger | 1 burger | 480 | n/a | 29 | 17 | 66 | 1509 | 32 | n/a | 23 |
| Quarter Pound Hamburger | 1 burger | 412 | n/a | 25 | 14 | 53 | 1264 | 32 | n/a | 20 |
| Roy's Real Roast Beef Sandwich | 1 sandwich | 329 | n/a | 10 | 3 | 62 | 875 | 29 | n/a | 31 |
| **SIDES** | | | | | | | | | | |
| Mashed Potatoes | as served | 92 | n/a | <1 | <1 | 0 | 320 | 2 | n/a | 2 |
| Regular French Fries | as served | 350 | n/a | 15 | 4 | 0 | 150 | 49 | n/a | 5 |

## Rubio's

| | SERVING SIZE | CAL | CAL FAT | TOT FAT (G) | SAT FAT (G) | CHOL (MG) | SOD (MG) | CARB (G) | FIBER (G) | PROT (G) |
|---|---|---|---|---|---|---|---|---|---|---|
| Baja Grill Chicken Burrito | 1 burrito | 630 | 250 | 28 | 11 | 95 | 1800 | 55 | 5 | 40 |
| Baja Grill Steak Burrito | 1 burrito | 720 | 340 | 38 | 16 | 100 | 2430 | 56 | 4 | 39 |
| Bean & Cheese Burrito | 1 burrito | 760 | 330 | 37 | 19 | 85 | 1860 | 78 | 11 | 30 |
| Big Especial Steak Burrito | 1 burrito | 900 | 350 | 38 | 12 | 65 | 2470 | 102 | 7 | 33 |
| Blackened Mahi Mahi Taco | 1 taco | 240 | 80 | 9 | 2 | 15 | 480 | 26 | 4 | 14 |
| Carnitas Enchilada | 1 enchilada | 380 | 210 | 23 | 13 | 80 | 810 | 24 | 3 | 23 |
| Carnitas Street Taco | 1 taco | 100 | 45 | 4.5 | 1.5 | 20 | 250 | 9 | 2 | 7 |
| Cheese Quesadilla | 1 quesadilla | 1120 | 630 | 70 | 30 | 130 | 1940 | 87 | 7 | 39 |
| Chicken Enchilada | 1 enchilada | 370 | 190 | 21 | 12 | 85 | 740 | 23 | 3 | 24 |
| Chicken Quesadilla | 1 quesadilla | 1200 | 630 | 70 | 30 | 175 | 2340 | 89 | 8 | 56 |
| Chile Lime Salmon Burrito | 1 burrito | 750 | 370 | 41 | 9 | 65 | 1260 | 62 | 5 | 31 |
| Fish Especial Taco | 1 taco | 330 | 160 | 18 | 4 | 50 | 520 | 32 | 5 | 14 |
| Fish Especial Flour Tortilla Taco | 1 taco | 380 | 190 | 21 | 5.5 | 50 | 860 | 32 | 4 | 15 |
| Grande Nachos | as served | 1270 | 710 | 78 | 27 | 120 | 1850 | 112 | 20 | 37 |
| Grande w/Chicken Nachos | as served | 1340 | 700 | 78 | 27 | 175 | 2260 | 114 | 22 | 54 |
| Grilled Chicken Taco | 1 taco | 250 | 110 | 12 | 3.5 | 35 | 380 | 23 | 4 | 13 |
| Grilled Steak Gourmet Taco | 1 taco | 350 | 180 | 21 | 8 | 55 | 790 | 24 | 3 | 19 |
| Grilled Veggie Burrito | 1 burrito | 680 | 250 | 27 | 11 | 35 | 1400 | 75 | 3 | 20 |
| HealthMex Chicken Taco | 1 taco | 130 | 10 | 1 | 0 | 20 | 240 | 22 | 3 | 10 |
| HealthMex Mahi Mahi Burrito | 1 burrito | 630 | 210 | 23 | 7 | 35 | 1400 | 67 | 6 | 39 |
| HealthMex Veggie Burrito | 1 burrito | 500 | 140 | 15 | 6 | 0 | 1380 | 74 | 8 | 12 |
| Steak Rajas Burrito | 2 burrito | 830 | 310 | 34 | 15 | 85 | 2280 | 76 | 3 | 36 |
| Steak Street Taco | 1 taco | 120 | 50 | 6 | 2 | 20 | 380 | 9 | 2 | 8 |

## Ruby Tuesday
### APPETIZERS

| | SERVING SIZE | CAL | CAL FAT | TOT FAT (G) | SAT FAT (G) | CHOL (MG) | SOD (MG) | CARB (G) | FIBER (G) | PROT (G) |
|---|---|---|---|---|---|---|---|---|---|---|
| Asian Sesame Wings | as served | 190 | 90 | 10 | n/a | n/a | 709 | 5 | 1 | n/a |
| Buffalo Chicken Minis | as served | 623 | 207 | 23 | n/a | n/a | 1703 | 64 | 5 | n/a |
| Crab Cake Minis | as served | 616 | 243 | 27 | n/a | n/a | 1411 | 60 | 6 | n/a |

| | SERVING SIZE | CAL | CAL FAT | TOT FAT (G) | SAT FAT (G) | CHOL (MG) | SOD (MG) | CARB (G) | FIBER (G) | PROT (G) |
|---|---|---|---|---|---|---|---|---|---|---|
| Four Way Sampler | as served | 311 | 153 | 17 | n/a | n/a | 864 | 14 | 2 | n/a |
| Ruby Minis | as served | 755 | 423 | 47 | n/a | n/a | 1438 | 48 | 2 | n/a |
| Wing Sampler | as served | 232 | 108 | 12 | n/a | n/a | 915 | 6 | 1 | n/a |
| **BURGERS & SANDWICHES** | | | | | | | | | | |
| Avocado Turkey Burger | 1 burger | 886 | 729 | 81 | n/a | n/a | 2961 | 62 | 6 | n/a |
| Bacon Cheeseburger | 1 burger | 1252 | 774 | 86 | n/a | n/a | 2270 | 61 | 6 | n/a |
| Chicken BLT | 1 sandwich | 798 | 594 | 66 | n/a | n/a | 2204 | 74 | 5 | n/a |
| Smokehouse Burger | 1 burger | 1461 | 873 | 97 | n/a | n/a | 2629 | 83 | 7 | n/a |
| Triple Prime Cheddar Burger | 1 burger | 1385 | 990 | 110 | n/a | n/a | 2264 | 45 | 2 | n/a |
| Turkey Burger Wrap | 1 wrap | 658 | 297 | 33 | n/a | n/a | 2514 | 45 | 3 | n/a |
| Ultimate Chicken | 1 sandwich | 1222 | 603 | 67 | n/a | n/a | 2477 | 60 | 6 | n/a |
| **ENTRÉES** | | | | | | | | | | |
| Asian Glazed Salmon | 1 entrée | 370 | 234 | 26 | n/a | n/a | 971 | 10 | 1 | n/a |
| Asian Sesame Glazed Full Rack | 1 entrée | 1077 | 567 | 63 | n/a | n/a | 1255 | 36 | 2 | n/a |
| Barbeque Grilled Chicken | 1 entrée | 310 | 27 | 3 | n/a | n/a | 1389 | 11 | 0 | n/a |
| Buffalo Shrimp | 1 entrée | 126 | 54 | 6 | n/a | n/a | 580 | 11 | 1 | n/a |
| California Club Quesadilla | 1 entrée | 1364 | 819 | 91 | n/a | n/a | 2546 | 42 | 6 | n/a |
| Chicken & Broccoli Pasta | 1 entrée | 1513 | 855 | 95 | n/a | n/a | 3177 | 85 | 7 | n/a |
| Chicken Piccata | 1 entrée | 1495 | 846 | 94 | n/a | n/a | 4194 | 90 | 9 | n/a |
| Chicken Tender Dinner | 1 entrée | 377 | 153 | 17 | n/a | n/a | 888 | 11 | 0 | n/a |
| Classic Barbeque Full Rack | 1 entrée | 970 | 423 | 47 | n/a | n/a | 1180 | 51 | 0 | n/a |
| Fresh Avocado Quesadilla | 1 entrée | 1065 | 675 | 75 | n/a | n/a | 1373 | 46 | 6 | n/a |
| Herb Crusted Tilapia | 1 entrée | 402 | 216 | 24 | n/a | n/a | 944 | 9 | 2 | n/a |
| Lobster Carbonara | 1 entrée | 1426 | 846 | 94 | n/a | n/a | 3206 | 77 | 7 | n/a |
| Louisiana Fried Shrimp | 1 entrée | 423 | 153 | 17 | n/a | n/a | 1709 | 38 | 2 | n/a |
| Memphis Dry Rub Full Rack | 1 entrée | 920 | 522 | 58 | n/a | n/a | 300 | 12 | 0 | n/a |
| Petite Sirloin | 1 entrée | 301 | 144 | 16 | n/a | n/a | 1157 | 1 | 0 | n/a |
| Plain Grilled Petite Sirloin | 1 entrée | 317 | 144 | 16 | n/a | n/a | 112 | 0 | 0 | n/a |
| Plain Grilled Salmon | 1 entrée | 167 | 81 | 9 | n/a | n/a | 30 | 0 | 0 | n/a |
| Ribs, Wings, & Shrimp | 1 entrée | 1034 | 450 | 50 | n/a | n/a | 2679 | 53 | 2 | n/a |
| Shrimp Scampi & Steak | 1 entrée | 1011 | 594 | 66 | n/a | n/a | 3151 | 39 | 4 | n/a |
| Southwestern Quesadilla | 1 entrée | 1574 | 963 | 107 | n/a | n/a | 3625 | 68 | 4 | n/a |
| Steak & Lobster Mac 'n Cheese | 1 entrée | 1055 | 576 | 64 | n/a | n/a | 2374 | 34 | 2 | n/a |
| **SOUPS & SALADS** | | | | | | | | | | |
| Carolina Chicken Salad | 1 salad | 707 | 630 | 70 | n/a | n/a | 2891 | 48 | 11 | n/a |
| Clam Chowder | 1 soup | 318 | 180 | 20 | n/a | n/a | 635 | 17 | 1 | n/a |
| Club House Salad | 1 salad | 926 | 531 | 59 | n/a | n/a | 2203 | 21 | 9 | n/a |

| | SERVING SIZE | CAL | CAL FAT | TOT FAT (G) | SAT FAT (G) | CHOL (MG) | SOD (MG) | CARB (G) | FIBER (G) | PROT (G) |
|---|---|---|---|---|---|---|---|---|---|---|
| Southwestern Beef Salad | 1 salad | 1139 | 729 | 81 | n/a | n/a | 2345 | 48 | 10 | n/a |
| White Bean Chicken Chili | as served | 233 | 72 | 8 | n/a | n/a | 1454 | 21 | 8 | n/a |

## Schlotzsky's
### PIZZAS

| | | | | | | | | | | |
|---|---|---|---|---|---|---|---|---|---|---|
| Combination Special | 1 slice | 640 | 226 | 25 | 10 | 54 | 1691 | 76 | 4 | 28 |
| Pepperoni & Double Cheese | 1 slice | 685 | 267 | 30 | 13 | 71 | 1741 | 74 | 3 | 31 |
| Vegetarian Special | 1 slice | 540 | 157 | 17 | 7 | 36 | 1370 | 74 | 4 | 22 |

### PANINIS, SANDWICHES, & WRAPS

| | | | | | | | | | | |
|---|---|---|---|---|---|---|---|---|---|---|
| Angus Roast Beef & Cheese | 1 sandwich | 785 | 292 | 33 | 15 | 119 | 2187 | 75 | 4 | 47 |
| Asian Chicken Wrap | 1 wrap | 538 | 101 | 11 | 2 | 51 | 2269 | 81 | 4 | 30 |
| BLT | 1 sandwich | 559 | 189 | 21 | 6 | 33 | 1353 | 73 | 4 | 21 |
| Cheese Original-Style | 1 sandwich | 791 | 338 | 38 | 20 | 105 | 1698 | 76 | 4 | 39 |
| Chicken Breast | 1 sandwich | 551 | 51 | 6 | 1 | 75 | 2023 | 82 | 4 | 42 |
| Deluxe Original-Style | 1 sandwich | 956 | 410 | 46 | 18 | 160 | 4084 | 80 | 5 | 55 |
| Fresh Veggie | 1 sandwich | 484 | 106 | 12 | 5 | 23 | 1159 | 76 | 6 | 19 |
| Grilled Chicken & Guacamole Wrap | 1 wrap | 691 | 317 | 35 | 9 | 84 | 1530 | 61 | 7 | 37 |
| Grilled Chicken Romano Pannini | 1 sandwich | 572 | 133 | 15 | 8 | 96 | 1693 | 63 | 1 | 43 |
| Ham & Cheese Original-Style | 1 sandwich | 733 | 239 | 27 | 12 | 113 | 2980 | 80 | 4 | 44 |
| Italiano Pannini | 1 sandwich | 736 | 286 | 32 | 15 | 114 | 2406 | 67 | 2 | 43 |
| Turkey Original-Style | 1 sandwich | 831 | 314 | 35 | 14 | 125 | 2529 | 79 | 4 | 47 |

### SOUPS & SALADS

| | | | | | | | | | | |
|---|---|---|---|---|---|---|---|---|---|---|
| Baby Spinach & Feta Salad | 1 salad | 113 | 66 | 7 | 5 | 27 | 448 | 6 | 3 | 8 |
| Greek Salad | 1 salad | 137 | 75 | 8 | 5 | 29 | 655 | 13 | 4 | 7 |
| Grilled Chicken Caesar Salad | 1 salad | 222 | 61 | 7 | 2 | 57 | 885 | 13 | 3 | 26 |
| Ham & Turkey Chef Salad | 1 salad | 254 | 121 | 13 | 6 | 60 | 1340 | 14 | 4 | 22 |
| Hearty Vegetable Beef Soup | 1 cup | 60 | 24 | 3 | 1 | 8 | 568 | 7 | 1 | 3 |
| Old Fashioned Chicken Noodle Soup | 1 cup | 83 | 14 | 2 | 1 | 22 | 1022 | 12 | 1 | 6 |
| Turkey Chef Salad | 1 salad | 309 | 158 | 18 | 7 | 67 | 1412 | 14 | 4 | 26 |
| Vegetarian Vegetable Soup | 1 cup | 98 | 6 | 1 | 0 | 0 | 1042 | 22 | 5 | 2 |

## Sizzler
### CHICKEN & RIB ENTRÉES

| | | | | | | | | | | |
|---|---|---|---|---|---|---|---|---|---|---|
| Grilled Chicken Fettuccine Alfredo | 1 entrée | 1018 | 531 | 59 | 36 | 278 | 2219 | 62 | 2 | 50 |
| Lemon Herb Chicken (Single) | 1 entrée | 220 | 108 | 12 | 3 | 112.5 | 624.5 | 2 | 0 | 26 |
| Ribs (Half Rack) | 1 order | 623 | 351 | 39 | 15 | 130 | 1105 | 37 | 0 | 28 |

### SANDWICHES & BURGERS

| | | | | | | | | | | |
|---|---|---|---|---|---|---|---|---|---|---|
| Grilled Chicken Club | 1 sandwich | 667 | 279 | 31 | 12 | 135 | 1339 | 48 | 3 | 45 |

| | SERVING SIZE | CAL | CAL FAT | TOT FAT (G) | SAT FAT (G) | CHOL (MG) | SOD (MG) | CARB (G) | FIBER (G) | PROT (G) |
|---|---|---|---|---|---|---|---|---|---|---|
| Malibu Chicken Sandwich | 1 sandwich | 704 | 333 | 37 | 13 | 61 | 1361 | 59 | 3 | 31 |
| Mega Bacon Cheeseburger (1/2 lb) | 1 burger | 1009 | 549 | 61 | 27 | 185 | 2475 | 48 | 3 | 64 |
| Burger (1/3 lb) | 1 burger | 619 | 270 | 30 | 12 | 96 | 1344 | 47 | 3 | 36 |
| **SEAFOOD** | | | | | | | | | | |
| Half Dozen Fried Shrimp | 1 entrée | 267 | 81 | 9 | 1 | 120 | 947 | 35 | 1 | 20 |
| Salmon, w/Rice Pilaf | 1 entrée | 532 | 180 | 20 | 6 | 101 | 921 | 40 | 1 | 47 |
| Shrimp Fettuccine Alfredo | 1 entrée | 986 | 495 | 55 | 35 | 381 | 2082 | 64 | 2 | 53 |
| Shrimp Fry Dozen | 1 entrée | 433 | 108 | 12 | 1 | 171 | 2263 | 48 | 2 | 29 |
| Shrimp, Shrimp, Shrimp | 1 entrée | 971 | 369 | 41 | 15 | 255 | 3192 | 92 | 5 | 51 |
| Shrimp Skewers, served on Rice Pilaf | 1 entrée | 545 | 234 | 26 | 11 | 209 | 1302 | 42 | 2 | 33 |
| Unlimited Shrimp (12 oz Shrimp) | 1 entrée | 720 | 171 | 19 | 3 | 284 | 3749 | 80 | 3 | 48 |
| **SIDES** | | | | | | | | | | |
| Baked Sweet Potato, w/Maple Topping | 1 potato | 442 | 144 | 16 | 7 | 0 | 244 | 69 | 8 | 5 |
| Cheese Toast | 1 slice | 238 | 171 | 19 | 9 | 5 | 395 | 13 | 1 | 5 |
| French Fries | 5 oz | 286 | 117 | 13 | 3 | 0 | 783 | 42 | 3 | 3 |
| **STEAKS & STEAK COMBOS** | | | | | | | | | | |
| Big Appetite Trio | 1 entrée | 1058 | 414 | 46 | 12 | 365 | 4511 | 69 | 2 | 82 |
| Chopped Steak (8 oz) | 1 entrée | 519 | 270 | 30 | 11 | 141 | 1402 | 17 | 1 | 42 |
| Classic (6 oz) | 1 entrée | 256 | 108 | 12 | 3 | 89 | 1475 | 2 | 0 | 32 |
| Classic Trio | 1 entrée | 836 | 360 | 40 | 12 | 254 | 2893 | 37 | 2 | 76 |
| Porterhouse (18 oz) | 1 entrée | 1363 | 963 | 107 | 42 | 347 | 1363 | 1 | 0 | 92 |
| Rib Eye (12 oz) | 1 entrée | 949 | 558 | 62 | 23 | 428 | 1278 | 1 | 0 | 91 |
| Steak & Colossal Shrimp, w/Rice Pilaf | 1 entrée | 625 | 171 | 19 | 5 | 305 | 2507 | 44 | 2 | 66 |
| Steak & Grilled Shrimp Skewers, w/Rice Pilaf | 1 entrée | 641 | 243 | 27 | 10 | 194 | 2495 | 43 | 2 | 51 |
| Steak & Half Dozen Fried Shrimp | 1 entrée | 523 | 189 | 21 | 4 | 209 | 2422 | 37 | 1 | 52 |
| Steak & Hibachi Chicken | 1 entrée | 457 | 171 | 19 | 4 | 196 | 2179 | 9 | 0 | 58 |
| Steak & Lemon Herb Chicken | 1 entrée | 476 | 216 | 24 | 6 | 202 | 2100 | 4 | 0 | 58 |
| Steak & Lobster Tail | 1 entrée | 369 | 117 | 13 | 2 | 89 | 1939 | 4 | 1 | 56 |
| Steak & Shrimp Fry Dozen | 1 entrée | 689 | 207 | 23 | 4 | 261 | 3738 | 50 | 2 | 61 |
| Steak & Unlimited Shrimp (12 oz Shrimp) | 1 entrée | 976 | 279 | 31 | 5 | 373 | 5224 | 82 | 3 | 80 |
| Ultimate Sizzlin' Trio | 1 entrée | 1414 | 774 | 86 | 33 | 311 | 4226 | 74 | 9 | 83 |
| **Sonic Drive In** | | | | | | | | | | |
| **BLASTS, MALTS, & SHAKES** | | | | | | | | | | |
| Butterfinger Blast | 14 fl oz | 730 | 350 | 38 | 26 | 130 | 410 | 87 | 0 | 11 |
| Chocolate Malt | 14 fl oz | 580 | 240 | 26 | 18 | 105 | 370 | 78 | 0 | 8 |
| Chocolate Cream Pie Shake | 14 fl oz | 710 | 260 | 29 | 20 | 100 | 370 | 103 | 0 | 8 |

# restaurants

| | SERVING SIZE | CAL | CAL FAT | TOT FAT (G) | SAT FAT (G) | CHOL (MG) | SOD (MG) | CARB (G) | FIBER (G) | PROT (G) |
|---|---|---|---|---|---|---|---|---|---|---|
| Coconut Cream Pie Shake | 14 fl oz | 600 | 260 | 29 | 20 | 100 | 330 | 78 | 0 | 8 |
| Cream Slushes Regular (average of all flavors) | 14 fl oz | 363 | 130 | 14 | 10 | 55 | 173 | 55 | >1 | 4 |
| Hot Fudge Shake | 14 fl oz | 590 | 280 | 31 | 22 | 100 | 340 | 70 | 1 | 8 |
| M&Ms Blast | 14 fl oz | 750 | 360 | 40 | 28 | 130 | 380 | 86 | 1 | 11 |
| Snickers Blast | 14 fl 0z | 680 | 330 | 37 | 25 | 135 | 400 | 76 | 0 | 11 |
| Strawberry Shake | 14 fl oz | 500 | 230 | 26 | 18 | 100 | 290 | 61 | 1 | 8 |
| Vanilla Malt | 14 fl oz | 480 | 240 | 26 | 18 | 105 | 290 | 53 | 0 | 8 |
| Vanilla Shake | 14 fl oz | 460 | 230 | 26 | 18 | 100 | 280 | 51 | 0 | 8 |
| **BREAKFAST** | | | | | | | | | | |
| Biscuit Dippers w/Gravy | 3 biscuits | 690 | 400 | 44 | 18 | 60 | 1170 | 57 | 0 | 16 |
| Breakfast Burrito, Bacon, Egg & Cheese | 1 burrito | 470 | 250 | 28 | 10 | 300 | 1470 | 37 | 1 | 19 |
| Breakfast Burrito, Sausage, Egg & Cheese | 1 burrito | 500 | 280 | 31 | 11 | 325 | 1380 | 37 | 1 | 18 |
| French Toast Sticks | 4 pieces | 500 | 280 | 31 | 5 | 15 | 490 | 49 | 2 | 7 |
| Steak & Egg Breakfast Burrito | 1 burrito | 590 | 290 | 33 | 11 | 320 | 1450 | 45 | 3 | 28 |
| **BURGERS & SANDWICHES** | | | | | | | | | | |
| Bacon Cheeseburger TOASTER Sandwich | 1 sandwich | 820 | 460 | 51 | 19 | 130 | 1500 | 51 | 3 | 39 |
| BLT TOASTER Sandwich | 1 sandwich | 490 | 280 | 31 | 7 | 40 | 960 | 39 | 2 | 14 |
| Breaded Pork Fritter Sandwich | 1 sandwich | 640 | 290 | 33 | 6 | 30 | 840 | 66 | 7 | 22 |
| Burger w/Mayonnaise | 1 burger | 800 | 440 | 49 | 15 | 110 | 740 | 55 | 5 | 36 |
| California Cheeseburger | 1 burger | 830 | 450 | 50 | 18 | 125 | 1000 | 56 | 5 | 39 |
| Chicken Club TOASTER Sandwich | 1 sandwich | 740 | 410 | 46 | 11 | 80 | 1160 | 54 | 4 | 30 |
| Fish Sandwich | 1 sandwich | 650 | 280 | 31 | 5 | 40 | 1160 | 71 | 7 | 22 |
| Super Jalapeno Cheeseburger | 1 burger | 1180 | 690 | 76 | 32 | 235 | 1660 | 54 | 5 | 67 |
| Western Chili Loaded Burger, Single | 1 burger | 960 | 490 | 55 | 21 | 140 | 1780 | 68 | 6 | 46 |
| **CHICKEN** | | | | | | | | | | |
| Chicken Strip Dinner, 4 piece | 1 entrée | 970 | 400 | 45 | 8 | 65 | 1970 | 106 | 7 | 37 |
| Crispy Chicken Wrap | 1 wrap | 490 | 210 | 23 | 5 | 40 | 1280 | 49 | 3 | 21 |
| Crispy Chicken Bacon Ranch | 1 sandwich | 610 | 310 | 35 | 9 | 75 | 1750 | 47 | 4 | 30 |
| Crispy Chicken Sandwich | 1 sandwich | 550 | 290 | 32 | 4.5 | 45 | 1070 | 46 | 4 | 22 |
| Fritos Chili Cheese Wrap | 1 wrap | 700 | 350 | 39 | 13 | 25 | 1600 | 66 | 4 | 21 |
| Grilled Chicken Wrap | 1 wrap | 390 | 130 | 14 | 3.5 | 80 | 1420 | 39 | 2 | 28 |
| Jumbo Popcorn Chicken, Small | 4 oz | 380 | 190 | 22 | 4 | 45 | 1250 | 27 | 3 | 18 |
| **Famous Slushes (average of all flavors)** | 14 fl oz | 196 | 0 | 0 | 0 | 0 | 31 | 53 | 0 | 0 |
| **FLOATS & SMOOTHIES** | | | | | | | | | | |
| Barq's Root Beer Float | 14 fl oz | 340 | 130 | 14 | 10 | 55 | 170 | 51 | 0 | 4 |
| Coca-Cola Float | 14 fl oz | 330 | 130 | 14 | 10 | 55 | 160 | 49 | 0 | 4 |

| | SERVING SIZE | CAL | CAL FAT | TOT FAT (G) | SAT FAT (G) | CHOL (MG) | SOD (MG) | CARB (G) | FIBER (G) | PROT (G) |
|---|---|---|---|---|---|---|---|---|---|---|
| Diet Coke Float | 14 fl oz | 260 | 130 | 14 | 10 | 55 | 160 | 29 | 0 | 4 |
| Java Chillers (average of all flavors) | 14 fl oz | 498 | 216 | 24 | 17 | 93 | 318 | 58 | 0 | 7 |
| Strawberry Fruit Smoothie | 14 fl oz | 420 | 0 | 0 | 0 | 0 | 115 | 106 | 4 | 3 |
| Tropical Fruit Smoothie | 14 fl oz | 440 | 0 | 0 | 0 | 0 | 125 | 109 | 3 | 3 |
| **HOT DOGS** | | | | | | | | | | |
| Corn Dog | 1 hot dog | 210 | 100 | 11 | 3.5 | 20 | 530 | 23 | 2 | 6 |
| Foot-Long Quarter-Pound Coney | 1 hot dog | 830 | 480 | 53 | 22 | 90 | 1980 | 55 | 4 | 32 |
| Regular Coney | 1 hot dog | 400 | 210 | 23 | 9 | 45 | 1210 | 32 | 2 | 16 |
| **ICE CREAM & SUNDAES** | | | | | | | | | | |
| Banana Fudge Sundae | 1 sundae | 540 | 230 | 26 | 19 | 80 | 280 | 71 | 2 | 6 |
| Banana Split | 1 split | 490 | 160 | 18 | 13 | 70 | 210 | 76 | 2 | 6 |
| Jr. Oreo Sundae | 1 sundae | 180 | 80 | 9 | 6 | 30 | 130 | 22 | 0 | 2 |
| Single Topping Hot Fudge Sundae | 1 sundae | 520 | 240 | 27 | 20 | 80 | 280 | 63 | 1 | 6 |
| Vanilla Dish, Regular | 1 serving | 240 | 120 | 13 | 9 | 55 | 140 | 26 | 0 | 4 |
| **Iced Latte (average of all flavors)** | 14 fl oz | 351 | 270 | 7.5 | 5 | 26 | 129 | 44 | 0 | 3 |
| **LIMEADES** | | | | | | | | | | |
| Cherry | 14 fl oz | 170 | 0 | 0 | 0 | 0 | 35 | 45 | 0 | 0 |
| Original | 14 fl oz | 140 | 0 | 0 | 0 | 0 | 30 | 38 | 0 | 0 |
| **Real Fruit Slushes (average of all flavors)** | 14 fl oz | 191 | 0 | 0 | 0 | 0 | 30 | 54 | 0 | 0 |
| **SIDES, MEDIUM** | | | | | | | | | | |
| French Fries | as served | 330 | 120 | 13 | 2.5 | 0 | 440 | 48 | 4 | 4 |
| Fritos Chili Pie | as served | 510 | 310 | 34 | 10 | 15 | 1000 | 36 | 3 | 14 |
| Mozzarella Sticks | as served | 440 | 200 | 22 | 9 | 45 | 1050 | 40 | 2 | 19 |
| Onion Rings | as served | 440 | 190 | 21 | 3.5 | 0 | 430 | 55 | 3 | 6 |
| Tots | as served | 200 | 120 | 13 | 2.5 | 0 | 440 | 20 | 2 | 2 |

## Starbucks
### BAKED GOODS

| | SERVING SIZE | CAL | CAL FAT | TOT FAT (G) | SAT FAT (G) | CHOL (MG) | SOD (MG) | CARB (G) | FIBER (G) | PROT (G) |
|---|---|---|---|---|---|---|---|---|---|---|
| Blueberry Scone | 1 Scone | 460 | 190 | 22 | 12 | 75 | 420 | 61 | 2 | 7 |
| Blueberry Streusel Muffin | 1 Muffin | 360 | 100 | 11 | 6 | 80 | 390 | 59 | 2 | 7 |
| Chocolate Chunk Cookie | 1 Cookie | 360 | 150 | 17 | 10 | 65 | 170 | 50 | 2 | 4 |
| Iced Lemon Pound Cake | 1 Cake | 490 | 200 | 23 | 13 | 135 | 520 | 68 | 1 | 5 |
| Multigrain Bagel | 1 Bagel | 320 | 40 | 4 | 4 | 0 | 220 | 62 | 4 | 12 |
| **FRAPPUCCINO BLENDED DRINKS** | | | | | | | | | | |
| Caffe Vanilla Frappuccino Light, Milk | 16 fl oz | 170 | 0 | 0 | 0 | 0 | 190 | 42 | 0 | 3 |
| Caffe Vanilla, Nonfat Milk | 16 fl oz | 280 | 0 | 0 | n/a | n/a | 21 | 67 | 0 | 3 |
| Caffe Vanilla, Whole Milk | 16 fl oz | 300 | 27 | 3 | 2 | 10 | 210 | 66 | 0 | 3 |

| | SERVING SIZE | CAL | CAL FAT | TOT FAT (G) | SAT FAT (G) | CHOL (MG) | SOD (MG) | CARB (G) | FIBER (G) | PROT (G) |
|---|---|---|---|---|---|---|---|---|---|---|
| Caramel, Whole Milk | 16 fl oz | 260 | 27 | 3 | n/a | n/a | n/a | 55 | 0 | 3 |
| Extra Coffee Caramel, Nonfat Milk | 16 fl oz | 240 | 0 | 0 | n/a | n/a | n/a | 53 | 0 | 3 |
| Extra Coffee Caramel, Whole Milk | 16 fl oz | 260 | 27 | 3 | n/a | n/a | n/a | 55 | 0 | 3 |
| Java Chip Frappuccino Light, Nonfat Milk | 16 fl oz | 200 | 31.5 | 3.5 | n/a | n/a | n/a | 42 | 2 | 5 |
| Java Chip, Nonfat Milk | 16 fl oz | 300 | 36 | 4 | n/a | n/a | n/a | 65 | 2 | 6 |
| Java Chip, Whole Milk | 16 fl oz | 320 | 63 | 7 | n/a | n/a | n/a | 65 | 2 | 5 |
| Mocha, Nonfat Milk | 16 fl oz | 230 | 9 | 1 | n/a | n/a | n/a | 55 | 1 | 4 |
| Mocha, Whole Milk | 16 fl oz | 260 | 31.5 | 3.5 | n/a | n/a | n/a | 54 | 1 | 4 |
| Tazo Chai Crème, Nonfat Milk | 16 fl oz | 220 | 0 | 0 | n/a | n/a | n/a | 50 | 0 | 5 |
| Tazo Chai Crème, Whole Milk | 16 fl oz | 250 | 36 | 4 | n/a | n/a | n/a | 50 | 0 | 4 |
| **HOT DRINKS** | | | | | | | | | | |
| Caffe Latte, Nonfat Milk | 16 fl oz | 130 | 54 | 6 | n/a | n/a | n/a | 11 | 0 | 7 |
| Caffe Latte, Whole Milk | 16 fl oz | 220 | 99 | 11 | n/a | n/a | n/a | 18 | 0 | 12 |
| Caffe Mocha, Nonfat Milk | 16 fl oz | 290 | 54 | 6 | n/a | n/a | n/a | 51 | 2 | 12 |
| Caffe Mocha, Whole Milk | 16 fl oz | 290 | 108 | 12 | n/a | n/a | n/a | 40 | 2 | 13 |
| Cappuccino, Nonfat Milk | 16 fl oz | 140 | 63 | 7 | n/a | n/a | n/a | 11 | 0 | 7 |
| Cappuccino, Whole Milk | 16 fl oz | 360 | 99 | 11 | n/a | n/a | n/a | 55 | 0 | 10 |
| Caramel Macchiato, Nonfat Milk | 16 fl oz | 270 | 90 | 10 | n/a | n/a | n/a | 34 | 0 | 10 |
| Caramel Macchiato, Whole Milk | 16 fl oz | 210 | 99 | 11 | n/a | n/a | n/a | 17 | 0 | 11 |
| Hot Chocolate, Made W/Nonfat Milk | 16 fl oz | 240 | 0 | 0 | n/a | n/a | n/a | 0 | 0 | 0 |
| Hot Chocolate, Made W/Whole Milk | 16 fl oz | 450 | 153 | 17 | n/a | n/a | n/a | 61 | 0 | 15 |
| Toffee Mocha, Nonfat Milk | 16 fl oz | 310 | 9 | 1 | n/a | n/a | n/a | 59 | 2 | 17 |
| Toffee Mocha, Whole Milk | 16 fl oz | 380 | 54 | 6 | n/a | n/a | n/a | 43 | 0 | 10 |
| **ICED** | | | | | | | | | | |
| Caffe Latte, Nonfat Milk | 16 fl oz | 90 | 0 | 0 | n/a | n/a | n/a | 13 | 0 | 8 |
| Caffe Latte, Whole Milk | 16 fl oz | 150 | 63 | 7 | n/a | n/a | n/a | 12 | 0 | 8 |
| Caffe Mocha Nonfat Milk | 16 fl oz | 170 | n/a | 2.5 | n/a | n/a | n/a | 36 | 2 | 9 |
| Caramel Macchiato, Nonfat Milk | 16 fl oz | 190 | 13.5 | 1.5 | n/a | n/a | n/a | 34 | 0 | 10 |
| Cinnamon Dolce, Nonfat | 16 fl oz | 210 | 0 | 0 | 0 | <5 | 135 | 41 | 0 | 11 |
| Flavored Latte, Nonfat Milk | 16 fl oz | 200 | 0 | 0 | n/a | n/a | n/a | 37 | 0 | 12 |
| Flavored Latte, Whole Milk | 16 fl oz | 220 | 54 | 6 | n/a | n/a | n/a | 34 | 0 | 7 |
| **Subway** | | | | | | | | | | |
| **6″ SANDWICHES** | | | | | | | | | | |
| Black Forest on Wheat | 1 sandwich | 290 | 40 | 4.5 | 1 | 25 | 1200 | 47 | 5 | 18 |
| Chicken & Bacon Ranch on Wheat | 1 sandwich | 570 | 250 | 28 | 10 | 95 | 1190 | 48 | 5 | 35 |
| Club on Wheat | 1 sandwich | 320 | 45 | 5 | 1.5 | 35 | 1140 | 47 | 5 | 26 |
| Cold Cut Combo on Wheat | 1 sandwich | 410 | 150 | 16 | 6 | 60 | 1450 | 48 | 5 | 21 |

| | SERVING SIZE | CAL | CAL FAT | TOT FAT (G) | SAT FAT (G) | CHOL (MG) | SOD (MG) | CARB (G) | FIBER (G) | PROT (G) |
|---|---|---|---|---|---|---|---|---|---|---|
| Italian B.M.T. on Wheat | 1 sandwich | 450 | 180 | 20 | 8 | 55 | 1730 | 48 | 5 | 22 |
| Meatball Marinara on Wheat | 1 sandwich | 580 | 200 | 23 | 9 | 45 | 1530 | 70 | 9 | 24 |
| Oven Roasted Chicken on Wheat | 1 sandwich | 320 | 40 | 4.5 | 1 | 25 | 750 | 49 | 5 | 23 |
| Roast Beef on Wheat | 1 sandwich | 310 | 40 | 4.5 | 1.5 | 25 | 800 | 45 | 5 | 26 |
| Spicy Italian on Wheat | 1 sandwich | 520 | 250 | 28 | 11 | 65 | 1830 | 47 | 5 | 22 |
| Sweet onion Chicken Teriyaki on Wheat | 1 sandwich | 380 | 40 | 4.5 | 1 | 50 | 1010 | 60 | 5 | 26 |
| Tuna on Wheat | 1 sandwich | 530 | 270 | 30 | 6 | 45 | 910 | 45 | 5 | 21 |
| Turkey Breast on Wheat | 1 sandwich | 280 | 30 | 3.5 | 1 | 20 | 920 | 47 | 5 | 18 |
| Veggie Delite on Wheat | 1 sandwich | 230 | 20 | 2.5 | .5 | 0 | 410 | 45 | 5 | 8 |
| **MUFFIN MELTS** | | | | | | | | | | |
| Black Forest Ham, Egg & Cheese | 1 sandwich | 180 | 60 | 7 | 2 | 95 | 650 | 18 | 5 | 15 |
| Double Bacon, Egg & Cheese | 1 sandwich | 220 | 90 | 10 | 3.5 | 95 | 640 | 18 | 4 | 16 |
| Egg & Cheese | 1 sandwich | 170 | 60 | 6 | 2 | 85 | 450 | 18 | 5 | 13 |
| Egg White & Cheese | 1 sandwich | 140 | 30 | 3.5 | 1 | 5 | 490 | 18 | 5 | 12 |
| Sausage, Egg & Cheese | 1 sandwich | 290 | 160 | 18 | 7 | 105 | 710 | 18 | 5 | 16 |
| Steak, Egg & Cheese | 1 sandwich | 190 | 60 | 7 | 2.5 | 95 | 600 | 19 | 6 | 16 |
| Western Egg w/Cheese | 1 sandwich | 460 | 60 | 7 | 2 | 200 | 650 | 19 | 6 | 15 |
| **OMELET SANDWICHES, 6" ON 9 GRAIN WHEAT** | | | | | | | | | | |
| Double Bacon Egg & Cheese | 1 sandwich | 520 | 220 | 25 | 11 | 210 | 1430 | 47 | 5 | 29 |
| Egg & Cheese | 1 sandwich | 420 | 160 | 18 | 7 | 190 | 1060 | 46 | 5 | 22 |
| Sausage, Egg & Cheese | 1 sandwich | 670 | 370 | 41 | 16 | 225 | 1580 | 46 | 5 | 30 |
| Western Egg w/Cheese | 1 sandwich | 450 | 170 | 19 | 7 | 20 | 1450 | 47 | 5 | 27 |
| **SALADS** | | | | | | | | | | |
| Turkey Breast | 1 salad | 110 | 20 | 2 | .5 | 20 | 570 | 11 | 4 | 12 |
| Veggie Delite | 1 salad | 50 | 10 | 1 | 0 | 0 | 65 | 9 | 4 | 3 |
| **Taco Bell** **BURRITOS & TACOS** | | | | | | | | | | |
| 7-layer Burrito | 1 burrito | 500 | 160 | 18 | 6 | 20 | 1270 | 68 | 12 | 18 |
| Bean Burrito | 1 burrito | 370 | 90 | 10 | 3.5 | 5 | 1150 | 56 | 11 | 14 |
| Beef Soft Taco | 1 taco | 210 | 80 | 9 | 4 | 30 | 560 | 21 | 3 | 10 |
| Cheesy Bean & Rice Burrito | 1 burrito | 490 | 190 | 21 | 5 | 10 | 1260 | 60 | 8 | 13 |
| Cheesy Double Beef Burrito | 1 burrito | 470 | 180 | 20 | 6 | 40 | 1580 | 54 | 6 | 18 |
| Chicken Supreme Burrito | 1 burrito | 400 | 110 | 12 | 5 | 40 | 1300 | 51 | 7 | 21 |
| Crunchy Taco | 1 taco | 170 | 90 | 10 | 3.5 | 30 | 330 | 12 | 3 | 8 |
| Fresco Bean Burrito | 1 burrito | 340 | 70 | 8 | 2.5 | 0 | 1170 | 56 | 11 | 12 |
| Fresco Crunchy Taco | 1 taco | 150 | 70 | 7 | 2.5 | 20 | 350 | 13 | 3 | 7 |

# restaurants

| | SERVING SIZE | CAL | CAL FAT | TOT FAT (G) | SAT FAT (G) | CHOL (MG) | SOD (MG) | CARB (G) | FIBER (G) | PROT (G) |
|---|---|---|---|---|---|---|---|---|---|---|
| Fresco Soft Chicken Taco | 1 taco | 180 | 60 | 7 | 3 | 20 | 580 | 22 | 3 | 8 |
| Fresco Supreme Chicken Burrito | 1 burrito | 340 | 70 | 8 | 2.5 | 25 | 1290 | 50 | 8 | 18 |
| **CHALUPAS & GORDITAS** | | | | | | | | | | |
| Beef Supreme Chalupa | 1 chalupa | 370 | 190 | 21 | 5 | 35 | 600 | 31 | 4 | 13 |
| Beef Supreme Gordita | 1 gordita | 300 | 120 | 13 | 5 | 35 | 590 | 31 | 4 | 13 |
| Chicken Nacho Cheese Gordita | 1 gordita | 270 | 90 | 10 | 1.5 | 25 | 760 | 30 | 2 | 15 |
| Chicken Supreme Chalupa | 1 chalupa | 350 | 160 | 18 | 4 | 35 | 640 | 30 | 3 | 17 |
| Steak Supreme Chalupa | 1 chalupa | 340 | 170 | 18 | 4 | 30 | 570 | 29 | 3 | 14 |
| **NACHOS** | | | | | | | | | | |
| BellGrande | as served | 770 | 380 | 42 | 7 | 30 | 1300 | 78 | 15 | 20 |
| Cheesy | as served | 280 | 150 | 17 | 1.5 | 0 | 300 | 28 | 2 | 4 |
| Original | as served | 330 | 190 | 21 | 2 | 0 | 520 | 31 | 2 | 4 |
| Supreme | as served | 440 | 220 | 24 | 5 | 30 | 800 | 42 | 8 | 13 |
| **SPECIALTIES** | | | | | | | | | | |
| Beef Enchirito | 1 enchirito | 370 | 150 | 17 | 8 | 45 | 1430 | 35 | 8 | 19 |
| Cheese Quesadilla | 1 item | 470 | 240 | 26 | 11 | 50 | 1120 | 40 | 4 | 19 |
| Chicken Ranch Taco Salad | 1 salad | 910 | 490 | 54 | 10 | 70 | 1660 | 71 | 9 | 35 |
| Crunchwrap Supreme | 1 item | 540 | 190 | 21 | 7 | 30 | 1400 | 71 | 6 | 16 |
| Mexican Pizza | 1 pizza | 540 | 270 | 30 | 8 | 45 | 1030 | 47 | 8 | 21 |
| Tostada | 1 tostada | 250 | 90 | 10 | 3.5 | 15 | 730 | 29 | 10 | 11 |

## Taco Del Mar
### ENCHILADAS & OTHERS

| | SERVING SIZE | CAL | CAL FAT | TOT FAT (G) | SAT FAT (G) | CHOL (MG) | SOD (MG) | CARB (G) | FIBER (G) | PROT (G) |
|---|---|---|---|---|---|---|---|---|---|---|
| Cheese Enchilada | 1 item | 820 | 240 | 27 | 11 | 55 | 2490 | 112 | 12 | 31 |
| Cheese Quesadilla | 1 item | 710 | 310 | 35 | 16 | 85 | 990 | 63 | 4 | 32 |
| Chicken Enchilada | 1 item | 990 | 300 | 33 | 13 | 115 | 2900 | 113 | 12 | 55 |
| Chicken Quesadilla | 1 item | 770 | 300 | 33 | 13 | 116 | 1220 | 34 | 5 | 49 |
| Nachos, Refried | as served | 1190 | 580 | 65 | 25 | 100 | 1800 | 110 | 12 | 37 |
| **REFRIED BAJA BOWLS** | | | | | | | | | | |
| Chicken | 1 bowl | 790 | 280 | 31 | 12 | 105 | 2230 | 79 | 9 | 44 |
| Fish | 1 bowl | 880 | 370 | 41 | 13 | 80 | 2330 | 95 | 9 | 31 |
| **REFRIED MONDO BURRITOS** | | | | | | | | | | |
| Cheese | 1 item | 870 | 220 | 24 | 8 | 30 | 1830 | 130 | 10 | 30 |
| Chicken | 1 item | 1030 | 280 | 32 | 9 | 90 | 2250 | 131 | 11 | 54 |
| Fish | 1 item | 840 | 270 | 30 | 5 | 35 | 1620 | 110 | 12 | 32 |
| **REFRIED TACO SALADS** | | | | | | | | | | |
| Chicken | 1 salad | 900 | 400 | 45 | 16 | 105 | 1870 | 73 | 11 | 47 |
| Fish | 1 salad | 1040 | 550 | 61 | 18 | 85 | 2050 | 89 | 11 | 34 |

| | SERVING SIZE | CAL | CAL FAT | TOT FAT (G) | SAT FAT (G) | CHOL (MG) | SOD (MG) | CARB (G) | FIBER (G) | PROT (G) |
|---|---|---|---|---|---|---|---|---|---|---|
| **TACOS** | | | | | | | | | | |
| Chicken, Hard Shell | 1 taco | 270 | 130 | 15 | 6 | 45 | 360 | 15 | 1 | 17 |
| Chicken, Soft Shell | 1 taco | 260 | 80 | 9 | 3.5 | 45 | 430 | 27 | 3 | 19 |
| Fish, Hard Shell | 1 taco | 270 | 130 | 14 | 5 | 45 | 370 | 17 | 1 | 15 |
| Fish, Soft Shell | 1 taco | 270 | 100 | 11 | 3.5 | 30 | 440 | 34 | 3 | 12 |
| **Taco Mayo** | | | | | | | | | | |
| **BURRITOS & TACOS** | | | | | | | | | | |
| Bean Burrito | 1 item | 496 | n/a | 16 | n/a | 15 | 1504 | 71 | 12 | 21 |
| Beef Burrito | 1 item | 492 | n/a | 23 | n/a | 56 | 1428 | 41 | 3 | 30 |
| Beef Super Burrito | 1 item | 539 | n/a | 23 | n/a | 44 | 1479 | 57 | 8 | 26 |
| Chicken Super Burrito | 1 item | 407 | n/a | 16 | n/a | 63 | 1089 | 39 | 2 | 25 |
| Crispy Beef Taco | 1 item | 161 | n/a | 9 | n/a | 20 | 243 | 10 | 1 | 9 |
| Soft Beef Taco | 1 item | 228 | n/a | 11 | n/a | 28 | 584 | 17 | 2 | 14 |
| Soft Chicken Taco | 1 item | 184 | n/a | 6 | n/a | 38 | 592 | 16 | 1 | 15 |
| Soft Steak Taco | 1 item | 204 | n/a | 7 | n/a | 33 | 577 | 16 | 1 | 17 |
| Steak Super Burrito | 1 item | 434 | n/a | 18 | n/a | 56 | 1069 | 39 | 2 | 27 |
| **NACHOS & QUESADILLAS** | | | | | | | | | | |
| Cheese Quesadilla | 1 item | 596 | n/a | 35 | n/a | 83 | 1174 | 45 | 4 | 25 |
| Chicken Quesadilla | 1 item | 676 | n/a | 37 | n/a | 123 | 1588 | 46 | 4 | 39 |
| Classic, Cheese Nachos | as served | 377 | n/a | 19 | n/a | 5 | 834 | 45 | 4 | 6 |
| Classic, Chicken Supreme Nachos | as served | 643 | n/a | 29 | n/a | 53 | 1716 | 69 | 11 | 28 |
| Classic, Steak Supreme Nachos | as served | 669 | n/a | 31 | n/a | 47 | 1696 | 69 | 11 | 30 |
| Steak Quesadilla | 1 item | 703 | n/a | 39 | n/a | 116 | 1568 | 46 | 4 | 41 |
| **SIDES** | | | | | | | | | | |
| Guac-N-Chips | as served | 399 | n/a | 22 | n/a | 0 | 371 | 45 | 7 | 4 |
| Potato Locos Small | as served | 379 | n/a | 24 | n/a | 0 | 1618 | 36 | 5 | 5 |
| Queso-N-Chips | as served | 449 | n/a | 22 | n/a | 44 | 1296 | 49 | 3 | 14 |
| **TACO SALADS** | | | | | | | | | | |
| Beef | 1 salad | 705 | n/a | 38 | n/a | 64 | 1766 | 57 | 13 | 37 |
| Chicken | 1 salad | 438 | n/a | 23 | n/a | 73 | 1169 | 30 | 3 | 27 |
| Steak | 1 salad | 444 | n/a | 25 | n/a | 56 | 1045 | 30 | 3 | 26 |
| **Taco Time** | | | | | | | | | | |
| **BREAKFAST** | | | | | | | | | | |
| Cheese Omelet | 1 item | 490 | 330 | 36 | 18 | 795 | 590 | 6 | 0 | 35 |
| Egg & Bacon Burrito | 1 item | 510 | 220 | 24 | 9 | 220 | 1110 | 49 | 8 | 25 |
| Nacho Omelet | 1 item | 740 | 430 | 48 | 23 | 840 | 2570 | 26 | 5 | 50 |
| Ultimate Burrito | 1 item | 860 | 520 | 58 | 17 | 425 | 1620 | 52 | 8 | 35 |

| | SERVING SIZE | CAL | CAL FAT | TOT FAT (G) | SAT FAT (G) | CHOL (MG) | SOD (MG) | CARB (G) | FIBER (G) | PROT (G) |
|---|---|---|---|---|---|---|---|---|---|---|
| **BURRITOS & TACOS** | | | | | | | | | | |
| Beef, Bean & Cheese Burrito | 1 item | 490 | 150 | 17 | 7 | 45 | 2310 | 55 | 11 | 26 |
| Casita Chicken Burrito | 1 item | 490 | 150 | 17 | 10 | 85 | 2350 | 42 | 5 | 34 |
| Casita Ground Beef Burrito | 1 item | 540 | 210 | 24 | 12 | 80 | 2570 | 46 | 6 | 29 |
| Chicken & Black Bean Burrito | 1 item | 490 | 140 | 16 | 6 | 60 | 1270 | 54 | 9 | 30 |
| Chicken B.L.T. Burrito | 1 item | 690 | 350 | 39 | 10 | 90 | 1600 | 43 | 8 | 39 |
| Crispy Chicken Ranchero Burrito | 1 item | 600 | 280 | 31 | 7 | 60 | 1250 | 51 | 7 | 29 |
| Crispy Ground Beef Burrito | 1 item | 430 | 190 | 21 | 6 | 45 | 830 | 36 | 4 | 22 |
| Crispy, Ground Beef Taco | 1 item | 260 | 150 | 17 | 5 | 35 | 460 | 12 | 2 | 14 |
| Soft Chicken Taco | 1 item | 360 | 80 | 9 | 4.5 | 50 | 860 | 40 | 7 | 28 |
| Soft Ground Beef Taco | 1 item | 420 | 140 | 16 | 7 | 45 | 1020 | 43 | 9 | 23 |
| **ENCHILADAS** | | | | | | | | | | |
| Chicken | 1 item | 230 | 50 | 5 | 3 | 50 | 610 | 17 | 1 | 23 |
| Ground Beef | 1 item | 290 | 110 | 12 | 5 | 45 | 830 | 21 | 3 | 18 |
| **SIDES** | | | | | | | | | | |
| Biscuits & Gravy—Small | as served | 410 | 210 | 23 | 5 | 20 | 1130 | 43 | 2 | 9 |
| Cheddar Fries—Medium | as served | 500 | 310 | 35 | 11 | 30 | 1170 | 39 | 4 | 11 |
| Mexi Fries—Medium | as served | 390 | 230 | 26 | 4.5 | 0 | 990 | 38 | 4 | 4 |
| Stuffed Fries—Medium | as served | 460 | 250 | 28 | 8 | 15 | 1020 | 42 | 4 | 11 |
| Taters & Gravy—Small | as served | 360 | 200 | 23 | 6 | 20 | 960 | 34 | 4 | 7 |
| **TACO SALADS** | | | | | | | | | | |
| Regular—Chicken | 1 salad | 310 | 120 | 13 | 4 | 50 | 680 | 22 | 2 | 25 |
| Regular—Ground Beef | 1 salad | 370 | 180 | 20 | 6 | 45 | 810 | 24 | 4 | 20 |
| **TOSTADA** | | | | | | | | | | |
| Bean | 1 item | 230 | 110 | 13 | 4 | 15 | 1320 | 21 | 3 | 8 |
| Chicken | 1 item | 380 | 180 | 20 | 6 | 0 | 1830 | 25 | 5 | 21 |
| **TCBY** | | | | | | | | | | |
| **BERIYO SMOOTHIES** | | | | | | | | | | |
| Berrylicious | 16 fl oz | 260 | 15 | 1.5 | 1 | 5 | 50 | 64 | 4 | 3 |
| Mondo Mango | 16 fl oz | 280 | 10 | 1 | 1 | 5 | 50 | 69 | 3 | 3 |
| Peach Palm | 16 fl oz | 300 | 40 | 4 | 3 | 5 | 85 | 67 | 3 | 3 |
| Pina Paradise | 16 fl oz | 320 | 90 | 10 | 8 | 5 | 150 | 57 | 3 | 3 |
| Pink Pineapple | 16 fl oz | 310 | 70 | 7 | 6 | 5 | 120 | 62 | 3 | 3 |
| Strawberry Banana | 16 fl oz | 300 | 15 | 1.5 | 1 | 5 | 50 | 72 | 3 | 3 |
| **FROZEN YOGURT & SORBET** | | | | | | | | | | |
| Average for Hand-Scooped Yogurt | 1/2 cup | 130 | 40 | 4 | 2.5 | 10 | 65 | 20 | 1 | 3 |
| Average for Soft Serve Yogurt | 1/2 cup | 105 | 10 | 1 | .5 | 2.5 | 70 | 23 | 3 | 4 |

| | SERVING SIZE | CAL | CAL FAT | TOT FAT (G) | SAT FAT (G) | CHOL (MG) | SOD (MG) | CARB (G) | FIBER (G) | PROT (G) |
|---|---|---|---|---|---|---|---|---|---|---|
| Mango Sorbet | 1/2 cup | 110 | 0 | 0 | 0 | 0 | 10 | 26 | 0 | 0 |
| Raspberry Sorbet | 1/2 cup | 100 | 0 | 0 | 0 | 0 | 10 | 25 | 0 | 0 |
| **PARFAITS** | | | | | | | | | | |
| Chocolate Dream | 1 parfait | 500 | 180 | 20 | 13 | 35 | 230 | 69 | 0 | 10 |
| Cookie Cookie Dough | 1 parfait | 500 | 160 | 18 | 9 | 35 | 250 | 76 | 1 | 11 |
| Caramel Crunch | 1 parfait | 700 | 220 | 24 | 8 | 35 | 330 | 108 | 1 | 13 |
| Fruity Fudge | 1 parfait | 600 | 230 | 25 | 16 | 40 | 240 | 85 | 1 | 12 |
| Triple Berry | 1 parfait | 440 | 150 | 17 | 13 | 35 | 170 | 63 | 2 | 10 |
| **SHIVERS, MEDIUM** | | | | | | | | | | |
| Banana Berry Super Split | 1 shiver | 650 | 90 | 10 | 7 | 35 | 340 | 133 | 15 | 20 |
| Berry Blend | 1 shiver | 980 | 240 | 27 | 17 | 95 | 470 | 158 | 2 | 26 |
| Candy Shoppe Reese's | 1 shiver | 1,020 | 300 | 33 | 15 | 40 | 620 | 169 | 16 | 29 |
| Chocolateberry | 1 shiver | 790 | 170 | 19 | 12 | 40 | 520 | 147 | 20 | 24 |
| Cookie Dough Monster | 1 shiver | 930 | 200 | 23 | 9 | 40 | 490 | 170 | 15 | 23 |
| M&M Peanut Butter Cup | 1 shiver | 1,020 | 290 | 32 | 16 | 45 | 690 | 176 | 19 | 29 |
| Nuts for Nuts | 1 shiver | 940 | 250 | 28 | 9 | 40 | 450 | 159 | 17 | 26 |
| PB & J | 1 shiver | 900 | 280 | 31 | 11 | 40 | 510 | 142 | 16 | 25 |
| Peanut Butter Perfection | 1 shiver | 990 | 300 | 33 | 15 | 40 | 570 | 159 | 17 | 28 |
| Strawberry Shortcake | 1 shiver | 730 | 130 | 15 | 9 | 45 | 430 | 141 | 15 | 22 |
| **SUNDAES & SPLITS** | | | | | | | | | | |
| Banana Split Mississippi Mud | 1 serving | 880 | 310 | 35 | 13 | 30 | 420 | 128 | 6 | 20 |
| Banana Split Monkey's Uncle | 1 serving | 790 | 260 | 29 | 12 | 35 | 270 | 123 | 4 | 15 |
| Black Forest Sundae | 1 sundae | 1,010 | 430 | 48 | 16 | 80 | 490 | 135 | 3 | 14 |
| Chocolate Chunk Cookie Sundae | 1 sundae | 580 | 200 | 22 | 13 | 40 | 330 | 87 | 1 | 9 |
| Hot Caramel Sundae | 1 sundae | 480 | 150 | 17 | 9 | 20 | 340 | 77 | 1 | 9 |
| Hot Fudge Strawberry Sundae | 1 sundae | 580 | 210 | 24 | 10 | 30 | 320 | 84 | 1 | 9 |
| Hot Fudge Brownie Sundae | 1 sundae | 710 | 300 | 33 | 12 | 55 | 330 | 93 | 2 | 11 |

# Uno Chicago Grill
### APPETIZERS

| | SERVING SIZE | CAL | CAL FAT | TOT FAT (G) | SAT FAT (G) | CHOL (MG) | SOD (MG) | CARB (G) | FIBER (G) | PROT (G) |
|---|---|---|---|---|---|---|---|---|---|---|
| 3 Way Buffalo Bites | 1/3 item | 430 | 190 | 21 | 2.5 | 60 | 1840 | 39 | 0 | 31 |
| 3 Way Buffalo Wings | 1/3 item | 430 | 310 | 65 | 8 | 135 | 470 | 3 | 0 | 21 |
| Buffalo Chicken Quesadillas | 1/3 item | 350 | 140 | 16 | 8 | 40 | 890 | 36 | 2 | 19 |
| Calamari | 1/3 item | 350 | 270 | 31 | 3.5 | 130 | 690 | 28 | 1 | 13 |
| House made Guacamole, w/Chips | 1/2 item | 230 | 100 | 11 | 1.5 | 0 | 230 | 32 | 6 | 4 |
| Muchos Nachos | 1/3 item | 460 | 190 | 21 | 8 | 45 | 810 | 54 | 5 | 13 |
| Onion Strings | 1/3 item | 600 | 380 | 42 | 7 | 5 | 630 | 50 | 5 | 6 |
| Pizza Skins | 1/5 item | 410 | 250 | 28 | 9 | 40 | 600 | 29 | 1 | 12 |

# restaurants

| | SERVING SIZE | CAL | CAL FAT | TOT FAT (G) | SAT FAT (G) | CHOL (MG) | SOD (MG) | CARB (G) | FIBER (G) | PROT (G) |
|---|---|---|---|---|---|---|---|---|---|---|
| Roasted Vegetable Quesadilla | 1/3 item | 300 | 120 | 13 | 5 | 20 | 730 | 36 | 2 | 11 |
| Shrimp & Crab Fondue | 1/5 item | 220 | 140 | 16 | 4.5 | 55 | 500 | 13 | 0 | 8 |
| **BURGERS** | | | | | | | | | | |
| BBQ w/Bacon & Cheddar | 1/2 burger | 700 | 420 | 46 | 18 | 130 | 1260 | 32 | 2 | 41 |
| Uno Original | 1/2 burger | 550 | 320 | 36 | 14 | 105 | 810 | 24 | 2 | 30 |
| Veggie | 1/2 burger | 310 | 70 | 8 | 2.5 | 5 | 1170 | 34 | 6 | 15 |
| **DEEP DISH PIZZAS** | | | | | | | | | | |
| Buffalo Chicken | 1 slice | 510 | 320 | 35 | 10 | 45 | 800 | 32 | 1 | 19 |
| Cheese & Tomato | 1 slice | 580 | 360 | 40 | 12 | 35 | 920 | 39 | 2 | 21 |
| Chicago Classic | 1 slice | 770 | 490 | 55 | 18 | 75 | 1640 | 40 | 2 | 33 |
| Four Cheese | 1 slice | 640 | 396 | 44 | 13 | 40 | 920 | 39 | 2 | 20 |
| Prima Pepperoni | 1 slice | 610 | 380 | 42 | 12 | 40 | 1040 | 39 | 2 | 30 |
| **ENTRÉES** | | | | | | | | | | |
| 8 oz Sirloin | 1/2 entrée | 200 | 60 | 7 | 2.5 | 50 | 310 | 0 | 0 | 33 |
| Baked Stuffed Chicken | 1/2 entrée | 180 | 80 | 9 | 3 | 60 | 640 | 3 | 1 | 27 |
| Brewmasters Grill NY Sirloin | 1/2 entrée | 260 | 60 | 7 | 2.5 | 90 | 790 | 12 | 0 | 43 |
| Cajun Blackened Salmon | 1/2 entrée | 310 | 200 | 22 | 5 | 75 | 500 | 5 | 1 | 22 |
| Chicken Broccoli Alfredo | 1/2 entrée | 620 | 310 | 35 | 11 | 85 | 820 | 53 | 3 | 28 |
| Chicken Penne w/White Wine Garlic Sauce | 1/2 entrée | 600 | 300 | 34 | 12 | 80 | 1050 | 54 | 4 | 24 |
| Romano Crusted Chicken Parmesan | 1/2 entrée | 560 | 170 | 19 | 4.5 | 65 | 1290 | 69 | 5 | 37 |
| Sirloin Steak Tips | 1/2 entrée | 290 | 120 | 14 | 4 | 85 | 1030 | 4 | 1 | 31 |
| The Chop House Classic | 1/2 entrée | 260 | 80 | 9 | 3.5 | 65 | 320 | 0 | 0 | 42 |
| **SALADS** | | | | | | | | | | |
| Asian Chicken | 1/2 salad | 560 | 250 | 28 | 3 | 90 | 1110 | 47 | 8 | 35 |
| Caesar | 1/2 salad | 250 | 200 | 22 | 5 | 25 | 430 | 9 | 3 | 7 |
| Chicken Caesar | 1/2 salad | 290 | 180 | 20 | 4.5 | 60 | 720 | 11 | 3 | 22 |
| Classic Cobb | 1/2 salad | 350 | 240 | 26 | 8 | 200 | 960 | 9 | 3 | 23 |
| House w/Grilled Chicken | 1/2 salad | 160 | 60 | 7 | 1 | 35 | 390 | 10 | 2 | 17 |
| **SIDES** | | | | | | | | | | |
| French Fries | as served | 450 | 290 | 33 | 3.5 | 0 | 1290 | 36 | 7 | 5 |
| Uno Breadstick | 1 item | 180 | 100 | 12 | 2 | 0 | 340 | 18 | 1 | 3 |
| **Wawa** | | | | | | | | | | |
| **HOT-TO-GO BOWLS** | | | | | | | | | | |
| Mac & Cheese w/Beef Stew | 1 bowl | 480 | 198 | 22 | 8 | n/a | 1660 | 48 | n/a | n/a |
| Mac & Cheese w/Chicken Strips | 1 bowl | 600 | 261 | 29 | 8.5 | n/a | 1910 | 56 | n/a | n/a |
| Mac & Cheese w/Chili | 1 bowl | 460 | 171 | 19 | 7 | n/a | 1620 | 52 | n/a | n/a |
| Mashed Potatoes, Medium | 1 bowl | 530 | 297 | 33 | 14 | n/a | 1400 | 52 | n/a | n/a |

| | SERVING SIZE | CAL | CAL FAT | TOT FAT (G) | SAT FAT (G) | CHOL (MG) | SOD (MG) | CARB (G) | FIBER (G) | PROT (G) |
|---|---|---|---|---|---|---|---|---|---|---|
| Mashed Potatoes w/Chicken Strips | 1 bowl | 760 | 405 | 45 | 16.5 | n/a | 2270 | 68 | n/a | n/a |
| Shepherd's Pie, Medium | 1 pie | 470 | 243 | 27 | 11 | n/a | 1880 | 41 | n/a | n/a |
| **SOUPS & SANDWICHES** | | | | | | | | | | |
| Beef Cheesesteak Classic | 1 hoagie | 730 | 225 | 25 | 11 | n/a | 2070 | 71 | n/a | n/a |
| Beef Stew, Medium | as served | 460 | 207 | 23 | 9 | n/a | 2630 | 35 | n/a | n/a |
| BLT Classic | 1 sandwich | 505 | 126 | 14 | 5 | n/a | 1650 | 74 | n/a | n/a |
| Chicken Cheesesteak Classic | 1 hoagie | 700 | 198 | 22 | 11 | n/a | 2070 | 71 | n/a | n/a |
| Chicken Salad Classic | 1 sandwich | 860 | 414 | 46 | 7 | n/a | 1810 | 80 | n/a | n/a |
| Chili, Medium | as served | 260 | 72 | 8 | 3 | n/a | 1670 | 33 | n/a | n/a |
| Clam Chowder, Medium | as served | 280 | 117 | 13 | 8 | n/a | 1340 | 29 | n/a | n/a |
| Egg Salad Classic | 1 sandwich | 860 | 450 | 50 | 10 | n/a | 1310 | 79 | n/a | n/a |
| Genoa Classic | 1 sandwich | 430 | 99 | 11 | 3 | n/a | 1250 | 71 | n/a | n/a |
| Grilled Chicken Breast | 1 hoagie | 35 | 9 | 1 | 0 | n/a | 460 | 1 | n/a | n/a |
| Ham Classic | 1 sandwich | 480 | 72 | 8 | 3 | n/a | 2020 | 73 | n/a | n/a |
| Home Style Roast Beef Classic | 1 hoagie | 820 | 279 | 31 | 12.5 | n/a | 3270 | 77 | n/a | n/a |
| Hot Turkey Classic | 1 hoagie | 760 | 234 | 26 | 11 | n/a | 2940 | 77 | n/a | n/a |
| Italian Classic | 1 sandwich | 595 | 171 | 19 | 6.5 | n/a | 2310 | 74 | n/a | n/a |
| Meatball Classic | 1 hoagie | 1030 | 495 | 55 | 21.5 | n/a | 3720 | 98 | n/a | n/a |
| Minestrone, Medium | as served | 140 | 36 | 4 | .5 | n/a | 1060 | 23 | n/a | n/a |
| Premium Turkey Classic | 1 sandwich | 460 | 36 | 4 | .5 | n/a | 1920 | 74 | n/a | n/a |
| Roast Beef Classic | 1 sandwich | 535 | 63 | 7 | .5 | n/a | 1470 | 74 | n/a | n/a |
| Tuna Classic | 1 sandwich | 925 | 495 | 55 | 9.5 | n/a | 1860 | 83 | n/a | n/a |
| Turkey Classic | 1 sandwich | 475 | 63 | 7 | .5 | n/a | 2340 | 77 | n/a | n/a |
| **Wendy's** | | | | | | | | | | |
| **BREADS** | | | | | | | | | | |
| Premium Bun | 1 bun | 190 | n/a | 2 | 0 | 0 | 360 | 36 | 1 | 6 |
| Sandwich Bun | 1 bun | 120 | n/a | 1 | 0 | 0 | 240 | 24 | 1 | 4 |
| Tortilla | 1 tortilla | 130 | n/a | 3.5 | 1 | 0 | 280 | 21 | 0 | 3 |
| **BURGERS & SANDWICHES** | | | | | | | | | | |
| Bacon Deluxe Single | 1 burger | 650 | 330 | 37 | 15 | 110 | 1380 | 46 | 2 | 34 |
| Baconator, Single | 1 burger | 610 | 310 | 34 | 14 | 105 | 1170 | 43 | 1 | 32 |
| Chicken Club Sandwich | 1 sandwich | 620 | 270 | 30 | 9 | 85 | 1400 | 55 | 2 | 35 |
| Crispy Chicken Sandwich | 1 sandwich | 350 | 140 | 16 | 3 | 30 | 710 | 39 | 2 | 14 |
| Double Jr. Bacon Cheeseburger | 1 burger | 440 | n/a | 25 | 11 | 80 | 730 | 28 | 2 | 25 |
| Double Stack | 1 burger | 360 | 160 | 18 | 8 | 70 | 760 | 27 | 1 | 23 |
| Double w/Everything & Cheese | 1 burger | 750 | n/a | 42 | 18 | 155 | 1370 | 44 | 2 | 49 |
| Homestyle Chicken Fillet Sandwich | 1 sandwich | 470 | n/a | 18 | 3.5 | 50 | 1160 | 52 | 3 | 26 |

# restaurants

| | SERVING SIZE | CAL | CAL FAT | TOT FAT (G) | SAT FAT (G) | CHOL (MG) | SOD (MG) | CARB (G) | FIBER (G) | PROT (G) |
|---|---|---|---|---|---|---|---|---|---|---|
| Jr. Cheeseburger Deluxe | 1 burger | 300 | n/a | 14 | 6 | 45 | 720 | 29 | 2 | 15 |
| Jr. Hamburger | 1 burger | 230 | n/a | 8 | 3 | 30 | 480 | 26 | 1 | 12 |
| Spicy Chicken Fillet Sandwich | 1 sandwich | 460 | n/a | 16 | 3 | 60 | 1330 | 54 | 3 | 26 |
| Ultimate Chicken Grill Sandwich | 1 sandwich | 370 | n/a | 7 | 1.5 | 90 | 1150 | 42 | 2 | 34 |
| **CHICKEN NUGGETS & WINGS** | | | | | | | | | | |
| Chicken Nuggets | 5 pieces | 230 | n/a | 14 | 3 | 35 | 430 | 13 | 0 | 12 |
| Honey BBQ Boneless Wings | as served | 620 | 190 | 21 | 3.5 | 85 | 1810 | 71 | 0 | 37 |
| Spicy Chipotle Boneless Wings | as served | 550 | 210 | 23 | 4 | 85 | 1510 | 50 | 1 | 37 |
| Sweet & Spicy Asian Boneless Wings | as served | 600 | 190 | 21 | 3.5 | 85 | 2350 | 64 | 1 | 37 |
| **DESSERTS** | | | | | | | | | | |
| Chocolate Frosty, Small | 1 frosty | 310 | 70 | 8 | 5 | 25 | 140 | 52 | 0 | 8 |
| **SALADS** | | | | | | | | | | |
| Apple Pecan Chicken Salad, Full | 1 salad | 350 | n/a | 12 | 7 | 110 | 1210 | 29 | 5 | 37 |
| Baja Salad, Full | 1 salad | 550 | n/a | 33 | 14 | 85 | 1610 | 36 | 12 | 33 |
| BLT Cobb Salad, Full | 1 salad | 460 | n/a | 26 | 12 | 285 | 1490 | 12 | 3 | 46 |
| Spicy Chicken Caesar Salad, Full | 1/2 salad | 450 | n/a | 25 | 11 | 100 | 1290 | 25 | 6 | 32 |
| **SNACKS & SIDES** | | | | | | | | | | |
| Plain Baked Potato | 1 potato | 270 | n/a | 0 | 0 | 0 | 25 | 61 | 7 | 7 |
| Small Chili | as served | 220 | n/a | 7 | 3 | 35 | 870 | 22 | 6 | 18 |
| Small French Fries | as served | 340 | 150 | 17 | 2.5 | 0 | 280 | 43 | 4 | 4 |
| Sour Cream & Chives Baked Potato | 1 potato | 320 | n/a | 3.5 | 2 | 10 | 50 | 63 | 7 | 8 |
| **Whataburger** | | | | | | | | | | |
| **BREAKFAST** | | | | | | | | | | |
| Biscuit Sandwich w/Bacon, Egg, & Cheese | 1 sandwich | 500 | 270 | 32 | 14 | 232 | 1231 | 33 | 1 | 16 |
| Biscuit w/Sausage | 1 sandwich | 540 | 320 | 37 | 17 | 23 | 1169 | 32 | 1 | 18 |
| Breakfast Platter w/Bacon | 1 sandwich | 730 | 390 | 45 | 14 | 460 | 1376 | 93 | 1 | 24 |
| Breakfast Platter w/Sausage | 1 sandwich | 920 | 550 | 63 | 21 | 475 | 1698 | 93 | 1 | 34 |
| Egg Sandwich | 1 sandwich | 310 | 150 | 17 | 5 | 224 | 604 | 25 | 1 | 12 |
| Taquito w/Bacon, Egg, & Cheese | 1 taquito | 420 | 220 | 24 | 9 | 355 | 1157 | 27 | 3 | 19 |
| **BURGERS** | | | | | | | | | | |
| Burger | 1 burger | 620 | 270 | 30 | 10 | 65 | 1262 | 58 | 2 | 26 |
| Double Meat | 1 burger | 870 | 440 | 49 | 18 | 129 | 1510 | 58 | 2 | 43 |
| Triple Meat | 1 burger | 1120 | 610 | 68 | 26 | 192 | 1759 | 58 | 2 | 61 |
| With bacon & cheese | 1 burger | 780 | 380 | 43 | 16 | 98 | 1997 | 59 | 2 | 36 |
| **CHICKEN & FISH** | | | | | | | | | | |
| Chicken Strips, 2 pieces | 2 pieces | 300 | 140 | 16 | 6 | 36 | 593 | 22 | 1 | 18 |
| Grilled Chicken Sandwich | 1 sandwich | 470 | 170 | 19 | 4 | 55 | 1018 | 49 | 3 | 27 |

| | SERVING SIZE | CAL | CAL FAT | TOT FAT (G) | SAT FAT (G) | CHOL (MG) | SOD (MG) | CARB (G) | FIBER (G) | PROT (G) |
|---|---|---|---|---|---|---|---|---|---|---|
| Honey Butter Chicken Biscuit | 1 sandwich | 560 | 290 | 34 | 13 | 27 | 1008 | 50 | 2 | 14 |
| Whatacatch Sandwich | 1 sandwich | 450 | 200 | 24 | 4 | 32 | 881 | 44 | 3 | 16 |

## SALADS

| | | | | | | | | | | |
|---|---|---|---|---|---|---|---|---|---|---|
| Chicken Strips | 1 salad | 350 | 140 | 16 | 6 | 36 | 606 | 33 | 5 | 19 |
| Garden | 1 salad | 50 | 0 | 0 | 0 | 0 | 13 | 11 | 4 | 1 |
| Grilled Chicken | 1 salad | 220 | 60 | 7 | 1.5 | 50 | 633 | 18 | 4 | 21 |
| Side Salad | 1 salad | 25 | 0 | 0 | 0 | 0 | 6 | 5 | 3 | 0 |

## SHAKES & MALTS

| | | | | | | | | | | |
|---|---|---|---|---|---|---|---|---|---|---|
| Medium Chocolate Malt | as served | 1050 | 230 | 25 | 18 | 97 | 460 | 188 | 3 | 21 |
| Medium Chocolate Shake | as served | 1000 | 240 | 26 | 18 | 102 | 439 | 171 | 3 | 22 |

## SIDES & ADD ONS

| | | | | | | | | | | |
|---|---|---|---|---|---|---|---|---|---|---|
| Biscuit | as served | 300 | 130 | 17 | 8 | 0 | 644 | 32 | 1 | 5 |
| Hash Brown Sticks | as served | 200 | 110 | 12 | .5 | 0 | 280 | 60 | 0 | 2 |
| Medium French Fries | as served | 480 | 250 | 27 | 4.5 | 0 | 347 | 55 | 7 | 5 |
| Medium Onion Rings | as served | 400 | 230 | 25 | 8 | 2 | 787 | 37 | 3 | 5 |

# White Castle
## BREAKFAST

| | | | | | | | | | | |
|---|---|---|---|---|---|---|---|---|---|---|
| Bacon, Egg, Cheese Sandwich | 1 sandwich | 190 | 100 | 11 | 4 | 225 | 430 | 13 | 1 | 12 |
| Bologna, Egg, Cheese Sandwich | 1 sandwich | 310 | 180 | 20 | 7 | 250 | 830 | 15 | 1 | 16 |
| Egg, Cheese Sandwich | 1 sandwich | 160 | 70 | 8 | 3 | 220 | 330 | 13 | 1 | 10 |
| French Toast Sticks | 1 sandwich | 460 | 270 | 31 | 4.5 | 0 | 410 | 39 | 2 | 5 |
| Hamburger, Egg, Cheese Sandwich | 1 sandwich | 230 | 120 | 14 | 6 | 225 | 350 | 13 | 1 | 14 |
| Huevos Rancheros w/Sausage Sandwich | 1 sandwich | 310 | 200 | 23 | 9 | 245 | 710 | 14 | 1 | 15 |
| Sausage, Egg, Cheese Sandwich | 1 sandwich | 320 | 200 | 22 | 9 | 245 | 640 | 13 | 1 | 15 |

## BURGERS & SANDWICHES

| | | | | | | | | | | |
|---|---|---|---|---|---|---|---|---|---|---|
| A1 Slider w/Cheese | 1 burger | 170 | 80 | 9 | 4 | 15 | 570 | 16 | 1 | 8 |
| Bacon Cheeseburger | 1 burger | 190 | 100 | 11 | 5 | 20 | 550 | 13 | 1 | 9 |
| Chicken Breast w/Cheese | 1 sandwich | 390 | 250 | 28 | 5 | 25 | 650 | 20 | 1 | 13 |
| Chicken Ring w/Cheese | 1 sandwich | 380 | 270 | 30 | 6 | 40 | 460 | 16 | 1 | 10 |
| Chicken Supreme | 1 sandwich | 420 | 280 | 31 | 6 | 30 | 750 | 20 | 1 | 14 |
| Double Burger | 1 burger | 240 | 110 | 12 | 5 | 20 | 660 | 21 | 1 | 12 |
| Double A1 Slider w/Cheese | 1 burger | 310 | 150 | 17 | 8 | 30 | 1070 | 26 | 1 | 15 |
| Double Bacon Cheeseburger | 1 burger | 350 | 200 | 22 | 10 | 40 | 1050 | 21 | 1 | 18 |
| Double Cheeseburger | 1 burger | 300 | 150 | 17 | 8 | 30 | 940 | 20 | 1 | 15 |
| Double Fish w/o Cheese | 1 sandwich | 550 | 390 | 43 | 6 | 30 | 420 | 24 | 23 | 17 |
| Fish w/Cheese | 1 sandwich | 340 | 220 | 24 | 4.5 | 20 | 410 | 18 | 12 | 11 |
| Pulled Pork BBQ | 1 sandwich | 170 | 40 | 4.5 | 1 | 25 | 460 | 25 | 1 | 9 |

# restaurants

| | SERVING SIZE | CAL | CAL FAT | TOT FAT (G) | SAT FAT (G) | CHOL (MG) | SOD (MG) | CARB (G) | FIBER (G) | PROT |
|---|---|---|---|---|---|---|---|---|---|---|
| Single Burger | 1 burger | 140 | 60 | 6 | 2.5 | 10 | 360 | 13 | 1 | 7 |
| Surf & Turf w/o Cheese | 1 sandwich | 480 | 300 | 33 | 8 | 35 | 720 | 26 | 13 | 19 |
| **CHICKEN & FISH** | | | | | | | | | | |
| Chicken Rings | 6 rings | 530 | 430 | 47 | 10 | 105 | 610 | 12 | 0 | 18 |
| Medium Fish Nibblers | as served | 320 | 140 | 16 | 2.5 | 10 | 700 | 28 | 1 | 16 |
| Regular Clam Strips | as served | 210 | 150 | 17 | 2 | 15 | 620 | 5 | 0 | 8 |
| **SIDES** | | | | | | | | | | |
| Hashbrowns | as served | 310 | 250 | 28 | 5 | 0 | 250 | 14 | 3 | 1 |
| Medium French Fries | as served | 370 | 230 | 25 | 4 | 0 | 50 | 33 | 3 | 3 |
| Medium Home-Style Onion Rings | as served | 480 | 290 | 33 | 4.5 | 0 | 580 | 40 | 2 | 6 |
| Medium Sweet Potato Fries | as served | 480 | 270 | 30 | 3 | 0 | 380 | 47 | 6 | 4 |
| Mozzarella Sticks | 5 sticks | 740 | 500 | 55 | 14 | 50 | 1420 | 36 | 2 | 21 |

## Zaxby's
### ENTRÉES

| | SERVING SIZE | CAL | CAL FAT | TOT FAT (G) | SAT FAT (G) | CHOL (MG) | SOD (MG) | CARB (G) | FIBER (G) | PROT |
|---|---|---|---|---|---|---|---|---|---|---|
| Big Zax Snak Meal Dealz | 1 entrée | 960 | 450 | 52 | 10 | 93 | 2100 | 83 | 8 | 40 |
| Boneless Wings Meal Dealz | 1 entrée | 850 | 460 | 50 | 9 | 57 | 1515 | 76 | 7 | 23 |
| Chicken Finger Plate | 1 entrée | 1280 | 620 | 71 | 13 | 151 | 2830 | 98 | 11 | 62 |
| Chicken Finger Sandwich Meal Dealz | 1 entrée | 1110 | 490 | 56 | 11 | 88 | 2100 | 107 | 9 | 45 |
| Chicken Parmesan Sandwich Meal Dealz | 1 entrée | 1120 | 510 | 58 | 11 | 94 | 2310 | 106 | 9 | 46 |
| Chicken Salad Sandwich Meal | 1 entrée | 1030 | 560 | 63 | 11 | 95 | 1320 | 81 | 7 | 28 |
| Nibbler Meal Dealz | 1 entrée | 1340 | 620 | 71 | 15 | 94 | 2430 | 138 | 10 | 50 |
| Wings & Things | 1 entrée | 1710 | 950 | 107 | 22 | 425 | 2735 | 86 | 8 | 73 |
| **ZALADS (NO DRESSING)** | | | | | | | | | | |
| Blue Zalad, No Chicken | 1 salad | 415 | 200 | 24 | 11 | 30 | 820 | 34 | 3 | 13 |
| Caesar Zalad, No Chicken | 1 salad | 380 | 200 | 21 | 8 | 46 | 845 | 29 | 4 | 13 |
| House, Grilled Chicken | 1 salad | 605 | 260 | 29 | 13 | 137 | 1580 | 34 | 3 | 47 |
| House, No Chicken | 1 salad | 415 | 210 | 24 | 11 | 30 | 710 | 34 | 3 | 12 |
| **MILKSHAKES** | | | | | | | | | | |
| Chocolate | 1 shake | 835 | 332 | 37 | 23 | 150 | 351 | 114 | 2 | 13 |
| **SIDES** | | | | | | | | | | |
| Boneless Wings | 5 pieces | 480 | 320 | 34 | 6 | 57 | 1135 | 24 | 2 | 18 |
| Buffalo Chicken Fingerz | 5 pieces | 750 | 500 | 55 | 12 | 332 | 635 | 3 | 0 | 33 |
| Buffalo Wings | 5 pieces | 750 | 500 | 55 | 12 | 332 | 635 | 3 | 0 | 33 |
| Crinkle Fries, Regular Size | as served | 370 | 140 | 16 | 3 | 0 | 380 | 52 | 5 | 5 |
| Fried White Cheddar Bites | as served | 470 | 260 | 27 | 11 | 45 | 960 | 38 | 1 | 16 |
| Onion Rings | as served | 840 | 560 | 61 | 11 | 21 | 1930 | 62 | 5 | 8 |
| Zestable Sauce | as served | 220 | 190 | 20 | 4 | 20 | 400 | 7 | 1 | 1 |